Prioritization & Clinical Judgment for NCLEX-RN®

THIRD EDITION

Prioritization & Clinical Judgment for NCLEX-RN®

Third Edition

Christi D. Doherty, DNP, MSN, RNC-OB, CNE, CHSE, CDP

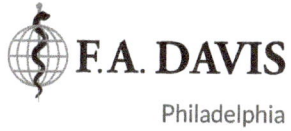

Philadelphia

F.A. Davis Company
1915 Arch Street
Philadelphia, PA 19103
www.fadavis.com

Copyright © 2025 by F.A. Davis Company

Copyright © 2025 by F.A. Davis Company. All rights reserved. This book is protected by copyright. No part of it may be reproduced, stored in a retrieval system, or transmitted in any form or by any means, electronic, mechanical, photocopying, recording, or otherwise, without written permission from the publisher.

Printed in the United States of America

Last digit indicates print number: 10 9 8 7 6 5 4 3 2 1

Sponsoring Editor: Haleahy Craven
Content Project Manager: Veronica Neff
Illustration and Design Manager: Carolyn O'Brien

As new scientific information becomes available through basic and clinical research, recommended treatments and drug therapies undergo changes. The author(s) and publisher have done everything possible to make this book accurate, up to date, and in accord with accepted standards at the time of publication. The author(s), editors, and publisher are not responsible for errors or omissions or for consequences from application of the book, and make no warranty, expressed or implied, in regard to the contents of the book. Any practice described in this book should be applied by the reader in accordance with professional standards of care used in regard to the unique circumstances that may apply in each situation. The reader is advised always to check product information (package inserts) for changes and new information regarding dose and contraindications before administering any drug. Caution is especially urged when using new or infrequently ordered drugs.

Library of Congress Cataloging-in-Publication Data

Names: Doherty, Christi D., author.
Title: Prioritization & clinical judgment for NCLEX-RN® / Christi D. Doherty.
Other titles: Prioritization and clinical judgment for NCLEX-RN®
Description: Third edition. | Philadelphia, PA : F.A. Davis, [2025] | Includes bibliographical references and index.
Identifiers: LCCN 2024060189 (print) | LCCN 2024060190 (ebook) | ISBN 9781719650977 (paperback) | ISBN 9781719654524 (epub) | ISBN 9781719654531 (pdf)
Subjects: MESH: Nursing Assessment | Clinical Decision-Making | Health Priorities | Nursing Care | Examination Questions
Classification: LCC RT48 (print) | LCC RT48 (ebook) | NLM WY 18.2 | DDC 616.07/5--dc23/eng/20250224
LC record available at https://lccn.loc.gov/2024060189
LC ebook record available at https://lccn.loc.gov/2024060190

Authorization to photocopy items for internal or personal use, or the internal or personal use of specific clients, is granted by F.A. Davis Company for users registered with the Copyright Clearance Center (CCC) Transactional Reporting Service, provided that the fee of $.25 per copy is paid directly to CCC, 222 Rosewood Drive, Danvers, MA 01923. For those organizations that have been granted a photocopy license by CCC, a separate system of payment has been arranged. The fee code for users of the Transactional Reporting Service is: 978-1-7196-5097-7/25 0 + $.25.

Thank you to all the nursing students, nursing faculty, and nursing colleagues I have had the privilege to work with during my career.

This book is dedicated to my husband and best friend, Kevin, thank you for all the support and encouragement in all my endeavors. You make everything worthwhile.

—Christi D. Doherty

Contributors

Loretta Aller, PhD, MSN, RN, CHSE
Assistant Professor
Kent State University, College of Nursing
Kent, Ohio

Kevin D. Doherty, BS, RDCS, RDMS, RVT
Cardiovascular Sonographer
UT Health East Texas
Gun Barrel City, Texas

Kris Skalsky, EdD, MSNEd, RN
Doctor of Nursing Practice (DNP) Chair
American Sentinel College of Nursing and Health Sciences at Post University
Waterbury, Connecticut

Nancy T. Wilkins, DNP, RN-BC
Duke Regional Hospital
Durham, North Carolina

Melodie Wong, DNP, MS, RN
West Coast University
Richardson, Texas

Table of Contents

1 Introduction to *Prioritization & Clinical Judgment for NCLEX-RN®* 1
    THE NATIONAL COUNCIL OF STATE BOARDS OF NURSING
TEST PLAN FOR QUESTIONS 1
    NCSBN CLINICAL JUDGMENT MEASUREMENT MODEL 2
    CLINICAL JUDGMENT GUIDE 2
    TYPES OF QUESTIONS 4
    PUTTING THE PIECES TOGETHER 7

2 Cardiovascular Management 9
    QUESTIONS 9
    CARDIAC CASE STUDY 23
    ANSWERS AND RATIONALES 27
    CASE STUDY ANSWERS 43

3 Peripheral Vascular Management 45
    QUESTIONS 45
    PERIPHERAL VASCULAR DISEASE CASE STUDY 57
    ANSWERS AND RATIONALES 61
    CASE STUDY ANSWERS 78

4 Respiratory Management 79
    QUESTIONS 79
    RESPIRATORY CASE STUDY 93
    ANSWERS AND RATIONALES 97
    CASE STUDY ANSWERS 114

5 Gastrointestinal Management 117
    QUESTIONS 117
    GASTROINTESTINAL CASE STUDY 130
    ANSWERS AND RATIONALES 135
    CASE STUDY ANSWERS 150

6 Renal and Genitourinary Management 153
    QUESTIONS 153
    RENAL AND GENITOURINARY CASE STUDY 164
    ANSWERS AND RATIONALES 169
    CASE STUDY ANSWERS 184

Table of Contents

7 Neurological Management ... 187
- QUESTIONS ... 187
- NEUROLOGICAL CASE STUDY ... 201
- ANSWERS AND RATIONALES ... 205
- CASE STUDY ANSWERS ... 221

8 Endocrine Management ... 223
- QUESTIONS ... 223
- ENDOCRINE CASE STUDY ... 237
- ANSWERS AND RATIONALES ... 241
- CASE STUDY ANSWERS ... 256

9 Integumentary Management ... 259
- QUESTIONS ... 259
- INTEGUMENTARY CASE STUDY ... 272
- ANSWERS AND RATIONALES ... 277
- CASE STUDY ANSWERS ... 292

10 Hematological and Immunological Management ... 295
- QUESTIONS ... 295
- HEMATOLOGICAL/IMMUNOLOGICAL CASE STUDY ... 307
- ANSWERS AND RATIONALES ... 312
- CASE STUDY ANSWERS ... 327

11 Women's Health Management ... 329
- QUESTIONS ... 329
- MATERNAL-CHILD CASE STUDY ... 340
- ANSWERS AND RATIONALES ... 343
- CASE STUDY ANSWERS ... 359

12 Pediatric Health Management ... 361
- QUESTIONS ... 361
- PEDIATRIC CASE STUDY ... 373
- ANSWERS AND RATIONALES ... 377
- CASE STUDY ANSWERS ... 391

13 Mental Health Management ... 393
- QUESTIONS ... 393
- MENTAL HEALTH CASE STUDY ... 407
- ANSWERS AND RATIONALES ... 413
- CASE STUDY ANSWERS ... 431

14 Case Studies ... 433
- CASE STUDY #1 ... 433
- CASE STUDY #2 ... 437
- CASE STUDY #3 ... 441
- CASE STUDY #4 ... 444

LABORATORY AND DIAGNOSTIC TEST INTENSIVE
QUESTIONS.. 447
CLINICAL SKILLS INTENSIVE QUESTIONS............................ 449
ANSWERS TO CASE STUDIES 452
CASE STUDY #1 452
CASE STUDY #2 454
CASE STUDY #3 456
CASE STUDY #4 457
LABORATORY SKILLS INTENSIVE ANSWERS 459
CLINICAL SKILLS INTENSIVE ANSWERS 459

15 Comprehensive Examination 463
QUESTIONS... 463
ANSWERS AND RATIONALES.. 483

BIBLIOGRAPHY 505
APPENDIX A: NORMAL LABORATORY VALUES 507
APPENDIX B: COMMON ABBREVIATIONS 509
GLOSSARY OF ENGLISH WORDS COMMONLY ENCOUNTERED
ON NURSING EXAMINATIONS 511
INDEX 515

Introduction to Prioritization & Clinical Judgment for NCLEX-RN®

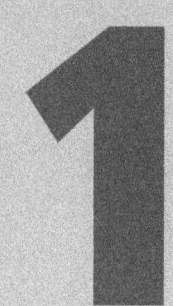

Each problem that I solved became a rule which served afterwards to solve other problems.

—Rene Descartes

This book is designed to assist students throughout nursing school and in taking nursing examinations, mainly the NCLEX-RN® exam, for registered nurse (RN) licensure. *Prioritization & Clinical Judgment for NCLEX-RN®* focuses on assisting students to improve and enhance their clinical judgment skills. Clinical judgment involves the nurse's ability to acquire information, analyze the data, recognize relevant findings, make inferences in a clinical situation, and implement appropriate nursing interventions. This ability requires a combination of knowledge, logical reasoning, and intuition. The nurse must implement appropriate nursing interventions and evaluate the client's response. Other aspects of applying clinical judgment involve complex nursing tasks such as setting priorities for client care, delegating nursing tasks, and managing clients and staff. Clinical judgment is necessary in all nursing practice areas, including medical, surgical, critical care, obstetric, pediatric, geriatric, rehabilitation, home health, mental health nursing, and inpatient and outpatient healthcare settings.

Clinical judgment questions involving critical thinking, management, prioritizing, and delegation are some of the most challenging questions for the student and new graduate because no reference book is available to find the correct answers for each scenario. Determining the answers to these questions requires knowledge of basic scientific principles, standards of care, pathophysiology, psychosocial behaviors, leadership qualities, and critical thinking. This book challenges students to sharpen their clinical judgment abilities in various nursing situations. Each question provides the student with detailed rationales for correct and incorrect responses. Many of the questions include a helpful tip, termed a "Clinical Judgment Guide," to assist the student with identifying what the questions are asking, recognizing the relevant data in the question stem, and selecting the correct response. It is considered poor test-taking to read rationales for incorrect answers. By doing this, students often will remember reading the rationale, but not whether the rationale was for the correct or incorrect answer.

Prioritization & Clinical Judgment for NCLEX-RN® contains numerous questions regarding various nursing areas and roles. The next 12 chapters (Chapters 2 to 13) present questions in a related field and a case study that requires detailed examination and assessment of clients with different illnesses or injuries in multiple healthcare settings. Also included is a comprehensive examination with answers and rationales. The test taker must note that practice questions and tests are valuable in preparing for an examination, but there is no substitute for studying the material.

THE NATIONAL COUNCIL OF STATE BOARDS OF NURSING TEST PLAN FOR QUESTIONS

The National Council of State Boards of Nursing (NCSBN) provides a test plan that helps test takers prepare for the examination and assists nursing faculty in developing test questions for the NCLEX-RN®. Table 1–1 indicates the breakdown of content on the NCLEX-RN®.

Table 1–1   Distribution of Content in NCLEX-RN® 2023

Client Needs Category	Percentage of Items
Safe and Effective Care Environment	
• Management of Care	15%–21%
• Safety and Infection Control	10%–16%
Health Promotion and Maintenance	6%–12%
Psychosocial Integrity	6%–12%
Physiological Integrity	
• Basic Care and Comfort	6%–12%
• Pharmacological and Parenteral Therapies	13%–19%
• Reduction of Risk Potential	9%–15%
• Physiological Adaptation	11%–17%

Source: National Council of State Boards of Nursing. (2023). *2023 NCLEX-RN® test plan.* https://www.ncsbn.org/publications/2023-nclex-rn-test-plan. Used with permission.

Clinical judgment skills are necessary for nurses to function competently in each content area. The Client Needs category of the Safe and Effective Care Environment section includes content on management of care, safety, and infection control. Content included in the management of care section guides and directs nursing care that enhances the healthcare delivery setting to protect clients and healthcare personnel. Specific content includes but is not limited to advance directives, advocacy, case management, client rights, collaboration with the interdisciplinary team, delegation, establishing priorities, ethical practice, informed consent, information technology, and performance improvement. Other topics are legal rights and responsibilities, referrals, resource management, staff education, supervision, confidentiality and information security, and continuity of care. Content provided in the Safety and Infection Control section is used to guide the nurse in the purposeful protection of the client and others from health and environmental risks. Specific content includes but is not limited to reporting requirements, security procedures, verification of appropriateness of treatment orders, and infection control measures. The questions in this book follow the NCLEX-RN® test plan.

NCSBN CLINICAL JUDGMENT MEASUREMENT MODEL

The goal of the NCLEX-RN® examination has always been to measure the knowledge and skills required by entry-level nurses to care for clients safely. With demographic shifts and technological advances, nurses must make increasingly complex decisions using clinical judgment and incorporate leadership, collaboration, and evidence-based practice into their nursing practice (NCSBN, 2023). The NCSBN has developed the Clinical Judgment Measurement Model (CJMM) as a framework for measuring clinical judgment within a standardized examination (Figure 1–1). Layer 3 of the CJMM outlines the six cognitive processes of clinical decision making and is the basis for the NCLEX case studies and test items. The six cognitive processes are recognizing cues, analyzing cues, prioritizing hypotheses, generating solutions, taking action, and evaluating outcomes.

CLINICAL JUDGMENT GUIDE

Nurses* base their decisions on many principles to determine a course of action. Among the basic guidelines to apply in nursing practice—and answering test questions—are the nursing process and Maslow's Hierarchy of Needs.

---

* In this book, the term "nurse," unless otherwise specified, refers to a licensed RN. An RN can assign tasks to a licensed practical nurse (LPN) or delegate to an unlicensed assistive personnel (UAP), a position that may be known under other terms such as "medical assistant" or "nurse's aide." An LPN can delegate tasks to a UAP. Each state will have specific regulations that govern what duties or tasks can be delegated or assigned to each of these types of personnel.

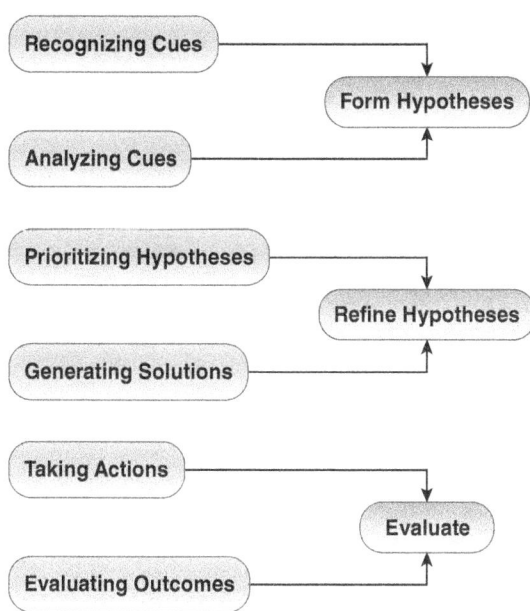

Figure 1–1. NCSBN Clinical Judgment Measurement Model. National Council of State Boards of Nursing, ©2019.

The Nursing Process

One of the basic guidelines to apply in nursing practice is the nursing process, which consists of five steps—assessment, nursing diagnosis, planning, intervention, and evaluation—usually completed systematically. Assessment is the first step. If a priority-setting question asks the test taker which steps to implement first, the test taker should first look at assessment.

EXAMPLE

> The nurse is caring for a client diagnosed with congestive heart failure who is currently reporting dyspnea. Which intervention should the nurse implement **first**?
> 1. Administer furosemide IV push (IVP).
> 2. Check the client for adventitious lung sounds.
> 3. Ask the respiratory therapist to administer a treatment.
> 4. Notify the healthcare provider[†] (HCP).
>
> Answer: 2
> Checking for adventitious lung sounds is assessing the client to determine the extent of the client's breathing difficulties causing the dyspnea.

† The term "healthcare provider," as used in this book, refers to a client's primary provider of medical care. It includes physicians (including osteopathic physicians), nurse practitioners (NPs), and physician assistants (PAs). Depending on state regulations, many NPs and some PAs have prescriptive authority for at least some categories of prescribed drugs.

Numerous words, such as "check," can be used to indicate assessment. The test taker should not discard an option because the word "assess" or "assessment" is not used. Alternatively, the test taker shouldn't assume an option is correct merely because the word "assess" is used. The test taker must also know that the assessment data must match the problem stated in the stem, regardless of terminology. The nurse must assess for the correct information. If option 2 in the previous example said, "Assess urinary output," it would not be a correct answer even though it includes the word "assess" because urinary output is not related to heart failure or breathing difficulties. In addition, the test taker should be aware that assessment is not always the correct answer when the question asks which should be done first. Suppose, for example, the previous question listed option 3 as "Apply oxygen via nasal cannula at 2 liters per minute." In that case, assessment would not come first. The nurse would first attempt to relieve the client's distress and then assess.

When a question asks what a nurse should do next, the test taker should determine from the information given in the question which steps in the nursing process have been completed and then choose an option that matches the next step in the nursing process.

The nurse has assessed the client and formulated a nursing diagnosis. The next step in the nursing process is implementation. The nurse should proceed to a nursing intervention appropriate for the situation. This type of question is designed to determine whether the test taker can set priorities in client care.

EXAMPLE

> The client diagnosed with peptic ulcer disease has a blood pressure of 88/42 mm Hg, an apical pulse of 132 bpm, and respirations of 28 per minute. Which intervention should the nurse implement **first**?
> 1. Notify the laboratory to draw a type and crossmatch.
> 2. Assess the client's abdomen for tenderness.
> 3. Insert an 18-gauge catheter and infuse lactated Ringer's solution.
> 4. Check the client's pulse oximeter reading.
>
> Answer: 3
> 1. Notifying the laboratory of a type and crossmatch would be an appropriate intervention because the client is showing signs of hypovolemia, but it is not the first intervention because it would not directly support the client's circulatory volume.
> 2. The stem of the question has provided enough assessment data to indicate the client's problem of hypovolemia. Further assessment data are not needed.
> 3. **The vital signs indicate hypovolemia, which is a life-threatening emergency that requires a nursing intervention to support the client's circulatory volume. The nurse can do this by infusing lactated Ringer's solution.**
> 4. A pulse oximeter reading would not support the client's circulatory volume.

Maslow's Hierarchy of Needs

If the test taker has looked at the question and the nursing process does not assist the test taker in determining the correct option, then a tool such as Maslow's Hierarchy of Needs (Fig. 1–2) should be utilized. Note that the bottom of the pyramid—physiological needs—is the top priority in instituting nursing interventions. If a question asks the test taker to determine the priority intervention and a physiological need is among the options, then that is the priority. Safety and security take priority if a physiological need is not listed, and so on up the pyramid.

TYPES OF QUESTIONS

Clinical judgment questions often involve prioritizing client care, delegating staff tasks, and managing issues related to clients and staff. These questions may include interpreting medication administration records (MARs) or laboratory values, determining when notifying the primary HCP is a priority, and choosing which tasks can be assigned to a licensed

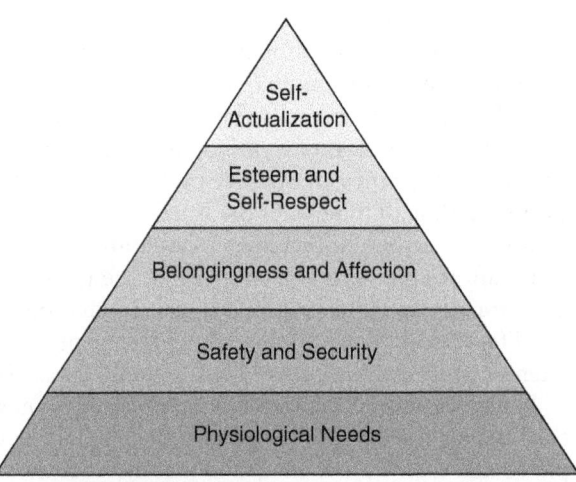

Figure 1–2. Maslow's Hierarchy of Needs.

practical nurse (LPN) or unlicensed assistive personnel (UAP) and which must be performed by an RN.

Some questions on the NCLEX-RN® are termed "alternate-format questions" and include choosing more than one option that correctly answers a question, ranking procedures or actions in correct order, drag-and-drop questions, and fill-in-the-blank questions.

EXAMPLE

> The nurse is assigning tasks to the UAP. Which is an appropriate delegation to the UAP?
> **Select all that apply.**
> 1. Check the area around an incisional wound for redness.
> 2. Help a client with an upper limb cast to eat.
> 3. Assist a client recovering from a hysterectomy to walk to the bathroom.
> 4. Explain to a client being discharged how to empty and clean the colostomy bag.
> 5. Transport a client with a suspected fractured tibia to the x-ray department.
>
> **Correct answers are 2, 3, and 5.**
> 1. Checking the area around a wound is an assessment. An RN cannot delegate assessment, teaching, evaluation, medications, or care of an unstable client to a UAP.
> 2. **The UAP can assist a client with a cast to eat.**
> 3. **The UAP can assist a stable client to the bathroom.**
> 4. Explaining colostomy care is a teaching intervention. An RN cannot delegate assessment, teaching, evaluation, medications, or care of an unstable client to a UAP.
> 5. **The UAP can transport a client to the x-ray department.**

Prioritizing Questions and Setting Priorities

In test questions asking the nurse which action to take first, two or more options will be appropriate nursing interventions for the situation described. When choosing the correct answer, the test taker must decide which intervention should occur *first* in a sequence of events or would directly impact the situation.

With a question that asks which client the nurse should assess first, the test taker should first look at each option and determine whether the signs or symptoms the client is exhibiting are typical or expected for the disease process; if so, the nurse does not need to assess that particular client first. Second, if two or more options state signs or symptoms that are not normal or expected for the disease process, then the test taker should select the option with the greatest potential for a poor outcome. The test taker should scrutinize each option to determine the priority by asking these questions:

- Is the situation life-threatening or life-altering? *If yes, this client is the highest priority.*
- Is the situation unexpected for the disease process? *If yes, then this client may be the priority.*
- Are the data presented abnormal? *If yes, then this client may be the priority.*
- Is the situation expected for the disease process and not life-threatening? *If yes, this client may be—but probably is not—the priority.*
- Is the situation or data normal? *If yes, this client can be seen last.*

On a computerized test, such as the NCLEX-RN® exam, the test taker must make a decision before advancing to the next question.

Delegating and Assigning Care

Although each state has its own Nurse Practice Act, some general guidelines apply to all professional nurses.

- When delegating to a UAP, the nurse may not delegate any activity that requires nursing clinical judgment. These activities include assessing, teaching, evaluating, administering medications, and caring for unstable clients.
- When assigning care to an LPN, the RN can assign the administration of some medications but cannot assign assessing, teaching, or evaluating any client and cannot delegate the care of an unstable client.

Management Decisions

The nurse is frequently called upon to make decisions about staffing, movement of clients from one unit to another, or handling conflicts as they arise. Some general guidelines for answering questions in this area include the following:

- The most experienced nurse gets the most critical client.
- A graduate nurse can care for any client with supervision.
- The most stable client can move or be discharged, whereas the most unstable client must move to the intensive care unit (ICU) or stay in the ICU.

When the nurse must make decisions regarding a conflict among nursing staff, involving the chain of command is a good rule to follow. The primary nurse should directly address a conflict with a peer (another primary nurse) or a subordinate unless the situation is illegal (such as stealing drugs). The primary nurse should use the chain of command in situations that address superiors (a manager or director of nursing). In this case, the nurse should discuss the situation with the next in command above the superior.

NGN Question Formats

The next-generation NCLEX (NGN) examination includes a variety of question types to address critical nursing skills such as recognizing cues, analyzing those cues, prioritizing hypotheses, generating solutions, taking action, and evaluating outcomes (NCSBN, 2023). The examination comprises single-answer questions, multiple-choice questions, and other alternate formats:

- *Fill-in-the-blank* questions require an answer; these questions often test math abilities.
- *"Select all that apply"* questions require the test taker to select one or more correct options. All answer options could be correct.
- *Extended multiple responses* are select-all-that-apply questions with more than the traditional five-answer options or questions requiring the learner to identify relevant or irrelevant items from a data set of no fewer than six options.
- *Enhanced hot spots* involve highlighting relevant information in a case study or identifying a specific body area as a correct answer.
- *CLOZE questions* are fill-in-the-blank questions with drop boxes that provide options for the test taker to select for the blank.
- *Drag-and-drop* questions originate from a brief client scenario or case study. In these questions, the test taker must complete several blanks within a sentence by selecting from a list of choices. Another format for extended drag-and-drop questions is the ranking or sequencing of interventions or processes.
- *Matrix items* involve reading a case study or passage and assigning a value to a group of responses, such as indicated or contraindicated.
- *Bowtie items* require the test taker to review a case study and select responses from three distinct yet intertwined categories, such as, for example, the condition the client is most likely experiencing, actions to take, and parameters to monitor.
- *Trend items* involve the evolution of vital signs or laboratory results over time and require an interpretation of the changes. Trends can incorporate cloze or matrix items.
- The *case study* is an unfolding narrative describing a client's situation. It contains assorted data, and the test taker must discern the relevant information. Then, additional data are revealed, culminating in a complete picture of the client's clinical presentation and associated interventions. The learner makes clinical judgment decisions throughout the case study, adapting the process to the evolving client information. The case study addresses all six cognitive processes outlined in the CJMM.

Examples of most of these types of questions are included in this book.

General Test-Taking Guidelines

A few standard test-taking guidelines should be utilized for the examination.

- Read the entire question and identify keywords, such as time frames, age, sex, marital status, disease or condition, symptoms, etc.
- All HCP orders needed to perform a listed intervention are already written unless otherwise stated.
- Make an educated guess.
- Absolutes, such as "all" or "every," are usually incorrect.
- When selecting an answer, choose a client-centered option before equipment.
- According to the NCSBN, "select-all-that-apply" questions can have one correct response, more than one correct response, or all responses are correct. No minimum or maximum number of responses is required. There are no partially correct answers.
- Answer "select-all-that-apply" questions by evaluating if each answer is true or false. Each option stands alone.
- The RN does not delegate assessment, teaching, evaluation, or an unstable client to an LPN or UAP. The RN does not assign a task to a staff member that is not within their scope of practice.
- If the client is in distress, do not assess; instead, do something.

For general information on how to prepare for an examination and on the types of questions used in nursing examinations, refer to *Fundamentals Success: A Q&A Review Applying Critical Thinking to Test Taking* by Patricia Nugent, RN, MA, MS, EdD, and Barbara Vitale, RN, MA.

PUTTING THE PIECES TOGETHER

The nurse is required to acquire information, analyze the data, and make inferences based on the available information. Sometimes, this process is relatively easy, and at other times, the available information and data pieces do not seem to fit. These challenges are precisely where clinical judgment guides decision making and nursing actions.

Cardiovascular Management

When you do the common things in life in an uncommon way, you will command the attention of the world.

—George Washington Carver

QUESTIONS

1. The nurse on the cardiac unit has received the shift report from the outgoing nurse. Which client should the nurse assess **first**?
    1. The client who has just been brought to the unit from the emergency department (ED) without any reported symptoms
    2. The client who received pain medication 30 minutes ago for chest pain that was a level 3 on a 1-to-10 pain scale
    3. The client who had a cardiac catheterization in the morning and has palpable pedal pulses bilaterally
    4. The client who has been turning on the call light frequently and stating her care has been neglected

2. The nurse on the cardiac unit is preparing to administer medications after receiving the morning change-of-shift report. Which medication should the nurse administer **first**?
    1. The cardiac glycoside to the client with an apical pulse of 58 bpm
    2. The loop diuretic to a client with a serum K+ level of 3.2 mEq/L
    3. The antidysrhythmic to the client diagnosed with ventricular fibrillation
    4. The calcium-channel blocker to the client with a blood pressure of 110/68 mm Hg

3. Which client should the RN telemetry nurse assess **first** after receiving the a.m. shift report?
    1. The client diagnosed with deep vein thrombosis with an edematous right calf
    2. The client diagnosed with mitral valve stenosis having heart palpitations
    3. The client diagnosed with arterial occlusive disease with intermittent claudication
    4. The client diagnosed with congestive heart failure (CHF) with pink, frothy sputum

4. The RN charge nurse is making assignments for clients on a cardiac unit. Which client should the RN charge nurse assign to a new graduate nurse (GN)?
    1. The 44-year-old client diagnosed with a myocardial infarction
    2. The 65-year-old client diagnosed with unstable angina
    3. The 75-year-old client scheduled for a cardiac catheterization
    4. The 50-year-old client reporting chest pain

5. The RN charge nurse is making assignments for a 30-bed cardiac unit staffed with three registered nurses (RNs), three licensed practical nurses (LPNs), and three unlicensed assistive personnel (UAPs). Which assignment is **most** appropriate by the charge nurse?
   1. Assign an RN to perform all sterile procedures.
   2. Assign an LPN to give all IV medications.
   3. Assign a UAP to complete the a.m. care.
   4. Assign an LPN to write the care plans.

6. The nurse on a cardiac unit is discussing a client with the case manager. Which information should the nurse share with the case manager?
   1. Discuss personal information the client shared with the nurse in confidence.
   2. Provide the case manager with any information required for continuity of care.
   3. Explain that client confidentiality prevents the nurse from disclosing information.
   4. Ask the case manager to get the client's permission before sharing information.

7. The RN staff nurse assesses erratic electrical activity on the telemetry reading while the client talks to the nurse on the intercom system. Which task should the nurse instruct the UAP to implement?
   1. Call a Code Blue immediately.
   2. Check the client's telemetry leads.
   3. Find the nurse to check the client.
   4. Remove the telemetry monitor.

8. The RN charge nurse on the cardiac unit must float a nurse to the emergency department for the shift. Which nurse should be floated to the emergency department?
   1. The nurse with 4 years of experience in the operating room
   2. The nurse recently transferred from critical care to the cardiac unit
   3. The nurse with 1 year of experience on the cardiac unit just returned from a week's sick leave
   4. The nurse with 2 years of experience in the gastrointestinal (GI) lab and 3 years in the cardiac unit

9. The cardiac nurse is preparing to administer 1 unit of blood to a client. Which interventions should the nurse implement? **Rank in order of priority.**
   1. Infuse the unit of blood at 20 gtt/min for the first 15 minutes.
   2. Check the unit of blood and the client's blood band with another nurse.
   3. Initiate Y-tubing with normal saline via an 18-gauge angiocatheter.
   4. Assess the client's vital signs and lung sounds and assess for a rash.
   5. Obtain informed consent for the blood administration from the client.

10. The RN charge nurse in the cardiac critical care unit is making rounds. Which client should the nurse see **first**?
    1. The client diagnosed with coronary artery disease reporting that the nurses are being rude and won't answer the call lights
    2. The client diagnosed with an acute myocardial infarction with an elevated creatine phosphokinase-cardiac muscle (CPK-MB) level
    3. The client diagnosed with atrial fibrillation on an oral anticoagulant and with an International Normalized Ratio (INR) of 2.8
    4. The client 2 days postoperative coronary artery bypass, now being transferred to the cardiac unit

11. The nurse is preparing to administer digoxin 0.25 mg IV push (IVP) to a client diagnosed with severe CHF, receiving D_5W/0.9 NaCl at 25 mL/hr. Rank in order of performance.
    1. Administer the medication over 5 minutes.
    2. Dilute the medication with normal saline.
    3. Draw up the medication in a tuberculin syringe.
    4. Check the client's identification band.
    5. Clamp the primary tubing distal to the port.

12. The client is in the cardiac intensive care unit (ICU) on dopamine when their BP increases to 210/130 mm Hg. Which intervention should the ICU nurse implement **first**?
    1. Discontinue the client's dopamine.
    2. Notify the client's healthcare provider (HCP).
    3. Administer hydralazine intravenously.
    4. Assess the client's neurological status.

13. The RN charge nurse is making client assignments in the cardiac critical care unit. Which client should be assigned to the **most** experienced nurse?
    1. The client diagnosed with acute rheumatic fever carditis refusing to stay on bedrest
    2. The client with the following arterial blood gas (ABG) values: pH 7.35; Pao$_2$ 88 mm Hg; Paco$_2$ 44 mm Hg; HCO$_3$ 22 mmol/L
    3. The client presenting with multifocal premature ventricular contractions (PVCs)
    4. The client diagnosed with angina and scheduled for a cardiac catheterization

14. The primary cardiac RN staff nurse is delegating tasks to the UAP. Which delegation task **warrants** intervention by the RN charge nurse of the cardiac unit?
    1. The UAP is instructed to bathe the client on telemetry monitoring.
    2. The UAP is requested to obtain a bedside glucometer reading.
    3. The UAP is asked to assist with a portable chest x-ray.
    4. The UAP is told to feed a client diagnosed with dysphagia.

15. The nurse is administering medications to clients in the cardiac critical care area. Which client should the nurse **question** before administering the medication?
    1. The client receiving a calcium-channel blocker and drinking a glass of grapefruit juice
    2. The client receiving a beta-adrenergic blocker with an apical heart rate of 62 bpm
    3. The client receiving nonsteroidal anti-inflammatory drugs (NSAIDs) immediately after breakfast
    4. The client receiving an oral anticoagulant with International Normalized Ratio (INR) of 2.8

16. The RN charge nurse on the cardiac unit is counseling a staff nurse because the nurse has clocked in late multiple times for the 7:00 a.m. to 7:00 p.m. shift. Which conflict resolution approach uses the **win-win** strategy?
    1. The charge nurse terminates the staff nurse per the hospital policy so that a new nurse can be transferred to the unit.
    2. The charge nurse discovers that the staff nurse is having problems with child care; therefore, the charge nurse allows the staff nurse to work a 9:00 a.m. to 9:00 p.m. shift.
    3. The charge nurse puts the staff nurse on probation, understanding that the next time the staff nurse is late to work, it will result in termination.
    4. The staff nurse asks another employer to talk to the charge nurse and explain that they are a valuable team member.

17. Which client warrants **immediate** intervention by the nurse?
    1. The client diagnosed with pericarditis having chest pain with inspiration
    2. The client diagnosed with mitral valve regurgitation and has a thready peripheral pulse
    3. The client diagnosed with Marfan syndrome and has pectus excavatum
    4. The client diagnosed with atherosclerosis having slurred speech and drooling

18. The UAP working in a long-term care facility notifies the RN staff nurse that the client on a low-sodium diet diagnosed with CHF is reporting that the food is inedible. Which intervention should the RN staff nurse implement **first?**
    1. Have the family bring food from home for the client.
    2. Check what the client has eaten in the past 24 hours.
    3. Tell the client that a low-sodium diet is essential for their diagnosis.
    4. Ask the dietitian to discuss food preferences with the client.

19. The RN charge nurse on the cardiac unit is making shift assignments. Which client should be assigned to the **most** experienced nurse?
    1. The client diagnosed with mitral valve stenosis
    2. The client diagnosed with asymptomatic sinus bradycardia
    3. The client diagnosed with fulminant pulmonary edema
    4. The client diagnosed with acute atrial fibrillation

20. The evening nurse in a long-term care facility is preparing to administer medications to a client diagnosed with atrial fibrillation.

    Client: Mr. A **Allergies:** Penicillin
    Date: Today **Diagnosis:** Atrial Fibrillation

Medication	0701–1900	1901–0700
Warfarin 5 mg PO daily		1800
		INR: 3.4 today
Metoclopramide 5 mg PO tid	0900 DN	1800
	1300 DN	
Docusate PO bid	0900 DN	1800
Atorvastatin PO daily		1800
Nurse Name/Initials	Day Nurse RN/DN	Night Nurse RN/NN

    Which medication should the nurse **question** administering?
    1. Warfarin
    2. Metoclopramide
    3. Docusate
    4. Atorvastatin

21. The RN staff nurse and the UAP enter the client's room and discover that the client is unresponsive. According to the American Heart Association (AHA) guidelines, which action should the RN staff nurse assign to the UAP **first?**
    1. Ask the UAP to check whether the client is asleep.
    2. Tell the UAP to perform cardiac compressions.
    3. Instruct the UAP to get the crash cart.
    4. Request the UAP to put the client in a recumbent position.

22. The elderly client on a cardiac unit has a do not resuscitate (DNR) order written. Which interventions should the nurse implement? **Select all that apply.**
    1. Continue to care for the client's needs as usual.
    2. Place a DNR identification armband on the client.
    3. Refer the client to a hospice organization.
    4. Limit visitors to two at a time to not tire the client.
    5. Remove telemetry monitors from the client.

23. The nurse is initiating discharge teaching for a 68-year-old male client recovering from quadruple coronary bypass surgery. Which **priority** question should the nurse ask the client?
    1. "Are you sexually active?"
    2. "Can you still drive your car?"
    3. "Do you have pain medications at home?"
    4. "Do you know when to call your HCP?"

24. The LPN informs the clinic RN that the client diagnosed with atrial fibrillation has an INR of 4.5. Which intervention should the clinic RN implement?
    1. Tell the LPN to notify the clinic HCP.
    2. Instruct the LPN to assess the client for abnormal bleeding.
    3. Obtain a STAT electrocardiogram (EKG) on the client.
    4. Take no action because this INR is within the normal range.

25. The RN staff nurse at a disaster site is triaging victims when an observer states, "I am a certified nurse aide. Can I do anything to help?" Which action should the RN staff nurse implement?
    1. Request the person to please leave the area.
    2. Ask the person to check the injured clients.
    3. Tell the person to try to keep the victim calm.
    4. Instruct the person to help the paramedics.

26. The cardiac clinic RN staff nurse hears the UAP tell the client, "You have gained over 15 pounds since your last visit." The scale is located in the open office area. Which action should the clinic RN staff nurse implement?
    1. Instruct the UAP in front of the client to not comment on the weight.
    2. Ask the UAP to put the client in the room and take no action.
    3. Privately explain to the UAP that this is an inappropriate comment and violates HIPAA.
    4. Report the UAP to the clinic's director of nurses.

27. The nurse on the cardiac unit is discussing case management with a client, asking "Why do I need a case manager for my heart disease?" Which statements are **most** appropriate for the nurse to respond? **Select all that apply.**
    1. "Case management helps contain your healthcare costs."
    2. "It will help enhance your quality of life with a chronic illness."
    3. "It decreases the fragmentation of care across many healthcare settings."
    4. "Case management is a form of health insurance for clients with chronic illnesses."
    5. "We try to provide quality care along the healthcare continuum."

28. The client diagnosed with arterial hypertension has been taking a calcium-channel blocker, a loop diuretic, and an angiotensin-converting enzyme (ACE) inhibitor for 3 years. Which statement by the client would **warrant** intervention by the nurse?
    1. "I go to the bathroom a lot during the morning."
    2. "I get up very slowly after sitting for a while."
    3. "I do not salt my food while cooking it but add it at the table."
    4. "I drink grapefruit juice every morning with my breakfast."

29. The RN director of nurses in the cardiac clinic is counseling a UAP for returning late from lunch break seven times in the past 2 weeks. Which conflict resolution uses the **win-lose** strategy?
    1. The UAP explains about checking on their ill mother during lunch, and the nurse director allows a longer lunch break and coming in earlier.
    2. The director of nurses offers the UAP a transfer to the emergency weekend clinic and to be off during the week.
    3. The director of nurses terminates the UAP, explaining that all staff must be on time so the clinic runs smoothly.
    4. The UAP is placed on a 1-month probation and told that any further occurrences will result in termination from this position.

30. The RN cardiac clinic nurse has told the UAP twice to change the sharps container in the examination room, but it has not been changed. Which action should the nurse implement **first?**
    1. Instruct the UAP to change it immediately.
    2. Ask the UAP why the sharps container has not been changed.
    3. Change the sharps container as per clinic policy.
    4. Document the situation and place a copy in the employee file.

31. The spouse of a client calls the clinic and tells the nurse the client is having chest pain but won't go to the hospital. Which action should the nurse implement **first?**
    1. Instruct the spouse to call 911 immediately.
    2. Tell the spouse to have the client chew an aspirin.
    3. Ask the spouse what the client had to eat recently.
    4. Request that the client talk to the clinic physician.

32. The home health nurse received phone messages from the agency secretary. Which client should the nurse contact **first?**
    1. The client diagnosed with hypertension reporting a BP of 148/92 mm Hg
    2. The client diagnosed with cardiomyopathy and a pulse oximeter reading of 93%
    3. The client diagnosed with congestive heart failure and edematous feet
    4. The client diagnosed with chronic atrial fibrillation having chest pain

33. The client is diagnosed with end-stage CHF. The nurse finds the client lying in bed, short of breath, unable to talk, and with buccal cyanosis. Which intervention should the nurse implement **first?**
    1. Assist the client to a sitting position.
    2. Assess the client's vital signs.
    3. Call 911 for the paramedics.
    4. Auscultate the client's lung sounds.

34. The home health nurse is visiting a client diagnosed with CHF. The client has an out-of-hospital DNR order, has stopped breathing, and has no pulse or blood pressure. The client's family is at the bedside. Which intervention should the home health nurse implement **first?**
    1. Contact the agency's chaplain.
    2. Pronounce the client's death.
    3. Ask the family to leave the bedside.
    4. Call the client's funeral home.

35. The cardiac nurse received laboratory results on the following clients. Which client warrants **immediate** intervention from the nurse?
    1. The client with an INR of 2.8
    2. The client with a serum potassium level of 3.8 mEq/L
    3. The client with a serum digoxin level of 2.6 mg/dL
    4. The client with a glycosylated hemoglobin of 6%

36. The home health nurse is completing the admission assessment for an obese client diagnosed with a myocardial infarction, comorbid type 1 diabetes, and arterial hypertension. Which **priority** intervention should the nurse implement?
    1. Encourage the client to walk 30 minutes a day.
    2. Request a home health registered dietitian to talk to the client.
    3. Refer the client to a cardiac rehabilitation unit.
    4. Discuss the client's need to lose 1 to 2 pounds a week.

37. The home health nurse is preparing for the initial visit to a client diagnosed with CHF. Which intervention should the nurse implement **first?**
    1. Prepare all the needed equipment for the visit.
    2. Call the client to arrange a time for the visit.
    3. Review the client's referral form and pertinent data.
    4. Make the necessary referrals for the client.

38. Which information should the experienced home health nurse discuss when orienting a new nurse to home health nursing? **Select all that apply.**
    1. If the client or family is hostile or obnoxious, call the police.
    2. Carry the home health agency identification in a purse or wallet.
    3. Visits can be scheduled at night with permission from the agency.
    4. Inform the agency of the times of the client's scheduled visits.
    5. Report unsafe environments to the agency.

39. The home health aide tells the home health nurse that the grandchild of the client they are caring for asked them out on a date. Which statement is the home health nurse's **best** response?
    1. "I am so excited for you; they seem like a very nice young person."
    2. "You should not date them while their grandmother is a client of our agency."
    3. "I think you should tell the director of the home health agency about this date."
    4. "You should never date someone you meet while caring for a client."

40. The cardiac nurse is teaching the client diagnosed with CHF. Which teaching interventions should the nurse discuss with the client? **Select all that apply.**
    1. Notify the HCP if the client gains more than 2 lb in 1 day.
    2. Keep the head of the bed elevated when sleeping.
    3. Take the loop diuretic once a day before going to sleep.
    4. Teach the client which foods are high in sodium and should be avoided.
    5. Perform isotonic exercises at least once a day.

41. The nurse is administering medications on a cardiac unit. Which medication should the nurse **question** administering?
    1. Warfarin to a client with a PT of 14 seconds and an INR of 1.6
    2. Digoxin to a client with a potassium level of 3.3 mEq/L
    3. Atenolol for the client with an aspartate aminotransferase (AST) of 18 U/L
    4. Lisinopril for the client with a serum creatinine level of 0.8 mg/dL

42. The nurse is providing end-of-life care to the client diagnosed with cardiomyopathy who is in hospice. Which **priority** assessment intervention should the hospice nurse implement?
    1. Assess the client's spiritual needs.
    2. Assess the client's financial situation.
    3. Assess the client's support system.
    4. Assess the client's medical diagnosis.

43. The spouse of the client diagnosed with infective endocarditis and a DNR order tells the nurse the client is not breathing. Which intervention should the RN staff nurse implement **first**?
    1. Contact the client's HCP.
    2. Notify the Rapid Response Team.
    3. Stay with the client and the spouse.
    4. Instruct the UAP to perform postmortem care.

44. The hospice nurse is triaging phone calls from clients. Which client should the nurse contact **first**?
    1. The client with family reporting the client is not eating
    2. The client asking to rescind the out-of-hospital DNR
    3. The client with pain uncontrolled with the current medications
    4. The client with urinary incontinence causing a stage 1 pressure injury

45. The hospice nurse is working with a volunteer. Which task could the nurse delegate to the volunteer? **Select all that apply.**
    1. Sit with the client as they reminisce about their life experiences.
    2. Give the client a sponge bath and rub lotion on the bony prominences.
    3. Provide spiritual support for the client and their family members.
    4. Check the home to see that all necessary medical equipment is available.
    5. Assist with light housekeeping chores and meal preparation.

46. The RN staff nurse delegates postmortem care to the UAP. The UAP tells the nurse they have never performed postmortem care. Which statement is the **best** response by the RN staff nurse to the UAP?
    1. "It can be uncomfortable. I will go with you and show you what to do."
    2. "The client is already dead. You cannot hurt them now."
    3. "There is nothing to it; it is just a bed bath and change of clothes."
    4. "Don't worry. You can skip it this time, but you must learn what to do."

47. The UAP tells the RN staff nurse the client is reporting chest pain. Which task should the RN staff nurse delegate to the UAP?
    1. Call the HCP and report the client's chest pain.
    2. Give the client some acetaminophen while the nurse checks the client.
    3. Bring the electronic health record (EHR) to the client's room.
    4. Notify the client's family of the onset of chest pain.

48. The RN and LPN are caring for a group of clients on a cardiac unit. Which nursing tasks can be assigned to the LPN? **Select all that apply.**
    1. Feed the client with an IV in both forearms.
    2. Assess the client diagnosed with stage IV heart failure.
    3. Perform discharge teaching for the client recovering from a cardiac catheterization.
    4. Administer the intravenous piggyback (IVPB) ceftriaxone.
    5. Contact the HCP for a prn acetaminophen order for a client.

49. The RN hospice nurse is discussing the client's care with the UAP. Which statement contains the **best** information about caring for a dying client diagnosed with end-stage heart failure?
    1. "Perform as much care for the client as possible to conserve their strength."
    2. "Do not get too attached to the client because it will hurt when they die."
    3. "You must not promise to withhold healthcare information from the team."
    4. "The client may want to talk about their life, but you should discourage that."

50. The client on telemetry is showing ventricular tachycardia. Which action should the telemetry RN staff nurse delegate to the UAP?
    1. Have the UAP call the operator and announce the code.
    2. Tell the UAP to answer the other call lights on the unit.
    3. Send the UAP to the room to start rescue breaths.
    4. Ask the family to step out of the room during the code.

51. The family member of the client experiencing a cardiac arrest refuses to leave the client's room. Which intervention should the administrative supervisor implement?
    1. Stay with the family member and explain what the team is doing.
    2. Call hospital security to escort the family member out of the room.
    3. Ask the HCP whether the family member can stay.
    4. Ignore the family member unless they become hysterical.

52. The client presents to the ED reporting chest pain but cannot pay for the services. Which action should the ED nurse implement **first**?
    1. Place the client on a telemetry monitor and assess the client.
    2. Call an ambulance to transfer the client to a charity hospital.
    3. Have the client sign a form agreeing to pay the bill.
    4. Ask the client why they chose to come to this hospital.

53. The nurse is caring for clients on a cardiac unit. Which client should the nurse assess **first**?
    1. The client diagnosed with angina reporting chest pain
    2. The client diagnosed with CHF having bilateral 4+ peripheral edema
    3. The client diagnosed with endocarditis and a temperature of 100°F
    4. The client diagnosed with aortic valve stenosis experiencing syncope

54. Which medication should the nurse administer **first** after receiving the morning shift report?
    1. The IVPB antibiotic to the client diagnosed with endocarditis admitted at 0530 today.
    2. The antiplatelet medication to the client diagnosed with myocardial infarction.
    3. The coronary vasodilator patch to the client diagnosed with coronary artery disease.
    4. The statin medication to the client diagnosed with atherosclerosis.

55. The nurse in a critical care cardiac unit is administering medications to a client. Which intervention should the nurse implement **first?**
    1. Check the radial pulse before administering digoxin.
    2. Monitor the amiodarone level for the client receiving amiodarone.
    3. Obtain the latest PTT results for the client with a heparin drip.
    4. Check the liver function panel for the client receiving a dopamine drip.

56. The surgical nurse is admitting a client having heart surgery to the operating room. Which information would require the nurse to call a time-out? **Select all that apply.**
    1. The client is drowsy from the preoperative medication and drifts off to sleep.
    2. The consent form states mitral valve replacement, and the client states aortic valve replacement.
    3. The EHR and client's armband state the client is allergic to the narcotic analgesic morphine.
    4. The client states their name and birth date as it appears on the EHR.
    5. The surgical procedure is beginning, and the team (surgeon, anesthesiologist, and nurse) is present.

57. The nurse is administering medications at 1800 to a client and uses the following medication administration record (MAR).

Client's Name: CC Diagnosis: Heart Failure	Allergies: NKDA Height: 68 inches	
Medication	0701–1900	1901–0700
Digoxin 0.125 mg PO daily	0900 DN	
Furosemide 40 mg IVP daily	0900 DN	
Cephalosporin 1800 500 mg PO every 6 hours	1200 DN	1800
Warfarin 5 mg PO daily		1800
Nurse Name/Initials	Day Nurse RN/DN	Night Nurse RN/NN

Which intervention should the nurse implement **first?**
    1. Assess the client's potassium and digoxin levels.
    2. Monitor the client's partial thromboplastin level.
    3. Check the client's International Normalized Ratio (INR).
    4. Verify the client's name and ID number with the MAR.

58. The nurse is administering medications to clients on a cardiac unit. Which medication should the nurse **question** administering?
    1. Furosemide to a client with 320 mL output in 4 hours
    2. Enoxaparin to a client recovering from open-heart surgery
    3. Ticlopidine to a client being prepared for surgery
    4. Captopril to a client who has a BP of 100/68 mm Hg

59. The RN ICU nurse and a UAP are caring for the client recovering from coronary artery bypass graft (CABG) surgery. Which nursing tasks should the RN staff nurse assign to the UAP? **Select all that apply.**
    1. Monitor the client's arterial blood gases.
    2. Reinfuse the client's blood using the cell saver.
    3. Assist the client to take a sponge bath.
    4. Change the client's saturated leg dressing.
    5. Empty the urinary catheter drainage bag.

60. The nurse is preparing to administer 2 units of packed red blood cells (PRBCs) to a client diagnosed with CHF. Which HCP order should the nurse **question?**
    1. Administer each unit over 2 hours.
    2. Administer furosemide IVP once.
    3. Restrict the client's fluids to 1,000 mL per 24 hours.
    4. Have a complete blood count (CBC) done the next morning.

61. The elderly client on the cardiac unit was found on the floor by their bed. Which information should the nurse document in the client's EHR?
    1. Fell. No injuries noted. Incident report completed. HCP notified.
    2. Found on floor. No reports of pain. Able to move all extremities.
    3. States no one answered call light, so attempted to get up without help.
    4. Got out of bed without assistance and fell by the bedside.

62. The RN home health nurse is caring for an elderly client. Which nursing task should the RN delegate to the home health aide?
    1. Cook and freeze meals for the client.
    2. Assist the client to sit on the front porch.
    3. Take the client for outings to the store.
    4. Monitor the client's mental status.

63. The client is admitted to determine whether they are experiencing a myocardial infarction. The client is reporting substernal chest pain radiating to the left arm and jaw. Which intervention should the nurse implement **first?**
    1. Take the client's pulse, respirations, and blood pressure.
    2. Call for a STAT electrocardiogram and a troponin level.
    3. Place sublingual nitroglycerin 0.3 mg under the tongue.
    4. Notify the HCP that the client has pain.

64. The client on the cardiac unit has a cardiac arrest. Which is the administrative supervisor nurse's **first** intervention during the code?
    1. Begin to take notes to document the code.
    2. Make sure all the jobs are being done.
    3. Arrange for an intensive care unit bed.
    4. Administer the emergency medications.

65. Which client should the cardiac nurse assess **first** after receiving the p.m. shift report?
    1. The client completing their second unit of PRBCs
    2. The crying client after being informed of a terminal diagnosis
    3. The client refusing to eat from the dietary tray but ate food from home
    4. The client experiencing shortness of breath ambulating in the hallway

66. The nurse is caring for a client on a telemetry unit. At 0830, the client reports chest pain.

Client Name: Mr. A.B. Weight in pounds: 202	Account Number: 1122337 Weight in kg: 91.82	Height: 72 in (182.9 cm) Date: Today
Medication	1901–0700	0701–1900
Morphine sulfate 2 mg IVP every 1 hour prn chest pain		
Oxycodone 7.5/acetaminophen 325 mg PO every 4 hours prn pain	0030 NN 0545 NN	
Aluminum Hydroxide; Magnesium Hydroxide; Simethicone 30 mL PO prn indigestion		
Nitroglycerin 0.4 mg SL every 5 minutes up to 3 tablets prn chest pain		
Nitroglycerin transdermal cream 1/2 inch	2100 Remove	0900 Apply
Signature/Initials	Night Nurse RN/NN	Day Nurse RN/DN

Which medication should the nurse administer?
1. One-half inch of nitroglycerin transdermally now
2. Morphine sulfate 2 mg IVP STAT
3. Oxycodone 7.5 mg/acetaminophen 325 mg PO now
4. Nitroglycerin 0.4 mg sublingual STAT

67. The charge nurse on a cardiac unit received laboratory reports to assess. Which laboratory report is a **priority** for the charge nurse to assess?
    1. The client, Ms. C.T., on a heparin drip

Client Name: C.T. Diagnosis: DVT Weight in kg: 60	Account Number: 2233669 Height: 66 in (167.6 cm) Weight in pounds: 132	Allergies: NKDA

Laboratory Report

Laboratory Test	Client Values	Reference Values
aPT	15	10–13 seconds
INR	1.4	2–3 (therapeutic value)
aPTT	56	25–35 seconds

2. The client, Mr. R.S., scheduled for a CABG this morning

Client Name: R.S.
Diagnosis: Coronary Artery Disease
Weight in kg: 112.73
Account Number: 8855992
Height: 73 in (185.4 cm)
Allergies: Sulfa
Weight in pounds: 248

Laboratory Report

Laboratory Test	Client Values	Reference Values
aPT	11	10–13 seconds
INR	1.0	2–3 (therapeutic value)
aPTT	34	25–35 seconds
White blood cell count	5.9	$4.5–11.1 \times 10^3$ cells/microL
Red blood cell count	4.9	Male: $4.51–6.01 \times 10^6$ cells/microL
		Female: $4.01–5.51 \times 10^6$ cells/microL
Hemoglobin	13.5	Male: 14–17.3 g/dL
		Female: 11.7–15.5 g/dL
Hematocrit	44.2	Male: 42%–52%
		Female: 36%–48%
Platelets	292	$150–450 \times 10^3$ platelets/microL

3. The client, Ms. T.R., who had a cardiac catheterization 18 hours ago

Client Name: T.R.
Diagnosis: Chest pain
Weight in kg: 90.9
Account Number: 6655774
Height: 62 inches
Allergies: Penicillin
Weight in pounds: 200

Laboratory Report

Laboratory Test	Client Values	Reference Values
aPT	12	10–13 seconds
INR	1.0	2–3 (therapeutic value)
aPTT	29	25–35 seconds

4. The client, Mr. J.E., who is being evaluated for a heart murmur

Client Name: J.E.
Diagnosis: R/O Gallbladder Disease
Weight in kg: 90
Account Number: 6251489
Height: 68 inches
Allergies: NKDA
Weight in pounds: 198

Laboratory Report

Laboratory Test	Client Values	Reference Values
aPT	9.8	10–13 seconds
INR	1.3	2–3 (therapeutic value)
aPTT	26	25–35 seconds
Platelets	392	$140–400 \times 10^3$/microL

68. The nurse on a medical unit is making rounds after receiving the shift report. Which client should the nurse see **first? Rank in order of priority.**
    1. The 45-year-old client reporting chest pain at midnight last night and receiving nitroglycerin (NTG) sublingually
    2. The 62-year-old client reporting that no one answered the call light for 2 hours yesterday
    3. The 29-year-old client diagnosed with septicemia calling to request more blankets because of being cold
    4. The 78-year-old client diagnosed with dementia with a daughter concerned because the client is more confused today
    5. The 37-year-old client diagnosed with a stage 4 pressure injury, needing the dressing to be changed this morning

69. Ambulating in the hallway with the nurse, the client diagnosed with myocardial infarction reports chest pain. Which interventions should the nurse implement? **Select all that apply.**
    1. Administer nitroglycerin 0.4 mg sublingual STAT.
    2. Have the client walk back to their room.
    3. Take the client's vital signs.
    4. Place the client on supplemental oxygen.
    5. Ask the unit secretary to call the HCP for orders.

70. The nurse received an aPTT report on a client receiving heparin via continuous drip infusion. According to the report, the client's drip rate should be decreased by 100 units per hour. The heparin comes prepared as 25,000 units in 500 mL of fluid. The current rate of infusion is 26 mL/hr. At what rate should the nurse set the pump?

    _____

71. Which client should the charge nurse assign to the **most** experienced RN on the unit?
    1. The elderly client diagnosed with atrial fibrillation receiving the first dose of dabigatran
    2. The 43-year-old client diagnosed with congestive heart failure coughing up pink, frothy sputum
    3. The 47-year-old client diagnosed with a myocardial infarction exhibiting occasional premature ventricular contractions
    4. The young adult client diagnosed with mitral valve prolapse reporting shortness of breath when sitting in their chair

72. The telemetry technician tells the RN primary nurse the 59-year-old client in room 420 has a flat line. Which intervention should the primary nurse implement **first?**
    1. Instruct the UAP to take the crash cart to room 420.
    2. Tell the telemetry technician to call the Rapid Response Team.
    3. Determine if the client has an apical pulse and blood pressure.
    4. Check to see if the client has the telemetry leads on their chest.

73. The RN primary nurse has instructed the UAP to assist an elderly client to the bathroom for a shower. Which action by the UAP **warrants** intervention by the RN primary nurse?
    1. The UAP did not notify the desk that the telemetry was being removed.
    2. The UAP did not remove the electrodes from the client's chest.
    3. The UAP placed a bath chair in the shower for the client.
    4. The UAP stayed in the client's bathroom while the client showered.

74. The RN charge nurse is looking over the morning laboratory results. Which client **warrants** the charge nurse notifying the HCP?
    1. The 65-year-old client receiving IVP digoxin with a digoxin level of 2.4 mg/dL
    2. The middle-age client receiving warfarin with an INR of 1.2
    3. The 56-year-old client receiving furosemide with a potassium level of 3.5 mEq/L
    4. The young adult client receiving nystatin and a cholesterol level of 205 mg/dL

75. Which client should the RN charge nurse assign to the LPN?
    1. The 19-year-old client just admitted from the emergency department to the unit
    2. The 72-year-old client exhibiting supraventricular tachycardia on telemetry
    3. The middle-age client recovering from a left femoral cardiac catheterization
    4. The 61-year-old client in need of teaching about coronary artery disease

76. The RN charge nurse is entering the HCP's admissions orders into the EHR for a 67-year-old client being admitted for R/O (rule out) myocardial infarction. Which HCP order should the RN charge nurse **question**?
    1. Draw cardiac isoenzymes every 6 hours.
    2. Provide a low-fat, low-cholesterol diet.
    3. Administer morphine IVP 2 mg every 5 minutes for chest pain.
    4. Schedule the client for endoscopy in the a.m.

77. Which nursing task is **most** appropriate for the RN charge nurse to delegate to the UAP?
    1. Request the UAP to obtain the newly admitted client's weight.
    2. Ask the UAP to clean the room for the client being discharged.
    3. Tell the UAP to take the vital signs on the hypovolemic client.
    4. Instruct the UAP to discuss the low-fat, low-cholesterol diet with the client.

78. The 79-year-old client is reporting severe chest pain of 10 on a 1-to-10 pain scale. Which intervention should the nurse implement **first**?
    1. Check the client's MAR for the last time medication was administered.
    2. Assess the client's apical pulse, blood pressure, and lung sounds.
    3. Administer sublingual nitroglycerin to the client.
    4. Place oxygen via nasal cannula at 6 L/min.

79. The 70-year-old client is in ventricular tachycardia. Which intervention should the nurse implement **first**?
    1. Defibrillate the client.
    2. Assess the carotid pulse.
    3. Administer epinephrine IVP.
    4. Start cardiopulmonary resuscitation.

80. The RN charge nurse is completing discharge teaching for the 56-year-old client diagnosed with angina. Which statement indicates the client needs **more** teaching?
    1. "I must always keep my nitroglycerin tablets in a dark bottle."
    2. "I should walk 30 minutes or more at least three times a week."
    3. "I will decrease the number of cigarettes I smoke daily."
    4. "I am going to take one baby aspirin daily."

CARDIAC CASE STUDY

(1500) A middle school student runs into the school to find the school nurse. The student states, "Mr. P. was cutting the grass and fell—he isn't moving!" The nurse runs to the client's location and finds the client unresponsive, diaphoretic, clammy, and with a very rapid heartbeat. The nurse asks another adult teacher to "call 911; then bring me the AED and my black bag." As the client begins to regain consciousness, the nurse instructs the client to lie still. The client denies pain but states shortness of breath. The school principal arrives with the client's employment file, which indicates a history of hypertension and long COVID. The ambulance arrives at the school as the nurse takes the client's vital signs.

Vital Signs	Client Values
Blood pressure	100/52 mm Hg
Heart rate	162 bpm
Respirations	22 breaths/min
Temperature	Not available
Spo_2	92%

1. **Recognize cues. What matters most?** The school nurse prepares to give report to the Emergency Medical System (EMS) responders upon arrival. Which **priority** client data should be reported? **Select all that apply.**
    1. Blood pressure
    2. Level of consciousness
    3. Heart rate
    4. Unknown allergies
    5. Shortness of breath
    6. Diaphoresis
    7. Past medical history
    8. Unknown medications

(1525) The ED triage nurse receives a call from EMS transporting an older adult male client with a syncopal episode while mowing the grass with a push mower. The client was initially unresponsive but regained consciousness before EMS arrival on the scene. The client is alert and oriented ×2, with vital signs as listed, oxygen at 2 L via face mask, and an IV solution of 0.9% NaCl to the right antecubital area (20-gauge).

Vital Signs	Client Values
Blood pressure	102/50 mm Hg
Heart rate	161 bpm
Respirations	21 breaths/min
Temperature	99.8°F (37.7°C)
Spo_2	90%
EKG	Sinus tachycardia

2. **Analyze cues. What could it mean?** Which issues most concern the triage nurse? **Select two answers.**
   1. Dysrhythmia
   2. Sunburn
   3. Infection
   4. Head injury
   5. Dehydration

(1540) The client arrives in the ED via stretcher. The nurse assesses the client and notes the following: alert and oriented ×2, pale and diaphoretic, skin flushed with circumoral pallor. The client states, "I feel like my heart is beating out of my chest!" The nurse documents the vital signs populated in the chart and contacts the ED physician. EKG reading shows atrial fibrillation.

Vital Signs	Client Values
Blood pressure	93/47 mm Hg
Heart rate	361 bpm
Respirations	25 breaths/min
Temperature	99.8°F (37.7°C)
Spo$_2$	90% on 2 L oxygen via mask

(1549) The ED physician visits the client and places the following orders:

PROVIDER ORDERS:

Albuterol 0.83 mg via nebulizer ×1 STAT then every 6 hours as needed for shortness of breath
Cardiology consult: New onset atrial fibrillation STAT
Central line placement STAT
Titrate oxygen via mask to maintain Spo$_2$ ≥94%
0.9% NaCl via IV @ 150 mL/hr

3. **Prioritize hypotheses. Where do I start?** Complete the sentence by choosing from the drop-down list of options. Based on the client's condition at the time, the nurse recognizes that the client is at the highest risk for _____

   Select ▼
   1. Fluid volume overload
   2. Decreased cardiac output
   3. Infection

and will require _____ .

   Select ▼
   1. Antibiotics
   2. Diuretic
   3. Central line placement

4. **Generate solutions. What can I do?** For each intervention, specify if the intervention is **indicated** or **not indicated** for the client's care at this time.

Potential Nursing Intervention	Indicated	Not Indicated
Offer the client PO fluids		
Send consult to cardiology STAT		
Send request for central line placement STAT		
Continuous EKG		
Increase oxygen to 5 L via nasal cannula		
Administer albuterol		
Assist the client to move to the chair		
Reduce IV rate to 75 mL/hr		

(1615) The cardiologist requests the client be transferred immediately to Interventional Radiology for cardioversion as soon as the central line is placed.

(1640) The IV team successfully placed a left subclavian triple lumen catheter. The client was transferred to Interventional Radiology and underwent a successful cardioversion. The client is transferred to Cardiovascular ICU (CVICU) with the following transfer orders:

PROVIDER ORDERS:

Admit to CVICU: atrial fibrillation requiring cardioversion
Continuous EKG and pulse oximetry
Maintain IV fluids of 0.9% NaCl @ 100 mL/hr
Call cardiology resident STAT for heart rate >120 bpm and/or suspected dysrhythmia
Diet and activity as tolerated; up with assistance only

(1830) Provider orders reviewed and report provided to ICU nurse. As client admitted, EKG now reading atrial fibrillation with a rate of 354 bpm. Vital signs populated in the chart. Client alert and oriented ×2, skin pale, clammy, and diaphoretic. Denies pain, stating, "It feels like my heart is racing again!" STAT call placed to cardiology resident.

Vital Signs	Client Values
Blood pressure	102/68 mm Hg
Heart rate	354 bpm
Respirations	22 breaths/min
Temperature	97.6°F (36.4°C)
Spo_2	92% on 3 L oxygen via nasal cannula

(1838) Cardiology resident at bedside. Explains to client that since a successful cardioversion ×1 was conducted today and rhythm autoconverted back to atrial fibrillation; will approach with medication and monitor closely. Provider informed client that chosen medication regimen is usually used for other dysrhythmias, but that protocol has been highly effective in treating atrial fibrillation. Client verbalized understanding and agreement. Provider issues new orders.

PROVIDER ORDERS:

Initiate amiodarone IV STAT:
• **Loading dose**: Infuse via central line:
  • 150 mg over the first 10 minutes (15 mg/min),
  • Then 360 mg over the next 6 hours (1 mg/min)
• **Then decrease to maintenance infusion**:
  • 0.5 mg/min for 12 hours, then call cardiology resident for further orders

Continuous EKG and pulse oximetry
Titrate oxygen to maintain ≥92%, up to 5 L via nasal cannula/mask as needed
Call cardiology resident STAT for heart rate <60 bpm or BP <80/50 mm Hg
IV 0.9% NaCl @ 125 mL/hr
Diet as tolerated
Activity as tolerated; up with assistance only

5. **Take action. What will I do?** Which admission orders should the unit nurse consider a priority action? **Select all that apply.**
   1. Initiate amiodarone IV.
   2. Maintain continuous EKG and pulse oximetry.
   3. Titrate oxygen to maintain ≥92%, up to 5 L via nasal cannula/mask as needed.
   4. Call cardiology resident STAT for heart rate <60 bpm or BP <80/50 mm Hg.
   5. Administer IV 0.9% NaCl @ 125 mL/hr.
   6. Provide diet as tolerated.
   7. Allow activity as tolerated; up with assistance only.

(2210) The unit nurse obtains an updated set of vital signs and prepares shift change report.

Vital Signs	Client Values
Blood pressure	112/78 mm Hg
Heart rate	130 bpm
Respirations	19 breaths/min
Temperature	97.6°F (36.4°C)
SpO_2	93% on 3 L oxygen via nasal cannula
EKG	Atrial fibrillation

6. **Evaluate outcomes. Did it help?** For each assessment finding, indicate if the client's condition has improved, declined, or showed no change.

Finding	Improved	Declined	No Change
Temperature			
Heart rate			
Respirations			
Blood pressure			
SpO_2			
EKG			

ANSWERS AND RATIONALES

The correct answer number and rationale are in **bold-face purple type.** Rationales for why other answer options are incorrect are also given.

1. 1. **This client may or may not be stable. The client may have no reported symptoms at this time, but the nurse must assess this client first to determine whether the issue that brought the client to the ED has stabilized. This client should be seen first.**
   2. It is essential for the nurse to assess for pain relief promptly, but this client has been medicated, and the pain was a 3. The nurse can evaluate the pain relief amount after ensuring the ED admission is stable.
   3. This client has been back from the procedure, and a bilateral pedal pulse indicates the client is stable; therefore, this client does need to be seen first.
   4. Psychological issues are important but not more so than a physiological issue, and the client admitted from the ED may have a physiological problem.

CLINICAL JUDGMENT GUIDE: The test taker should use some tool as a reference to guide the decision-making process. In this situation, Maslow's Hierarchy of Needs should be applied. Physiological needs have priority over psychosocial ones.

2. 1. The cardiac glycoside, such as digoxin, should not be administered unless the apical pulse is 60 bpm or above.
   2. The nurse should question administering a loop diuretic because the client's serum K+ level is already low.
   3. **The client in ventricular fibrillation is in a life-threatening situation; therefore, an antidysrhythmic, such as amiodarone, should be administered first.**
   4. The client's BP is above 90/60 mm Hg, so the calcium-channel blocker can be administered, but it is not a priority over a client in a life-threatening situation.

CLINICAL JUDGMENT GUIDE: The test taker should know which medications are a priority, such as life-sustaining medications, insulin, and mucolytics (Carafate). These medications should be administered first by the nurse.

3. 1. The nurse would expect the client diagnosed with a deep vein thrombosis to have an edematous right calf, so the nurse would not need to assess this client first.
   2. The nurse would expect the client diagnosed with mitral valve stenosis to have heart palpitations (sensations of rapid, fluttering heartbeat).
   3. The nurse would expect the client diagnosed with arterial occlusive disease to have intermittent claudication (leg pain), so the nurse would not need to assess this client first.
   4. **The nurse would not expect the client diagnosed with CHF to have pink, frothy sputum because this is a sign of pulmonary edema. This client should be assessed first.**

CLINICAL JUDGMENT GUIDE: The test taker must determine which sign or symptom is not expected for the disease process. If the sign or symptom is unexpected, the nurse should assess the client first. This type of question determines whether the nurse knows signs or symptoms of various disease processes.

4. 1. This client is at high risk for complications related to necrotic myocardial tissue and will need extensive teaching; therefore, this client should not be assigned to a new graduate.
   2. Unstable angina means this client is at risk for life-threatening complications and should not be assigned to a new graduate.
   3. **A new graduate should be able to complete a preprocedural checklist and get this client to the catheterization laboratory.**
   4. Chest pain means this client could be having a myocardial infarction and should not be assigned to a new graduate.

CLINICAL JUDGMENT GUIDE: When deciding which client should be assigned to a new graduate, the test taker should give the most stable client to the least experienced nurse.

5. 1. An LPN can perform sterile procedures such as inserting indwelling catheters and IV lines. An RN should perform the functions that require nursing judgment, such as planning and evaluating the care of the clients.
   2. Although an LPN could administer most IVPB medications, only qualified RNs may administer IVP medications and chemotherapy.
   3. **A UAP is capable of performing the morning care. This is an appropriate nursing task to delegate.**
   4. Writing a care plan for a client requires nursing judgment; therefore, an RN should be assigned this function.

CLINICAL JUDGMENT GUIDE: An RN cannot delegate assessment, teaching, evaluation, medications, or an unstable client to a UAP. Tasks that require nursing clinical judgment cannot be delegated. Remember, in most instances, options with the word "all" (options 1 and 2) can be eliminated because if the test taker can think of one time when some other level of licensure could safely perform the task, the option automatically becomes wrong.

6. 1. The nurse should not share confidential information with anyone else unless the information shared is directly connected to healthcare issues. The nurse should inform clients that information will be shared on a need-to-know basis only.
   2. The case manager's job is to ensure continuity and adequacy of care for the client. This individual has a "need to know."
   3. The case manager is part of the healthcare team; therefore, information should be shared.
   4. The client gave permission when admitted to the hospital for information to be shared among those providing care. The case manager does not need to obtain further consent.

CLINICAL JUDGMENT GUIDE: The test taker must know the role of each member of the multidisciplinary healthcare team as well as the HIPAA rules and regulations. The NCLEX-RN® exam has questions on these topics.

7. 1. The telemetry strip indicates an artifact, so there is no need for the UAP or any staff member to call a Code Blue.
   2. The UAP should be instructed to check the telemetry lead placement; this reading cannot be ventricular fibrillation because the client is talking to the nurse over the intercom system. This telemetry is an artifact; therefore, the leads should be checked, and the UAP can do this because the client is stable.
   3. The UAP can take care of this problem; there is no need for the primary nurse to check the client based on the information provided.
   4. The strip indicates an artifact, but there is no indication to remove the client from telemetry monitoring.

CLINICAL JUDGMENT GUIDE: An RN cannot delegate assessment, teaching, evaluation, medications, or an unstable client to a UAP. Tasks that cannot be delegated are nursing interventions requiring nursing clinical judgment.

8. 1. The nurse with only surgical nursing experience would not be the choice to float to the ED.
   2. The nurse with critical care experience would be the best choice to float to the ED.
   3. The nurse just returning from sick leave would not be a good choice to send to the ED, which may be very busy at times.
   4. This nurse has no experience in critical care; therefore, this nurse would not be the best choice to float to the ED.

CLINICAL JUDGMENT GUIDE: The test taker needs to know management issues for the NCLEX-RN®. The nurse with experience in certain areas of nursing would be most appropriate to float to the areas with related types of clients, such as critical care and the ED.

9. Correct order is 5, 4, 3, 2, 1.
   5. The nurse must first obtain informed consent before administering the blood product.
   4. The nurse needs to complete the pre-transfusion assessment including assessing for any signs of allergic reaction before administering the unit of blood.
   3. The blood must be hung with Y-tubing and normal saline; an 18-gauge angiocatheter is preferred.
   2. The nurse must check the unit of blood from the laboratory with another nurse and with the client's blood band.
   1. During the first 15 minutes, the blood transfusion must be administered slowly to determine whether the client will have an allergic reaction.

CLINICAL JUDGMENT GUIDE: This is an alternate type of question included in the NCLEX-RN® test plan. The nurse must be able to perform skills in the correct order. Obtaining informed consent and assessment should always be the first interventions.

10. 1. The charge nurse is responsible for all clients. At times it is necessary to see clients diagnosed with a psychosocial need before other clients who have situations that are expected and are not life-threatening.
    2. An elevated CPK-MB (cardiac isoenzyme) level is expected in a client diagnosed with an acute myocardial infarction; therefore, the charge nurse would not see this client first.
    3. The INR is within the normal limits of 2 to 3; therefore, this client does not need to be assessed first.
    4. This client is being transferred to the cardiac unit; therefore, the client is stable and does not require the charge nurse to see this client first.

CLINICAL JUDGMENT GUIDE: The test taker must determine whether any of the assessment data are normal or abnormal for the client's diagnosis. If the data are abnormal, then this client should be seen first. If the physiological data are normal, then a client diagnosed with a psychosocial problem is the client the nurse should assess first.

11. Correct order is 3, 2, 4, 5, 1.
    3. Because this amount is lower than 1 mL, the nurse should draw this medication up in a 1-mL tuberculin syringe to ensure dosage accuracy.
    2. The nurse should dilute the medication with normal saline to help decrease pain during administration and maintain the IV site longer. Administering 0.25 mg of digoxin in 0.5 mL is difficult, if not impossible, to push over 5 full minutes, which is the manufacturer's recommended administration rate. If the medication is diluted, it is easier for the nurse to administer it over 5 minutes.
    4. The nurse must check two identifiers according to The Joint Commission (2024) safety guidelines.
    5. The nurse should clamp the tubing between the port and the primary IV line so that the medication will enter the vein, not ascend the IV tubing.
    1. Cardiovascular and narcotic medications are administered over 5 minutes.

CLINICAL JUDGMENT GUIDE: This is an alternate type of question included in the NCLEX-RN® test plan. The nurse must be able to perform skills in the correct order.

12. 1. The nurse should first discontinue the medication dopamine, a vasoconstrictor, which is causing the increase in the client's blood pressure, before doing anything else.
    2. The nurse should notify the HCP, but not before taking care of the client's elevated blood pressure.
    3. The client may need a vasopressor hydralazine medication to decrease the blood pressure, but the nurse should first discontinue the medication that is causing the elevated blood pressure.
    4. The nurse must first decrease the client's blood pressure before assessing the client.

CLINICAL JUDGMENT GUIDE: The test taker should remember that when the client is in distress, do not assess. The nurse must intervene and take care of the client. If any options are assessment data the HCP will need or an intervention that will help the client, then the test taker should not select the option to notify the HCP.

13. 1. The client diagnosed with rheumatic heart fever is expected to have carditis and should be on bedrest. The nurse needs to talk to the client about the importance of being on bedrest, but this client is not in a life-threatening situation and does not need the most experienced nurse.
    2. These ABG values are within normal limits; therefore, a less experienced nurse could care for this client.
    3. Multifocal PVCs are an emergency and are possibly life-threatening. An experienced nurse should care for this client.
    4. A cardiac catheterization is a routine procedure and would not require the most experienced nurse.

CLINICAL JUDGMENT GUIDE: The test taker must determine which client is the most unstable and would require the most experienced nurse, thus making this type of question an "except" question. Three clients are either stable or have non-life-threatening conditions.

14. 1. All clients in the ICU are on telemetry, and the UAP could bathe the client. This would not warrant intervention by the charge nurse.
    2. The UAP can perform glucometer checks at the bedside, and nothing indicates the client is unstable. This would not warrant intervention by the charge nurse.
    3. The UAP can assist with helping the client sit up for a portable chest x-ray if the UAP is not pregnant and wears a shield.
    4. This client is at risk for choking and is not stable; therefore, the charge nurse should intervene and not allow the UAP to feed this client.

CLINICAL JUDGMENT GUIDE: This is an "except" question. The test taker could ask which task is appropriate to delegate to the UAP; three options would be appropriate to delegate and one would not be. Remember, the RN cannot delegate assessment, teaching, evaluation, medications, or an unstable client to the UAP.

15. 1. The client receiving a calcium-channel blocker (CCB) should avoid grapefruit juice because it can cause the CCB to rise to toxic levels. Grapefruit juice inhibits cytochrome P450-3A4 found in the liver and the intestinal wall. This inhibition affects the metabolism of some drugs and can, as

is the case with CCBs, lead to toxic levels. For this reason, the nurse should investigate any medications the client is taking if the client drinks grapefruit juice.
2. The apical heart rate should be greater than 60 bpm before administering the medication; therefore, the nurse would not question administering this medication.
3. NSAIDs should be taken with foods to prevent gastric upset; therefore, the nurse would not question administering this medication.
4. The INR therapeutic level for warfarin (Coumadin), an anticoagulant, is 2 to 3; therefore, the nurse would not question administering this medication.

CLINICAL JUDGMENT GUIDE: The test taker must know medications. In most scenarios, there is no test-taking hint to help the test taker when answering medication questions except common nursing interventions, such as do not administer cardiac medications if the client has an apical pulse lower than 60 bpm or BP lower than 90/60 mm Hg, do not administer medications with grapefruit juice or antacids, or administer most medications with food to prevent GI distress.

16. 1. This is a win-lose strategy wherein, during the conflict, one party (charge nurse) exerts dominance, and the other (staff nurse) submits.
    2. **This is a win-win strategy that focuses on goals and attempts to meet the needs of both parties. The charge nurse keeps an experienced nurse, and the staff nurse keeps their position. Both parties win.**
    3. This is a negotiation in which the conflicting parties give and take on the issue. The staff nurse gets one more chance, and the charge nurse's authority remains intact.
    4. This is not an example of a win-win strategy and is not an appropriate action for the staff nurse. The opinion of the staff should not influence the charge nurse's action.

CLINICAL JUDGMENT GUIDE: Management questions will be on the NCLEX-RN®. There is often no test-taking strategy; the nurse must be knowledgeable of management issues.

17. 1. The client diagnosed with pericarditis is expected to have chest pain with inspiration; therefore, this client does not warrant immediate intervention.
    2. The client diagnosed with mitral valve regurgitation is expected to have thready peripheral pulses and cool, clammy extremities. Therefore, this client does not warrant immediate intervention.
    3. The client diagnosed with Marfan syndrome is expected to have a chest that sinks in or sticks out, known as funnel chest or pectus excavatum; therefore, this client does not warrant immediate intervention.
    4. **Slurred speech and drooling are signs of a cerebrovascular accident (stroke) and are not normal for a client diagnosed with atherosclerosis; therefore, this client should be assessed first.**

CLINICAL JUDGMENT GUIDE: The test taker should ask, "Are the assessment data normal for the disease process?" If they are normal for the disease process, the nurse would not need to intervene; if they are not normal for the disease process, then this warrants intervention by the nurse.

18. 1. The family may be allowed to bring in food occasionally from home, but what they bring may not adhere to a low-sodium diet, and the family should not be required to provide three meals per day for the client. Providing meals is the facility's responsibility.
    2. **Assessing the client's intake will help the nurse determine the extent of the client's dissatisfaction with the food. This is the first intervention.**
    3. This may be true, but does not help the client adjust to a lack of sodium in the diet.
    4. The nurse should assess the situation before making a referral to the dietitian.

CLINICAL JUDGMENT GUIDE: Assessment is the first step of the nursing process, and the test taker should use the nursing process or some other systematic process to assist in determining priorities.

19. 1. The client diagnosed with mitral valve stenosis can live with this diagnosis; it is not life-threatening.
    2. The client diagnosed with asymptomatic sinus bradycardia is stable, and because the client is not exhibiting any signs or symptoms, this client does not need to be assigned to the most experienced nurse.
    3. **A client diagnosed with fulminant pulmonary edema is experiencing an acute, life-threatening problem. The most experienced nurse should be assigned to this client.**
    4. A client diagnosed with acute atrial fibrillation is not in a life-threatening situation; therefore, this client would not be assigned to the most experienced nurse.

CLINICAL JUDGMENT GUIDE: The test taker must determine which client is the most unstable and would require the most experienced nurse, thus making this type of question an "except" question. Three clients are either stable or have non-life-threatening conditions.

20. 1. The client's INR is 3.4. The therapeutic range is 2 to 3 for a client diagnosed with atrial fibrillation. This client is at risk for bleeding. The nurse should hold the medication and discuss the warfarin (Coumadin) with the HCP.
    2. Metoclopramide (Reglan) is used to stimulate gastric emptying. Nothing in the stem or the MAR indicates a problem with administering this medication. The nurse would administer this medication.
    3. Docusate (Colace) is a stool softener. Nothing in the stem or the MAR indicates a problem with administering this medication. The nurse would administer this medication.
    4. Atorvastatin (Lipitor) is a lipid-lowering medication. Nothing in the stem or the MAR indicates a problem with administering this medication. The nurse would administer this medication.

CLINICAL JUDGMENT GUIDE: This is an alternate type question included in the NCLEX-RN® test plan. The test taker must be able to read a medication administration record (MAR), be knowledgeable of medications, and be able to decide on the nurse's most appropriate intervention.

21. 1. According to the AHA guidelines, the first step in CPR is to establish unresponsiveness by "shaking and shouting." If the client does not respond to being shaken, the nurse can proceed to the next step, "look, listen, and feel" for breaths. According to AHA guidelines, this is assessment, and the UAP could perform this function if alone. However, the nurse should assess the client before a UAP.
    2. Chest compressions are administered after establishing unresponsiveness and lack of respiration.
    3. **The nurse can tell the UAP to get the crash cart while the nurse assesses the client. This is the best task to assign the UAP because this client may be unstable; until that is determined, the nurse should not delegate any client care.**
    4. The nurse should place the client in the recumbent position before attempting to perform chest compressions; the nurse should send the UAP for the crash cart and for help.

CLINICAL JUDGMENT GUIDE: This is an "except" question. The test taker could ask which task is appropriate to delegate to the UAP; three options would be appropriate to delegate and one would not be. Remember, the RN cannot delegate assessment, teaching, evaluation, medications, or an unstable client to the UAP.

22. Correct answers are 1 and 2.
    1. The nurse should care for the client as if the DNR order was not on the EHR. A DNR order does not mean the client no longer wishes treatment. It means the client does not want CPR or to be placed on a ventilator if the client's heart stops beating.
    2. The information about the DNR status should be communicated to other healthcare personnel by placement of a special armband on the client or a similar form of designation.
    3. The client has a DNR order, but this does not imply that there may be 6 months or less life expectancy for the client. (Hospice care may be requested for clients with a life expectancy of fewer than 6 months.) An order for hospice must be written by the attending HCP before making this referral.
    4. The client should be allowed as many visitors as the hospital policy allows.
    5. A DNR order does not indicate that the client does not want cardiac telemetry monitoring or other diagnostic procedures.

CLINICAL JUDGMENT GUIDE: This is an alternate type of question included in the NCLEX-RN®. The NCLEX-RN® test plan includes nursing care that is guided by legal requirements. The nurse must be knowledgeable of these issues.

23. 1. The nurse should be aware that sexual activity is vital to most adults and should not decide that the client is not sexually active because of the client's age. The nurse should provide instructions regarding sexual activity before the client is discharged. This question should be asked because many clients may be embarrassed to bring up the subject.
    2. The client should not drive a motor vehicle until released to do so by the HCP. This is not an appropriate question at this time.
    3. The client should be discharged with a prescription for oral pain medications to be taken as directed by the surgeon. The nurse should not encourage the client to use old medications the client may have at home. This is not an appropriate question.

4. The nurse is providing discharge instructions and should tell the client when to call the HCP. This is not an appropriate question.

CLINICAL JUDGMENT GUIDE: The NCLEX-RN® test plan includes sexuality under Health Promotion and Maintenance to assist the client in achieving optimal health. The nurse should assess and educate the client on sexuality issues following surgery.

24. 1. The LPN can give pertinent information to the HCP. The INR is high (therapeutic range is 2 to 3), and the HCP should be informed.
    2. The RN cannot assign the assessment to an LPN.
    3. The INR is elevated but will not affect the client's atrial fibrillation. The client is at risk for abnormal bleeding, not a life-threatening dysrhythmia.
    4. The normal INR range is 2 to 3; therefore, some action should be implemented.

CLINICAL JUDGMENT GUIDE: The nurse cannot assign assessment, teaching, evaluation, or an unstable client to an LPN. The LPN can transcribe HCP orders and can call them on the phone to obtain orders for a client.

25. 1. In a disaster, the nurse should utilize as many individuals as possible to help control the situation; therefore, this intervention is inappropriate.
    2. The UAP cannot assess clients; therefore, this is inappropriate.
    3. The UAP can keep the victims calm; therefore, this is an appropriate action. This action is not critical to the safety of the victims.
    4. The paramedics do not need civilians assisting them as they stabilize and transport the victims. This is not an appropriate action.

CLINICAL JUDGMENT GUIDE: The test taker must know the role of each member of the multidisciplinary healthcare team as well as HIPAA rules and regulations. The NCLEX-RN® examination tests these topics.

26. 1. The clinic nurse should not correct the UAP in front of the client. This is embarrassing to the UAP and makes the client uncomfortable.
    2. The clinic nurse must correct the UAP's behavior. The client's weight gain should not be announced in the office area so that all staff, clients, and visitors can hear. This is a violation of confidentiality.
    3. The clinic nurse should correct the UAP's behavior, but privately, with an explanation as to why the action is inappropriate. The UAP's action is a violation of confidentiality because the scale is located in the office area, and any client or visitor passing by, as well as other staff members, can hear the comment.
    4. The clinic nurse should handle this situation. If the UAP's behavior shows a pattern of behavior, then it should be reported to the director of nurses.

CLINICAL JUDGMENT GUIDE: In any business, including a healthcare facility, arguments or discussions of confidential information should not occur among staff of any level where the customers—in this case, the clinic clients—can hear it or see it.

27. Correct answers are 1, 2, 3, and 5.
    1. Case managers help coordinate healthcare between multiple sources of healthcare attempting to contain healthcare cost.
    2. The case manager is a client advocate and helps with communication between the client and HCPs, which enhances the client's quality of life.
    3. The case manager coordinates outpatient and inpatient care and helps with referrals for the client.
    4. Case management is not a form of health insurance.
    5. The case manager is involved in assessing, planning, facilitating, and advocating for health services for a client. Coordinating care is often exhausting and frustrating for the client and family.

CLINICAL JUDGMENT GUIDE: The test taker must know the role of each member of the multidisciplinary healthcare team as well as HIPAA rules and regulations. The NCLEX-RN® examination will have test questions on this topic.

28. 1. If the client takes the loop diuretic in the morning, then going to the bathroom frequently in the morning would not warrant intervention.
    2. Rising from a sitting position slowly helps prevent orthostatic hypotension, a potential side effect of all the medications. This statement would not warrant intervention.
    3. This statement indicates the client is adhering to a low-sodium diet, as they should be. No intervention is warranted.

4. Grapefruit juice can cause calcium-channel blockers to rise to toxic levels. Grapefruit juice inhibits cytochrome P450-3A4 found in the liver and intestinal wall. This statement warrants intervention by the nurse.

CLINICAL JUDGMENT GUIDE: The test taker must be knowledgeable of medications. In most scenarios, there is no test-taking hint to help the test taker when answering medication questions except common nursing interventions, such as do not administer cardiac medications if the client has an apical pulse less than 60 bpm or BP less than 90/60 mm Hg, do not administer medications with grapefruit juice or antacids, or administer most medications with food to prevent GI distress.

29. 1. This is a win-win strategy that focuses on goals (to have adequate staff) and attempts to meet the needs of both parties. The director of nurses keeps an experienced nurse, and the UAP maintains their position. Both parties win.
    2. This is a possible win-win strategy in which both parties win. The UAP keeps their job, and the director of nurses can hire a UAP who can work the assigned hours.
    3. This is a win-lose strategy during which the conflict shows that one party (the director of nurses) exerts dominance and the other (UAP) must submit and lose.
    4. This is a negotiation in which the conflicting parties give and take on the issues. The UAP gets one more chance, and the director of nurse's authority is still intact.

CLINICAL JUDGMENT GUIDE: Management questions will be on the NCLEX-RN®. There is often no test-taking strategy; the nurse must be knowledgeable of management issues.

30. 1. A full sharps container violates Occupational Health and Safety Administration (OSHA) regulations, and because the UAP has not changed it after being asked twice, a third request is unnecessary.
    2. The nurse should discuss why the sharps container has not been changed, but it is not the first intervention.
    3. A full sharps container violates OSHA regulations and may result in a $25,000 fine. The nurse should take care of this situation immediately and then discuss it with the UAP, modeling appropriate behavior.
    4. The situation must be documented because the UAP was told twice, but documentation is not the first intervention.

CLINICAL JUDGMENT GUIDE: The NCLEX-RN® test plan includes nursing care that is ruled by legal requirements. The nurse must be knowledgeable of these issues. The nurse may have to take action first and then take further action if necessary.

31. 1. The spouse should call 911, but the AHA recommends chewing a baby aspirin at the onset of chest pain.
    2. The AHA recommends that the client with chest pain chew an aspirin to help decrease platelet aggregation. This is the first intervention the clinic nurse should tell the spouse to do. The client is in distress; therefore, the nurse should have the spouse do something.
    3. This question could be asked to determine whether the pain is secondary to a gallbladder attack or gastric irritation, but this is not the first intervention.
    4. The clinic physician could talk to the client while the spouse is getting an aspirin, but this is not the first intervention.

CLINICAL JUDGMENT GUIDE: The test taker should apply the nursing process when asked, "Which intervention should be implemented first?" If the client is in distress, do not assess; if the client is in distress, do something.

32. 1. This BP—148/92 mm Hg—is elevated, but it would not be life-threatening for someone diagnosed with hypertension; therefore, the nurse would not contact this client first.
    2. A pulse oximeter reading of 93% is low but still within normal limits, and a client diagnosed with cystic fibrosis, a chronic respiratory condition, would be expected to have a chronically low oxygen level. This client would not need to be contacted first.
    3. The client diagnosed with CHF would be expected to have edematous feet; this client would not need to be contacted first.
    4. The client diagnosed with chronic atrial fibrillation is at risk for pulmonary emboli, a potentially life-threatening complication. Chest pain is a common symptom of pulmonary embolism. The nurse should contact this client first.

CLINICAL JUDGMENT GUIDE: When deciding which client to assess first, the test taker should determine whether the signs or symptoms the client exhibits are normal or expected for the client's situation. After eliminating the expected option, the test taker should determine which situation is more life-threatening.

33. 1. The nurse's first intervention is to assist the client to a sitting position to decrease the heart's workload by decreasing venous return and maximizing lung expansion. The goal is to help relieve the client's respiratory distress.
    2. The nurse should assess the client's vital signs, but the first intervention is to help the client breathe.
    3. The nurse should contact the paramedics if the client does not improve after being placed in a sitting position, but this is not the nurse's first intervention.
    4. The nurse should auscultate the client's lungs, but the first intervention is to help the client breathe more easily.

CLINICAL JUDGMENT GUIDE: The nurse should remember that if a client is in distress and the nurse can do something to relieve the distress, that action should be done first, before assessment. The test taker should select an option that helps the client's condition directly.

34. 1. The home health nurse can contact the agency's chaplain to provide spiritual support for the client's family, but the first intervention is to pronounce the client's death.
    2. Nurses in home health have the authority to pronounce death for clients who are on service and if death is imminent. This intervention should be implemented first.
    3. The family should be able to stay at the bedside, but if they need to leave for some reason, the nurse asking them to leave is not the first intervention. The nurse can assess the apical pulse with the family at the bedside.
    4. The client's funeral home needs to be contacted, but it is not the nurse's first action, and often the family will call the funeral home.

CLINICAL JUDGMENT GUIDE: The NCLEX-RN® test plan includes nursing care ruled by legal requirements. The nurse must be knowledgeable of these issues. The nurse must be aware of the rules and regulations of the various areas of nursing.

35. 1. The therapeutic range for INR is 2 to 3; therefore, this client would not need to be contacted first.
    2. The client's serum potassium level is within the normal range—3.5 to 5.3 mEq/L. Therefore, this client would not need to be contacted first.
    3. The client's digoxin level is higher than the therapeutic level for digoxin, which is 0.5 to 2 ng/dL. This client should be contacted first to assess for signs or symptoms of digoxin toxicity.
    4. The glycosylated hemoglobin, the average blood glucose level over 3 months, should not be more than 8%. This client, with a level of 6%, does not need to be contacted.

CLINICAL JUDGMENT GUIDE: The test taker must know normal laboratory data.

36. 1. The client should be encouraged to exercise, but it should be in a supervised setting, such as a cardiac rehabilitation unit, because the client has diabetes and hypertension.
    2. The client should adhere to a low-fat, low-cholesterol, carbohydrate-counting diet, which is not the priority intervention. The client needs to be supervised, and diet teaching is included in cardiac rehabilitation.
    3. Cardiac rehabilitation includes progressive exercise, diet teaching, and classes on modifying risk factors. This supervised setting would be the priority intervention for this client when discharged from home health.
    4. The client should lose weight slowly, but the priority intervention for this client would be a referral to a supervised setting where the client can lose weight slowly and safely.

CLINICAL JUDGMENT GUIDE: The test taker must know the role of each member of the multidisciplinary healthcare team as well as HIPAA rules and regulations. These topics will be tested on the NCLEX-RN® examination.

37. 1. The nurse should prepare the needed equipment, but it is not the nurse's first intervention.
    2. The nurse should call and arrange a time convenient for the visit, but the nurse should first review the client referral so the nurse is aware of the need for the visit.
    3. Before taking any further steps, the nurse should review the client's referral form and other pertinent data concerning the client's condition. The nurse may need to contact the referring agency if the information is unclear or important information is missing. This action is assessment.
    4. The nurse will not know which referrals are needed until after the first visit.

CLINICAL JUDGMENT GUIDE: Assessment is the first step of the nursing process, and the test taker should use the nursing process or some other systematic process to assist in determining priorities. The client is not in distress because they are at home.

38. Correct answers are 4 and 5.
    1. If the client or family is intoxicated, hostile, or obnoxious, the nurse should leave and reschedule the visit. There is no need to call the police unless the nurse thinks they will be hurt.
    2. The home health nurse should wear the agency identification on the shirt or blouse; it should be visible to anyone talking to the nurse.
    3. To be eligible for home health visits, the client must be homebound, and all visits should be done during daylight hours as a safety precaution.
    4. **The agency should be informed of the schedule so the nurse can be located if the nurse does not return when expected.**
    5. **The home health nurse should report unsafe work environments to the agency. The agency should be proactive in providing support for nurses caring for clients in an unsafe situation.**

CLINICAL JUDGMENT GUIDE: This is an alternate type of question included in the NCLEX-RN®. The test taker must be knowledgeable of all the various areas of nursing, the role of each member of the multidisciplinary healthcare team, and HIPAA rules and regulations. These topics will be tested on the NCLEX-RN® examination.

39. 1. This is professional boundary crossing. Even though the grandchild is not the client, they are related to the client. The home health aide should not go out with them.
    2. **This statement protects the home health aide. This is professional boundary crossing. The employee should not date the client's relatives because this may pose a conflict of interest. The aide should wait until the client is no longer on service.**
    3. The nurse's best response is to tell the home health aide the facts about dating clients' relatives. The director would tell the aide the same information.
    4. The home health aide could date the grandchild when the client is no longer on service. So this statement is not the nurse's best response.

CLINICAL JUDGMENT GUIDE: Management questions will be on the NCLEX-RN®. There is often no test-taking strategy; the nurse must be knowledgeable of management issues. Boundary crossing is a critical area of which every nurse must be aware.

40. Correct answers are 1, 2, 4, and 5.
    1. A 2-lb weight gain indicates the client is retaining fluid and should contact the HCP. This teaching intervention is appropriate.
    2. Keeping the head of the bed elevated will help the client breathe easier; therefore, this is an appropriate teaching intervention.
    3. The loop diuretic should be taken in the morning to prevent nocturia. This teaching intervention is inappropriate.
    4. Sodium retains water. Telling the client to avoid eating foods high in sodium is an appropriate teaching intervention.
    5. Isotonic exercise, such as walking or swimming, helps tone the muscles; discussing this with the client is an appropriate teaching intervention.

CLINICAL JUDGMENT GUIDE: This is an alternate type of question included in the NCLEX-RN®. Each answer option should be evaluated independently.

41. 1. The INR is not therapeutic yet; the nurse should administer warfarin (Coumadin), an anticoagulant medication.
    2. This potassium level is very low. Hypokalemia potentiates dysrhythmias in clients receiving digoxin (Lanoxin), a cardiac glycoside. This nurse should discuss potassium replacement with the HCP before administering this medication.
    3. An AST test measures the amount of this enzyme in the blood. The enzyme is part of the liver function panel. The normal range is 14 to 20 U/L for males and 10 to 36 U/L for females.
    4. Creatinine level is reflective of renal status. The normal range is 0.61 to 1.21 mg/dL (males) and 0.51 to 1.04 mg/dL (females).

CLINICAL JUDGMENT GUIDE: The test taker must know normal laboratory data.

42. 1. Assessment of the client's spiritual needs in end-of-life issues is a key consideration but is the chaplain's responsibility when they are a hospice team member.
    2. The client's financial situation can be assessed, but it is not a priority over the client's spiritual needs when death is near.

3. The client's support system is the priority assessment for the hospice nurse. The client will be cared for in the home, and the nurse must know who can help the client.
4. The client's medical diagnosis is important when addressing the grieving process. Still, there is nothing the nurse can do about the medical diagnosis, so assessing, supporting, and addressing the client's spiritual needs will be carried out before the medical diagnosis.

CLINICAL JUDGMENT GUIDE: The test taker must be knowledgeable of all the various areas of nursing, the role of each member of the multidisciplinary healthcare team, and HIPAA rules and regulations. The NCLEX-RN® examination tests these topics.

43. 1. The client's HCP will need to determine the time of death, but it is not the nurse's first intervention.
    2. The Rapid Response Team would not be notified because the client has a DNR order.
    3. The nurse should stay with the client and their spouse and not make any life-rescuing interventions while the client is dying. The spouse should not be left alone.
    4. The UAP can perform postmortem care, but it is not the first intervention when the client's spouse tells the nurse the client has quit breathing.

CLINICAL JUDGMENT GUIDE: A DNR order is a written physician's order instructing HCPs not to attempt CPR. A new term introduced is "allow natural death" (AND), which may be more acceptable to clients and their families. The nurse cannot legally perform CPR on a client with a DNR order.

44. 1. This client should be seen, but a terminally ill client refusing to eat is not an emergency situation.
    2. The client has a right to rescind the out-of-hospital DNR, but paperwork is not a priority over a client in pain.
    3. One of the main goals of hospice is pain and symptom control. This client should be seen first so that appropriate pain control can be obtained immediately.
    4. A stage 1 pressure injury must be assessed and treatment started, but this is not a priority over pain control.

CLINICAL JUDGMENT GUIDE: The nurse can use Maslow's Hierarchy of Needs to determine which client to assess first. Pain is a physiological need.

45. Correct answers are 1 and 5.
    1. Encouraging the client to review their life experiences assists the client in coming to a closure of their life. This is an important intervention the volunteer can perform.
    2. This is the job of the UAP, not the volunteer.
    3. This is the job of the chaplain, not the volunteer.
    4. This is the job of the nurse or occupational therapist, not the volunteer.
    5. The hospice volunteer can assist with light housekeeping chores, meal preparation, running errands, and other tasks.

CLINICAL JUDGMENT GUIDE: When the test taker is deciding which options are appropriate tasks to delegate or assign, the test taker should choose the tasks that allow each staff member to function within their full scope of practice. Do not assign a task to a staff member that falls outside the staff member's or volunteer's expertise.

46. 1. The nurse should provide instruction and support to the UAP. This response is the best.
    2. This is a callous statement and does not help the UAP learn to provide postmortem care.
    3. This does not address the UAP's concern.
    4. The nurse should assist the UAP to learn to perform the duties of a UAP, not circumvent the workload.

CLINICAL JUDGMENT GUIDE: The nurse cannot delegate any task the UAP admits to being unable to perform. Delegation means the nurse is responsible for the UAP's actions; therefore, the nurse must also intervene if the UAP is performing unsafely.

47. 1. If the HCP is called, the nurse, not the UAP, should perform this task. A UAP cannot take a telephone order; only a licensed nurse can take telephone orders.
    2. The UAP cannot administer medication, not even acetaminophen (Tylenol).
    3. The nurse should immediately go to the client's room and assess the client. Sometimes, the nurse may need to access the client's EHR and review the MAR to assist in assessing findings. The UAP can bring a computer or tablet that contains the EHR to the client's room.
    4. The UAP should not be asked to relay such information. This is the nurse's or HCP's responsibility.

CLINICAL JUDGMENT GUIDE: When the test taker is deciding which option is the most appropriate task to delegate or assign, the test taker should choose the task that allows each staff member to function within their full scope of practice. Do not assign a task to a staff member that requires a higher level of expertise than that staff member has. Conversely, do not assign a task to a staff member when that task could be performed by a staff member with a lower level of expertise.

48. Correct answers are 1, 4, and 5.
    1. The LPN can feed a stable client unable to feed themselves because of medical equipment. This is an appropriate task to assign.
    2. The nurse cannot assign assessment. This is an inappropriate task for to the LPN.
    3. The LPN should not perform discharge teaching for a client. This task is inappropriate to assign to the LPN.
    4. The LPN can administer a routine IVPB antibiotic ceftriaxone (Rocephin) medication.
    5. The LPN can contact the HCP for a PRN analgesic medication for a client. This is an appropriate task to assign.

CLINICAL JUDGMENT GUIDE: The nurse cannot assign assessment, teaching, evaluation, or an unstable client to an LPN. The LPN can call HCPs on the phone to obtain orders for a client.

49. 1. The UAP should encourage the client to remain independent as long as possible. If the client cannot perform activities of daily living (ADLs), then the UAP should perform the tasks.
     2. This may be true, but the UAP cannot and should not distance themselves from the clients. The UAP should maintain a professional relationship with the clients.
     3. This is an essential statement for the UAP to understand. If information revealed to the UAP is necessary to provide appropriate care to the client, then the information must be shared on a need-to-know basis with the healthcare team.
     4. Clients should be encouraged to discuss their life because life review may help clients accept their death.

CLINICAL JUDGMENT GUIDE: The test taker must know the role of each member of the multidisciplinary healthcare team as well as HIPAA rules and regulations. These topics will be tested on the NCLEX-RN® examination.

50. 1. The nurse in the client's room notifies the hospital operator of a code situation.
     2. Answering the call lights of the other clients on the unit can be delegated to the UAP.
     3. In a hospital, the respiratory therapist is responsible for ventilation.
     4. The nursing supervisor is responsible for requesting the family to leave the room. The UAP does not have the authority to make this request.

CLINICAL JUDGMENT GUIDE: When the test taker is deciding which option is the most appropriate task to delegate or assign, the test taker should choose the task that allows each member of the staff to function within their full scope of practice. Do not assign a task to a staff member that requires a higher level of expertise or that a staff member with a lower level of expertise could perform.

51. 1. If the family member is not disrupting the care, they should be allowed to stay in the room with the supervisor remaining near the family member, explaining why the interventions are being implemented. The supervisor should be ready to escort the family member out of the room if they become disruptive.
     2. This will cause ill will on the part of the family and could result in the filing of a needless lawsuit.
     3. The HCP is busy caring for the client. This is not the time to ask an HCP a question the supervisor can handle.
     4. Ignoring the family member could cause a problem; the supervisor should proactively manage the situation.

CLINICAL JUDGMENT GUIDE: The nurse should always try to support the client or the family's request if it does not violate any local, state, or federal rules and regulations. If unsure of the correct answer, this is the test taker's best decision.

52. 1. Federal law requires that clients presenting to an ED must be assessed and treated without regard to payment. The nurse should initiate steps to assess the client.
     2. The nurse must assess the client. If a transfer is made, it will be after the client has been stabilized and the receiving hospital has accepted the transfer.
     3. Federal law requires that clients presenting to an ED must be assessed and treated without regard to payment. The hospital will attempt to recover the costs after the client has been treated.
     4. This is irrelevant information.

CLINICAL JUDGMENT GUIDE: The NCLEX-RN® test plan includes nursing care ruled by legal requirements. The nurse must be knowledgeable of these issues.

53. 1. The client diagnosed with angina should be asymptomatic; when the client is reporting chest pain, this is abnormal data. Therefore, this client should be assessed first. Remember, Maslow's Hierarchy of Needs identifies physiological needs, and pain is a priority.
    2. In a client diagnosed with CHF, 4+ edema is expected. The nurse would not need to assess this client first.
    3. The client diagnosed with endocarditis is expected to have a fever. The nurse would not need to assess this client first.
    4. The client diagnosed with aortic valve stenosis has the classic triad of syncope, angina, and exertional dyspnea; therefore, this client would not be assessed first.

    CLINICAL JUDGMENT GUIDE: The test taker must determine which sign or symptom is not expected for the disease process. If the sign or symptom is unexpected, the nurse should assess that client first. This type of question is posed to determine whether the nurse knows the clinical manifestations of various disease processes.

54. 1. First-dose IV antibiotic medications are priority medications and should be administered within 1 to 2 hours of being ordered. This should be the first medication administered.
    2. Antiplatelet medication, aspirin, is not a priority medication.
    3. A coronary vasodilator patch, nitroglycerin, is not a priority medication.
    4. Most statin medications that decrease cholesterol levels should be administered in the evening when the enzyme for cholesterol metabolism is at its highest peak.

    CLINICAL JUDGMENT GUIDE: The test taker should know priority medications, such as life-sustaining medications, insulin, and mucolytics (Carafate). As the rationale explains, antibiotic therapy should be initiated as soon as possible; a delay could cause the death of the client.

55. 1. The nurse checks an apical pulse, not a radial pulse, before administering digoxin, a cardiac glycoside.
    2. There is no serum amiodarone level; therefore, the nurse cannot implement this intervention.
    3. IV heparin increases the client's partial thromboplastin time and causes an anticoagulant effect. The nurse should always be aware of the client's most current PTT levels when administering therapeutic heparin.
    4. The nurse should monitor the client's renal function and creatinine level, not the liver function.

    CLINICAL JUDGMENT GUIDE: The nurse must be aware of interventions that must be implemented before administering medications. The nurse must know what to monitor before administering medications because untoward reactions and possibly death can occur.

56. Correct answers are 2 and 5.
    1. The client would be expected to be drowsy after a narcotic preoperative medication. The nurse would not need to call a time-out for this client.
    2. Whenever there is a discrepancy in the EHR or with what the client says, the nurse should call an immediate time-out until the situation has been resolved.
    3. The client's allergy must be documented on the client's EHR and identification band; therefore, this would not warrant a time-out.
    4. Because this is what is supposed to happen, the nurse would not need to call a time-out.
    5. A time-out is standard before surgical procedures and should include vital team members such as the surgeon, anesthesiologist, and nurse.

    CLINICAL JUDGMENT GUIDE: The NCLEX-RN® test plan includes nursing care ruled by the current safety measures and familiarization with the National Patient Safety Goals. The nurse must be knowledgeable of these goals.

57. 1. The day shift nurse should check the client's potassium and digoxin levels before administering the digoxin (Lanoxin). The digoxin has been administered for the day.
    2. A PTT is monitored for IV heparin, not warfarin (Coumadin).
    3. **The nurse should monitor the INR before administering warfarin (Coumadin). The therapeutic INR level for warfarin is 2 to 3.**
    4. This task should be done immediately before administering the medication at the bedside.

    CLINICAL JUDGMENT GUIDE: This is an alternate type question included in the NCLEX-RN® test plan. The test taker must be able to read a medication administration record (MAR), be knowledgeable of medications, and be able to decide on the nurse's most appropriate intervention.

58. 1. The loop diuretic furosemide (Lasix) should be administered to the client with adequate urinary output.
    2. The anticoagulant enoxaparin (Lovenox) is prescribed to prevent deep vein thromboses (DVT) for immobile clients, such as a postsurgical client.
    3. **The nurse should not administer ticlopidine (Ticlid), an antiplatelet medication, to a client undergoing surgery because this will increase postoperative bleeding. The nurse should hold this medication and discuss this with the surgeon.**
    4. The client's blood pressure is within an acceptable range. The nurse should administer the ACE inhibitor captopril (Capoten).

    CLINICAL JUDGMENT GUIDE: The nurse must know specific interventions when administering medications to clients undergoing surgery; for example, the client should not receive most PO medications or any medications that could increase bleeding.

59. Correct answers are 3 and 5.
    1. The nurse and respiratory therapist, not the UAP, are responsible for monitoring the ABGs.
    2. Infusion of blood and blood products, even the client's own, cannot be delegated to a UAP.
    3. **The UAP can assist with hygiene needs; this is one of the main tasks that may be delegated to UAPs.**
    4. The nurse must assess the surgical site for bleeding, infection, and healing. The UAP cannot perform assessments.
    5. **The UAP can perform repetitive tasks such as emptying the urinary catheter drainage (Foley) bag.**

    CLINICAL JUDGMENT GUIDE: This is an alternate type of question included in the NCLEX-RN®. An RN cannot delegate assessment, teaching, evaluation, medications, or an unstable client to a UAP. Tasks that cannot be delegated are nursing interventions requiring nursing clinical judgment.

60. 1. **The nurse should administer a unit of blood over the greatest length of time possible (4 hours) to a client diagnosed with CHF to prevent fluid volume overload. The nurse should question this order.**
    2. Administering the loop diuretic furosemide (Lasix) to a client diagnosed with CHF receiving blood is an appropriate order. The nurse would not question this HCP order.
    3. Restricting fluids to a client diagnosed with CHF is appropriate, depending on the severity of the client's condition. The nurse would not question this order, especially when administering IV fluids to the client.
    4. The HCP should evaluate the effects of the 2 units of blood. The nurse would not question this HCP order.

    CLINICAL JUDGMENT GUIDE: When the stem asks the nurse to determine which HCP order to question, the test taker must realize this is an "except" question. Three of the options are appropriate for the HCP to prescribe, and one is not appropriate for the client's disease process or procedure.

61. 1. The nurse should not document that the client fell unless the nurse observed the client fall. The nurse should never write "incident report" in an EHR. An incident report can be called an occurrence report. This is a red flag to a lawyer.
    2. **The nurse should document exactly what was observed. This statement is the correct documentation.**
    3. This statement is not substantiated and should not be placed in the EHR.
    4. This statement documents a fall that the nurse did not observe.

    CLINICAL JUDGMENT GUIDE: The nurse must be able to document nursing care safely. It includes accurate, timely documentation; it meets professional, legislative, and agency standards; it facilitates communication between nurses and other HCPs; and it is comprehensive.

62. 1. Cooking and cleaning can be arranged through some home health agencies, but these jobs would be done by a housekeeper, not by the UAP.
    2. **The home health aide is responsible for assisting the client with activities of daily living and transferring from the bed to the chair. Sitting outside is good for the client and is a task that can be delegated to the home health aide.**
    3. This is boundary crossing by the UAP and could create legal difficulties if the UAP had an accident.
    4. This is assessment and cannot be delegated to a UAP.

    CLINICAL JUDGMENT GUIDE: When deciding on the most appropriate task to delegate or assign, the test taker should choose the task that allows each staff member to function within their full scope of practice. Do not assign a task to a staff member that falls outside the staff member's or volunteer's expertise. Remember, the RN cannot delegate assessment, teaching, evaluation, medications, or an unstable client to the UAP.

63.
    1. If the client is in distress, assessment is not the first intervention if there is an action the nurse can take to relieve the distress. The nurse should administer the nitroglycerin first.
    2. Calling for an EKG and troponin level should be implemented, but not before administering the nitroglycerin.
    3. Placing nitroglycerin under the client's tongue may relieve the client's chest pain and provide oxygen to the heart muscle. This is the nurse's first intervention.
    4. The HCP can be notified after the nurse has stabilized the client.

CLINICAL JUDGMENT GUIDE: The nurse should remember that if a client is in distress and the nurse can do something to relieve the distress, that action should be done first before assessment. The test taker should select an option that helps the client's condition directly.

64.
    1. The supervisor can take notes documenting the code until relieved, but the supervisor needs to be free to supervise the code and coordinate room assignments and staffing.
    2. The first intervention for the supervisor is ensuring that all the jobs in the code are filled.
    3. This is the supervisor's responsibility, but it is not the first intervention.
    4. The supervisor can administer medications, but the supervisor needs to be flexible to complete the supervisor's duties.

CLINICAL JUDGMENT GUIDE: The test taker must know the role of each member of the multidisciplinary healthcare team as well as HIPAA rules and regulations. The NCLEX-RN® examination will have questions on these topics. The administrative manager is responsible for the other members of the healthcare team.

65.
    1. This client is being treated, and if the blood is almost finished, then it can be assumed that the client is tolerating the blood without incident.
    2. The client has been given devastating news. When all the information in the options is expected and not life-threatening, then psychological issues have priority. This client should be seen first.
    3. The client has eaten. The nurse could arrange for the dietitian to consult with the client about food preferences, but this client does not need to be assessed first.
    4. Dyspnea on exertion is not a priority if the client is exerting themselves.

CLINICAL JUDGMENT GUIDE: The test taker must determine whether the assessment data are normal or abnormal for the client's diagnosis or situation. If the data are abnormal, then this client should be seen first. If the data are normal, then a client diagnosed with a psychosocial problem is the client the nurse should assess first.

66.
    1. This medication could be administered, but it will not have as rapid an impact as the sublingual dose.
    2. Nitroglycerin (NTG) is administered first because it will dilate the vessels and resolve the cause of the chest pain. If the chest pain is still present after 3 NTG tablets, then morphine should be administered.
    3. Oxycodone and acetaminophen will not address the chest pain specifically.
    4. The nurse should administer the medication with the most rapid onset and directly resolve the problem. Nitroglycerin is a potent vasodilator and will dissolve rapidly under the tongue (sublingually).

CLINICAL JUDGMENT GUIDE: This is an alternate type question included in the NCLEX-RN® test plan. The test taker must be able to read a MAR, be knowledgeable of medications, and be able to decide on the nurse's most appropriate intervention.

67.
    1. A client diagnosed with a DVT on a heparin drip should have an aPTT in this range. The charge nurse should ensure that the drip maintains the client in the therapeutic range, but the safety of the client going to surgery is the first priority.
    2. This client is scheduled for surgery this morning; therefore, the charge nurse must make sure they are stable for the procedure and notify the surgeon if there is any reason to question the safety of the client having the procedure this morning.
    3. This client is postprocedure, so unless a situation arises from the nurse's assessment, this client is not a priority.
    4. A heart murmur is not life-threatening but can be associated with other disease processes. This client is not a priority.

CLINICAL JUDGMENT GUIDE: This is an alternate type of question included in the NCLEX-RN® test plan. The test taker must be able to read an EHR, be knowledgeable of laboratory data, and decide on the nurse's most appropriate action.

68. Correct order is 3, 1, 4, 2, 5.
    3. This client may be chilling, indicating a potential temperature rise. The nurse should assess the client and the temperature to see if interventions should be initiated based on a progression of the septicemia.
    1. This client should be assessed to be sure that the client is stable because there was chest pain during the last shift.
    4. The nurse should assess this client next because although confusion is expected, the nurse must determine whether any new situation is occurring.
    2. This client has a psychosocial need, but it must be addressed, and steps must be implemented to resolve the problem.
    5. A dressing change can take some time to complete. This is a physiological but not life-threatening situation; the nurse should see this client when they have time to perform the dressing change.

CLINICAL JUDGMENT GUIDE: This is an alternate type of question that requires the nurse to assess clients in order of priority. This requires the nurse to evaluate each client's situation and determine which situations are life-threatening, which situations are expected for the client's situation, or which client has a psychosocial problem.

69. Correct answers are 1, 3, and 4.
    1. Nitroglycerin tablets are vasodilators administered to dilate the coronary vessels and provide oxygen to the heart muscle.
    2. The client should be made to sit down immediately. Exercise is the probable cause of the chest pain; therefore, the activity should immediately stop.
    3. The nurse should assess the client's vital signs as part of assessing the client's current situation.
    4. Supplemental oxygen will assist in getting higher concentrations of oxygen to the heart muscle.
    5. A unit secretary cannot take orders; only a nurse should discuss the client with the HCP.

CLINICAL JUDGMENT GUIDE: This is an alternate type of question included in the NCLEX-RN®. The nurse must be able to select all the options that answer the question correctly. There are no partially correct answers.

70. Answer: 24 mL/hr.
    25,000 divided by 500 mL = 50 units of heparin per mL.
    26 (current rate) × 50 = 1,300 units of heparin currently infusing.
    1,300 − 100 = 1,200 units of heparin needed as new infusion rate.
    1,200 divided by 50 = 24 mL/hr to infuse.

CLINICAL JUDGMENT GUIDE: This is an alternate type of question included in the NCLEX-RN®. The nurse must know how to perform math calculations.

71. 1. Dabigatran (Pradaxa) is a medication prescribed to prevent clotting in clients diagnosed with atrial fibrillation. Any nurse could administer the first dose of the medication; it would not have to be the most experienced nurse.
    2. Pink, frothy sputum indicates pulmonary edema, a serious complication of CHF; therefore, the most experienced nurse should be assigned to this client.
    3. Most individuals experience occasional PVCs; this client would not require the most experienced nurse.
    4. Clients diagnosed with mitral valve prolapse exhibit signs of CHF; therefore, shortness of breath is expected, and the most experienced nurse should not be assigned to this client.

CLINICAL JUDGMENT GUIDE: The test taker must determine which client is the most unstable and would require the most experienced nurse, thus making this type of question an "except" question. Three clients are either stable or have non-life-threatening conditions.

72. 1. The crash cart would need to be brought to the room if the client was coding, but first the nurse should determine whether the client's leads are on the chest.
    2. The Rapid Response Team is called if the client is in a potentially life-threatening situation and the nurse must first determine whether the leads are on the client.
    3. The nurse should assess the client's vital signs, but because the telemetry technician reports the client is flatlined the nurse should first check whether the leads are in place on the chest.
    4. The RN primary nurse should first determine whether the client's telemetry leads are in place on the chest. If the leads are

off, it will show as a flat line at the telemetry station. The telemetry technician cannot leave the station.

CLINICAL JUDGMENT GUIDE: Assessment is the first step of the nursing process, and the test taker should use the nursing process or some other systematic process to assist in determining priorities.

73. 1. This warrants intervention because the telemetry technician needs to know if the client's telemetry is being removed so the technician won't think the client is in asystole.
    2. The electrodes attached to the client's chest do not have to be removed when the client showers, so this would not warrant intervention. The telemetry must be removed, not the electrodes.
    3. Placing a bath chair in the shower is an appropriate intervention so the client won't get tired during the shower; this would not warrant intervention.
    4. The UAP should stay near the client in the shower in case the client needs assistance; this would not warrant intervention.

CLINICAL JUDGMENT GUIDE: The test taker must know that delegating tasks to the UAP means the RN should evaluate the tasks to determine whether they are being done appropriately. The RN should intervene if the client's safety is at risk.

74. 1. The therapeutic digoxin level is 0.5 to 2.0 mg/dL; therefore, the charge nurse should notify the client's HCP because this is above the therapeutic level.
    2. The therapeutic INR is 2 to 3; therefore, the charge nurse would not notify the HCP.
    3. The normal potassium level is 3.5 to 5.3 mEq/L, so the charge nurse would not notify the HCP.
    4. Normal cholesterol level is below 200 mg/dL, but 205 mg/dL is not life-threatening and would not warrant notifying the HCP.

CLINICAL JUDGMENT GUIDE: The test taker should know normal laboratory levels and which ones are life-threatening, requiring notification of the HCP.

75. 1. This client must have an admission assessment completed and the charge nurse cannot assign assessment to an LPN.
    2. The client diagnosed with supraventricular tachycardia will need IV adenosine; therefore, this client should not be assigned to an LPN.
    3. The LPN could care for the client after a diagnostic test; this would be an appropriate client assignment.
    4. The charge nurse cannot assign teaching to the LPN.

CLINICAL JUDGMENT GUIDE: The nurse cannot assign assessment, teaching, evaluation, or an unstable client to an LPN. The LPN can transcribe HCP orders and can call them on the phone to obtain orders for a client.

76. 1. The client would need to have cardiac isoenzymes to determine whether a myocardial infarction has occurred; therefore, this HCP order would not be questioned.
    2. The client probably has coronary artery disease, and a low-fat, low-cholesterol diet would be expected.
    3. IV morphine is the drug of choice for chest pain; therefore, this order would not be questioned.
    4. An endoscopy is not a usual diagnostic test for a client diagnosed with R/O myocardial infarction; therefore, the charge nurse should question this order.

CLINICAL JUDGMENT GUIDE: The test taker should be familiar with laboratory and diagnostic tests commonly associated with disease processes.

77. 1. The UAP can obtain the client's weight. The nurse cannot delegate assessment, teaching, evaluation, medications, or an unstable client.
    2. The custodial or housekeeping department is responsible for cleaning the room, not the UAP.
    3. The nurse cannot delegate assessment, teaching, evaluation, medications, or an unstable client. A client diagnosed with hypovolemia is not stable; therefore, this task cannot be delegated.
    4. The nurse cannot delegate assessment, teaching, evaluation, medications, or an unstable client. Discussing the diet is teaching, which cannot be delegated to a UAP.

CLINICAL JUDGMENT GUIDE: The test taker should be familiar with the role of each healthcare team member and their scope of practice to delegate tasks appropriately.

78. 1. The nurse can check the MAR, but it is not the first intervention when the client is having acute chest pain. Remember, the nurse does not treat paperwork.

2. When the client is in distress the nurse should not assess. The nurse should treat the client's pain immediately; therefore, this is not the first intervention.
3. The nurse should treat the pain, so administering sublingual nitroglycerin, a coronary vasodilator, is the nurse's first intervention.
4. The nurse should administer oxygen but not before addressing the client's chest pain first.

CLINICAL JUDGMENT GUIDE: The test taker should first address the client in distress. If the client is in distress, do not assess; if the client is in distress, do something.

79. 1. The nurse must first determine whether the client has a pulse. If the client does not have a pulse, the nurse must defibrillate the client. If the client has a pulse, the nurse should not defibrillate the client.
2. **The nurse must determine whether the client has a pulse or not before taking any further action; therefore, this is the nurse's first intervention.**
3. This is the first medication administered during a code, but the nurse first determines whether the client has a pulse.
4. This is appropriate intervention if the client has no pulse, but the nurse first determines whether the client has a pulse.

CLINICAL JUDGMENT GUIDE: The test taker should know when assessment is critical. The care of the client in ventricular tachycardia is guided by the presence or absence of a pulse.

80. 1. Nitroglycerin tablets lose efficacy when exposed to sunlight; therefore, keeping the tablets in a dark bottle indicates the client understands the teaching.
2. A sedentary lifestyle is a modifiable risk factor for atherosclerosis, which causes angina, so walking three times a week is an appropriate intervention.
3. **This is a modifiable risk factor; the client must stop smoking altogether. Decreasing the number of cigarettes per day indicates the client needs more teaching.**
4. A daily aspirin will help prevent platelet aggregation, indicating the client understands the discharge teaching.

CLINICAL JUDGMENT GUIDE: The test taker should be able to recognize when a client understands the teaching provided and correct any misinterpretations of the information.

CASE STUDY ANSWERS

1. Correct answers are 1, 2, 3, 4, 5, 6, 7, and 8. A BP of 100/52 mm Hg is slightly lower than expected for an adult and should be reported. The client's level of consciousness changed from unconscious when the nurse first arrived to regaining consciousness, and this information should be reported. The client is tachycardic, short of breath, and diaphoretic, and the nurse has no information regarding allergies or medications, which should be reported. The client's past medical history includes hypertension and long COVID. While aspects of long COVID continue to evolve, there is evidence that it can cause cardiovascular complications such as increased incidence of dysrhythmias, inflammatory and ischemic heart disease, heart failure, and thromboembolic disease. The documented history of long COVID should be reported.

2. Correct answers are 1 and 5.
   1. The client's history of long COVID and current tachycardia indicate an increased potential for dysrhythmia such as atrial fibrillation.
   2. While the client was outside mowing the grass at the time of the syncope, there is no assessment information to indicate that the client is at risk for sunburn.
   3. The client has a slightly elevated temperature, the only known indicator of infection. At the time of the incident, the client was outside mowing, which may account for the slight elevation in temperature. Since there is another ABC answer that makes sense, it takes priority over temperature.
   4. While the client's level of consciousness and the fall could indicate a head injury, the risk for dehydration is most likely.
   5. The client is showing signs of dehydration (hypotension, tachycardia, change in level of consciousness).

CLINICAL JUDGMENT GUIDE: Consider airway (A), breathing (B), and circulation (C) issues as life-threatening when asked to identify priority assessments or actions.

3. Correct answers are 2 and 3.
   Based on the client's condition, the nurse recognizes that the client is at the highest risk for

   | 2. Decreased cardiac output |

   and will require

   | 3. Central line placement |

   2. The client's hypotension, tachycardia, recent syncopal episode, and new-onset atrial fibrillation place the client at high risk for poor perfusion due to decreased cardiac output. There are no signs of fluid volume overload or infection other than a slightly elevated temperature.
   3. The nurse anticipates the cardiologist will likely recommend cardioversion and an amiodarone infusion requiring central line placement. There are no indications for antibiotics or diuretics, especially given the client's hypotensive status.

4. Correct answers are marked.

Potential Nursing Intervention	Indicated	Not Indicated
Offer the client PO fluids		X
Send consult to cardiology STAT	X	
Send STAT request for central line placement	X	
Continuous EKG	X	
Increase oxygen to 5 L via nasal cannula		X
Administer albuterol	X	
Assist the client to move to the chair		X
Reduce IV rate to 75 mL/hr		X

   1. The client should not be given PO fluids.
   2. A cardiologist should see this client to provide specialized care.
   3. A cardiologist will likely order a STAT cardioversion and/or amiodarone infusion, which requires a central line for administration.
   4. Continuous monitoring via EKG is indicated.
   5. While the client's most recent vital signs indicate the need to increase the oxygen, moving from 2 L to 5 L is too much; the rate should be increased incrementally unless ordered otherwise.
   6. The nurse should administer albuterol for the client's shortness of breath and to improve oxygenation.
   7. The client should remain in bed and take nothing by mouth due to the potential need for immediate cardioversion.
   8. The IV flow rate should not be decreased due to the client's underlying dehydration.

5. Correct answers are 1, 2, and 5.
   1. Initiate amiodarone IV because this is a STAT order.
   2. Continuous EKG and pulse oximetry are necessary for a client with these symptoms.
   3. Titrate oxygen to maintain SpO_2 92% or higher, up to 5 L via nasal cannula/mask as needed. This option is not needed as the client's last set of vital signs indicated a pulse oximeter reading of 92% on an acceptable oxygen flow rate.
   4. Call cardiology resident STAT for heart rate <60 bpm or BP <80/50 mm Hg. The cardiology resident was on the unit and provided orders based on an elevated heart rate.
   5. Administer IV 0.9% NaCl @ 125 mL/hr. This order is indicated because the client's BP is still borderline low.
   6. Provide diet as tolerated. This order is not a priority.
   7. Allow activity as tolerated; up with assistance only. This order is not a priority.

6. Correct answers are given in the box.

Finding	Improved	Declined	No Change
Temperature			X
Heart rate	X		
Respirations	X		
Blood pressure	X		
SpO_2	X		
EKG			X

   At this point, the client's heart rate, respirations, blood pressure, and pulse oximetry readings have improved. There has been no change in temperature from the previous set of vital signs and the client remains in atrial fibrillation. Note: While the EKG will include the heart rate and there has been significant improvement, this value is captured in the "improved" heart rate; the EKG reading remains atrial fibrillation.

Peripheral Vascular Management

3

Not everything that can be counted counts, and not everything that counts can be counted.

—Albert Einstein

QUESTIONS

1. The nurse has finished receiving the morning change-of-shift report. Which client should the nurse assess **first**?
   1. The client diagnosed with arterial occlusive disease and intermittent claudication
   2. The client on strict bedrest reporting calf pain and a reddened calf
   3. The client reporting low back pain when lying supine in bed
   4. The upset client saying the food doesn't taste good and is cold all the time

2. The nurse is caring for clients on a vascular disorder unit. Which laboratory data warrant **immediate** intervention by the nurse?
   1. The partial thromboplastin time (PTT) of 98 seconds for a client diagnosed with deep vein thrombosis (DVT)
   2. The hemoglobin of 14.4 g/dL for a client diagnosed with Raynaud's phenomenon
   3. The white blood cell (WBC) count of 11,000/microL for a client diagnosed with a stasis venous ulcer
   4. The triglyceride level of 312 mmol/L in a client diagnosed with hypertension (HTN)

3. The unlicensed assistive personnel (UAP) informs the RN staff nurse the client has a blood pressure of 78/46 mm Hg and a pulse of 116 bpm using a vital signs machine. Which intervention should the nurse implement **first**?
   1. Notify the healthcare provider (HCP) immediately.
   2. Have the UAP recheck the client's vital signs manually.
   3. Place the client in the Trendelenburg position.
   4. Assess the client's cardiovascular status.

4. The RN charge nurse on a vascular unit is working with a new unit secretary. Which statement concerning laboratory data is **most** important for the charge nurse to tell the unit secretary?
   1. "Be sure to inform me of any lab information called into the unit."
   2. "Make sure to confirm all lab reports are in the EHR."
   3. "Do not take any laboratory reports over the telephone."
   4. "Verify all telephone reports by calling back to the lab."

5. The nurse is preparing to administer medications to clients on a vascular unit. Which medication should the nurse **question** administering?
   1. Vitamin K to a client with an International Normalized Ratio (INR) of 2.8
   2. Propranolol to a client diagnosed with arterial hypertension
   3. Nifedipine to a client diagnosed with Raynaud's disease
   4. Enalapril to a client with a sodium level of 138 mEq/L

6. The nurse has received the shift report. Which client should the nurse assess **first**?
   1. The client diagnosed with a DVT reporting dyspnea and coughing
   2. The client diagnosed with Buerger's disease and intermittent claudication
   3. The client diagnosed with an aortic aneurysm and an audible bruit
   4. The client diagnosed with acute arterial ischemia and bilateral palpable pedal pulses

7. The client diagnosed with atherosclerosis tells the clinic nurse their stomach hurts after taking morning medications. The client is taking a calcium-channel blocker, a daily acetylsalicylic acid, and a statin. The medications have not changed during the past year. Which intervention should the nurse implement **first**?
   1. Assess the client for abnormal bleeding.
   2. Instruct the client to stop taking the acetylsalicylic acid.
   3. Recommend the client take an enteric-coated acetylsalicylic acid.
   4. Instruct the client to notify the HCP.

8. The RN nurse educator on a vascular unit is discussing delegation guidelines with a group of new graduate nurses. Which statement from the group indicates the need for **more** teaching?
   1. "The UAP will be practicing on my brand-new nursing license."
   2. "I will still retain accountability for what I delegate to the UAP."
   3. "I must make sure the UAP I delegate to is competent at performing the task."
   4. "When I delegate, I must follow up with the UAP and evaluate the task."

9. The nurse is reviewing the literature to identify evidence-based practice research that supports a new procedure for using a new product when changing the central line catheter dressing. Which research article would **best** support the nurse's proposal for a change in the procedure?
   1. The article in which the study was conducted by the manufacturer of the product used
   2. The research article that included 10 subjects participating in the study
   3. The review-of-literature article that cited ambiguous statistics about the product
   4. The review-of-literature article that cited numerous studies supporting the product

10. The RN staff nurse and the UAP are caring for clients on a vascular unit. Which task is **most** appropriate for the nurse to delegate?
    1. Provide indwelling catheter care to a client on bedrest.
    2. Evaluate the client's 8-hour intake and output.
    3. Give a bath to the client diagnosed with third-spacing.
    4. Administer a cation-exchange resin enema to a client.

11. The RN staff nurse asks the UAP to apply the sequential compression devices (SCDs) to a client on strict bedrest. The UAP tells the nurse they have never done this procedure. Which action would be a **priority** for the RN to take?
    1. Tell another UAP to put the SCDs on the client.
    2. Demonstrate the procedure for applying the SCDs.
    3. Perform the task and apply the SCDs to the client.
    4. Request the UAP watch the video demonstrating this task.

12. The RN staff nurse in the vascular critical care unit is working with an LPN pulled to the unit because of a high census. Which task is **most** appropriate for the nurse to assign to the LPN?
    1. Assess the client being transferred to the medical unit in the morning.
    2. Administer a unit of blood to the recovering client now 1 day postoperative.
    3. Hang a bag of heparin for the client diagnosed with a pulmonary embolism.
    4. Assist the HCP with the insertion of a client's Swan-Ganz catheter.

13. The nurse is administering 1 unit of packed red blood cells to a client. Fifteen minutes after initiating the blood transfusion, the client becomes restless and reports itching on the trunk and arms. Which intervention should the nurse implement **first?**
    1. Assess the client's vital signs.
    2. Notify the HCP.
    3. Maintain a patent IV line.
    4. Stop the transfusion at the hub.

14. The staff nurse on a vascular disorder unit asks the RN charge nurse, "What should I be looking for when I read a research article?" Which response indicates the charge nurse understands how to read a nursing research article? **Select all that apply.**
    1. "You should be able to determine why the research was done."
    2. "You should find out how much money was used for the research study."
    3. "You should evaluate which research method was used for the study."
    4. "You should read the method section to find out what setting was used."
    5. "You should find information about how the data were collected for the study."

15. The nurse calls the HCP for an order of pain medication for a client now 2 days postoperative aortic aneurysm repair. The HCP gives the nurse an order for "meperidine 50 mg IVP now and then every 4 hours as needed." Which action should the nurse implement **first?**
    1. Enter the order in the EHR with the words "per telephone order (TO)."
    2. Request another nurse to verify the HCP's order on the phone.
    3. Read back the order to the HCP before hanging up the phone.
    4. Call the pharmacy to add the medication to the medication administration record (MAR).

16. The charge nurse on the vascular unit is reviewing laboratory blood work. Which result **warrants** intervention by the charge nurse?
    1. The client has an INR of 2.3.
    2. The client has Hgb 11 g/dL and Hct 36%.
    3. The client's platelet count is 65,000/mL of blood.
    4. The client's red blood cell count is 4.8×10^6 cells/microL.

17. A client on the vascular unit tells the day shift primary nurse that the night nurse did not answer the call light for almost 1 hour. Which statement would be **most** appropriate by the day shift primary nurse?
    1. "The night shift often has trouble answering the lights promptly."
    2. "I am sorry that happened, and I will answer your lights promptly today."
    3. "I will notify my charge nurse to come and talk to you about the situation."
    4. "There might have been an emergency situation so your light was not answered."

18. The nurse is preparing to administer a unit of packed red blood cells to a postoperative elderly client 1 day after abdominal aortic aneurysm surgery. Which interventions should the nurse implement? **Rank in order of performance.**
    1. Obtain the unit of blood from the blood bank.
    2. Start an IV access with normal saline at a keep-open rate.
    3. Have the client sign the permit to receive blood products.
    4. Check the unit of blood with another nurse at the bedside.
    5. Initiate the transfusion at a slow rate for 15 minutes.

19. The elderly client diagnosed with DVT is reporting chest pain during inhalation. Which intervention should the nurse implement **first?**
    1. Ask the HCP to order a STAT lung scan.
    2. Place oxygen on the client via nasal cannula.
    3. Prepare to administer IV heparin.
    4. Tell the client not to ambulate and remain in bed.

20. Which laboratory data should the nurse in the long-term care unit notify the HCP about?
    1. The client receiving digoxin with a digoxin level of 2.6 ng/mL
    2. The client receiving enoxaparin with a prothrombin time (PT) of 12.9 seconds
    3. The client receiving ticlopidine with a platelet count of 160,000/microL
    4. The client receiving furosemide with a potassium level of 4.2 mEq/L

21. The occupational nurse is caring for the client presenting with two severed fingers from their right hand. Which intervention should the occupational nurse implement **first**?
    1. Place the severed fingers in a sterile cloth and then in an ice chest.
    2. Instruct the client to elevate their right arm over the heart.
    3. The nurse should put on their nonsterile gloves.
    4. Apply direct pressure to the right radial pulse.

22. The RN clinic charge nurse is making assignments for the staff. Which assignment or delegation is **most** appropriate?
    1. Request the LPN to escort the client to the examination room.
    2. Ask the UAP to prepare the room for the next client.
    3. Instruct the RN to administer a tetanus shot to the client.
    4. Tell the clinic secretary to call in a new prescription for a client.

23. The client tells the RN charge nurse that the UAP did not know how to take a blood pressure (BP) reading. Which action should the charge nurse implement **first**?
    1. Discuss the client's comment with the UAP.
    2. Retake the BP and inform the client of the BP reading.
    3. Explain that the UAP knows how to take a BP reading.
    4. Ask the UAP to demonstrate taking a BP reading.

24. Which medication is **most** appropriate for the RN staff nurse to assign for the LPN to administer?
    1. The IV push (IVP) antiemetic to the client with nausea and vomiting
    2. The subcutaneous low-molecular-weight heparin to the client diagnosed with a pulmonary embolus
    3. The oral pentoxifylline to the client diagnosed with intermittent claudication
    4. The sublingual nitroglycerin to the client reporting chest pain

25. The clinic nurse is assessing a client reporting right leg calf pain. The right calf is edematous and warm to the touch. Which intervention should the nurse implement **first**?
    1. Notify the clinic HCP immediately.
    2. Ask the client how long their leg has been hurting.
    3. Complete a neurovascular assessment on the leg.
    4. Place the client's right leg on two pillows.

26. The fire alarm is activated in the family practice clinic. Which action should the nurse take **first**?
    1. Determine whether there is a fire in the clinic.
    2. Evacuate all the people from the clinic.
    3. Immediately call 911 and report the fire.
    4. Instruct clients to stay in their rooms and close the doors.

27. The UAP informs the RN clinic nurse, "One of the medical interns asked me out on a date. I told them no, but the intern keeps asking." Which statement is the nurse's **best** response?
    1. "I will talk to the intern and tell them to stop."
    2. "Did anyone hear the intern asking you out?"
    3. "That intern asks everyone out; it is just their way."
    4. "You should inform the clinic's director of nurses."

28. The clinic nurse overhears another staff nurse telling the pharmaceutical representative, "If you bring us lunch from the best place in town, I will make sure you get to see the HCP." Which action should the clinic nurse take?
    1. Tell the pharmaceutical representative the staff nurse's statement was inappropriate.
    2. Report this behavior to the clinic's director of nurses immediately.
    3. Do not take any action and wait for the food to be delivered.
    4. Inform the HCP of the staff nurse's and pharmaceutical representative's behavior.

29. The home health nurse in the office is notified the client on warfarin has an INR of 3.8. Which action should the home health nurse implement **first**?
    1. Document the result of the INR in the client's EHR.
    2. Contact the client and ask whether they have any abnormal bleeding.
    3. Notify the client's HCP of the INR results.
    4. Schedule an appointment with the client to draw another INR.

30. The home health nurse is caring for a client diagnosed with arterial hypertension recovering from a cerebrovascular accident. Which **priority** intervention should the nurse discuss with the client when teaching about arterial hypertension?
    1. Discuss the importance of the client adhering to a low-salt diet.
    2. Explain the need for the client to take antihypertensive medications as prescribed.
    3. Tell the client to check and record their blood pressure readings daily.
    4. Encourage the client to walk at least 30 minutes three times a week.

31. Which action by the UAP indicates to the RN staff nurse the UAP **understands** the correct procedure for applying compression stockings to the client recovering from a pulmonary embolus? **Select all that apply.**
    1. The UAP instructs the client to sit in the chair when applying the stockings.
    2. The UAP can insert one finger under the proximal end of the stocking.
    3. The UAP ensures the toe opening is placed on the top side of the feet.
    4. The UAP ensures the client's toes are warm after applying the stockings.
    5. The UAP applies lotion to the legs immediately before applying the stockings.

32. The home health nurse enters a client's yard and is bitten on the leg by the client's dog. Which intervention should the nurse implement **first**?
    1. Clean the dog bite with soap and water, then apply antibiotic ointment.
    2. Obtain the phone number and contact the client's veterinarian.
    3. Contact the home healthcare agency and complete an occurrence report.
    4. Ask the client whether the dog has had all the required vaccinations.

33. The nurse on the vascular unit is caring for a client diagnosed with arterial occlusive disease. Which statement by the client warrants **immediate** intervention by the nurse?
    1. "My legs start to hurt when I walk to check the mail."
    2. "My legs were so cold I had to put a heating pad on them."
    3. "I hang my legs off the side of the bed when I sleep."
    4. "I noticed that the hair on my feet and up my leg is gone."

34. The home health nurse has completed a home assessment on a client and discovers no smoke detectors in the home. The client tells the nurse they cannot afford them. Which action should the nurse implement **first**?
    1. Purchase at least one smoke detector for the client's home.
    2. Notify the home healthcare agency social worker to discuss the situation.
    3. Ask the client whether a family member could buy a smoke detector.
    4. Contact the local fire department to see whether they can provide smoke detectors for the client.

35. The nurse is admitting a 72-year-old client and notes multiple bruises on their face, arms, and legs along with possible cigarette burns on the upper arms. The client claims to have fallen on an ashtray and does not want to discuss it. Which nursing intervention is the **priority?**
    1. Document the objective findings in the client's EHR.
    2. Tell the client they must discuss the situation with the nurse.
    3. Report the situation to the Adult Protective Services.
    4. Take photographs of the bruises and cigarette burns.

36. The nurse is admitting a client diagnosed with DVT in the right leg. Which statement by the client warrants **immediate** intervention by the nurse?
    1. "I take a baby acetylsalicylic acid daily at breakfast."
    2. "I have ordered myself a medical alert bracelet."
    3. "I eat spinach and greens at least twice weekly."
    4. "I got a new recliner so I can elevate my legs."

37. The client diagnosed with peripheral vascular disease tells the nurse, "I know my foot is really bad. My doctor told me I don't have any choice, and I must have an amputation, but I don't want one." Which action supports the nurse being a client advocate?
    1. Support the medical treatment and recommend the client have the amputation.
    2. Recommend the client discuss this decision with their spouse and children.
    3. Explain to the client they have the right to a second opinion.
    4. Offer to go with the client to discuss this decision with the doctor.

38. The RN charge nurse observes the UAP crying after the death of a client. Which is the charge nurse's **best** response to the UAP?
    1. "If you cry every time a client dies, you won't last long on the unit."
    2. "It can be difficult when a client dies. Would you like to take a break?"
    3. "You need to stop crying and go on about your responsibilities."
    4. "Did you not realize that clients die in a healthcare facility?"

39. The nursing staff confronts the hospice nurse overseeing the care of a client in a long-term care facility. The nursing staff wants to send the client diagnosed with gangrene of the left leg, secondary to peripheral occlusive disease, to the hospital for treatment. Which intervention should the nurse implement **first?**
    1. Check with the client to see if they want to go to a hospital.
    2. Explain that the client can be kept comfortable at the long-term care facility.
    3. Discuss the hospice concept of comfort measures only with the staff.
    4. Call a client care conference immediately to discuss the conflict.

40. The client diagnosed with an abdominal aortic aneurysm died unexpectedly, and the nurse must notify the significant other. Which statement by the nurse is the **best** over the telephone?
    1. "I am sorry to tell you, but your loved one has died."
    2. "Could you come to the hospital? The client is not doing well."
    3. "The HCP has asked me to tell you of your family member's death."
    4. "Do you know whether the client wished to be an organ donor?"

41. The nurse has been pulled from a medical unit to work on the vascular unit for the shift. Which client should the charge nurse assign to the medical unit nurse?
    1. The client with the femoral-popliteal bypass and paresthesia of the foot
    2. The client diagnosed with an abdominal aortic aneurysm reporting low back pain
    3. The client newly diagnosed with chronic venous insufficiency, requiring teaching
    4. The client diagnosed with varicose veins reporting deep, aching pain of the legs

42. The charge nurse in the vascular intensive care unit (ICU) assigns three clients to the staff nurse. The staff nurse thinks this is an unsafe assignment. Which action should the staff nurse implement **first?**
    1. Refuse to take the assignment and leave the hospital immediately.
    2. Tell the supervisor they are concerned about the unsafe assignment.
    3. Document their concerns in writing and give it to the supervisor.
    4. Take the assignment for the shift but turn in a resignation letter.

43. At 2230, the nurse is preparing to administer pain medication to a client reporting pain as a 4 on the numeric pain scale.

Client: M. C. Date: Today	Allergies: Ibuprofen Diagnosis: Chronic vein insufficiency	
Medication	0701–1900	1901–0700
Morphine sulfate 2 mg IVP every 2 hours PRN	0930 DN	
Promethazine 12.5 mg IVP every 4 hours PRN	1845 DN	
Prochlorperazine 5 mg PO tid PRN		
Hydrocodone 5 mg PO every 4–6 hours PRN	1730 DN	
Ibuprofen 600 mg PO every 3–4 hours PRN		
Nurse Name/Initials	Day Nurse RN/DN	Night Nurse RN/NN

    Which medication should the nurse administer?
    1. Administer morphine 2 mg IVP.
    2. Administer promethazine 12.5 mg IVP.
    3. Administer hydrocodone 5 mg PO.
    4. Administer ibuprofen 600 mg PO.

44. The matriarch of a family has died in the vascular unit. The family tells the nurse the daughter is coming to the hospital from a nearby city to see the body. Which intervention should the nurse implement?
    1. Plan to allow the daughter to see the client in the room.
    2. Take the client to the morgue for the daughter to view.
    3. Request the family call the daughter and tell them not to come.
    4. Explain to the daughter that the unit is too busy for family visitation.

45. The unit manager on the vascular unit is planning a change in how postmortem care is provided. Which is the **first** step in the change process?
    1. Collect data.
    2. Identify the problem.
    3. Select an alternative.
    4. Implement a plan.

46. The nurse is preparing to administer the third unit of packed red blood cells (PRBCs) to a client diagnosed with a ruptured aortic aneurysm. Which interventions should the nurse implement? **Select all that apply.**
    1. Hang a bag of D_5NS to keep open (TKO).
    2. Change the blood administration set.
    3. Check the client's current vital signs.
    4. Assess for allergies to blood products.
    5. Obtain a blood warmer for the blood.

47. The RN staff nurse and the UAP are caring for clients in a vascular unit. Which task should the nurse delegate to the UAP?
    1. Apply bilateral sequential compression devices to the client diagnosed with DVT.
    2. Accompany the client diagnosed with thromboangiitis obliterans outside to smoke a cigarette.
    3. Elevate the leg of the client now 1 day postoperative femoral-popliteal bypass.
    4. Perform Doppler studies on the client diagnosed with right upper extremity lymphedema.

48. The RN charge nurse on a vascular postsurgical unit observes a new graduate nurse telling an elderly client's spouse not to push the client's patient-controlled analgesia (PCA) pump button. Which action should the charge nurse implement?
    1. Encourage the visitor to push the button for the client.
    2. Ask the nurse to step into the hallway to discuss the situation.
    3. Discuss the hospital protocol for the use of PCA pumps.
    4. Continue to perform the charge nurse's other duties.

49. Which client should the nurse assess **first** after receiving the shift report?
    1. The client with a right above-the-knee amputation reporting right foot pain
    2. The client diagnosed with arterial hypertension reporting a severe headache
    3. The client diagnosed with lymphedema and 4+ pitting edema of the left lower leg
    4. The client diagnosed with gangrene of the right foot with a foul-smelling discharge

50. The RN staff nurse observes an LPN crushing nifedipine XL before administering the medication to a client diagnosed with arterial hypertension and has difficulty swallowing pills. Which intervention should the nurse implement **first?**
    1. Request the LPN to take the client's blood pressure.
    2. Take no action because this is appropriate behavior.
    3. Show the LPN where to find pudding for the client.
    4. Tell the LPN this medication cannot be crushed.

51. A 90-year-old client was recently widowed after more than 60 years of marriage. The client was admitted to a long-term care facility and is refusing to eat. Which intervention is an example of the ethical principle of autonomy?
    1. Place a nasogastric feeding tube and feed the client.
    2. Discuss why the client does not want to eat anymore.
    3. Arrange for the family to bring food for the client.
    4. Allow the client to refuse to eat if they want to.

52. The nurse is admitting a client diagnosed with an abdominal aortic aneurysm. The client is a Church of Jesus Christ of Latter-Day Saints (Mormon) member. Which action by the nurse indicates **cultural sensitivity** to the client?
    1. The nurse does not insist on administering a blood transfusion.
    2. The nurse pins the client's amulet to the client's pillow.
    3. The nurse keeps the client's undershirt on during the bath.
    4. The nurse notifies the client's curandero of the admission.

53. Which client should the nurse on the vascular unit assess **first** after receiving the shift report?
    1. The client diagnosed with lymphedema and arterial blood gas (ABG) results pH 7.33, Pao$_2$ 89 mm Hg, Paco$_2$ 47 mm Hg, and HCO$_3$ 25 mmol/L
    2. The client diagnosed with Raynaud's phenomenon reporting bluish cold upper extremities
    3. The client diagnosed with chronic venous insufficiency and an ulcerated area on the right foot
    4. The client receiving IV heparin infusion with a PTT of 78 seconds

54. The RN charge nurse of a long-term care facility is making assignments. Which client should be assigned to the **most** experienced UAP?
    1. The client diagnosed with arterial occlusive disease requiring them to dangle the legs off the side of the bed
    2. The client diagnosed with congestive heart failure expressing anger about their family not visiting
    3. The client with an above-the-knee amputation needing full body lift to get in the wheelchair
    4. The client diagnosed with Buerger's disease needing things done in a particular way

55. The client reports chest pain on deep inspiration. Which intervention should the nurse implement **first?**
    1. Place the client on oxygen.
    2. Assess the client's lungs.
    3. Notify the respiratory therapist.
    4. Assess the client's pulse oximeter reading.

56. Which of the staff nurse's attributes are important for the unit manager when considering the selection of an experienced nurse as a preceptor for new graduates? **Select all that apply.**
    1. The nurse's need for the monetary stipend
    2. The nurse's ability to organize the work
    3. The ability of the nurse to interact with others
    4. The quality of care the nurse provides
    5. The nurse's willingness to be a preceptor

57. The nurse just received the a.m. shift report. Which client should the nurse assess **first?**
    1. The client now 6 hours postoperative vein ligation with absent pedal pulses
    2. The client diagnosed with deep vein thrombosis (DVT) reporting calf pain
    3. The client diagnosed with Raynaud's disease reporting throbbing and tingling in the extremities
    4. The client diagnosed with Buerger's disease and intermittent claudication of the feet and arms

58. The ICU nurse is calculating the total fluid intake for a client diagnosed with hypertensive crisis. The client has received 950 mL of D_5W (5% dextrose in water), 2 IV piggyback infusions of 100 mL of 0.9% NS, 16 oz of water, 8 oz of milk, and 6 oz of chicken broth. The client has had a urinary output of 2,200 mL. What is the total intake for this client? _____

59. The nurse is teaching the client diagnosed with arterial occlusive disease. Which statement indicates the client needs **more** teaching?
    1. "I will wash my legs and feet daily in warm water."
    2. "I should buy my shoes in the afternoon."
    3. "I must wear knee-high stockings."
    4. "I should not elevate my legs."

60. The RN staff nurse is caring for clients on a vascular unit. Which nursing task is **most** appropriate to delegate to the UAP?
    1. Tell the UAP to obtain the glucometer reading of the client reporting being dizzy and lightheaded.
    2. Request the UAP to elevate the feet of the client diagnosed with chronic venous insufficiency.
    3. Ask the UAP to take the vital signs of the client with numbness of the right arm.
    4. Instruct the UAP to administer a tap water enema to the client diagnosed with an aortic aneurysm.

61. A client is 2 days postoperative abdominal aortic aneurysm (AAA) repair. Which data require **immediate** intervention from the nurse?
    1. The client refuses to take deep breaths and cough.
    2. The client's urinary output is 300 mL (10.1 oz) in 8 hours.
    3. The client has hypoactive bowel sounds.
    4. The client's vital signs are T 98°F (36.7°C), P 68 bpm, R 16 breaths/min, and BP 110/70 mm Hg.

62. The nurse is caring for clients on a vascular surgical floor. Which client should be assessed **first**?
    1. The client now 2 days postoperative after a right below-the-knee amputation with phantom pain in the right foot
    2. The client 1 day postoperative abdominal aortic aneurysm repair reporting numbness and tingling of both feet
    3. The client diagnosed with superficial thrombophlebitis of the left arm reporting tenderness to the touch
    4. The client diagnosed with arterial occlusive disease reporting calf pain when ambulating down the hall

63. The nurse is caring for a client receiving heparin sodium via constant infusion. The heparin protocol reads to increase the IV rate by 100 units/hour if the PTT is less than 50 seconds. The current PTT is 46 seconds. The heparin comes in 500 mL of D_5W with 25,000 units of heparin added. The current rate on the IV pump is 20 mL/hr. At what rate should the nurse set the pump? _____

64. The UAP is caring for a client diagnosed with chronic venous insufficiency. Which action would warrant **immediate** intervention from the RN staff nurse?
    1. The UAP assists the client in applying compression stockings.
    2. The UAP elevates the client's leg while sitting in the recliner.
    3. The UAP assists the client to the bathroom for a.m. care.
    4. The UAP cuts the client's toenails after soaking the feet in tepid water.

65. The nurse has just received the a.m. shift report. Which client would the nurse assess **first**?
    1. The client diagnosed with a venous stasis ulcer refusing to eat a high-protein meal
    2. The client diagnosed with varicose veins refusing to wear thromboembolic hose
    3. The client diagnosed with arterial occlusive disease refusing to elevate their legs
    4. The client diagnosed with deep vein thrombosis (DVT) refusing to stay in the bed

66. At 1000 a client is reporting severe right upper quadrant pain of 10 out of 10 on the pain scale after femoral-popliteal bypass surgery on the right leg.

Client Name: B.A.	Account Number: 0101223	Height: 72 in (182.9 cm)
Weight: 220 lb (99.8 kg)	Date: Today	

Medication	1901–0700	0701–1900
Morphine sulfate 2 mg IVP every 4 hours PRN pain	0445 NN	0845 DN
Oxycodone 7.5/acetaminophen 325 mg PO every 3 hours PRN pain	0030 NN 0545 NN	
Aluminum hydroxide; magnesium hydroxide; simethicone 30 mL PO PRN indigestion		
Nitroglycerin 0.4 mg SL every 5 minutes up to 3 tablets PRN chest pain		
Signature/Initials	Night Nurse RN/NN	Day Nurse RN/DN

    Based on the information in the chart, what should the nurse do for the client?
    1. Administer the oxycodone and acetaminophen PO.
    2. Help the client to practice guided imagery for the pain.
    3. Call the surgeon for an increase in pain medication.
    4. Administer a dose of morphine to the client.

67. The client on a surgical unit is scheduled to receive an antibiotic piggyback for 1 hour. The piggyback is prepared in 150 mL of solution. At what rate should the nurse set the piggyback if the administration set delivers 20 drops/mL? _____

68. The client in the day surgical unit is scheduled to have vein ligation on the right leg. The client states, "I am having surgery on my left leg." Which intervention should the nurse implement **first?**
    1. Have the client sign the surgical operative permit.
    2. Assess the client's neurological status.
    3. Ask when the client last took a drink of water or ate anything.
    4. Call a time-out until clarifying which leg is having the vein ligation.

69. The 63-year-old client is diagnosed with an abdominal aortic aneurysm. On which area of the figure should the nurse place a stethoscope to assess for a bruit?

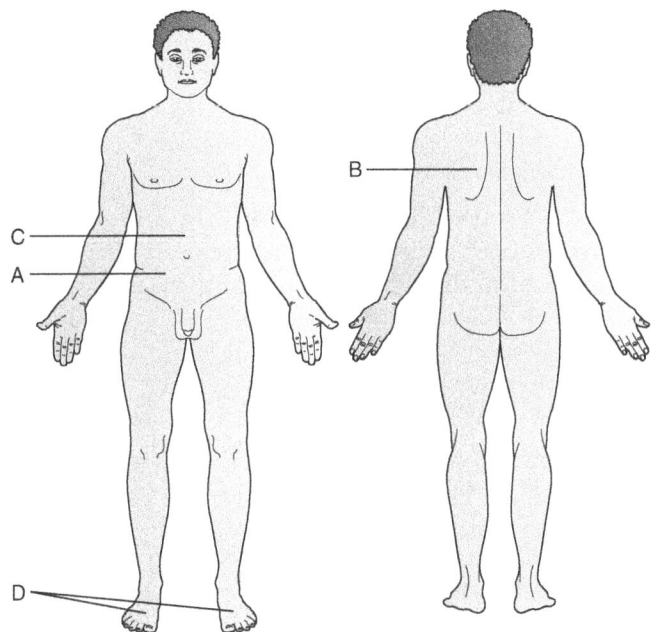

    1. A
    2. B
    3. C
    4. D

70. The client recovering from femoral-popliteal bypass notifies the desk via the intercom system that they have fallen and are now bleeding. Which interventions should the nurse implement? **Rank in order of performance.**
    1. Apply pressure directly to the bleeding site.
    2. Notify the surgeon of the fall and the bleeding.
    3. Redress the site with a sterile dressing.
    4. Assist the client to a recumbent position in the bed.
    5. Make out an occurrence report and document the fall.

71. The RN just received the a.m. shift report. Which client should the nurse assess **first?**
    1. The noncompliant middle-aged client diagnosed with coronary artery disease and has BP of 170/100 mm Hg
    2. The obese young adult client diagnosed with deep vein thrombosis (DVT) reporting calf pain
    3. The client with tobacco addiction diagnosed with arterial occlusive disease and intermittent claudication
    4. The disruptive elderly client diagnosed with aortic abdominal aneurysm reporting low back pain

72. Which assessment data would warrant **immediate** intervention by the RN charge nurse for the middle-aged client diagnosed with arterial occlusive disease?
    1. The client has decreased hair on their calf.
    2. The client has no palpable dorsal pedal pulse.
    3. The client has paralysis and paresthesia.
    4. The client hangs their legs off the side of the bed.

73. The RN and the UAP are caring for an elderly client now 4 hours postoperative right femoral-popliteal bypass surgery. Which nursing task should the RN delegate to the UAP?
    1. Check the client's pedal pulse with the Doppler ultrasound.
    2. Assist the client to ambulate down the hall.
    3. Review the client's neurovascular assessment.
    4. Elevate the client's leg on two pillows.

74. Which interventions should the RN charge nurse discuss with the elderly client diagnosed with atherosclerosis? **Select all that apply.**
    1. Take a low dose of acetylsalicylic acid daily.
    2. Eat a low-fat, low-cholesterol diet.
    3. Maintain a sedentary lifestyle as much as possible.
    4. Decrease all foods high in fiber.
    5. Walk 30 minutes a day at least 3 days a week.

75. The client is 2 days postoperative abdominal aortic aneurysm. Which intervention should the nurse implement **first** when making initial rounds?
    1. Auscultate the client's bowel sounds.
    2. Assess the client's surgical dressing.
    3. Encourage the client to splint the incision.
    4. Monitor the client's IV therapy.

76. The middle-aged client is diagnosed with a small abdominal aortic aneurysm. Which statement by the client indicates to the RN that the client needs **more** discharge teaching?
    1. "I should not lift more than 5 pounds for at least 4 to 6 weeks."
    2. "I attend a support group to help me quit smoking."
    3. "I must wear a truss at all times after the surgery."
    4. "If I get a temperature of 101°F (38.3°C) or higher, I will call my doctor."

77. The RN is assigned the following clients. Which client should the RN assess **first?**
    1. The client, now 4 days postoperative abdominal surgery, reporting abdominal pain when ambulating
    2. The client 1 day postoperative femoral-popliteal repair and a 3+ posterior tibial pulse
    3. The client after an abdominal aortic repair with urine output of 150 mL (5.1 oz) in the last 8 hours
    4. The client diagnosed with DVT reporting being unable to get out of bed

78. The nurse is caring for a client receiving heparin sodium via constant infusion. The heparin protocol reads to decrease the IV rate by 100 units/hr if the PTT is between 78 and 90 seconds. The current PTT level is 85 seconds. The heparin comes in 500 mL of D_5W with 25,000 units of heparin added. The current rate on the IV pump is 18 mL/hr. At what rate should the nurse set the pump? _____

79. The UAP is caring for the middle-aged client diagnosed with chronic venous insufficiency. Which action would warrant **immediate** intervention by the nurse?
    1. The UAP is elevating the client's legs on two pillows.
    2. The UAP is massaging the client's calf muscles.
    3. The UAP is instructing the client to stay in the bed.
    4. The UAP is calculating the client's shift intake and output (I&O).

80. An 80-year-old client is being discharged home after having surgery to débride a chronic venous ulcer on the right ankle. Which referral is appropriate for the RN charge nurse to make?
    1. Hospice
    2. Home health
    3. Physical therapist
    4. Cardiac rehabilitation

PERIPHERAL VASCULAR DISEASE CASE STUDY

(1100) A 42-year-old female arrives at the emergency department (ED) complaining of sudden, sharp pain and swelling in her right calf. She states the pain began about 2 days ago after a long overseas flight she took for work.

(1115) Upon assessment, the triage nurse finds an alert and oriented female. Skin is pink, warm, and dry. Mucous membranes are moist. Lung sounds are clear throughout all fields. Heart sounds are normal. Abdomen is soft and flat with bowel sounds present ×4. Upon examination of the legs, the right calf is red, warm, and tender to the touch, and there is significant swelling in the right calf. Pedal pulses are bounding bilaterally.

Vital Signs	Client Values
Heart rate	80 bpm
Respirations	12 breaths/min
Temperature	98.7°F (38.1°C)
Spo$_2$	99% (room air)
Pain level	6 out of 10

The nurse takes a complete medical history, reviews the client's medications, and places this information in the EHR.

Medical History. The client is generally healthy with no major past medical illnesses. The client does not smoke.

Weight: 195 lb (88.5 kg)

Height: 62 inches (157.5 cm)

Allergies: Penicillin

Social History. The client works as a marketing manager for a travel agency, which requires frequent air travel. She is married with no children.

Family History. No significant history of blood clots or clotting disorders in the family.

Medication List

Medication	Time Taken
Ethinyl estradiol	1 tab every day

1. **Recognize cues. What matters most?** The nurse prepares to call the ED physician. Which **priority** client data should be reported to the HCP? **Select all that apply.**
    1. Heart rate of 80 bpm
    2. Pain level of 6
    3. Respiratory assessment
    4. Travel history
    5. Redness in right leg

6. Temperature of 98.7°F (37.1°C)
7. Spo₂ 99% on room air
8. Edema in right leg
9. Bowel sounds
10. Respirations 12 breaths/min

2. **Analyze cues. What could it mean?** What at-risk issues should the nurse be concerned for the client developing? **Select three answers.**
   1. Decreased tissue perfusion
   2. Malnutrition
   3. Decreased skin integrity
   4. Impaired gas exchange
   5. Decreased cardiac output

(1145) The physician visits the client and orders a complete blood count (CBC), basic metabolic panel (BMP), and a D-dimer test to be done STAT. The physician orders are populated in the chart.

PROVIDER ORDERS:

CBC, BMP, and D-dimer test STAT
Chest x-ray
Duplex ultrasound of the leg veins
Saline IV lock
Compression stockings

(1830) Diagnostic and laboratory results are posted.

Laboratory Test	Client Values	Reference Values
Hemoglobin (Hgb)	13.4 g/dL	Male 14 to 18 g/dL
		Female 12 to 16 g/dL
Hematocrit (Hct)	40%	Male 40% to 54%
		Female 36% to 48%
White blood cell (WBC) count	6.0×10^9/L	4.5 to 11.0×10^9/L
Platelets	300×10^3/microL	150 to 450×10^3/microL
Creatinine	0.65 mg/dL	Male 0.7 to 1.3 mg/dL
		Female 0.6 to 1.1 mg/dL
Glucose	150 mg/dL	Fasting: Less than 100 mg/dL
		Random: Less than 200 mg/dL
Potassium	3.9 mEq/L	3.5 to 5.3 mEq/L or mmol/L
Sodium	144 mEq/L	135 to 145 mEq/L or mmol/L
Blood urea nitrogen	10 mg/dL	8 to 21 mg/dL
		Adult over 90 years: 10 to 31 mg/dL
D-dimer	Positive	Negative

3. **Prioritize hypotheses. Where do I start?** Complete the sentence by choosing from the drop-down list of options. Based on the client's condition at the time, the nurse recognizes that the client is at the **highest** risk for _____

> *Select* ▼
> 1. Gangrene
> 2. Stroke
> 3. Congestive heart failure

and will require_____.

> *Select* ▼
> 1. Antibiotics
> 2. Total parental nutrition
> 3. Anticoagulants

(1300) The ultrasound of the leg veins confirms the presence of a blood clot in the deep veins of the right calf.

4. **Generate solutions. What can I do?** For each intervention, specify whether the intervention is **indicated** or **not indicated** for the client's care.

Potential Nursing Intervention	Indicated	Not Indicated
Encourage hydration		
Elevate right leg		
Bed rest		
Ice right leg		
Bleeding precautions		
Restrict visitors		
Sequential compression device to left leg		

5. **Take action. What will I do?** The client is admitted to the hospital. Which admission orders should the nurse consider a **priority** action? **Select all that apply.**
   1. Repeat CBC and BMP in a.m.
   2. Regular diet
   3. PT/PTT every 4 hours
   4. Darvocet-N 100 mg every 4 hours PRN pain greater than 6 out of 10
   5. Referral to social work
   6. Heparin 10,000 U bolus IV followed by heparin 900 U IV per hour

(0800) The client is awake, alert, and oriented. Skin is pink, warm, and dry. Mucous membranes are pink and moist. Lungs are clear throughout all fields. Abdomen is soft with bowel sounds present ×4. Upon examination of the legs, the right calf is pink, warm, and tender to touch, and there is swelling in the right calf. Pedal pulses are bounding bilaterally. The client states that pain in the right leg is a 4 out of 10.

Vital Signs	Client Values
Heart rate	77 bpm
Respirations	12 breaths/min
Temperature	98.7°F (37.1°C)
Spo$_2$	99% on room air
Pain level	4 out of 10

6. **Evaluate outcomes. Did it help?** For each assessment finding, indicate whether the client's condition has **improved**, **declined**, or **not changed**.

Finding	Improved	Declined	No Change
Temperature			
Heart rate			
Respirations			
Respiratory assessment			
Spo$_2$			
Pain level			

Four days later, the client is ready for discharge. Skin is pink, warm, and dry. Mucous membranes are pink and moist. Lungs are clear throughout all fields. The abdomen is soft, with bowel sounds present ×4. Upon examination of the legs, the right calf is pink, warm, and dry without edema. Pedal pulses are bounding bilaterally. The client states that pain in the right leg is a 0 out of 10. The client is excited to go home and get back to work.

Vital Signs	Client Values
Heart rate	78 bpm
Respirations	16 breaths/min
Temperature	98.6°F (37.0°C)
Spo$_2$	100% on room air
Pain level	0 out of 10

ANSWERS AND RATIONALES

The correct answer number and rationale are in **boldface purple type.** Rationales for why other answer options are incorrect are also given.

1. 1. Intermittent claudication is a symptom of arterial occlusive disease; therefore, this client does not need to be assessed first.
   2. **The client diagnosed with calf pain could be experiencing DVT, a complication of immobility, which may be fatal if a pulmonary embolus occurs; therefore, this client should be assessed first.**
   3. The client experiencing low back pain when lying in bed should be assessed, but not before the client diagnosed with suspected DVT.
   4. The nurse should address the client's concern about the food, but it is not a priority over a physiological problem.

   CLINICAL JUDGMENT GUIDE: When deciding which client to assess first, the test taker should determine whether the signs or symptoms the client is exhibiting are normal or expected for the client's situation. After eliminating the expected options, the test taker should determine which situation is more life-threatening.

2. 1. **Therapeutic levels for PTT should be 1.5 to 2 times the normal value, which is 39 seconds; therefore, this client is at risk for bleeding. The prolonged PTT indicates the client is receiving heparin (the drug of choice to treat DVT). The nurse should stop the infusion and follow the facility protocol.**
   2. The hemoglobin is within normal range, and the client diagnosed with Raynaud's disease does not have a problem with bleeding.
   3. The WBC count is elevated (normal is 4,500 to 11,100/microL), but it would be elevated in a client diagnosed with an infection such as venous stasis ulcer.
   4. The nurse should notify the HCP on rounds of abnormal laboratory data that are not immediately life-threatening. The triglyceride level is high, but it will take weeks to months of a heart healthy diet, exercise, and possibly medications to lower this level.

   CLINICAL JUDGMENT GUIDE: When a question asks for immediate intervention, the test taker must decide whether there is an intervention the nurse can implement immediately or whether the HCP must be notified. If the data are abnormal, but not life-threatening, then the option can be eliminated as a possible correct answer.

3. 1. The nurse should first assess the client to determine the status before notifying the HCP.
   2. The UAP has notified the nurse of a potentially serious situation. The nurse must first assess the client before taking any action.
   3. The nurse might place the client in the Trendelenburg position once cardiovascular shock is determined.
   4. **The nurse should immediately go to the client's room to assess the client.**

   CLINICAL JUDGMENT GUIDE: Any time the nurse receives information about a client experiencing a complication from another staff member, the nurse must assess the client. The nurse should not decide about the client's needs based on another staff member's information.

4. 1. **Because laboratory values called into a unit usually include critical values, the charge nurse should tell the unit secretary to "inform me of any laboratory information immediately." The charge nurse must evaluate this information immediately.**
   2. Posting laboratory results in the EHR is the responsibility of the laboratory staff, not the unit secretary.
   3. This is unrealistic because laboratory data are important information that must be called into a unit when there is a critical value so that immediate action can be taken for the client's welfare. The secretary must know how to process the information.
   4. The unit secretary should verify the information by repeating back the information at the time of the call, not by making a second telephone call to the laboratory.

   CLINICAL JUDGMENT GUIDE: The test taker must know the roles of all members of the multidisciplinary healthcare team, as well as HIPAA (Health Insurance Portability and Accountability Act) rules and regulations. The nurse must ensure the healthcare team member knows the appropriate actions to take in specific situations. These will be tested on the NCLEX-RN®.

5. 1. **Vitamin K (AquaMephyton), a vitamin, is the antidote for warfarin (Coumadin) overdose and is administered to a client when their INR level is above the therapeutic 2 to 3; therefore, the nurse should question administering this medication.**

61

2. Propranolol (Inderal), a beta-adrenergic agent, is administered to clients diagnosed with hypertension; therefore, the nurse would not question administering this medication.
3. Nifedipine (Procardia), a calcium-channel blocker, reduces the number of vasospastic attacks in clients diagnosed with Raynaud's disease; therefore, the nurse would not question administering this medication.
4. Enalapril (Vasotec), an angiotensin-converting enzyme (ACE) inhibitor, is administered to clients diagnosed with diabetes to help prevent diabetic nephropathy. The nurse would not question administering this medication.

CLINICAL JUDGMENT GUIDE: The nurse must be aware of interventions that must be implemented before administering medications. The nurse should know what to monitor before administering medications because untoward reactions and possibly death can occur.

6. 1. **This client is exhibiting signs and symptoms of a potentially fatal complication of DVT—pulmonary embolism. The nurse should assess this client first.**
   2. Intermittent claudication of the feet, hands, and arms is a symptom of Buerger's disease; therefore, this client should not be assessed first.
   3. The client diagnosed with an aortic aneurysm is expected to have an audible bruit, which does not indicate any life-threatening condition; therefore, this client does not need to be assessed first.
   4. The client diagnosed with acute arterial ischemia should have unpalpable pedal pulses to be considered a medical emergency; therefore, this client does not need to be assessed first.

CLINICAL JUDGMENT GUIDE: The test taker must determine which sign or symptom is not expected for the disease process. If the sign or symptom is unexpected, the nurse should assess the client first. This type of question determines whether the nurse is knowledgeable of the signs or symptoms of various disease processes.

7. 1. Because the client has been on the daily acetylsalicylic acid (aspirin) for more than a year, the nurse should assess for bleeding by asking questions such as, "Do your gums bleed after brushing your teeth?" or "Do you notice blood when you blow your nose?"

2. Because acetylsalicylic acid (aspirin) can cause gastric distress, the nurse could instruct the client to stop taking it; however, because this is a daily medication being used as an antiplatelet agent, the nurse should provide information that would allow the client to continue the medication.
3. The nurse should realize the stomach discomfort is probably secondary to daily acetylsalicylic acid (aspirin), and enteric-coated acetylsalicylic acid (aspirin) would be helpful to decrease the stomach discomfort and allow the client to stay on the medication, but the nurse should first assess the client for bleeding.
4. Because acetylsalicylic acid (aspirin) is not a prescription medication, the nurse can recommend a different form of acetylsalicylic acid (aspirin), such as an enteric-coated one. However, if the enteric-coated acetylsalicylic acid (aspirin) does not relieve the pain, the HCP should be notified.

CLINICAL JUDGMENT GUIDE: Assessment is the first step of the nursing process, and the test taker should use the nursing process or some other systematic process to determine priorities.

8. 1. **This statement indicates the new graduate needs more teaching because the nurse is responsible for delegating the right task to the right individual. Absolutely no one works on the nurse's license except the nurse holding the license.**
   2. The nurse does retain accountability for the task delegated; therefore, the new graduate does not need more teaching.
   3. The nurse must make sure the UAP can perform the task safely and competently; therefore, the new graduate does not need more teaching.
   4. The nurse must ensure the delegated task was completed correctly; therefore, the new graduate does not need more teaching.

CLINICAL JUDGMENT GUIDE: An RN cannot delegate assessment, teaching, evaluation, medications, or an unstable client to a UAP. Tasks that cannot be delegated are nursing interventions requiring nursing clinical judgment. The nurse must be aware of delegation rules and regulations.

9. 1. The product manufacturer would provide biased information and not provide the best data to support a change proposal.
   2. Research studies with limited participants indicate the need for further research and would not be the best research to support a change proposal.

3. Research should provide clear statistical data that support the research problem or hypothesis.
4. The more research articles that support a change proposal, the more valid the information, which increases the possibility for change to be considered by the healthcare facility.

CLINICAL JUDGMENT GUIDE: The NCLEX-RN® test plan includes nursing care based on evidence-based practice. The nurse must be knowledgeable of nursing research.

10. 1. The UAP can clean the perineal area of a client on bedrest with an indwelling catheter. Because the client is stable, the nurse could delegate this nursing task to the UAP.
    2. The UAP can obtain the client's intake and output, but the nurse must evaluate the data to determine whether interventions are needed or effective.
    3. A client diagnosed with third-spacing is unstable and in a life-threatening situation; therefore, the nurse cannot delegate the UAP to bathe this client.
    4. This is a medication enema, and the UAP cannot administer medications. In addition, if a cation-exchange resin enema is ordered, the client is unstable and has an excessively high serum potassium (K^+) level.

CLINICAL JUDGMENT GUIDE: An RN cannot delegate assessment, teaching, evaluation, medications, or an unstable client to a UAP. Tasks requiring clinical judgment cannot be delegated.

11. 1. Although the nurse could request another UAP to perform the task, this is not the best action because the nurse should demonstrate applying SCDs so that the UAP can learn how to complete the task.
    2. **This is the priority action because the nurse will ensure the UAP knows how to apply SCDs correctly, enabling the nurse to delegate the task to the UAP successfully in the future.**
    3. The nurse could do the task, but if the UAP is not shown how to do it, then the UAP will not be able to perform the task the next time it is delegated.
    4. The UAP could watch a video demonstrating this task, but the priority action is for the nurse to demonstrate SCD application to the UAP.

CLINICAL JUDGMENT GUIDE: The nurse cannot delegate any task the UAP admits to being unable to perform. It is the nurse's responsibility to know what can be delegated and when. The nurse may have to complete the task if the UAP is not competent.

12. 1. The nurse should not assign assessment of a client to an LPN even if the client is stable.
    2. The LPN cannot initiate the administration of blood; therefore, the nurse must complete this task.
    3. **The LPN can administer medications; therefore, the LPN could hang a bag of heparin on an IV pump for this client.**
    4. The nurse must assess for dysrhythmias during the insertion, and the nurse assisting the HCP should be experienced in inserting the line. An LPN pulled from another unit should not be assigned this task.

CLINICAL JUDGMENT GUIDE: The nurse cannot assign assessment, teaching, evaluation, or an unstable client to an LPN. The LPN can call HCPs on the phone to obtain orders for a client.

13. 1. The client is having signs or symptoms of a blood transfusion reaction. The nurse must immediately stop the transfusion and assess the client's vital signs.
    2. The HCP needs to be notified, but not before the nurse stops the blood transfusion.
    3. The nurse should maintain a patent IV line to administer medications, but this is not the first intervention.
    4. **Any time the nurse suspects the client is having a reaction to blood or blood products, the nurse should stop the infusion at the spot closest to the client and not allow any more of the blood to enter the client's body. This is the nurse's first intervention.**

CLINICAL JUDGMENT GUIDE: The nurse should remember: If a client is in distress and the nurse can do something to relieve the distress, it should be done first, before assessment. The test taker should select an option that helps the client's condition directly.

14. **Correct answers are 1, 3, 4, and 5.**
    1. A research article should answer the question, "Why?" Why was the research done? This statement indicates the charge nurse understands how to read a research article.
    2. The cost of the research is not pertinent when reading a research article and determining whether the research supports

evidence-based practice. This statement indicates the charge nurse does not understand how to read a research article.
3. A research article should answer the question "What?" What research method was used? This statement indicates the charge nurse understands how to read a research article.
4. A research article should answer the question "Where?" In what setting was the research conducted? This statement indicates the charge nurse understands how to read a research article.
5. A research article should explain how the data were collected. This statement indicates the charge nurse understands how to read a research article.

CLINICAL JUDGMENT GUIDE: The NCLEX-RN® test plan includes nursing care based on evidence-based practice. The nurse must be knowledgeable of nursing research.

15. 1. The nurse should enter the order in the EHR and document "per telephone order," but this is not the nurse's first intervention.
    2. The nurse does not need another nurse to verify the HCP's telephone order.
    3. The Joint Commission has implemented this requirement for all telephone orders. The nurse should document on the HCP's order for meperidine (Demerol) "repeat order verified."
    4. The nurse should send electronic or written confirmation of the order to the pharmacy, but this is not the first intervention.

CLINICAL JUDGMENT GUIDE: The NCLEX-RN® test plan includes nursing care that is ruled by legal requirements as well as rules and regulations of The Joint Commission, Centers for Medicare & Medicaid Services, Centers for Disease Control and Prevention, and the Occupational Safety and Health Administration. The nurse must be knowledgeable regarding these standards.

16. 1. The therapeutic level for a client on warfarin (Coumadin) is an INR of 2 to 3; therefore, this client does not warrant intervention.
    2. These hemoglobin and hematocrit levels are a little low but not so critical that this would warrant intervention by the charge nurse.
    3. A platelet count of fewer than 100,000/mL of blood indicates thrombocytopenia; therefore, this client warrants intervention by the charge nurse.
    4. This is a normal red blood cell count; therefore, the charge nurse would not need to intervene.

CLINICAL JUDGMENT GUIDE: The nurse must be knowledgeable of normal laboratory values. The nurse must be able to determine whether the laboratory value is normal for the client's disease process or medications the client is taking.

17. 1. This statement does not support the night shift and makes the unit look bad. The nurse should not "bad-mouth" the night shift.
    2. The nurse has no idea what happened that delayed answering the call light; it could have been a code or other type of life-threatening situation. The day shift primary nurse may be unable to answer the light in certain situations and should not falsely reassure the client.
    3. The nurse should have someone in a position to investigate what happened on the night shift talk to the client and determine why this happened. The day shift primary nurse does not have this authority.
    4. This negates the client's feeling, and the client does not need to know what was happening in the critical care unit.

CLINICAL JUDGMENT GUIDE: There will be management questions on the NCLEX-RN®. There is often no test-taking strategy for these questions; the nurse must be knowledgeable of management issues.

18. Correct order is 3, 2, 1, 4, 5.
    3. The client must agree to the risks and benefits of a blood transfusion before the nurse can administer the blood product. This is the first intervention.
    2. The nurse has only 30 minutes from when the blood is retrieved from the blood bank until the transfusion is initiated. The nurse should ensure the client has patent IV access before obtaining the blood from the blood bank.
    1. The nurse can obtain the unit of packed cells when the client has signed the permit and has patent IV access.
    4. The nurse should always check the blood product with another nurse at the client's bedside against the client's hospital identification band and blood bank crossmatch band.

5. After the nurse has followed the procedure to ensure the correct blood product is being administered, a second nurse can initiate the transfusion of packed cells. The blood is initiated at a slow rate—10 mL/hr for the first 15 minutes—so that the nurse can observe the client for potential complications.

CLINICAL JUDGMENT GUIDE: This is an alternate type of question included in the NCLEX-RN® test plan. The nurse must be able to perform skills in the correct order. Obtaining informed consent and conducting an assessment should always be the first interventions.

19. 1. This should be an anticipated order if the nurse suspects a pulmonary embolus, but it is not the first intervention.
    2. **The nurse should suspect the client has a pulmonary embolus, a complication of the thrombophlebitis. Pulmonary emboli decrease the oxygen supply to the body, and the nurse should immediately administer oxygen to the client.**
    3. An anticoagulant infusion will be ordered for the client once it is determined that the client is experiencing a pulmonary embolus.
    4. Getting oxygen to the body is a priority; telling the client not to ambulate can be done after initiating the oxygen.

CLINICAL JUDGMENT GUIDE: Physiological problems have the highest priority when deciding on a course of action. If the client is distressed, the nurse must intervene with a nursing action that attempts to alleviate or control the problem. The test taker should not choose a diagnostic test if there is an option that directly treats the client.

20. 1. **The therapeutic level for digoxin is 0.5 to 2 ng/mL, which warrants notifying the HCP.**
    2. There is no serum blood level to monitor enoxaparin (Lovenox), a low-molecular-weight heparin administered to prevent DVT.
    3. The platelet level is within the normal level of 150,000 to 450,000/microL, so this would not warrant notifying the HCP.
    4. The normal potassium level is 3.5 to 5.3 mEq/L, so this result would not warrant notifying the HCP.

CLINICAL JUDGMENT GUIDE: The nurse must be knowledgeable of normal laboratory values. The nurse must be able to determine whether the laboratory value is normal for the client's disease process or for the medications the client is taking.

21. 1. This is the correct procedure to help preserve the fingers so the surgeon can reattach the fingers, but is not the first intervention.
    2. Elevating the right arm will help decrease bleeding, but it is not the first intervention.
    3. **The nurse should first put on nonsterile gloves to protect from getting any blood-borne diseases.**
    4. Applying direct pressure is an appropriate intervention, but the first intervention is to apply gloves to protect the nurse.

CLINICAL JUDGMENT GUIDE: The test taker must remember: If the client is in distress, do not assess, but Standard Precautions take priority. The nurse must always make Standard Precautions a priority when caring for all clients, especially when blood and body fluids are present.

22. 1. The UAP could escort the client to the room so that the LPN could be assigned tasks within the LPN's scope of practice.
    2. **The UAP can ensure the room is clear of the previous client's gown and equipment. The UAP can also make sure there are gowns, tongue blades, and additional equipment in the examination room.**
    3. The LPN can administer medication; therefore, it would be more appropriate to assign this task to the LPN so that the RN could be assigned tasks that are beyond the scope of practice of an LPN and within the RN's scope of practice.
    4. The clinic secretary is unlicensed personnel and does not have the authority to call in a new prescription for a client.

CLINICAL JUDGMENT GUIDE: When the test taker decides which option is the most appropriate task to delegate or assign, the test taker should choose the task that requires each staff member to function within their full scope of practice. Do not assign a task to a staff member that requires a higher level of expertise than the staff member has, and do not assign a task to a staff member when the task could be delegated or assigned to a staff member with a lower level of expertise.

23. 1. The nurse should discuss the client's comment, but it is not the nurse's first intervention.
    2. **The nurse should first take the client's BP correctly and address the client's concern.**
    3. If the nurse's BP reading and the UAP's BP reading are close to the same, the nurse could reassure the client that the UAP does know

how to take BP readings. However, this is not the nurse's first intervention.
4. This is an appropriate action, but it is not the first intervention. The nurse is responsible for ensuring the UAP can perform delegated tasks correctly.

CLINICAL JUDGMENT GUIDE: The nurse should address the client's needs first, including answering the client's questions, verifying the client's vital signs, or assessing the client if the client is not in distress.

24. 1. IV push medications cannot be assigned to an LPN. It is the most dangerous route for administering medication, and only an RN (or HCP) can perform this task.
    2. The client diagnosed with a pulmonary embolus is not stable; therefore, this medication is not the best medication to be assigned to the LPN.
    3. **Pentoxifylline (Trental) is a PO medication explicitly prescribed to treat intermittent claudication. It increases erythrocyte flexibility and reduces blood viscosity.**
    4. The client may be having a myocardial infarction; therefore, this client is unstable and should not be assigned to an LPN.

CLINICAL JUDGMENT GUIDE: The test taker must determine which option is included within the LPN's scope of practice. LPNs are not routinely taught how to administer IV push medications. The test taker must also determine which client is the most stable, which makes this an "except" question. Three clients are either unstable or have potentially life-threatening conditions and should not be assigned to an LPN.

25. 1. **The nurse should realize the client probably has DVT, a medical emergency. The HCP should be notified immediately so the client can be started on IV heparin and admitted to the hospital.**
    2. This information may be needed, but the nurse should notify the HCP based on the signs or symptoms alone.
    3. A neurovascular assessment should be completed, but not before notifying the HCP. The signs or symptoms alone indicate a potentially life-threatening condition.
    4. The client's leg should be elevated, but this is a potentially life-threatening emergency and the nurse should first call the HCP.

CLINICAL JUDGMENT GUIDE: The test taker must read all the options carefully before choosing the option that says, "Notify the HCP." If any of the options will provide information the HCP needs to know to make a decision, the test taker should choose that option. If the HCP does not need any additional information to make a decision and the nurse suspects the condition is serious or life-threatening, the priority intervention is to call the HCP.

26. 1. **The nurse should first determine whether there is a fire or someone accidentally or purposefully pulled the fire alarm. Because this is a clinic, not a hospital, the nurse should keep calm and determine the situation before acting.**
    2. The nurse should not evacuate clients, visitors, and staff without a real fire.
    3. The nurse should assess the situation before contacting the fire department.
    4. This is an appropriate intervention but not the first one. The nurse should first assess to determine whether there is a fire.

CLINICAL JUDGMENT GUIDE: The nurse must be knowledgeable of emergency preparedness. Employees receive this information in employee orientation and are responsible for implementing procedures correctly. The NCLEX-RN® test plan includes questions on a safe and effective care environment.

27. 1. The clinic nurse should allow the director to address sexual harassment allegations. This is a matter that should be handled legally.
    2. This is an appropriate question when investigating sexual harassment allegations, but the clinic nurse should allow the director of nurses to pursue this situation.
    3. The clinic nurse is responsible for taking the appropriate action when sexual allegations are reported. This statement shows that the clinic nurse is not taking the allegations seriously, which could result in disciplinary action against the nurse.
    4. **This is the most appropriate response because sexual harassment allegations are a legal matter. The clinic nurse implemented the correct action by ensuring the UAP reported the allegation to the director of nurses.**

CLINICAL JUDGMENT GUIDE: There will be management questions on the NCLEX-RN®. In many instances, there is no test-taking strategy for these questions. The nurse must know which management issues must comply with local, state, and federal requirements.

28. 1. The clinic nurse should not discuss the staff nurse's statement with the pharmaceutical representative because the staff member's behavior is unethical and could have repercussions. The clinic nurse should notify the director of nurses.
    2. **This behavior is unethical and is making promises that the staff nurse may or may not be able to keep. Because this situation includes the HCP, an outside representative, and the staff nurse, this situation should be reported to the director of nurses for further action.**
    3. This behavior must be reported. This situation involves bribing the pharmaceutical representative and using a meeting with the HCP as a reward.
    4. The clinic nurse should maintain the chain of command and report this to the nursing supervisor, not the HCP.

CLINICAL JUDGMENT GUIDE: There will be management questions on the NCLEX-RN®. In many instances, there is no test-taking strategy for these questions. The nurse must be knowledgeable of management issues.

29. 1. The nurse should document the results in the client's EHR, but this is not the nurse's first intervention.
    2. **The therapeutic value for INR is 2 to 3; levels higher than that increase the risk of bleeding. The nurse should first contact the client and determine whether they have any abnormal bleeding and then instruct the client not to take any more warfarin (Coumadin), an oral anticoagulant.**
    3. The nurse should notify the client's HCP, but the nurse should first determine whether the client has any abnormal bleeding to report it to the HCP.
    4. The client must have another INR drawn, but it is not the nurse's first intervention.

CLINICAL JUDGMENT GUIDE: Any time the nurse receives information from another source about a client experiencing a complication, the nurse must assess the client. In this scenario, the nurse assesses the client by talking to them on the phone. The nurse should not make decisions about the client's needs unless the nurse talks to the client.

30. 1. A low-salt diet is used to treat arterial hypertension, but it is not the priority intervention.
    2. **The priority intervention for the client diagnosed with arterial hypertension is to take antihypertensive medications.**
    3. Taking and documenting blood pressure readings is important but does not treat arterial hypertension; therefore, it is not the priority intervention.
    4. Walking will help decrease the client's high blood pressure in some situations, but it is not a priority.

CLINICAL JUDGMENT GUIDE: All options are plausible in questions that ask the test taker to identify a priority intervention. The test taker must determine the most important intervention.

31. Correct answers are 2 and 4.
    1. Stockings should be applied after the legs have been elevated for some time—when the amount of blood in the leg vein is at its lowest. Applying the stockings when the client is sitting in a chair indicates the UAP does not understand the correct procedure for applying compression stockings.
    2. If the UAP cannot insert a finger under the proximal end of the stocking, the compression hose is too tight. By performing this test, the UAP demonstrated an understanding of the correct procedure for applying the stockings.
    3. The toe opening should be placed on the plantar side of the foot. Placing the toe opening on the top side of the foot indicates the UAP does not understand the correct procedure for applying compression stockings.
    4. Warm toes mean the stockings are not too tight, and there is good circulation. Checking that the toes are warm indicates the UAP understands the correct procedure for applying the compression stockings.
    5. Lotions should not be applied immediately before putting on compression stockings. This indicates the UAP does not understand the correct procedure for applying compression stockings.

CLINICAL JUDGMENT GUIDE: The nurse must ensure the UAP can perform any delegated tasks. The nurse is responsible for evaluating the task, demonstrating it, or teaching the UAP how to perform the task.

32. 1. The nurse should first take care of the bite and then determine whether the dog is current on the required vaccinations. The nurse should be concerned about the possibility of rabies.

2. If the dog is not current on the required vaccinations, the veterinarian should be notified to quarantine the dog to check for rabies.
3. The nurse should complete an occurrence report and document the dog bite. If the nurse must pay for anything concerning the dog bite, it should be covered by workers' compensation.
4. Besides an infection of the dog bite, the worst complication would be the nurse contracting rabies. If the dog is current on the required vaccinations, this should not be a concern.

CLINICAL JUDGMENT GUIDE: The test taker should apply the nursing process when the question asks, "Which intervention should be implemented first?" If the client is in distress, do not assess; if the client is in distress, take action.

33.
1. This would not warrant immediate intervention because intermittent claudication, pain when walking, is the hallmark sign of arterial occlusive disease.
2. This comment warrants immediate intervention because the client's legs have decreased sensation secondary to the arterial occlusive disease, and a heating pad could burn the client's legs without the client realizing it. The client should not use a heating pad to keep the legs warm.
3. Hanging their legs off the bed helps increase the arterial blood supply to the legs, which, in turn, helps decrease leg pain. This comment would not warrant immediate intervention by the nurse.
4. Hair growth requires oxygen, and the client has decreased oxygen to the legs; therefore, decreased hair growth would be expected and not require immediate intervention.

CLINICAL JUDGMENT GUIDE: When the question asks, "Which warrants immediate intervention?" it is an "except" question. Three of the comments indicate the client understands the teaching, and one suggests the client does not understand the teaching.

34.
1. The nurse cannot purchase supplies for the client. This is crossing a professional boundary.
2. The social worker does assist with financial concerns and referrals for the client, but purchasing smoke detectors is not within the social worker's scope of practice.
3. The nurse should not encourage the client to depend on family members to purchase supplies for the client's home. This may be a possibility when all other avenues have been pursued.
4. The nurse should contact the fire department. Many fire departments will supply and install smoke detectors for people unable to afford them. The nurse should investigate this option first because it is the most immediate response to the safety need.

CLINICAL JUDGMENT GUIDE: The nurse must know about hospital and community emergency preparedness. Employees receive this information in employee orientation and are responsible for implementing procedures correctly. The NCLEX-RN® test plan includes questions on a safe and effective care environment.

35.
1. The nurse should document the objective findings in the EHR, but this is not the priority intervention.
2. The nurse cannot force the client to discuss the situation.
3. The bruises and burns should make the nurse suspect elder abuse, and the nurse is mandated by law to report this to Adult Protective Services.
4. The nurse should let Adult Protective Services take pictures of the suspected abuse because a legal chain of custody must be followed if the case goes to court.

CLINICAL JUDGMENT GUIDE: The NCLEX-RN® test plan includes nursing care ruled by legal requirements. The nurse is legally obligated to report possible child abuse and adult abuse. The nurse must be knowledgeable of these issues.

36.
1. Acetylsalicylic acid (aspirin), an antiplatelet agent, puts the client at risk for bleeding. The client diagnosed with DVT will be on warfarin (Coumadin), an anticoagulant, which puts the client at risk for bleeding; therefore, this comment requires immediate intervention by the nurse.
2. The client should wear a medical alert bracelet to notify any emergency HCP of the client's condition and medication. This statement would not warrant immediate intervention.
3. Most books recommend not eating green, leafy vegetables high in vitamin K because doing so is the antidote to Coumadin toxicity. The client would have to eat green, leafy vegetables more than twice a week to counteract

the Coumadin; therefore, this comment would not warrant immediate intervention as much as taking daily acetylsalicylic acid (aspirin).
4. Elevating the client's legs would not warrant intervention by the nurse.

CLINICAL JUDGMENT GUIDE: This question asks the nurse to identify which statement warrants immediate intervention; this indicates three options are appropriate for the disease process or disorder, and one is inappropriate. This is an "except" question, but it does not say all the options are correct "except."

37. 1. The nurse should be a client advocate and support the client's wishes, not support the HCP's recommendation, even if it is best for the client.
2. Recommending the client talk to their family may be appropriate, but it does not support the nurse being a client advocate.
3. The client has a right to a second opinion, but this action does not support the client's decision not to have an amputation and thus is not client advocacy.
4. **This action shows the nurse being the client's advocate. Offering to talk to the HCP about the amputation and making sure the HCP hears the client's opinion is being a client advocate. Another discussion may change the client's decision, but either way, client advocacy supports the client's decision.**

CLINICAL JUDGMENT GUIDE: There will be management questions on the NCLEX-RN® addressing client advocacy. A client advocate acts as a liaison between clients and HCPs to help improve or maintain a high quality of healthcare.

38. 1. Crying at a death is a universal human response. Although the statement may be true, the nurse should recognize the UAP's need for a short time to compose themself.
2. **Hospital personnel are not immune to human emotions. The UAP needs a short time to compose themself. The nurse should offer the UAP compassion. If this occurred with every death, the UAP could be counseled to transfer to a different hospital area.**
3. This is not accepting the UAP's feelings.
4. This is not accepting the UAP's feelings.

CLINICAL JUDGMENT GUIDE: There will be management questions on the NCLEX-RN®. In many instances, there is no test-taking strategy for these questions. The nurse must be knowledgeable regarding management issues.

39. 1. **Clients receiving hospice can discontinue the service and resume standard healthcare practices and treatments whenever they wish. The nurse should assess the client's wishes before continuing.**
2. This is true, but if the client wants to be treated, it is the client's decision. If the client does not want treatment, the nurse should discuss the client's wishes with the long-term care facility staff.
3. If the client does not want treatment, the nurse should discuss the client's wishes with the long-term care facility staff.
4. A client conference should be called if the staff continues to try to get the client to accept futile treatment, but this is not the first action for the hospice nurse because a client conference is a scheduled event and does not occur immediately.

CLINICAL JUDGMENT GUIDE: This question requires the test taker to have a basic knowledge of hospice and hospice goals. The nurse must also be aware of appropriate referrals.

40. 1. Telling the family over the telephone could cause the client's significant other to have an accident while driving to the hospital. The nurse should avoid disclosing this type of information over the phone.
2. **This response lets the family or significant other know there has been some incident, but it does not disclose the death. It is the best statement for the nurse at this time. The family will be able to arrive safely at the hospital before hearing the news their loved one has died.**
3. Telling the family over the telephone could cause the client to have an accident while driving to the hospital. The nurse should avoid disclosing this type of information over the phone.
4. The nurse should avoid this backward way of telling the family that the client died.

CLINICAL JUDGMENT GUIDE: There will be management questions on the NCLEX-RN®. In many instances, there is no test-taking strategy for these questions. The nurse must be knowledgeable regarding management issues.

41. 1. The client is experiencing a surgical procedure complication and should be assigned to a nurse more experienced in caring for clients diagnosed with vascular complications.
    2. Low back pain could indicate a leaking abdominal aortic aneurysm and should not be assigned to a floating nurse. A more experienced vascular nurse should care for this client.
    3. Because this client needs extensive teaching, this client should not be assigned to a floating nurse but to a more experienced vascular nurse.
    4. The client diagnosed with varicose veins would be expected to have deep aching pain in the legs; therefore, the nurse floated to the vascular unit could be assigned to this client.

    CLINICAL JUDGMENT GUIDE: The nurse should assign the most stable client to the least experienced nurse.

42. 1. Leaving the facility will make client care even more strained.
    2. The nurse should notify the supervisor that the nurse is concerned that the assignment will not allow the nurse to provide adequate care to any of the three clients. It is the first step the nurse should implement.
    3. This is the second step. The nurse should write their concerns and present the documentation to the supervisor. In states with a "safe harbor" clause in the Nurse Practice Act, this will prevent the nurse from losing their license should a poor outcome result from the assignment.
    4. If the staffing continues to be unsafe, the nurse may choose to resign, but the resignation should follow accepted business practices.

    CLINICAL JUDGMENT GUIDE: There will be management questions on the NCLEX-RN®. There is often no test-taking strategy for these questions; the nurse must be knowledgeable of management issues. If the nurse thinks the assignment violates the state's Nurse Practice Act, then the nurse must notify the supervisor immediately.

43. 1. Morphine is a potent narcotic analgesic. A 4 on the 1-to-10 pain scale is considered moderate pain and should be treated with a less potent pain medication.
    2. Promethazine (Phenergan) is administered for nausea.
    3. Hydrocodone (Vicodin) is a narcotic analgesic that is less potent than morphine. It has been 5 hours since the hydrocodone was last administered, and the client has required no other pain medication. This is the best medication for moderate pain.
    4. Ibuprofen (Motrin) may be effective for moderate pain, but the client is allergic to ibuprofen. The nurse should tag the MAR and EHR to notify the HCP to discontinue this medication.

    CLINICAL JUDGMENT GUIDE: This is an alternate type question included in the NCLEX-RN® test plan. The test taker must be able to read an MAR, know the medications, and decide the most appropriate intervention.

44. 1. The daughter lives in a "nearby" city. The client should not be moved until the daughter arrives.
    2. A morgue is a difficult place to view a body. This could be appropriate if the daughter were to take hours or days to get to the hospital.
    3. Many people feel it is necessary to view the body. Not allowing the daughter time to view the body before transfer to a funeral home or the morgue could cause hurt feelings and impede the grieving process.
    4. Many people feel it is necessary to view the body. Not allowing the daughter time to view the body before transfer to a funeral home or the morgue could cause hurt feelings and impede the grieving process.

    CLINICAL JUDGMENT GUIDE: The nurse should always try to support the client's or family's request if it does not violate any local, state, or federal rules and regulations.

45. 1. The change process can be compared to the nursing process. The first step of each is to assess the problem. Assessment involves collecting the pertinent data that support the need for a change.
    2. The second step is to identify the problem, similar to identifying possible nursing diagnoses.
    3. The third step is to select an alternative to implement to fix the problem, similar to choosing a specific nursing diagnosis.
    4. The fourth step is to implement a plan of action, similar to implementing the nursing care plan.

CLINICAL JUDGMENT GUIDE: Assessment is the first step of the nursing process, and the test taker should use the nursing process or some other systematic process to assist in determining priorities.

46. Correct answers are 2 and 3.
    1. The only solution compatible with blood is normal saline. Dextrose causes the blood to coagulate.
    2. The blood administration set is changed after every 2 units.
    3. The nurse must assess the client's vital signs before every unit of blood is administered.
    4. The nurse should assess for allergies before administering medications. Before administering blood products, the nurse should assess compatibility with the client's blood type. The client may have an incompatible blood type, but this is not an allergy.
    5. A blood warmer is used when the client has identified cold agglutinins, which is not in the question's stem.

CLINICAL JUDGMENT GUIDE: This is an alternate type of question included in the NCLEX-RN®. The nurse must be able to select all the options that answer the question correctly.

47. 1. The client diagnosed with a DVT is placed on strict bedrest and should not have any pressure on their calf, which may cause the clot to dislodge and cause a pulmonary embolus. This task should not be delegated to a UAP.
    2. The number one intervention for a client diagnosed with thromboangiitis obliterans (Buerger's disease) is to stop smoking; therefore, this task should not be delegated. The UAP should be on the unit caring for clients, not outside for a client to smoke.
    3. **The leg should be elevated to prevent postoperative edema; therefore, this task could be delegated to the UAP.**
    4. The UAP cannot perform Doppler studies; a trained technician must perform this test.

CLINICAL JUDGMENT GUIDE: An RN cannot delegate assessment, teaching, evaluation, medications, or an unstable client to a UAP. Tasks that cannot be delegated are nursing interventions requiring nursing clinical judgment.

48. 1. Only the client should activate the PCA pump. Allowing family or significant others to push the button places the client at risk for an overdose.
    2. The nurse is acting appropriately; there is no reason to discuss the instructions further.
    3. The nurse is acting appropriately; there is no reason to discuss the instructions further.
    4. **The nurse is acting appropriately, and there is no reason to discuss the instructions further. The charge nurse should continue with other duties.**

CLINICAL JUDGMENT GUIDE: There will be management questions on the NCLEX-RN®. In many instances, there is no test-taking strategy for these questions; the nurse must be knowledgeable regarding management issues concerning personnel. The nurse is responsible for evaluating the behavior of subordinates when caring for clients.

49. 1. **This client may be having phantom pain, but it must be assessed, and the client must be medicated. The nurse should assess this client first.**
    2. The client's blood pressure must be taken to determine whether the headache is because of hypertensive crisis, but it is not a priority for postoperative surgical pain.
    3. The client diagnosed with lymphedema would be expected to have lower leg edema; therefore, the nurse would not assess this client first.
    4. The client diagnosed with gangrene would be expected to have a foul-smelling discharge; therefore, this client would not be assessed first.

CLINICAL JUDGMENT GUIDE: When deciding which client to assess first, the test taker should determine whether the signs or symptoms the client is exhibiting are normal or expected for the client's situation. After eliminating the expected option, the test taker should determine which situation is more life-threatening.

50. 1. The LPN should not administer the medication if the client's BP is lower than 90/50 mm Hg, but this is not the first action the nurse should take.
    2. This medication cannot be crushed, and the nurse needs to intervene and correct the LPN's behavior.
    3. The LPN should be shown where to find pudding or applesauce to mix in crushed medications, but this medication should not be crushed.
    4. **The XL in the name of the medication nifedipine (Procardia XL) indicates that this medication is a sustained-release formulation and should not be crushed. The nurse should speak directly with the LPN to correct the behavior.**

CLINICAL JUDGMENT GUIDE: The nurse should be aware of interventions that must be implemented before administering medications. The nurse must know which medications cannot be crushed. The nurse is responsible for evaluating the behavior and actions of their subordinates.

51.
    1. This action is an example of paternalism or beneficence.
    2. This action is an example of beneficence.
    3. This action is an example of nonmalfeasance or beneficence.
    4. This action is an example of autonomy.

CLINICAL JUDGMENT GUIDE: The NCLEX-RN® test plan includes nursing care that addresses ethical principles, including autonomy, beneficence, justice, and veracity, to name a few.

52.
    1. This would be culturally sensitive to a Jehovah's Witness client.
    2. Mormons do not wear amulets.
    3. The devout Mormon client wears a religious undershirt that should not be removed; this action indicates cultural sensitivity on the part of the nurse.
    4. Mormons do not consult curanderos. Some Hispanic cultures consult curanderos.

CLINICAL JUDGMENT GUIDE: The NCLEX-RN® test plan includes nursing care that addresses cultural diversity. The nurse needs to be aware of cultural differences.

53.
    1. These ABGs show respiratory acidosis, which needs immediate intervention; therefore, this client should be assessed first.
    2. The client diagnosed with Raynaud's phenomenon would be expected to have bluish, cold upper extremities; therefore, the nurse would not need to assess the client first.
    3. The client diagnosed with chronic venous insufficiency has ulceration on the feet; therefore, this nurse would not need to assess the client first.
    4. The PTT is 1.5 to 2 times the normal; therefore, the nurse would not need to assess this client first. Normal PTT is 39 seconds; therefore, the therapeutic PTT is 58 to 78.

CLINICAL JUDGMENT GUIDE: The test taker must determine which sign or symptom is not expected for the disease process. If the sign or symptom is unexpected, the nurse should assess the client first. This type of question determines if the nurse knows the signs and symptoms of various disease processes.

54.
    1. The client diagnosed with arterial occlusive disease dangles the feet off the side of the bed to increase the blood supply to the legs; therefore, a less experienced unlicensed assistive personnel (UAP) could care for this client.
    2. The nurse should be assigned to care for this client, who is angry about the family's not visiting, because the client requires assessment, nursing judgment, and therapeutic communication and intervention, which are not within the UAP's scope of practice.
    3. This client requires an experienced UAP skilled in client lifts so the client is lifted safely and the UAP is not injured in the process. The most experienced UAP should be assigned to this client.
    4. The experienced UAP could care for this client, but other UAPs would not learn to care for the client. This client should be rotated through the UAPs so that all the UAPs can learn to care for the client who is particular about the way things are done.

CLINICAL JUDGMENT GUIDE: When the test taker is deciding which option is the most appropriate task to delegate or assign, the test taker should choose the task that allows each staff member to function within their full scope of practice. Remember: The RN cannot delegate assessment, teaching, evaluation, medications, or an unstable client to the UAP.

55.
    1. Chest pain on deep inspiration is a symptom of pulmonary embolism. The nurse should first place the client on oxygen.
    2. The first intervention is to provide the client with oxygen. The test taker should not assess when the client is in distress.
    3. The respiratory therapist can be notified, but it is not the nurse's first intervention. The nurse should first address the client's needs.
    4. The nurse should not select equipment over addressing the client's needs.

CLINICAL JUDGMENT GUIDE: The nurse should remember: If a client is in distress and the nurse can do something to relieve the distress, that should be done first, before assessment. The test taker should select an option that helps the client's condition directly.

56. Correct answers are 2, 3, 4, and 5.
    1. Monetary need is not a good reason to select a nurse to become a preceptor.
    2. The nurse should be able to organize their workload before becoming a role model for a new nurse. If the nurse is not

organized, taking on new responsibilities will be very frustrating for the preceptor and the preceptee.
3. The nurse acting as a preceptor should have good people skills and be approachable.
4. The nurse should consistently provide quality care that others should emulate.
5. The nurse should be willing to take on this responsibility of being a preceptor, or the nurse will resent the new graduate.

CLINICAL JUDGMENT GUIDE: This is an alternate type of question included in the NCLEX-RN®. The nurse must be able to select all the options that answer the question correctly.

57. 1. This client is experiencing neurovascular compromise and requires immediate attention. The client diagnosed with venous problems should have palpable pedal pulses. This procedure is for clients diagnosed with varicose veins.
2. The calf pain is expected with a client diagnosed with DVT; therefore, the nurse would not assess this client first.
3. The client diagnosed with Raynaud's phenomenon has coldness and numbness in the vasoconstriction phase followed by throbbing, aching pain, tingling, and swelling in the hyperemic phase. The nurse would not see this client first because these are expected signs and symptoms.
4. Buerger's disease (thromboangiitis obliterans) is often confused with peripheral arterial disease (PAD). As the disease progresses, rest pain develops along with color and temperature changes in the affected limb or limbs.

CLINICAL JUDGMENT GUIDE: The test taker must determine which sign or symptom is not expected for the disease process. If the sign or symptom is unexpected, the nurse should assess the client first. This type of question determines if the nurse is knowledgeable regarding the signs and symptoms of various disease processes.

58. Answer: 2,050 mL total intake. The urinary output is not used in this calculation. The nurse must add up both IV fluids and oral fluids to obtain the total intake for this client: 950 + 200 = 1,150 mL IV fluids. Because 1 oz = 30 mL, multiply intake in ounces by 30: 16 oz × 30 mL = 480 mL; 8 oz × 30 mL = 240 mL; 6 oz × 30 mL = 180 mL; 480 + 240 + 180 = 900 mL oral fluids. Therefore, total intake = 1,150 + 900 = 2,050 mL.

CLINICAL JUDGMENT GUIDE: This is an alternate type question included in the NCLEX-RN®. The nurse must be knowledgeable on how to perform math calculations.

59. 1. Cold water causes vasoconstriction, and hot water may burn the client's feet; therefore, warm water should be used, and the feet should be cleaned daily. This statement indicates the client understands the teaching.
2. Shoes should be purchased in the afternoon when the feet are the largest. This statement indicates the client understands the teaching.
3. This statement indicates the client needs more teaching because knee-high stockings will further decrease leg circulation.
4. The client should not elevate their legs because it further decreases arterial blood flow to the legs. The client should dangle their legs off the side of the bed, which increases arterial blood flow to the lower extremities. This statement indicates that the client understands the teaching.

CLINICAL JUDGMENT GUIDE: When the question says "needs more teaching," it is an "except" question. Three of the comments indicate the client understands the teaching, and one suggests the client does not understand the teaching.

60. 1. The nurse cannot delegate an unstable client to the unlicensed assistive personnel (UAP). The client is experiencing hypoglycemia and is not stable.
2. The client is stable, and elevating the feet is an appropriate intervention for a client diagnosed with venous problems; therefore, the UAP could assist this client.
3. The nurse cannot delegate an unstable client to the UAP. The client has numbness of the right arm and should be assessed by the nurse.
4. The client diagnosed with an abdominal aortic aneurysm should not have any increased pressure in the abdomen because it may cause the aneurysm to rupture; therefore, this should not be implemented by anyone.

CLINICAL JUDGMENT GUIDE: This is an "except" question. The test taker could ask which task is appropriate to delegate to the UAP; three options would be appropriate to delegate, and one would not be. Remember: The RN cannot delegate assessment, teaching, evaluation, medications, or an unstable client to the UAP.

61. 1. The nurse needs to intervene because the client is at high risk for developing pneumonia, primarily because of the abdominal incision.
    2. The client must have 30 mL of urinary output every hour, and 300 mL in 8 hours is adequate urinary output. Clients postoperative AAA repair are at high risk for renal failure because of the anatomical location of the AAA near the renal arteries.
    3. The client should have hypoactive bowel sounds on the second day postoperative. The client was NPO (nothing by mouth) before surgery and NPO until bowel sounds returned, so hypoactive bowel sounds would be expected.
    4. These vital signs are within normal limits and would not warrant immediate intervention by the nurse.

    CLINICAL JUDGMENT GUIDE: The test taker should ask, "Are the assessment data normal for the disease process?" If they are normal for the disease process, then the nurse would not need to intervene; if they are not normal for the disease process, then this warrants intervention.

62. 1. The nurse should assess the client's right foot pain, but not before a potentially life-threatening situation.
    2. Paresthesia (numbness and tingling) indicates a graft occlusion from the surgical procedure, a potentially life-threatening complication; therefore, the nurse should assess this client first.
    3. The most common cause of superficial thrombophlebitis is IV therapy, and tenderness to the touch, redness, and warmth are expected. This is not a medical emergency; therefore, the nurse would not assess this client first.
    4. The client diagnosed with arterial occlusive disease would be expected to have pain in the calf when ambulating, which is called intermittent claudication.

    CLINICAL JUDGMENT GUIDE: When deciding which client to assess first, the test taker should determine whether the signs or symptoms the client is exhibiting are normal or expected for the client's situation. After eliminating the expected option, the test taker should determine which situation is more life threatening.

63. Answer: 22 mL/hr. To determine the rate, the test taker must first determine how many units are in each mL of fluid: 25,000 divided by 500 = 50 units of heparin in each mL of fluid, and 50 divided into 100 = 2, and 2 + 20 = 22 mL/hr.

    CLINICAL JUDGMENT GUIDE: This is an alternate type of question included in the NCLEX-RN®. The nurse must know how to perform math calculations.

64. 1. Compression stockings are used to treat chronic venous insufficiency; therefore, this action does not warrant intervention by the nurse.
    2. The client's legs should be elevated; therefore, this action would not warrant immediate intervention.
    3. The client can ambulate with assistance; therefore, this action does not warrant intervention.
    4. The client should have a podiatrist cut their toenails. The unlicensed assistive personnel (UAP) should not do this because if the UAP accidentally cuts the skin, it could cause a sore that may not heal and then result in amputation of the extremity.

    CLINICAL JUDGMENT GUIDE: The nurse cannot delegate any task the UAP admits to being unable to perform. Delegation means the nurse is responsible for the UAP's actions; therefore, the nurse must intervene if the UAP performs unsafely.

65. 1. The client diagnosed with a venous stasis ulcer should eat a diet high in protein (meat, beans, cheese, tofu), vitamin A (green, leafy vegetables), vitamin C (citrus fruits, tomatoes, cantaloupe), and zinc (meat, seafood). The nurse needs to talk to this client, but it is not a life-threatening condition or a complication; therefore, the client is not assessed first.
    2. The client should wear thromboembolic hose, but this is not a life-threatening condition or a complication; therefore, the client does not have to be assessed first.
    3. The client diagnosed with arterial occlusive disease should not elevate the feet because it further decreases oxygen to the extremity; therefore, this action is not required to be assessed by the nurse.
    4. The nurse should assess this client first because if the client does not stay in the bed, the clot in the calf muscle may dislodge and result in a pulmonary embolus. The client diagnosed with a DVT must be on bedrest.

CLINICAL JUDGMENT GUIDE: The nurse must determine whether the client's behavior is potentially unsafe for the client's disease process. If the client is putting themselves at risk, then the nurse must assess this client first.

66. 1. Oral pain medications relieve mild to moderate pain. A 10 is considered to be severe pain.
    2. Guided imagery will not alleviate severe pain.
    3. If the current pain regimen is not working for this client, the nurse should notify the surgeon for an adjustment in the pain medication.
    4. It has only been 1 hour and 15 minutes since the pain medication was administered. It is too soon for the nurse to administer the morphine.

CLINICAL JUDGMENT GUIDE: This is an alternate type of question included in the NCLEX-RN® test plan. The test taker must be able to read an MAR, know medications, and decide the most appropriate intervention.

67. Answer: 50 drops/min
    150 mL ÷ 60 = 2.5 mL/min to infuse
    2.5 × 20 = 50 drops/min

CLINICAL JUDGMENT GUIDE: This is an alternate type question included in the NCLEX-RN®. The nurse must know how to perform math calculations.

68. 1. The nurse needs to have the surgical operative permit signed by the client, but not until the discrepancy between what the operative permit says and what the client said is resolved.
    2. The nurse can assess the client's neurological status, but not before calling a time-out. Calling a time-out is the priority intervention.
    3. Determining if the client had anything by mouth is an appropriate intervention, but it is not a priority over clarifying which leg will have the surgical procedure.
    4. **The nurse must stop everything and clarify which leg will have the surgical procedure. This is the first and priority intervention the nurse must implement.**

CLINICAL JUDGMENT GUIDE: The NCLEX-RN® test plan includes nursing care administered by the current National Patient Safety Goals. The nurse must be knowledgeable regarding these goals.

69. 1. The abdominal bruit is located at the midabdominal area above the umbilicus.
    2. The midscapula area is not appropriate to auscultate an abdominal aortic aneurysm.
    3. An abdominal aortic aneurysm is diagnosed when the client has an abdominal bruit. An abdominal bruit is a murmur that corresponds to the cardiac cycle. It is heard best with the stethoscope's diaphragm, usually over the abdominal aorta.
    4. The nurse cannot auscultate a bruit on the feet.

CLINICAL JUDGMENT GUIDE: This is an alternate type question included in the NCLEX-RN®. It is a picture, and the nurse must be able to point the cursor at the appropriate area. It is called a hot spot.

70. Correct order is 1, 4, 3, 2, 5.
    1. The bleeding must be stopped. The nurse should don nonsterile gloves and apply pressure to the bleeding site for at least 5 minutes.
    4. When the bleeding has stopped, the client can be assisted back to bed so a thorough assessment of the injuries can be performed.
    3. When possible, the site should be redressed to protect the wound from infectious organisms.
    2. Once the nurse can assess the client and has the client in a safe environment, the nurse should notify the surgeon.
    5. The occurrence should be noted on a report form, and the appropriate hospital personnel should be notified, but this can be done after caring for the client.

CLINICAL JUDGMENT GUIDE: This is an alternate type question included in the NCLEX-RN®. The nurse must be able to prioritize interventions. The nurse can use Maslow's Hierarchy of Needs to prioritize the interventions. Written documentation is the last action taken in an emergency or life-threatening situation.

71. 1. The client has elevated blood pressure, which is not life-threatening; therefore, the client does not need to be seen first.
    2. The client diagnosed with a DVT would be expected to be reporting calf pain; therefore, this client would not be seen first.
    3. The client diagnosed with peripheral vascular disease would be expected to have intermittent claudication; therefore, this client would not be seen first.
    4. The client diagnosed with an AAA reporting low back pain could have a leak, which could be life-threatening; therefore, this client should be assessed first.

CLINICAL JUDGMENT GUIDE: When deciding which client to assess first, the test taker should determine whether the signs or symptoms the client is exhibiting are normal or expected for the client's situation. After eliminating the expected options, the test taker should determine which situation is more life-threatening.

72. 1. Increased hair loss occurs because of decreased oxygen to the lower extremities, but this is not life-threatening; therefore, this information would not warrant immediate intervention.
    2. The client diagnosed with arterial occlusive disease would be expected to have an absent dorsal pedal pulse; therefore, this would not warrant immediate intervention.
    3. Numbness, tingling, and inability to move their toes warrant immediate intervention by the nurse. These findings indicate no arterial blood flow to the extremities.
    4. The client hangs their legs off the bed to help increase arterial oxygen blood flow to the lower extremities. This intervention would not warrant immediate intervention.

CLINICAL JUDGMENT GUIDE: When a question asks for immediate intervention, the test taker must decide whether there is an intervention the nurse can implement immediately or whether the HCP must be notified.

73. 1. The nurse cannot delegate assessment, teaching, evaluation, medications, or an unstable client to the UAP. Checking the pedal pulse is an assessment.
    2. The client, 4 hours postoperative leg surgery, could not ambulate down the hall. The client will be on bedrest for longer.
    3. The nurse cannot delegate assessment, teaching, evaluation, medications, or an unstable client to the UAP.
    4. The leg should be elevated to help decrease edema secondary to surgery; this can be delegated to a UAP.

CLINICAL JUDGMENT GUIDE: An RN cannot delegate assessment, teaching, evaluation, medications, or an unstable client to a UAP. Tasks that cannot be delegated are nursing interventions requiring nursing clinical judgment. The nurse must be aware of delegation rules and regulations.

74. Correct answers are 1, 2, and 5.
    1. A daily acetylsalicylic acid (aspirin) is recommended as an anticoagulant for clients diagnosed with atherosclerosis.
    2. A low-fat, low-cholesterol diet is recommended to help decrease vessel plaque formation.
    3. Sedentary lifestyle is not recommended for clients diagnosed with atherosclerosis.
    4. The client should eat foods high in fiber to help decrease their cholesterol level.
    5. Walking is an excellent isotonic exercise recommended to help lose weight, develop collateral circulation, and decrease stress.

CLINICAL JUDGMENT GUIDE: This is an alternate type of question included in the NCLEX-RN®. The nurse must be able to select all the options that answer the question correctly.

75. 1. The nurse should auscultate the bowel sounds, but the nurse should first assess the client's surgical incision because the client is 2 days postoperative.
    2. The nurse should first assess the surgical dressing to assess for bleeding or any drainage, then continue with the rest of the assessment, including bowel sounds, vital signs, and IV therapy.
    3. The nurse should assess first because it is the first part of the nursing process when the client is not in distress.
    4. The nurse should monitor the IV therapy, but assessment is the first intervention.

CLINICAL JUDGMENT GUIDE: Assessment is the first step of the nursing process, and the test taker should use the nursing process or some other systematic process to assist in determining priorities.

76. 1. The client should not lift more than 5 pounds; doing so might cause the surgical incision to have dehiscence. This statement indicates the client understands the teaching.
    2. The number one factor for developing atherosclerosis and increased blood pressure is smoking cigarettes; therefore, the client must quit. This statement indicates the client understands the teaching.
    3. A truss is a surgical appliance for clients diagnosed with a hernia. It supports the herniated area using a pad and belt arrangement to hold it in the correct position. This client would not be prescribed a truss; therefore, the client needs more discharge teaching.
    4. The client should notify the HCP if there is an elevated temperature because this indicates that the client has a postoperative infection. This statement indicates the client understands the teaching.

CLINICAL JUDGMENT GUIDE: When the question says "needs more teaching," it is an "except" question. Three of the comments indicate the client understands the teaching, and one suggests the client does not understand the teaching.

77. 1. The nurse would expect the client to have pain in the surgical area, and though this client's pain needs to be assessed, it would not be assessed before a client with renal failure.
    2. The 3+ posterior tibial pulse indicates the blood supply to the foot is adequate and would not require the client to be seen first by the nurse.
    3. The client is going into renal failure (should be 30 mL/hr), which is a potentially life-threatening complication of AAA surgery; therefore, this client must be assessed first.
    4. The client report needs to be addressed, but not before a physiological, potentially life-threatening complication.

CLINICAL JUDGMENT GUIDE: When deciding which client to assess first, the test taker should determine whether the signs or symptoms the client is exhibiting are normal or expected for the client's situation. After eliminating the expected options, the test taker should determine which situation is more life-threatening.

78. Answer: 16 mL/hr. To determine the rate, the test taker must first determine how many units are in each mL of fluid: 25,000 ÷ 500 = 50 units of heparin in each mL of fluid, and 50 divided into 100 = 2; 18 − 2 = 16 mL/hr.

CLINICAL JUDGMENT GUIDE: This is an alternate type of question included in the NCLEX-RN®. The nurse must know how to perform math calculations.

79. 1. The client should elevate the lower extremities to help decrease the edema and help the unoxygenated blood go up the inferior vena cava.
    2. Massaging the legs would not warrant intervention for this client; it would be inappropriate for a client diagnosed with DVT. Varicose veins will not dislodge a clot.
    3. The client diagnosed with varicose veins should not be on bedrest. The client should have bathroom privileges and be allowed up ad lib (as desired).
    4. The UAP can calculate the client's I&O, not evaluate the I&O.

CLINICAL JUDGMENT GUIDE: The nurse is responsible for the UAP's actions and must evaluate their actions and intervene if the UAP performs incorrect or unsafe actions.

80. 1. Hospice is for clients an HCP determines have fewer than 6 months to live. This client does not have this diagnosis.
    2. The home health nurse is an appropriate charge nurse referral for this client. The client's home should be assessed to determine whether the client needs assistance.
    3. The physical therapist addresses gait training and transferring.
    4. Cardiac rehabilitation helps clients after myocardial infarctions, cardiac bypass surgery, or congestive heart failure to recover.

CLINICAL JUDGMENT GUIDE: The test taker must be knowlegeable about the roles of the multidisciplinary healthcare team members and make referrals approrpiately.

CASE STUDY ANSWERS

1. **Correct answers are 2, 4, 5, and 8.**
   A pain level of 6 is not normal. Assessment data of a redness and edema to the right leg, and the client's history of long travel is pertinent to the client's clinical findings and should be reported.

   CLINICAL JUDGMENT GUIDE: The test taker should examine each answer option individually. Alternative question formats, such as this extended multiple response or select all that apply question, can have one to all correct answers.

2. **Correct answers are 1, 3, and 4.**
   1. The client is experiencing swelling in the right leg. Swelling can push on the arteries putting the client at risk for decreased tissue perfusion.
   2. No assessment information indicates this client is at risk for malnutrition.
   3. The client is experiencing swelling in the right leg. Swelling can put the client at risk for decreased skin integrity.
   4. The client is experiencing signs of a DVT. This puts the client at risk for a pulmonary embolism and impaired gas exchange.
   5. No assessment information indicates this client is at risk for decreased cardiac output.

3. **Correct answers are 2 and 3.**
   Based on the client's condition, the nurse recognizes that the client is at the highest risk for

   | 1. Stroke |

   and will require

   | 2. Anticoagulants |

4. Correct answers are marked to show interventions that are indicated or not indicated.

Potential Nursing Intervention	Indicated	Not Indicated
Encourage hydration	X	
Elevate right leg	X	
Bed rest	X	
Ice to right leg		X
Bleeding precautions	X	
Restrict visitors		X
Sequential compression device to left leg	X	

   The client has a DVT. Hydration should be encouraged to help decrease the viscosity of the client's blood. The affected leg should be elevated to enhance venous and lymph return. Bed rest is appropriate to ensure the client does not dislodge a portion of the clot while putting weight on the right leg. To decrease the pain and swelling the nurse should apply heat, not ice. The client will be placed on anticoagulation therapy, so bleeding precautions are appropriate. There is no reason to limit visitors. Sequential compression devices applied to the left leg would be an appropriate action to ensure a clot does not form in the left leg.

5. **Correct answers are 3, 4, and 6.**
   1. Scheduling routine blood work is not a priority for this client.
   2. Ensuring nutrition is important but is not a priority for this client.
   3. Ensuring a PT/PTT is drawn every 4 hours is a priority for this client because heparin is titrated based on these laboratory results.
   4. Pain control is always a priority.
   5. A social work referral is not a priority for this client.
   6. Starting the anticoagulant protocol is a priority for this client.

6. Correct answers are marked.

Finding	Improved	Declined	No Change
Temperature			X
Heart rate			X
Respirations			X
Respiratory assessment			X
SpO$_2$			X
Pain level	X		

   The client's pain level is lower than on admission. This indicates that the client's condition has improved. The remaining findings indicate that the client's condition has not changed or deteriorated.

Respiratory Management

The best way to predict your future is to create it.
—Peter Drucker

QUESTIONS

1. The nurse on a medical unit has a client diagnosed with adventitious breath sounds, but the nurse cannot determine the exact nature of the situation. Which multidisciplinary team member should the nurse consult **first**?
    1. The healthcare provider (HCP)
    2. The unit manager
    3. The respiratory therapist
    4. The case manager

2. The registered nurse (RN) staff nurse is working with a licensed practical nurse (LPN) and an unlicensed assistive personnel (UAP) to care for a group of clients. Which nursing tasks can the RN delegate or assign? **Select all that apply.**
    1. The routine oral medications for the clients
    2. The bed baths and oral care
    3. Evaluating the client's progress
    4. Transporting a client to dialysis
    5. Administering scheduled vaccinations

3. Which client should the RN charge nurse assign to the new graduate nurse on the respiratory unit?
    1. The client diagnosed with lung cancer having rust-colored sputum and chest pain of 10 on a scale of 1 to 10
    2. The client diagnosed with atelectasis experiencing shortness of breath and difficulty breathing
    3. The client diagnosed with tuberculosis having a nonproductive cough and orange urine
    4. The client diagnosed with pneumonia, a pulse oximeter reading of 91%, and a capillary refill time greater than 3 seconds

4. Which tasks are appropriate for the RN to assign to the UAP? **Select all that apply.**
    1. Perform mouth care on the client diagnosed with pneumonia.
    2. Apply oxygen via nasal cannula to the client.
    3. Empty the trash cans in the clients' rooms.
    4. Take the empty blood bag back to the laboratory.
    5. Show the client how to ambulate on the walker.

5. Which client should the medical unit nurse assess **first** after receiving the shift report?
   1. The 84-year-old client diagnosed with pneumonia and afebrile but getting restless
   2. The 25-year-old client diagnosed with influenza and febrile with a headache
   3. The 56-year-old client diagnosed with a left-sided hemothorax and tidaling in the water-seal compartment of the chest drainage system
   4. The 38-year-old client diagnosed with a sinus infection having green drainage from the nose

6. The client 2 days postoperative after a left pneumonectomy has an apical pulse rate of 128 bpm and a blood pressure (BP) of 80/50 mm Hg. Which intervention should the nurse implement **first?**
   1. Notify the HCP.
   2. Assess the client's incisional wound.
   3. Prepare to administer dopamine.
   4. Increase the client's IV rate.

7. The client, 1 day postoperative after chest surgery, is having difficulty breathing, has bilateral rales, is confused, and is restless. Which intervention should the nurse implement **first?**
   1. Assess the client's pulse oximeter reading.
   2. Notify the Rapid Response Team.
   3. Place the client in the Trendelenburg position.
   4. Check the client's surgical dressing.

8. The postanesthesia care unit (PACU) client has noisy and irregular respirations with a pulse oximeter reading of 89%. Which intervention should the PACU nurse implement **first?**
   1. Increase the client's oxygen rate via nasal cannula.
   2. Notify the respiratory therapist to draw arterial blood gases (ABGs).
   3. Tilt the client's head back and push forward on the angle of the lower jaw.
   4. Obtain an intubation tray and prepare for emergency intubation.

9. The day surgery admission nurse is obtaining operative permits for clients having surgery. Which client should the nurse **question** signing the consent form?
   1. The 16-year-old married client diagnosed with an ectopic pregnancy
   2. The 39-year-old client diagnosed with paranoid schizophrenia
   3. The 50-year-old client who admitted to being a recovering alcoholic
   4. The 84-year-old client diagnosed with chronic obstructive pulmonary disease (COPD)

10. The intensive care unit (ICU) nurse is caring for a client on a ventilator exhibiting respiratory distress. The ventilator alarms are going off. Which intervention should the nurse implement **first?**
    1. Notify the respiratory therapist.
    2. Ventilate with a manual resuscitation bag.
    3. Check the ventilator to resolve the problem.
    4. Auscultate the client's lung sounds.

11. The charge nurse on the critical care respiratory unit is evaluating several clients' ABG values. Which client would require an **immediate** intervention by the charge nurse?

   1. The client diagnosed with COPD

   Client Name: C.T.   **Account Number:** 2156669

   ### Arterial Blood Gas Report

Parameter	Client Values	Normal Range
pH	7.34	7.35–7.45
Po_2	70	80–95 mm Hg
Pco_2	55	35–45 mm Hg
HCO_3	24	22–26 mmol/L

   2. The client diagnosed with acute respiratory distress syndrome (ARDS)

   Client Name: L.D.   **Account Number:** 2377699

   ### Arterial Blood Gas Report

Parameter	Client Values	Normal Range
pH	7.35	7.35–7.45
Po_2	75	80–95 mm Hg
Pco_2	50	35–45 mm Hg
HCO_3	26	22–26 mmol/L

   3. The client diagnosed with reactive airway disease

   Client Name: P.C.   **Account Number:** 3004863

   ### Arterial Blood Gas Report

Parameter	Client Values	Normal Range
pH	7.48	7.35–7.45
Po_2	80	80–95 mm Hg
Pco_2	30	35–45 mm Hg
HCO_3	23	22–26 mmol/L

   4. The client diagnosed with a pneumothorax

   Client Name: R.W.   **Account Number:** 2758931

   ### Arterial Blood Gas Report

Parameter	Client Values	Normal Range
pH	7.41	7.35–7.45
Po_2	98	80–95 mm Hg
Pco_2	43	35–45 mm Hg
HCO_3	25	22–26 mmol/L

12. The primary nurse in the critical care respiratory unit is very busy. Which nursing task should be the nurse's **priority?**
    1. Assist the HCP with a sterile dressing change for a client with a left pneumonectomy.
    2. Obtain a tracheostomy tray for a client exhibiting air hunger.
    3. Review orders for a client diagnosed with cystic fibrosis transferring from the emergency department (ED).
    4. Assess the upset, angry, and crying client diagnosed with mesothelioma.

13. The nurse is caring for a client diagnosed with flail chest and requiring a chest tube for 3 days. The nurse notes there is no tidaling in the water-seal compartment. Which **initial** action should be taken by the nurse?
    1. Check the tubing for any dependent loops.
    2. Auscultate the client's posterior breath sounds.
    3. Prepare to remove the client's chest tubes.
    4. Notify the HCP that the lungs have re-expanded.

14. The client diagnosed with a right-sided pneumothorax had chest tubes inserted 2 hours ago. There is no fluctuation in the water-seal chamber of the chest drainage system. Which intervention should the nurse implement **first?**
    1. Assess the client's lung sounds.
    2. Check for any kinks in the tubing.
    3. Ask the client to take deep breaths.
    4. Turn the client from side to side.

15. Which client requires the **immediate** attention of the ICU nurse?
    1. The client diagnosed with histoplasmosis and having excessive diaphoresis and neck stiffness
    2. The client diagnosed with ARDS and experiencing difficulty breathing
    3. The client diagnosed with pulmonary sarcoidosis and having a dry cough and mild chest pain
    4. The client diagnosed with asbestosis and experiencing a productive cough and chest tightness

16. The client in the ICU is on a ventilator. Which interventions should the nurse implement? **Select all that apply.**
    1. Ensure there is a manual resuscitation bag at the bedside.
    2. Monitor the client's pulse oximeter reading every shift.
    3. Assess the client's respiratory status every 2 hours.
    4. Check the ventilator settings every 4 hours.
    5. Collaborate with the respiratory therapist.

17. The UAP is bathing the client diagnosed with adult ARDS on a ventilator. The bed is in a high position with the opposite side rail elevated. Which action should the ICU RN take?
    1. Demonstrate the correct technique when giving a bed bath.
    2. Encourage the UAP to put the bed in the lowest position.
    3. Explain that the client on a ventilator should not be bathed.
    4. Give the UAP praise for performing the bath safely.

18. The charge nurse on the respiratory unit tells another nurse, "You are really cute and have a great body. Do you work out?" Which action should be taken by the other nurse if they think they are being sexually harassed?
    1. Document the comment in writing and tell another staff nurse.
    2. Ask the charge nurse to stop making comments such as this.
    3. Notify the clinical manager of the sexual harassment.
    4. Report this to the corporate headquarters office.

19. The client diagnosed with abdominal pain of unknown etiology has a nasogastric (NG) tube draining green bile and reports abdominal pain of 8 on a scale of 1 to 10. The client's ABG values are reported in the accompanying table.

    Arterial Blood Gas Report

Parameter	Client Values	Normal Range
pH	7.48	7.35–7.45
Po_2	98	80–95 mm Hg
Pco_2	36	35–45 mm Hg
HCO_3	28	22–26 mmol/L

    Which intervention should the nurse implement based on the client's ABGs?
    1. Assess the client to rule out complications secondary to the client's pain.
    2. Determine the last time the client was medicated for abdominal pain.
    3. Check the amount of suction on the client's NG tube.
    4. Administer IV sodium bicarbonate to the client.

20. The RN charge nurse in the ICU asks a nurse to float from the medical/surgical unit to the ICU. Which client should the charge nurse assign to the float nurse?
    1. The 3 hours postoperative lung transplant client
    2. The client with a central venous pressure (CVP) of 13 cm H_2O
    3. The client diagnosed with bacterial pneumonia
    4. The client diagnosed with hantavirus pulmonary syndrome

21. The client has ABG values of pH 7.38, Pao_2 77 mm Hg, $Paco_2$ 40 mm Hg, HCO_3 24 mmol/L. Which intervention should the critical care nurse implement?
    1. Administer oxygen 6 L/min via nasal cannula.
    2. Encourage the client to take deep breaths.
    3. Administer IV sodium bicarbonate.
    4. Assess the client's respiratory status.

22. The spouse of a client diagnosed with terminal lung cancer asks the nurse, "How am I going to take care of my spouse when we go home?" Which action by the nurse is **most** appropriate?
    1. Notify the social worker about the spouse's concerns.
    2. Contact the hospital chaplain to talk to the spouse.
    3. Leave a note on the electronic health record (EHR) for the HCP to talk to the spouse.
    4. Reassure the spouse that everything will be all right.

23. The clinic nurse is scheduling a chest x-ray for a female client experiencing clinical manifestations of pneumonia. Which question is **most** important for the nurse to ask the client?
    1. "Have you ever had a chest x-ray before?"
    2. "Can you hold your breath for a minute?"
    3. "Do you smoke or have you ever smoked cigarettes?"
    4. "Is there any chance you may be pregnant?"

24. The clinic nurse is returning phone messages from clients. Which client should the nurse contact **first**?
    1. The elderly client diagnosed with pneumonia reporting dizziness when getting up
    2. The client diagnosed with cystic fibrosis needing a prescription for pancreatic enzymes
    3. The client diagnosed with lung cancer on chemotherapy reporting nausea
    4. The client diagnosed with pertussis reporting coughing spells so severe that they cause vomiting

25. The client diagnosed with active tuberculosis tells the public health nurse, "I am not going to take any more medications. I am tired of them." Which statement is the nurse's **best** response?
    1. "You are tired of taking your tuberculosis medications."
    2. "You must take your tuberculosis medications. It is not an option."
    3. "You must discuss this with your healthcare provider."
    4. "As long as you wear a mask, you do not have to take the meds."

26. The RN staff nurse is working in an outpatient clinic along with an LPN. Which clients should the RN staff nurse assign to the LPN? **Select all that apply.**
    1. The client with a purified protein derivative (PPD) induration on the left arm of 14 mm
    2. The client diagnosed with pneumonia and a pulse oximeter reading of 90%
    3. The client diagnosed with acute bronchitis exhibiting a chronic cough with clear mucus and low fever
    4. The client diagnosed with reactive airway disease wheezing bilaterally
    5. The client diagnosed with influenza reporting generalized muscle aches

27. The UAP informs the RN clinic nurse that the client in Room 4 is "really breathing hard and can't seem to catch their breath." Which instruction should the nurse give to the UAP?
    1. Give 4 mL oxygen to the client.
    2. Sit the client upright in a chair.
    3. Go with the nurse to the client's room.
    4. Take the client's vital signs.

28. The clinic nurse is scheduling a 14-year-old client for a tonsillectomy. Which intervention should the clinic nurse implement?
    1. Obtain informed consent from the client.
    2. Send a throat culture to the laboratory.
    3. Discuss the need to cough and deep breathe.
    4. Request the laboratory to draw a PT and a PTT.

29. The client calls the clinic nurse and asks, "What is the best way to prevent getting influenza?" Which statement is the nurse's **best** response?
    1. "Take prophylactic antibiotics for 10 days after being exposed to influenza."
    2. "Stay away from large crowds and wear a scarf over your mouth during cold weather."
    3. "The best way to prevent getting influenza is to get a yearly flu vaccine."
    4. "You must eat three well-balanced meals daily and exercise daily to prevent influenza."

30. The clinic nurse evaluates vital signs for clients seen in the outpatient clinic. Which client would require **immediate** nursing intervention?
    1. The 10-month-old infant with a pulse rate of 140 bpm
    2. The 3-year-old toddler with a respiratory rate of 28 breaths per minute
    3. The 24-week gestational woman with a BP of 142/96 mm Hg
    4. The 42-year-old client with a temperature of 100.2°F (37.8°C)

31. The nurse is accidentally stuck with a needle used to administer an intradermal injection of a purified protein derivative (PPD). Which intervention should the nurse implement **first**?
    1. Complete the accident/occurrence report.
    2. Wash the area thoroughly with soap and water.
    3. Ask the client whether they have AIDS or hepatitis.
    4. Place an antibiotic ointment and bandage on the site.

32. The clinic nurse is reviewing laboratory results for clients seen in the clinic. Which clients require additional assessment by the nurse? **Select all that apply.**
    1. The client with a hemoglobin of 9 g/dL and a hematocrit of 29%
    2. The client with a white blood cell (WBC) count of 9×10^3/microL
    3. The client with a serum potassium level of 4.8 mEq/L
    4. The client with a serum sodium level of 125 mEq/L
    5. The client with a cholesterol of 175 mg/dL and triglycerides of 125 mg/dL

33. A client diagnosed with bacterial pneumonia is being admitted to the medical unit. The client's spouse answers questions even though the nurse directly asks the client. The nurse suspects this may be because of a cultural issue. Which action should the nurse take?
    1. Ask the spouse to allow the client to answer the questions.
    2. Request the spouse to leave the examination room.
    3. Continue to allow the spouse to answer the client's questions.
    4. Do not ask any further questions until the client starts answering.

34. The clinic nurse encounters a client not responding to verbal stimuli and initiates CPR. What should the nurse do? **Rank in order of performance.**
    1. Open the client's airway.
    2. Check the client's carotid pulse.
    3. Assess the client for unresponsiveness.
    4. Perform compressions at a 30:2 rate.
    5. Give two breaths with a CPR mask/face shield.

35. The RN home health nurse is visiting the client diagnosed with end-stage COPD while the UAP is providing care. Which action by the UAP would **warrant** intervention by the RN home health nurse?
    1. Keeping the bedroom at a warm temperature.
    2. Maintaining the client's oxygen rate at 2 L/min.
    3. Helping the client sit in the orthopneic position.
    4. Allowing the client to sleep in the recliner.

36. Which task is **most** appropriate for the RN home health nurse to delegate to the UAP?
    1. Changing the client's subclavian dressing
    2. Reinserting the client's Foley catheter
    3. Demonstrating ambulation with a walker
    4. Getting the client up in a chair three times a day

37. In the local restaurant, the nurse overhears another hospital staff member talking to a friend about a client. The staff member disclosed that the client was just diagnosed with lung cancer. What is the **most** appropriate action by the nurse?
    1. Do not approach the staff member in the restaurant.
    2. Ask the staff member not to discuss anything about the client.
    3. Contact the staff member's clinical manager and report the behavior.
    4. Tell the client that the staff member was discussing confidential information.

38. A 92-year-old client has a hospital bed in their home and is on strict bedrest. The UAP cares for the client in the morning 5 days a week. Which statement indicates that the UAP **needs additional** education by the RN staff nurse?
    1. "I do not give the client a lot of fluids to prevent bed wetting."
    2. "I perform passive range-of-motion exercises every morning."
    3. "I put the client on their side to relieve pressure on their butt."
    4. "I do not pull the client across the sheets when moving them in bed."

39. The home health client is diagnosed with COPD. The UAP informs the RN home health nurse that the client has trouble breathing when the client lies in a supine position. Which **priority** instruction should the RN provide to the UAP?
    1. To ensure the client's oxygen is in place correctly
    2. To allow the client to sleep in a recliner
    3. To allow a fan to blow on the client when lying in bed
    4. To have the client take slow, deep breaths

40. The spouse of a client diagnosed as terminal is concerned that the client is not eating or drinking. Which is the home health nurse's **best** response?
    1. "I will start an IV if the client continues to refuse to eat or drink."
    2. "You should discuss placing a feeding tube in your partner with the HCP."
    3. "This is normal at the end of life; the dehydration produces euphoria."
    4. "You are right to be concerned. Would you want to talk about your worry?"

41. The client has just been told a medical condition cannot be treated successfully, and the client has a life expectancy of about 6 months. To which resource should the nurse refer the client at this time?
    1. A home health nurse
    2. The client's pastor
    3. A hospice agency
    4. The social worker

42. The hospice client asks the nurse, "What should I do about my house? My son and daughter are fighting over it." Which statement is the nurse's **best** response?
    1. "I think you should tell your children that you will leave the house to a charity."
    2. "I would sell the house and go on an extended vacation to spend the money."
    3. "What do you want to happen to your house? It is your decision."
    4. "Wait and let your children fight over the house after you are gone."

43. The nurse manager is communicating the results of the yearly performance evaluation with a nurse employee. Which information regarding communication styles is important to consider when talking with the employee? **Select all that apply.**
    1. Some nurses see the work from a global perspective, focusing on feelings.
    2. Some nurses see the work environment from a logical, focused perspective.
    3. Some nurses ask many more questions than others and require specific answers.
    4. All nurses communicate similarly in a nursing environment.
    5. All nurses should keep an open mind when communicating with others.

44. The newly hired nurse unit manager has identified that the entire unit has a bad day whenever a specific staff member is unhappy with an assignment. Which action should the unit manager take to correct this problem?
    1. Determine why the staff member is unhappy.
    2. Discuss the staff member's attitude and how it affects the unit.
    3. Place the staff member on a counseling record for the behavior.
    4. Suspend the staff member until the behavior improves.

45. The healthcare facility where the nurse works uses e-mail to notify the staff of in-services and mandatory requirements. Which important information should the nurse manager remember when using e-mail to disseminate information?
    1. Give as much information as possible in each e-mail.
    2. Use e-mail for all communications with the staff.
    3. Use capital letters to get the point across with emphasis.
    4. Make the e-mail notices quick and easy to read.

46. At 1700, the HCP yells at the nursing staff because the early morning lab work is unavailable in the client's EHR. Which is the **most** appropriate response by the charge nurse?
    1. Call the lab and have the lab supervisor talk with the HCP.
    2. Discuss the HCP's concerns with the nursing supervisor.
    3. Form a lab and nursing personnel committee to fix the problem.
    4. Tell the HCP to stop yelling and calm down.

47. The nurse is caring for a client with a chest tube. What actions should the nurse implement? **Rank in order of performance.**
    1. Assess the client's lung sounds.
    2. Note the amount of suction being used.
    3. Check the chest tube dressing for drainage.
    4. Make sure that the chest tube is securely taped.
    5. Place a bottle of sterile saline at the bedside.

48. The nurse is assessing clients in a respiratory unit. Which client should be the nurse's **first** priority?
    1. The client diagnosed with bronchiectasis and clubbing of the fingernails
    2. The client diagnosed with byssinosis reporting chest tightness
    3. The client diagnosed with cystic fibrosis with a pulse oximeter reading of 91%
    4. The client diagnosed with pneumoconiosis experiencing shortness of breath

49. The nurse assists with inserting a chest tube in a client diagnosed with a spontaneous pneumothorax. Which data indicate that the treatment has been **effective?**
    1. The chest x-ray indicates consolidation.
    2. The client has bilateral breath sounds.
    3. The suction chamber has vigorous bubbling.
    4. The client has crepitus around the insertion site.

50. The HCP ordered bumetanide to be administered STAT to a client diagnosed with pulmonary edema. After 4 hours, which assessment data indicate the client may be experiencing a **complication** of the medication?
    1. The client develops jugular vein distention.
    2. The client has bilateral rales and rhonchi.
    3. The client reports painful leg cramps.
    4. The client's output is greater than their intake.

51. The client involved in a motor vehicle accident is being prepped for surgery when the client asks the ED nurse, "What happened to my child?" The nurse knows the child is dead. Which statement is an example of the ethical principle of nonmaleficence?
    1. "I will find out for you and let you know after surgery."
    2. "I am sorry, but your child died at the scene of the accident."
    3. "You should concentrate on your surgery right now."
    4. "You are concerned about your child. Do you want to talk?"

52. The new graduate nurse has accepted a position at a facility that The Joint Commission accredits. Which statement describes the purpose of this organization?
    1. The Commission reviews facilities for compliance with standards of care.
    2. Accreditation by The Commission guarantees reimbursement for care provided.
    3. Accreditation by The Commission reduces liability in a legal action against the facility.
    4. The Commission eliminates the need for Medicare to survey a hospital.

53. The client in a critical care unit has died. What action should the nurse implement **first**?
    1. Stay with the significant other.
    2. Gather the client's belongings.
    3. Perform postmortem care.
    4. Ask about organ donation.

54. The nurse caring for client B.C. is preparing to administer medications.

    Client Name: B.C. **Account Number:** 55678-78 **Allergies:** Sulfa
    Diagnosis: Deep Vein Thrombosis **Height:** 70 in (177.8 cm) **Weight:** 150 lb (68.0 kg)

    ### Laboratory Report

Laboratory Test	Client Values	Reference Values
PT	19.3	10–13 seconds
INR	1.7	2.0–3.0 (therapeutic)
PTT	53	34 seconds

    Based on the laboratory data given in the table, which intervention should the nurse implement?
    1. Administer warfarin IV push (IVP).
    2. Continue the heparin drip.
    3. Hold the next dose of warfarin.
    4. Administer the daily acetylsalicylic acid.

55. In the ICU, the critical care nurse assesses a client diagnosed with an asthma attack and a respiration rate of 10 breaths/min with oxygen saturation of 88%. Which intervention should the nurse implement **first**?
    1. Call a Rapid Response Team.
    2. Increase the oxygen to 10 L/min.
    3. Check the client's ABG results.
    4. Administer the fast-acting inhaler.

56. The client in the ICU has been on a ventilator for 2 weeks with an endotracheal (ET) tube in place. Which intervention should the nurse prepare the client for **next**?
    1. Transfer to a long-term care facility
    2. Daily ABGs
    3. Removal of life support
    4. Placement of a tracheostomy

57. The nurse is teaching the parents of a child diagnosed with cystic fibrosis. Which information is the **priority** to teach the parents?
    1. Explain that the child's skin tastes salty.
    2. Observe the consistency of the stools daily.
    3. Give pancreatic enzymes with every meal.
    4. Increase the intake of salt in the child's diet.

58. The UAP enters the elderly client's room to bathe them, but the client is watching a favorite soap opera and shakes their head "no." Which instructions should the RN staff nurse give to the UAP?
    1. Tell the UAP to complete the bath at this time.
    2. Have the UAP skip the client's bath for the day.
    3. Instruct the UAP to give the bath after the program.
    4. Document the attempt to give the bath as refused.

59. The nurse has been made a quality improvement committee chairperson. Which statement is an example of an **effective** group process?
    1. The nurse involves all committee members in the discussion.
    2. The nurse makes sure all group members agree with the decisions.
    3. The nurse asks two committee members to do the work.
    4. The nurse does not allow deviation from the agenda to occur.

60. The ventilator alarm sounds while the nurse is caring for a client on a ventilator. What is the **first** action taken by the nurse?
    1. Determine the ventilator alarm sounding.
    2. Notify the respiratory therapist.
    3. Assess the client's respiratory status.
    4. Ventilate the client using a manual resuscitation bag.

61. The client diagnosed with ARDS is having increased difficulty breathing. The ABG indicates an arterial oxygen level of 54% on O_2 at 10 L/min. Which intervention should the ICU nurse implement **first?**
    1. Prepare the client for intubation.
    2. Bag the client with a bag/mask device.
    3. Call a Code Blue and initiate CPR.
    4. Start an IV with an 18-gauge catheter.

62. The nurse is reviewing a client's ABG results.

    Client Name: A.W.   **Account Number:** 3785690

    Arterial Blood Gas Report

Parameter	Client Values	Normal Range
pH	7.34	7.35–7.45
Po_2	87	80–95 mm Hg
Pco_2	50	35–45 mm Hg
HCO_3	24	22–26 mmol/L

    Which intervention should the nurse implement **first?**
    1. Have the client turn, cough, and deep breathe.
    2. Place the client on oxygen via nasal cannula.
    3. Check the client's pulse oximeter reading.
    4. Notify the HCP of the ABG results.

63. The client is admitted to the ED with an apical pulse of 134 bpm, respiration is 28 breaths/min, BP is 92/56 mm Hg, and the skin is pale and clammy. What action should the nurse perform **first?**
    1. Type and crossmatch the client for packed red blood cells.
    2. Start two IV lines with large-bore catheters.
    3. Obtain the client's history and perform the physical examination.
    4. Check the client's allergies to medications.

64. The charge nurse of the respiratory care unit is making assignments. Which clients should be assigned to the ICU nurse working on the respiratory care unit for the day? **Select all that apply.**
    1. The client recovering from four coronary artery bypass grafts 3 days ago
    2. The client with anterior and posterior chest tubes after a motor vehicle accident
    3. The client being moved to the ICU when a bed is available
    4. The client with a do not resuscitate order requesting to see a chaplain
    5. The client on multiple IV drip medications that need to be titrated

65. The ED nurse is preparing to assist the surgeon in inserting a chest tube in a client diagnosed with a right hemothorax. Which position is appropriate for the procedure?
    1. Have the client sit upright and bend over the bed table.
    2. Place the client in the left lateral recumbent position.
    3. Have the client sit on the side of the bed with their back arched like a Halloween cat.
    4. Place the client lying on their back with the head of the bed up 45 degrees.

66. The nurse is admitting a client diagnosed with pneumonia. Which HCP order should be implemented **first**?
    1. 1,000 mL normal saline (NS) at 125 mL/hr
    2. Obtain sputum for Gram stain and culture
    3. Ceftriaxone 1,000 mg IV piggyback (IVPB) every 12 hours
    4. Ultrasonic nebulization treatment every 6 hours

67. The nurse is preparing to make rounds after receiving shift report. Which client should the nurse assess **first**?
    1. The client diagnosed with end-stage COPD reporting shortness of breath after ambulating to the bathroom
    2. The client diagnosed with a deep vein thrombosis requesting an antianxiety medication
    3. The client diagnosed with cystic fibrosis and has a sputum specimen to be taken to the laboratory
    4. The client diagnosed with an empyema and a temperature of 100.8°F (38.2°C), pulse of 118 bpm, respiration of 26 breaths/min, and BP of 148/64 mm Hg

68. The respiratory unit nurse is calculating the shift intake and output for a client with a right-sided chest tube. The client has received 1,500 mL of D_5W, IVPB of 100 mL of 0.9% NS, 12 oz of water, 6 oz of milk, and 4 oz of chicken broth. The client has had a urinary output of 800 mL and chest drainage of 125 mL. What is the total intake and output for this client? _____

69. Which client should the RN charge nurse on the respiratory unit assign to the graduate nurse having just completed orientation?
    1. The client diagnosed with bronchiolitis experiencing a wheezy cough and rapid breathing
    2. The client diagnosed with pneumonia and dull percussion and vocal fremitus
    3. The client diagnosed with a flail chest and paradoxical movement of the chest wall
    4. The client diagnosed with reactive airway disease experiencing bilateral wheezing

70. The charge nurse is making shift assignments. Which client should be assigned to the **most** experienced RN?
    1. The elderly client diagnosed with pneumonia having bilateral crackles and a pulse oximeter reading of 96%
    2. The client with decreasing pulse oximeter readings after receiving high levels of oxygen via nasal cannula
    3. The client recovering from a Caldwell-Luc procedure 1 day ago with purulent drainage on the drip pad
    4. The teenage client after a tonsillectomy this morning reporting throat pain rated 8 on a pain scale of 1 to 10

71. The nursing home client diagnosed with community-acquired pneumonia is being admitted to the unit. Which HCP order should be implemented **first**?
    1. Administer ceftriaxone 50 mg IVPB every 24 hours.
    2. Apply oxygen 2 L via nasal cannula.
    3. Obtain a sputum specimen for culture and sensitivity.
    4. Place the elderly client in respiratory isolation.

72. The 50-year-old client diagnosed with an exacerbation of COPD and tobacco abuse is in respiratory distress. Which intervention should the nurse implement **first?**
    1. Place the client in the orthopneic position.
    2. Administer 6 L oxygen via nasal cannula.
    3. Assess the client's pulse oximeter reading.
    4. Notify the respiratory therapist.

73. Which client should the RN charge nurse assign to the LPN?
    1. The obese client recovering from a laryngectomy 2 days ago with crepitus
    2. The client diagnosed with respiratory difficulty acting confused and climbing out of bed
    3. The client with a productive cough newly diagnosed with active tuberculosis needing medication teaching
    4. The young adult client diagnosed with asthma with a pulse oximeter reading of 90%

74. The RN charge nurse and the UAP are caring for the following clients. Which information provided by the UAP requires **immediate** intervention by the charge nurse?
    1. The client with a productive cough diagnosed with active tuberculosis, in respiratory isolation, and with orange urine in the urinary catheter
    2. The middle-age client recovering from a right upper lobectomy, on a patient-controlled analgesia (PCA) pump, with level 4 pain on a scale of 1 to 10
    3. The client recovering from a fall diagnosed with a left-sided pneumothorax and 200 mL of blood in the collection chamber of the chest drainage system
    4. The 65-year-old client diagnosed with bacterial pneumonia having an elevated temperature and chills

75. One of the RN charge nurse's staff nurses is preparing to administer a.m. medications to clients. Which medication should the nurse **question** administering to the client?
    1. Sucralfate for the diabetic client before breakfast
    2. Digoxin to the elderly client with a digoxin level of 1.9 mg/dL
    3. Hanging the heparin bag for a client with a PT/PTT of 12.9/78 seconds
    4. The aminoglycoside antibiotic to the client with an elevated trough level

76. The edematous client is getting out of bed, becomes very anxious, and has a feeling of impending doom. The nurse reports these findings to the RN charge nurse. Which intervention should the charge nurse tell the nurse to implement **first** after placing the client in the high Fowler's position?
    1. Administer oxygen via nasal cannula.
    2. Prepare the client for a computed tomographic angiography.
    3. Notify the client's healthcare provider.
    4. Auscultate the client's lung sounds.

77. The postoperative client with a right-sided chest tube is reporting pain rated 6 on a pain scale of 1 to 10. Which intervention should the nurse implement **first?**
    1. Document the client's pain report in the EHR nurse's notes.
    2. Instruct the client to take slow, deep breaths and exhale slowly.
    3. Assess the client's respiratory status and chest tube insertion site.
    4. Check the client's MAR to determine when the last pain medication was administered.

78. The RN charge nurse is discussing, with a graduate nurse, the care of a client with a right-sided chest tube secondary to a pneumothorax. Which interventions should the charge nurse discuss with the graduate nurse? **Select all that apply.**
    1. Place the client in the high Fowler's position.
    2. Assess the chest tube drainage system every shift.
    3. Maintain strict bedrest for the client.
    4. Ensure the tubing has no dependent loops.
    5. Mark the collection chamber for drainage every shift.

79. The RN charge nurse is making client assignments. Which client should the charge nurse assign to the LPN?
    1. The morbidly obese client suspected of having acute respiratory distress syndrome (ARDS)
    2. The recovering motor vehicle accident client diagnosed with a hemothorax needing 2 units of blood
    3. The postoperative client with chest tubes, jugular vein distention, and BP 96/60 mm Hg
    4. The client with dyspnea scheduled for a bronchoscopy to rule out lung cancer

80. The nurse assesses tachypnea, intercostal and suprasternal retractions, and a change in mental status in the client. Which **priority** interventions should the nurse perform? **Select all that apply.**
    1. Prepare to place the client on a ventilator.
    2. Administer oxygen using a high-flow system.
    3. Place the client in the supine position.
    4. Address nutritional needs.
    5. Continuously monitor oxygen saturation.

81. The nurse assists the provider with the endotracheal intubation of a client. Which **priority** interventions should be performed to determine the correct ET tube placement? **Select all that apply.**
    1. Obtain ABG readings.
    2. Auscultate the lungs bilaterally.
    3. Perform a chest x-ray.
    4. Check capillary refill.
    5. Suction secretions from the ET tube.

82. The nurse is preparing to perform endotracheal suctioning on a client. Which interventions should the nurse implement? **Rank in order of performance.**
    1. Provide mouth care to the client.
    2. Apply suction while withdrawing the catheter.
    3. Hyperoxygenate the client as needed.
    4. Determine the measurement of length to suction.
    5. Lubricate the catheter tip with saline solution.

83. Which alternate methods should the nurse use to communicate with the client intubated with an ET tube and on a ventilator? **Select all that apply.**
    1. Usage of an electrolarynx
    2. Communication boards
    3. Hand gestures
    4. Eye blinks for yes or no questions
    5. Augmented communication device

84. Which interventions should the nurse implement when caring for a client on the ventilator? **Select all that apply.**
    1. Collaborate with the respiratory therapist.
    2. Continuously monitor the pulse oximeter reading.
    3. Ensure a manual resuscitation bag is at the bedside.
    4. Assess the ventilator settings throughout the shift.
    5. Confirm ventilator alarms are set to silence.

RESPIRATORY CASE STUDY

(0800) Security noticed an older adult wandering around in the hospital lobby. The client is lethargic and disoriented, her appearance disheveled, and she is unable to describe the reason she is in the lobby. She cannot recall her name. The client was assisted to a wheelchair and transported to the ED.

(0825) Triage nurse receives situational data and moves the client to an ED bed. The client is very unsteady and unable to answer questions stating, "I don't know why or how I got here." Initial vital signs are populated in the following chart. Skin is grayish with cyanosis and pale, dry mucous membranes. Hair is tangled and dirty/greasy, and clothes smell of urine and alcohol. Lungs are bilaterally diminished with crackles in bases posteriorly, nonproductive coarse cough. Heart rate regular, S_1 and S_2. Peripheral pulses present 2+, capillary refill >5 seconds in all four extremities. Bilateral hand grasps and feet push/pull are equal but weak. Abdomen is soft with hypoactive bowel sounds ×4. The client denies pain. Side rails up ×4. The nurse finds the client's wallet in her sweater pocket and asks the unit clerk to look her up in the EHR.

Vital Signs	Client Values
Blood pressure	80/53 mm Hg
Heart rate	114 bpm
Respirations	32 breaths/min
Temperature	103.8°F (39.9°C)
Spo_2	88% on room air

1. **Recognize cues. What matters most?** The nurse prepares to call the ED physician. Which **priority** client data should be reported to the HCP? **Select all that apply.**
    1. Respirations
    2. Blood pressure
    3. Level of consciousness
    4. Lung sounds
    5. Location client found
    6. Heart rate
    7. Temperature
    8. Spo_2
    9. Cyanosis
    10. Homelessness

2. **Analyze cues. What could it mean?** For each client finding, indicate whether it is consistent with the disease process of COVID (+), urinary tract infection (UTI), or cerebrovascular accident (CVA). Each finding may support more than one condition.

Finding	COVID (+)	UTI	CVA
Respirations			
Blood pressure			
Level of consciousness			
Lung sounds			
Location client found			
Heart rate			
Temperature			
Spo_2			
Cyanosis			
Physical appearance			

(0900) The physician visits the client and orders a complete blood count (CBC), basic metabolic panel (BMP), polymerase chain reaction (PCR), and chest x-ray STAT; oxygen to maintain oximetry readings of 93% or higher; and to start an IV of 0.9% NaCl at 100 mL/hr. The client's identity has been confirmed in the EHR; however, the last list of medications and medical history are dated 6 years ago. The nurse asks the care coordinator to contact the last known contact.

(0915) Successful IV insertion of #20 gauge catheter in the right forearm; saline infusing as ordered. Oxygen via nasal cannula started at 2 L. The client tolerated well.

(0940) Diagnostic and laboratory results received.

Chest x-ray report: Bilateral multifocal airspace opacities and consolidations throughout lower half of lung fields.

Laboratory Test	Client Values	Reference Values
Hemoglobin (Hgb)	12 g/dL	Male: 14–17.3 g/dL
		Female: 11.7–15.5 g/dL
Hematocrit (Hct)	35%	Male: 42%–52%
		Female: 36%–48%
White blood cell (WBC) count	14.6	4.5 to 11.1 × 10^3/microL
Platelets	160	140 to 400 × 10^3/microL
Creatinine	0.8 mg/dL	Male: 0.61 to 1.21 mg/dL
		Female: 0.51 to 1.11 mg/dL
Glucose	217 mg/dL	Fasting: Less than 100 mg/dL
		Random: Less than 200 mg/dL
Potassium	3.7 mEq/L	0.5 to 5.3 mEq/L or mmol/L
Sodium	132 mEq/L	135 to 145 mEq/L or mmol/L
Blood urea nitrogen	23 mg/dL	8 to 21 mg/dL
		Adult over 90 years: 10 to 31 mg/dL
PCR	SARS-CoV-2 positive	Negative

EHR history: Past medical history of osteoporosis, breast cancer with bilateral mastectomy 7 years ago. Allergies: Penicillin, pet dander, mold, and dust. ED bed weight 92.4 lb (42 kg).
Home medications: None listed.

(1010) Repeat vital signs obtained as follows and oxygen increased to 3 L via nasal cannula.

Vital Signs	Client Values
Blood pressure	90/68 mm Hg
Heart rate	104 bpm
Respirations	28 breaths/min
Temperature	103.6°F (39.8°C)
SpO_2	90% on 2 L oxygen

(1120) The physician speaks to the client's daughter via telephone; the daughter agrees with admission. States that the client has been living alone in a subsidized apartment for seniors and that she and her siblings live out of state. Provider orders are entered in the chart:

PROVIDER ORDERS:

Admit to medical unit—Diagnosis: COVID (+)
COVID precautions
Albuterol sulfate 0.83% STAT then every 6 hours via aerosol
Titrate oxygen to maintain SpO_2 >93%
Hydrocortisone sodium succinate 100 mg IVP every 12 hours
0.9% NaCl via IV @ 100 mL/hr
Acetaminophen 1,000 mg PO PRN temperature >100.5°F (38.2°C)
Urinalysis
Sputum culture
Regular diet as tolerated
Bedrest—may use bedside commode with assist

(1200) The nurse on the medical unit receives the client and begins the admission process.

3. **Prioritize hypotheses. Where do I start?** Complete the sentence by choosing from the drop-down list of options. Based on the client's condition at this time, the nurse recognizes that the client is at the highest risk for _____

   Select... ▼
   1. Injury (falls)
   2. Impaired gas exchange
   3. Bleeding

   and will require _____

   Select... ▼
   1. Oxygen therapy
   2. Anticoagulants
   3. Four-extremity restraints

4. **Generate solutions. What can I do?** For each intervention, specify whether the intervention is **indicated** or **not indicated** for the client's care.

Potential Nursing Intervention	Indicated	Not Indicated
Ensure the client's code status is known		
Instruct staff on COVID personal protective equipment.		
Apply wrist and ankle restraints		
Increase oxygen to 4 L via nasal cannula		
Start remdesivir IVPB		
Reorient the client as needed		
Place the client in a high Fowler's position.		
Request UAP to ambulate client in hall		
Notify the social worker that the client is homeless		

5. **Take action. What will I do?** Which admission orders should the nurse consider a priority action? Select all that apply.
    1. Initiate droplet precautions
    2. Albuterol sulfate 0.83% STAT then every 6 hours via aerosol
    3. Titrate oxygen to maintain Spo$_2$ >93%
    4. Hydrocortisone sodium succinate 100 mg IVP every 12 hours
    5. 0.9% NaCl via IV @ 100 mL/hr
    6. Remdesevir 100 mg IV STAT ×1 then daily
    7. Acetaminophen 1,000 mg PO PRN temperature >100.5°F (38.2°C)
    8. Urinalysis
    9. Sputum culture
    10. Regular diet as tolerated
    11. Bedrest—may use bedside commode with assist

(1445) The nurse prepares to give the oncoming shift report, including the following assessment data and vital signs. The client is awake and remains disoriented but pleasantly confused. Color is pale, skin warm and dry. Lungs with crackles bilaterally posterior lower to midback. Abdomen soft with bowel sounds ×4. Hand grasps and pedal pushes equal but weak. Pedal pulses (+2) bilaterally. IV right forearm #20 gauge with normal saline @ 100 mL/hr without redness, edema, or coolness. Side rails up. The daughter called and will take the next available flight in and will be in to see the client tonight or tomorrow a.m.

Vital Signs	Client Values
Blood pressure	94/72 mm Hg
Heart rate	108 bpm
Respirations	28 breaths/min
Temperature	100.5°F (38.1°C)
Spo$_2$	93% (4 L)

6. **Evaluate outcomes. Did it help?** For each assessment finding, indicate whether the client's condition has improved, declined, or shows no change.

Finding	Improved	Declined	No Change
Temperature			
Heart rate			
Respirations			
Blood pressure			
Spo$_2$			
Level of consciousness			

ANSWERS AND RATIONALES

The correct answer number and rationale are in **bold-face purple type.** Rationales for why other answer options are incorrect are also given.

1. 1. The client's HCP should be consulted if the nurse determines a need, but at this time, the nurse should discuss the client with the respiratory therapist.
   2. The unit manager may or may not be capable of helping the nurse assess a client diagnosed with adventitious breath sounds; therefore, this is not the first person the nurse should consult.
   3. **Respiratory therapists assess and treat clients diagnosed with lung problems multiple times every day. Therefore, this is the best person to consult when the nurse needs help identifying a respiratory problem.**
   4. The case manager can usually maneuver through the maze of healthcare referrals, but is not necessarily an expert in lung sounds.

   CLINICAL JUDGMENT GUIDE: The test taker must be knowledgeable about the roles of all members of the multidisciplinary healthcare team as well as HIPAA (Health Insurance Portability and Accountability Act) rules and regulations. These will be tested on the NCLEX-RN® examination.

2. **Correct answers are 1, 2, 4, and 5.**
   1. **The LPN may be assigned to administer routine oral medications to the clients.**
   2. **The UAP can perform bed baths and oral care.**
   3. The nurse cannot delegate or assign tasks that require nursing judgment, such as evaluating a client's progress.
   4. **The UAP can transport a client to dialysis.**
   5. **The LPN may administer scheduled vaccinations.**

   CLINICAL JUDGMENT GUIDE: This is an alternate type of question included in the NCLEX-RN®. The nurse cannot delegate assessment, evaluation, teaching, or administration of medications to any client or the care of an unstable client to a UAP. Also, the nurse cannot assign assessment, evaluation, teaching, or tasks that require nursing judgment to an LPN.

3. 1. The client diagnosed with lung cancer is expected to have rust-colored sputum; however, reporting pain rated as a 10 warrants a more experienced nurse to assess the cause of the pain and medicate as needed.
   2. The client diagnosed with atelectasis (collapsed lung) and having difficulty breathing needs a more experienced nurse to assess the client. This client is not stable.
   3. **The orange urine is secondary to rifampin, an antitubercular medication, and a nonproductive cough is expected. Therefore, this client is stable and should be assigned to a new graduate nurse.**
   4. The client is exhibiting respiratory compromise and is not stable. The pulse oximeter reading should be greater than 93% and the capillary refill time should be less than 3 seconds.

   CLINICAL JUDGMENT GUIDE: The charge nurse should assign the most stable client to the new graduate nurse. The test taker must determine which client is exhibiting expected clinical manifestations, and this client should be assigned to the new graduate nurse. Clients exhibiting signs or symptoms not expected for the client should be assigned to a more experienced nurse.

4. **Correct answers are 1 and 4.**
   1. **The UAP can perform mouth care on a stable client.**
   2. Oxygen is a medication, and the nurse cannot delegate medication administration to the UAP.
   3. The housekeeping staff members empty trash cans; the UAP does not. Remember not to assign tasks that another hospital department should do.
   4. **The UAP can take the empty blood bag to the laboratory.**
   5. The nurse cannot delegate teaching to the UAP.

   CLINICAL JUDGMENT GUIDE: This is an alternate type of question included in the NCLEX-RN®. The nurse should not delegate assessment, teaching, evaluation, medications, or an unstable client to the UAP.

5. 1. **Elderly clients diagnosed with pneumonia may not present with the "normal" symptoms, such as fever. The client's increased restlessness may indicate decreased oxygen to the brain. This client should be seen first.**
   2. The client diagnosed with influenza would be expected to have an elevated temperature and a headache; therefore, this client would not need to be assessed first.
   3. Tidaling in the water-seal compartment is expected; therefore, the nurse would not need to assess this client first.
   4. Sinus drainage is expected in a client diagnosed with a sinus infection.

CLINICAL JUDGMENT GUIDE: The test taker must determine which sign or symptom is not expected for the disease process. If the sign or symptom is unexpected, the nurse should assess the client first. This type of question determines whether the nurse is knowledgeable about clinical manifestations of various disease processes.

6. 1. The HCP should be notified, but this is not the first intervention. The HCP will require other information, such as how the incision looks and whether any bleeding can be seen, before making any decisions. The nurse, therefore, should first provide emergency care to the client—in this case, support the client's circulatory system by increasing the IV rate—and then assess the client before reporting to the HCP.
   2. The incisional wound should be assessed, but the priority is maintaining circulatory status because the client's vital signs indicate shock.
   3. The client may require medication, such as dopamine, a vasopressor, to increase the blood pressure, but the client's circulatory system needs immediate support, which increasing the IV rate will provide. That, then, is the priority.
   4. Increasing the IV rate will immediately give the client circulatory volume. Therefore, this is the first intervention.

CLINICAL JUDGMENT GUIDE: Remember: If the client is in distress, do not assess. Situations such as those in this question require the nurse to intervene to prevent the client's status from deteriorating. The test taker must examine the other three options before selecting "notify the HCP" as the correct answer. If any options will relieve the client's distress, prevent a life-threatening situation, or provide information the HCP will need to make an informed decision, then the test taker should eliminate the "notify the HCP" option.

7. 1. The client is in distress; therefore, the nurse should do something to help the client.
   2. The Joint Commission mandated the Rapid Response Team (RRT), which is a team of healthcare professionals that responds to breathing clients the nurse thinks are in an emergency. A code is called if the client is not breathing.
   3. The Trendelenburg position is used for a client in hypovolemic shock, so this would not be appropriate for a client in respiratory distress.
   4. The question's stem provides enough information to indicate the client is in distress, and assessing the surgical dressing will not help the client.

CLINICAL JUDGMENT GUIDE: The nurse must determine whether the client is in distress; remember: if in distress do not assess. The nurse must intervene to help the client. Do not select equipment over the client's body. The NCLEX-RN® test plan includes nursing care that is ruled by the current National Patient Safety Goals. The nurse must be knowledgeable regarding these goals.

8. 1. Increasing the oxygen rate will not help open the client's airway, which is the first intervention. Oxygen can be increased after the airway is patent.
   2. The respiratory therapist could be notified and ABGs drawn if positioning does not increase the pulse oximeter reading, but this is not the first intervention.
   3. The client is exhibiting clinical manifestations of hypopharyngeal obstruction, and this maneuver pulls the tongue forward and opens the air passage.
   4. The client may need to be intubated if positioning does not open the airway, but this is not the first intervention.

CLINICAL JUDGMENT GUIDE: Physiological problems have the highest priority when deciding on a course of action. If the client is in distress, then the nurse must intervene with a nursing action that attempts to alleviate or control the problem. The test taker should not choose a diagnostic test if there is an option that directly treats the client.

9. 1. An emancipated minor under 18 but married or independently earning their own living would not warrant the nurse's questioning whether they should sign the permit. "Married" indicates an independently functioning individual.
   2. An incompetent client cannot sign the consent form. An incompetent client is an individual who is not autonomous and cannot give or withhold consent, i.e., individuals cognitively impaired, mentally ill, neurologically incapacitated, or under the influence of mind-altering drugs. The client may be able to sign the permit, but the nurse should question the client's ability to sign the permit because paranoid schizophrenia is a mental illness.

3. A recovering alcoholic is not considered incapacitated. If the client is currently under the influence of alcohol, then the permit could not legally be signed by the client.
4. The elderly client is considered competent until deemed incompetent in a court of law or meets the criteria to be considered incompetent.

CLINICAL JUDGMENT GUIDE: The NCLEX-RN® test plan includes nursing care ruled by legal requirements. The nurse must be knowledgeable regarding these issues.

10. 1. The nurse must first address the client's acute respiratory distress and then notify other multidisciplinary team members.
    2. If the ventilator system malfunctions, the nurse must ventilate the client with a manual resuscitation (Ambu) bag until the problem is resolved. The nurse should determine whether they can remedy the situation by assessing the ventilator before beginning manual ventilations.
    3. **The client is having respiratory distress, and the ventilator is sounding an alarm; therefore, the nurse should first assess the ventilator to determine the cause of the problem and correct it because the client is dependent on the ventilator for breathing. This is one of the few situations wherein the nurse would assess the equipment before assessing the client.**
    4. In most situations, assessing the client is the first intervention. Still, because the client is dependent on the ventilator for breathing, the nurse should first assess the ventilator to determine the cause of the alarms.

CLINICAL JUDGMENT GUIDE: The nurse must determine whether the client is in distress; remember: if in distress, do not assess. The nurse must intervene to help the client. In most situations, the nurse should not select equipment over the client's body, but because the ventilator is breathing for the client, the ventilator should be assessed first.

11. 1. Although these ABG values are abnormal, indicating respiratory acidosis, they are expected in a client diagnosed with COPD; therefore, the nurse would not need to see this client first.
    2. The client diagnosed with ARDS would be expected to have a low arterial oxygen level; therefore, the nurse would not assess this client first.
    3. **The ABG report shows respiratory alkalosis; therefore, the nurse should assess this client first to determine whether the client is hyperventilating, in pain, or has an elevated temperature.**
    4. These ABG values are normal; therefore, the nurse would not need to assess this client first.

CLINICAL JUDGMENT GUIDE: The nurse must be knowledgeable about normal laboratory values and determine whether the laboratory value is expected for the client's disease process or the medications the client is taking.

12. 1. Changing the dressing is not a priority over a client in respiratory distress.
    2. **The client exhibiting air hunger indicates respiratory distress; therefore, a tracheostomy tray should be obtained first.**
    3. Reviewing orders is essential, but not more important than a client in respiratory distress.
    4. The angry and upset client needs to be assessed but is not a priority over the client in respiratory distress.

CLINICAL JUDGMENT GUIDE: The nurse should use some tool to guide the decision-making process. In this situation, Maslow's Hierarchy of Needs is applied. Physiological needs have priority over psychosocial ones.

13. 1. After 3 days, the nurse should suspect that the lung has re-expanded. The nurse should not expect dependent loops to have caused this situation.
    2. After 3 days, the nurse should assess the lung sounds to determine whether the lungs have re-expanded. This would be the nurse's first intervention.
    3. The chest tubes will be removed if it is determined the lungs have re-expanded, but it is not the first intervention.
    4. The nurse should notify the HCP if it is determined the lungs have re-expanded; a chest x-ray can be taken before removing the chest tubes.

CLINICAL JUDGMENT GUIDE: The nurse must determine whether the client is in distress; remember: if in distress, do not assess. If the client is not in distress, the nurse should assess, the first part of the nursing process.

14. 1. The nurse should assess the client's breath sounds but not before determining why there is no tidaling in the water-seal chamber.

2. The nurse should first determine why there is no tidaling in the water-seal chamber. Because the client just had the chest tubes inserted, it is probably a kink or a dependent loop, or the client is lying on the tubing. The nurse should first check for this before taking any other action.
3. The nurse should encourage the client to take deep breaths and cough, which may push a clot through the tubing, but should not do so before checking for a kink.
4. Turning the client side to side will not help determine why there is no tidaling in the water-seal compartment of the chest drainage system.

CLINICAL JUDGMENT GUIDE: When the test question asks the test taker to determine which intervention should be implemented first, all the options are possible. This is one of the few times the nurse should check equipment before assessing the client.

15. 1. The client diagnosed with histoplasmosis would be expected to have excessive sweating and neck stiffness; therefore, this client would not be seen first. Histoplasmosis is an infection in the lungs caused by inhaling the spores of a fungus.
2. The client diagnosed with ARDS is expected to have difficulty breathing, but of these four clients, the client diagnosed with breathing difficulty has priority. Apply Maslow's Hierarchy of Needs. ARDS is the sudden failure of the respiratory system. A person diagnosed with ARDS has rapid breathing, difficulty getting enough air into the lungs, and low blood oxygen levels.
3. The client diagnosed with pulmonary sarcoidosis would be expected to have a dry cough and mild chest pain; therefore, this client would not be seen first. In pulmonary sarcoidosis, small patches of inflamed cells can appear on the lungs' small alveoli, bronchioles, or lymph nodes. The lungs can become stiff and may not be able to hold as much air as healthy lungs.
4. The client diagnosed with asbestosis would be expected to have a productive cough and chest tightness; therefore, this client would not be seen first. Asbestosis is a disease involving lung tissue scarring because of breathing in asbestos fibers.

CLINICAL JUDGMENT GUIDE: The nurse should determine whether the clinical manifestations the client is experiencing are expected or normal; if they are, then the client would not warrant immediate intervention. If all the clients have expected signs or symptoms, then apply Maslow's Hierarchy of Needs and oxygenation is a priority.

16. Correct answers are 1, 3, 4, and 5.
1. A manual resuscitation bag must be at the bedside in case the ventilator does not work appropriately. The nurse must use this to bag the client.
2. The pulse oximeter reading should be done more often than every shift.
3. The client's respiratory status should be assessed frequently—every 2 hours.
4. The ventilator's settings should be monitored throughout the shift.
5. The respiratory therapist is the multidisciplinary team member responsible for ventilators.

CLINICAL JUDGMENT GUIDE: This is an alternate type of question included in the NCLEX-RN®.

17. 1. This is the correct technique when bathing a client; therefore, the nurse does not need to demonstrate the proper method to give a bath.
2. The bed should be at a comfortable height for the UAP to bathe the client, not in the lowest position.
3. All clients should receive a bath; therefore, this would not be an appropriate action for the nurse to take.
4. Part of the delegation process is to evaluate the UAP's performance, and the nurse should praise any action on the part of the UAP that ensures the client's safety.

CLINICAL JUDGMENT GUIDE: The nurse must ensure the UAP can perform delegated tasks. The nurse is responsible for evaluating the task, demonstrating it, or teaching the UAP how to perform it.

18. 1. The nurse should document the comment and tell other people, such as family, friends, and staff, but this is not the nurse's first intervention.
2. The first action is to ask the person directly to stop. The harasser must be told clearly that the behavior makes the nurse uncomfortable and that they want it to stop immediately.

3. The nurse could take this action, but it is not the first action.
4. This nurse could take this action, but only if direct contact and the chain of command at the hospital do not stop the charge nurse's behavior.

CLINICAL JUDGMENT GUIDE: There will be management questions on the NCLEX-RN®. There is often no test-taking strategy; the nurse must be knowledgeable about management issues that comply with local, state, and federal requirements.

19. 1. The client is in metabolic alkalosis, so this intervention is not appropriate for the client's ABGs.
    2. The client is in metabolic alkalosis, so this intervention is not appropriate for the client's ABGs.
    3. The ABGs indicate metabolic alkalosis, which could be caused by too much hydrochloric acid being removed via the NG tube. Therefore, the nurse should check the NG wall suction.
    4. Sodium bicarbonate is administered for metabolic acidosis, not metabolic alkalosis.

CLINICAL JUDGMENT GUIDE: The nurse must be knowledgeable about normal laboratory values. The nurse must determine whether the laboratory value is normal for the client's disease process or medications the client is taking.

20. 1. This client is critical, and organ rejection is possible; therefore, this client should not be assigned to a float nurse.
    2. The normal CVP is 4 to 10 cm H_2O and an elevated CVP indicates right ventricular failure or volume overload; therefore, this client should not be assigned to a float nurse.
    3. The float nurse from the medical unit can administer antibiotic therapy and complete respiratory assessments; therefore, this client would be the most appropriate client to assign to the float nurse.
    4. Hantavirus pulmonary syndrome (HPS) is a disease that results from contact with infected rodents or their urine, droppings, or saliva. HPS is potentially deadly; there is no specific treatment, and there is no cure. This client should be assigned to a more experienced nurse.

CLINICAL JUDGMENT GUIDE: The test taker must determine the most stable client and assign that client to a float nurse. The more critical clients should be assigned to more experienced ICU nurses.

21. 1. The client's PaO_2 is below the normal level of 80 to 100 mm Hg; therefore, the nurse should administer oxygen.
    2. The client should take deep breaths if the client's $PaCO_2$ is greater than 45 mm Hg.
    3. The nurse should administer sodium bicarbonate if the client's HCO_3 is lower than 22 mmol/L.
    4. The client needs oxygen because of the low arterial oxygen level and does not need a respiratory assessment.

CLINICAL JUDGMENT GUIDE: The nurse must be knowledgeable about normal laboratory values. The nurse must be able to determine whether the laboratory value is normal for the client's disease process or medications the client is taking.

22. 1. A social worker is qualified to assist the client with referrals to any agency or personnel needed after the client is discharged home.
    2. The chaplain should be contacted if spiritual guidance is required, but the question stem did not specify this need.
    3. The HCP can talk to the spouse but cannot address the concerns of taking care of the client when discharged home.
    4. This is false reassurance and does not address the spouse's concern after the client is discharged home. The nurse does not know whether everything is going to be all right.

CLINICAL JUDGMENT GUIDE: The test taker must be knowledgeable about the roles of all members of the multidisciplinary healthcare team as well as HIPAA rules and regulations. These will be tested on the NCLEX-RN® examination.

23. 1. The nurse could ask this question because the radiologist may need to compare the previous chest x-ray with the current one, but this is not the most important question.
    2. The client will have to hold her breath when the chest x-ray is taken, but this is not the most important question.
    3. Smoking or a history of smoking is pertinent to the diagnosis of pneumonia, but it is not the most important question.
    4. This is the most important question because if the client is pregnant, the x-rays can harm the fetus.

CLINICAL JUDGMENT GUIDE: The test taker should realize that for any female client of childbearing age, the most important questions or concerns will probably address the chance of pregnancy. Most medications and many diagnostic tests and treatments can harm the fetus.

24. 1. The elderly client should be called first so that the nurse can determine whether the dizziness when getting up is the result of medication or some other reason. Orthostatic hypotension can be life-threatening; therefore, this client may need to be assessed immediately.
    2. Ordering a prescription is not a priority over a client diagnosed with a physiological problem.
    3. Nausea is often expected with chemotherapy; therefore, this client's phone call would not be returned before calling a client diagnosed with a potentially life-threatening problem.
    4. Pertussis—whooping cough—is a serious, contagious disease that causes severe, uncontrollable coughing fits. The coughing makes breathing difficult and often ends with a "whoop" noise. Because coughing spells are expected, the nurse would not call this client first.

CLINICAL JUDGMENT GUIDE: The test taker should apply some systematic approach when answering priority questions. All the clients are experiencing physiological problems, the first priority according to Maslow's Hierarchy of Needs. Once that is established, then the test taker should determine which physiological problem is most life-threatening—in this case, dizziness when standing because of its possible cause, hypotension, which can be life-threatening.

25. 1. The therapeutic response is to have the client vent their feelings. This statement not appropriate for the client's comment. The nurse must give factual information.
    2. The client diagnosed with active tuberculosis must take the medication as prescribed for 9 to 12 months. If the client refuses to take the medication, a court order will be obtained to make the client take the medication because tuberculosis is a community threat.
    3. The nurse should provide factual information when possible and not shift the responsibility to the HCP.
    4. This is not a true statement. The client must be on the prescribed medications.

CLINICAL JUDGMENT GUIDE: The nurse must be knowledgeable about diseases that pose a threat to the community and provide factual information to the client.

26. Correct answers are 3 and 5.
    1. An induration greater than 10 mm is positive for tuberculosis. This client needs to be assessed and followed up to rule out tuberculosis. This client should not be assigned to an LPN.
    2. A pulse oximeter reading lower than 93% is life-threatening; therefore, this client should not be assigned to an LPN.
    3. Acute bronchitis is an inflammation of the bronchial tubes, the major airways into the lungs. The client is exhibiting expected clinical manifestations; therefore, the LPN could care for this client.
    4. The client is exhibiting wheezing, an acute exacerbation of reactive airway disease. This client should not be assigned to an LPN.
    5. Influenza is a viral infection of the respiratory system. The client is exhibiting generalized muscle aches, an expected symptom; therefore, the LPN could care for this client.

CLINICAL JUDGMENT GUIDE: This is an alternate type of question included in the NCLEX-RN®. The nurse should assign the LPN to the clients with the lowest level of need, making sure that the task remains in the LPN's scope of practice. The nurse cannot assign assessing, teaching, evaluating, or an unstable client to an LPN.

27. 1. The UAP cannot administer oxygen to a client. Oxygen is considered a medication.
    2. The nurse should not depend on the UAP to care for the client experiencing a potentially life-threatening condition.
    3. This is the first intervention because the nurse must assess the client. Asking the UAP to accompany the nurse will allow the nurse to stay with the client while the UAP obtains any needed equipment.
    4. The nurse should immediately assess the client. The UAP does not have the knowledge or skills to care for the client experiencing shortness of breath.

CLINICAL JUDGMENT GUIDE: Any time the nurse receives information from another staff member about a client experiencing a new problem, complication, or life-threatening problem, the nurse must assess the client. The nurse should not make decisions about client needs based on another staff member's information.

28. 1. The parent or guardian must sign the consent for surgery because the client is under 18.
    2. The client has already been diagnosed with tonsillitis; therefore, a throat culture is not needed before surgery.

3. The client should not cough after this surgery because it could cause bleeding from the incision site.
4. A PT/PTT will assess the client for any bleeding tendencies and is a priority before this surgery because bleeding is a life-threatening complication.

CLINICAL JUDGMENT GUIDE: The NCLEX-RN® test plan includes perioperative nursing care. The nurse must be knowledgeable about preoperative and postoperative care that is generic for all clients undergoing surgery.

29. 1. Influenza, or the flu, is a serious respiratory illness caused by a virus. Antibiotics are not prescribed to treat influenza.
    2. Staying away from large crowds and wearing a scarf over the mouth are not the best ways to prevent getting influenza.
    3. Influenza, or flu, is a serious respiratory illness. It is easily spread from person to person and can lead to severe complications, even death. The best way to prevent influenza is to get a yearly flu vaccine. The influenza virus is constantly changing. Each year, scientists work together to identify the virus strains they believe will cause the most illness and a new vaccine is made based on their recommendations.
    4. Three meals a day and daily exercise will help the client stay healthy, but it is not the best way to prevent getting influenza.

CLINICAL JUDGMENT GUIDE: The nurse must know about immunizations for children and adults. This question is knowledge-based, which is included on the NCLEX-RN® examination.

30. 1. The normal pulse rate for a 1- to 11-month-old is 100 to 150 bpm. This client would not warrant immediate intervention.
    2. The normal respiratory rate for a toddler is 20 to 30 breaths/min. This client would not warrant immediate intervention.
    3. A 24-week gestational woman with a BP of 142/96 mm Hg would warrant intervention because the average systolic BP should be between 90 and 140 mm Hg and the diastolic BP should be between 60 and 85 mm Hg. This BP could indicate gestational hypertension.
    4. This is an elevated temperature, but it would not warrant intervention from the nurse. This is not a potentially life-threatening temperature.

CLINICAL JUDGMENT GUIDE: The nurse must be knowledgeable about vital signs. This is basic nursing care that is tested on the NCLEX-RN®.

31. 1. The documentation of the accident must be completed, but it is not a priority over caring for the wound first.
    2. The nurse should wash the area with soap and water and attempt to squeeze the area to make it bleed.
    3. The nurse should not ask the client this question directly. The nurse could ask the client to have blood drawn for testing but not directly ask whether the client has AIDS or hepatitis.
    4. The puncture site would not require antibiotic ointment unless it is infected, and it wouldn't be infected immediately after the incident.

CLINICAL JUDGMENT GUIDE: The NCLEX-RN® test plan includes adhering to Standard Precautions when providing nursing care to clients. Remember: The nurse should always address the problem directly before completing documentation.

32. Correct answers are 1 and 4.
    1. The normal hemoglobin level is 11.7 to 15.5 g/dL (female) and 14 to 17.2 g/dL (male). Normal hematocrit is 36% to 48% (female) and 42% to 52% (male). This client's Hgb and Hct values are low. The nurse should contact the client and make an immediate appointment.
    2. The normal WBC count is 4.5 to 11.1 × 10^3/microL. This client's WBC count is within normal range and does not warrant intervention from the clinic nurse.
    3. The normal serum potassium level is 3.5 to 5.3 mEq/L. This client's level is within normal range and does not warrant intervention from the clinic nurse.
    4. The normal serum sodium level is 135 to 145 mEq/L. This client's level is 125 mEq/L, which is low. The nurse should contact the client and make an appointment.
    5. The normal cholesterol is lower than 200 mg/dL. The normal triglyceride value is lower than 150 mg/dL. This client's cholesterol and triglyceride levels are within the normal range and do not warrant intervention from the clinic nurse.

CLINICAL JUDGMENT GUIDE: This is an alternate type of question included in the NCLEX-RN®. The nurse must be able to select all the options that answer the question.

33. 1. In some cultures, the husband speaks for the wife and family. Requesting them not to speak may be insulting. This action may cause the wife to leave as well.
    2. In some cultures, the husband is the spokesperson and often makes decisions for the wife and family. Asking them to leave the room may also cause the client to leave.
    3. This behavior may be cultural, and the nurse should continue to allow the husband to answer the questions while the nurse looks at the client. The nurse must be respectful of the client's culture. The nurse can, however, ask whether the client agrees with the answers.
    4. This is disrespectful to the client's culture. Often, the nurse must honor the client's culture while caring for the client.

    CLINICAL JUDGMENT GUIDE: The NCLEX-RN® test plan includes nursing care addressing cultural diversity. The nurse needs to be aware of cultural differences.

34. Correct order is 3, 4, 1, 5, 2.
    3. The nurse must determine whether the client is unresponsive before taking action. If the client is unresponsive, then compressions are performed.
    4. The American Heart Association recommends 30 compressions followed by two breaths.
    1. After completing compressions, open the client's airway to ensure a patent airway.
    5. Next, the nurse should administer two breaths with a CPR mask and face shield or bag-valve-mask device.
    2. The nurse then must determine whether the client's heart is pumping by checking the carotid pulse.

    CLINICAL JUDGMENT GUIDE: This is an alternate type of question included in the NCLEX-RN® test plan. The nurse must be able to perform skills in the correct order.

35. 1. The client diagnosed with end-stage COPD usually prefers a cool climate, with fans to help ease breathing. A warm area would increase the effort to breathe for the client. This action would warrant intervention by the nurse.
    2. The client diagnosed with end-stage COPD should be maintained on a low oxygen rate, such as 2 L/min, to prevent depression of the hypoxic drive. High levels of oxygen will depress the client's ability to breathe. This action would not warrant intervention by the nurse.
    3. The client will usually sit in the orthopneic position, slumped over a bedside table, to help ease breathing. This position is called the three-point stance and would not warrant intervention by the nurse.
    4. The client in end-stage COPD has great difficulty breathing; therefore, sitting in a recliner is sometimes the only way the client can sleep. This action would not warrant intervention by the nurse.

    CLINICAL JUDGMENT GUIDE: The nurse only delegates tasks the UAP has been trained to perform. Delegation means the nurse is responsible for the UAP's actions; therefore, the nurse must evaluate the UAP's understanding of the procedure the UAP is asked to perform.

36. 1. The UAP cannot perform sterile dressing changes.
    2. The UAP cannot perform sterile procedures.
    3. The UAP cannot teach the client.
    4. The UAP can transfer the client from the bed to the chair three times a day.

    CLINICAL JUDGMENT GUIDE: The nurse cannot delegate assessment, evaluation, teaching, medication administration, or an unstable client to a UAP.

37. 1. The staff member is violating HIPAA, and the nurse should take action immediately.
    2. The nurse should first ask the staff member not to discuss the client with a friend. Discussing any information about a client is a violation of HIPAA.
    3. The nurse should address the staff member in the restaurant. The nurse could tell the clinical manager, but the nurse must stop the conversation in the restaurant immediately.
    4. The nurse should not tell the client about the breach of confidentiality.

    CLINICAL JUDGMENT GUIDE: There will be management questions on the NCLEX-RN®. There is often no test-taking strategy; the nurse must be knowledgeable regarding management issues. HIPAA was passed into law in 1996 to standardize the exchange of information between HCPs and to ensure client record confidentiality.

38. 1. This statement warrants intervention because fluids will help prevent dehydration and renal calculi. The nurse should explain the client needs to increase fluids.
    2. Range-of-motion exercises help prevent deep vein thrombosis. This statement does not

require intervention by the nurse. The UAP can perform skills if taught and the nurse evaluates performance.
3. Keeping the client off their buttocks is an appropriate intervention for a client on strict bedrest. This comment does not require intervention by the nurse.
4. Pulling the client across the sheets will cause skin breakdown. Because the UAP is not doing this, no intervention by the nurse is needed.

CLINICAL JUDGMENT GUIDE: Delegation means the nurse is responsible for the UAP's actions and performance. The nurse must correct the UAP's performance to ensure the client is cared for safely in the hospital or the home.

39. 1. The client's oxygen should always be placed correctly, but it is not the priority intervention for difficulty breathing.
    2. **Because the client has difficulty breathing while lying in bed, allowing the client to sit in a recliner will help the client; therefore, this is the priority intervention.**
    3. Often, clients report a fan blowing on the face helps with difficulty breathing but this is not a priority intervention.
    4. Slow, deep breaths will not help the client diagnosed with difficulty breathing as much as sitting in a recliner.

CLINICAL JUDGMENT GUIDE: In questions that ask the test taker to identify a priority intervention, all the options are something a nurse can implement. The test taker must identify the most important intervention.

40. 1. The body naturally begins to slow down, and clients may not wish to take in liquids or nourishment. This can produce a natural euphoria and make the dying process easier for the client. IV fluids would interfere with this process and would increase secretions the client cannot handle, thus making the client more uncomfortable.
    2. A percutaneous endoscopic gastrostomy (PEG) feeding tube increases intake for the client but would increase secretions the client cannot handle. This can require suctioning the client and further augmenting the client's discomfort.
    3. **Refusal to take in food and liquids produces a natural euphoria, making the dying process easier for the client. This is an appropriate teaching statement.**
    4. This is a therapeutic response, but factual information is needed to accept the process.

CLINICAL JUDGMENT GUIDE: The NCLEX-RN® addresses questions concerned with end-of-life care, which is included in the Psychosocial Integrity section of the test plan.

41. 1. The home health nurse is possible if a hospice organization is unavailable, but hospice is the best referral.
    2. The nurse would not refer the client to their own pastor. The nurse could place a call to notify the pastor at the client's request, but this would not be a referral.
    3. **One of the guidelines for admission to a hospice agency is a terminal process with a life expectancy of 6 months or less. These organizations assist the client and family to live life to its fullest while providing comfort measures and a peaceful, dignified death.**
    4. The hospital social worker is not an appropriate referral at this time.

CLINICAL JUDGMENT GUIDE: The nurse must be knowledgeable about appropriate referrals and refer to the most suitable person or agency.

42. 1. This is advising and crossing professional boundaries. The nurse should not try to influence the client on these concerns.
    2. This is advising and crossing professional boundaries. The nurse should not try to influence the client on these concerns.
    3. **This response allows the client to make their own decision. It validates that the nurse heard the concern but does not advise the client.**
    4. This is advising and crossing professional boundaries. The nurse should not try to influence the client on these concerns.

CLINICAL JUDGMENT GUIDE: The nurse must never forget that they have positions of authority in a healthcare environment. Nurses must maintain professional boundaries at all times and never cross professional boundaries.

43. **Correct answers are 1, 2, 3, and 5.**
    1. Some nurses see the big picture and seek solutions based on what makes people comfortable rather than logic.
    2. Some nurses see the world logically and focus on a specific intervention.
    3. Some nurses ask fewer questions, especially if they perceive that asking the question will make them look foolish or ignorant.
    4. Different nurses communicate differently. The manager should recognize these differences to arrive at a common goal.

5. All nurses should keep an open mind when communicating with others. Open-mindedness correlates with flexibility and teamwork.

CLINICAL JUDGMENT GUIDE: This is an alternate type of question included in the NCLEX-RN®. The nurse must be able to select all the options that answer the question correctly. There are no partially correct answers.

44. 1. The staff member's attitude changes from one day to the next. The "why" is not important for the manager to know. The important thing for the manager to know is whether the staff member can control their attitude.
    2. The first step is an informal meeting with the staff member to discuss their inappropriate attitude and how it affects the staff. The manager should document the conversation informally with the date and time (the staff member does not need to see this documentation) for future reference. If the situation is unresolved, formal counseling must take place.
    3. This step would follow the informal discussion if their attitude did not improve.
    4. This is a step sometimes used to get the staff member's attention when formal counseling has not been effective. This step occurs just before termination.

CLINICAL JUDGMENT GUIDE: There will be management questions on the NCLEX-RN®. There is often no test-taking strategy; the nurse must be knowledgeable regarding management issues.

45. 1. E-mails should be easy to read and concise. Individuals may not read and understand poorly worded, lengthy e-mails.
    2. When discussing a problem with an individual, it is best to use face-to-face communication in which both parties can give and receive feedback.
    3. Capital letters in e-mails may be interpreted as shouting or yelling at the receiver.
    4. E-mail communication should be concise and easy to read. E-mails with a lot of information should have bullet points to separate information.

CLINICAL JUDGMENT GUIDE: There will be management questions on the NCLEX-RN®. There is often no test-taking strategy; the nurse must be knowledgeable regarding management issues.

46. 1. This is not a nursing problem. The HCP should discuss this with an individual from the department who "owns" the problem.
    2. This is not a nursing problem.
    3. This is not a nursing problem.
    4. This will make the HCP angrier. The HCP should be directed to discuss the problem with the department that can "fix" the problem.

CLINICAL JUDGMENT GUIDE: There will be management questions on the NCLEX-RN®. There is often no test-taking strategy; the nurse must be knowledgeable regarding management issues.

47. Correct order is 1, 4, 3, 2, 5.
    1. The nurse should begin the care by assessing the client. Remember the nursing process.
    4. The nurse should have the client's chest and dressing exposed, and check to ensure the chest tube is securely taped.
    3. The nurse then follows the chest tube to the drainage system and assesses the system.
    2. The suction system is the last part of the chest tube drainage system to assess.
    5. The nurse should ensure emergency supplies are at the bedside last.

CLINICAL JUDGMENT GUIDE: This is an alternate type of question included in the NCLEX-RN® test plan. The nurse must be able to perform skills in the correct order. Assessment should always be the first intervention if the client is not in distress.

48. 1. Bronchiectasis is when the lungs' airways are abnormally stretched and widened, often caused by mucus blockage, which allows bacteria to grow and leads to infection. Clinical manifestations include coughing, abnormal breath sounds, and clubbing; therefore, the nurse would not assess this client first.
    2. Byssinosis (brown lung disease) is a lung disease caused by exposure to dust from cotton processing, hemp, and flax. Clinical manifestations include chest tightness, cough, and wheezing; therefore, this client would not be assessed first.
    3. Cystic fibrosis (CF) is an inherited disease that causes thick, sticky mucus in the lungs, pancreas, and other organs. In the lungs, this mucus blocks the airways, causing lung damage and making breathing hard. A pulse oximeter reading of 90% equates to approximately 60% arterial saturation. The nurse should assess this client first.
    4. Pneumoconiosis, or black lung disease, is an occupational lung disease caused by inhaling

coal dust. The clinical manifestations are shortness of breath and chronic cough; therefore, this client would not be assessed first.

CLINICAL JUDGMENT GUIDE: The test taker must determine which sign or symptom is not expected for the disease process. If the sign or symptom is unexpected, the nurse should assess the client first. This type of question determines whether the nurse is knowledgeable about clinical manifestations of various disease processes.

49. 1. Consolidation indicates fluid or exudates in the lung—pneumonia, and this would not indicate the client is improving.
    2. **Bilateral breath sounds indicate the left lung has re-expanded and the treatment is effective.**
    3. Vigorous bubbling in the suction chamber indicates a leak in the system, but this does not indicate the treatment is effective.
    4. Crepitus (subcutaneous emphysema) indicates that oxygen is escaping into the subcutaneous layer of the skin, but this does not indicate the lung has re-expanded, which is the goal of the treatment.

CLINICAL JUDGMENT GUIDE: The nurse should realize that a normal finding indicates the effective medical treatment. If the nurse is vacillating between two options and one option is equipment, the nurse should select the client's body as the correct answer.

50. 1. Jugular vein distention would indicate the client has congestive heart failure, but is not a complication of a loop diuretic.
    2. Rales and rhonchi are pulmonary edema symptoms, not a loop diuretic complication.
    3. **Leg cramps may indicate a low serum potassium level, which can occur because of the administration of the loop diuretic, bumetanide (Bumex).**
    4. This would indicate the loop diuretic, bumetanide (Bumex), is effective and is not a complication of the medication.

CLINICAL JUDGMENT GUIDE: The nurse must know the medication's expected actions and the assessment data indicating the medication is effective or causing a side effect or an adverse effect.

51. 1. **Nonmaleficence means to do no harm. This statement lets the client know that the concern has been heard but does not give the client bad news before surgery. The nurse is aware that someone having surgery should be of sound mind, and** finding out your child is dead would be horrific.
    2. This is an example of veracity.
    3. This is an example of paternalism, telling the client what they should do.
    4. This is a therapeutic response, not an example of nonmaleficence.

CLINICAL JUDGMENT GUIDE: The NCLEX-RN® test plan includes nursing care that addresses ethical principles, including autonomy, beneficence, justice, and veracity, to name a few.

52. 1. **The Joint Commission is an organization that monitors healthcare facilities for compliance with standards of care. Accreditation is voluntary, but most third-party payers will not reimburse a facility that is not accredited by some outside organization.**
    2. Accreditation does not guarantee reimbursement, although most third-party payers require some accreditation by an outside organization.
    3. Accreditation does not reduce the hospital's liability.
    4. Medicare or Medicaid will not review a facility routinely if The Joint Commission has accredited the facility, but a representative will review the facility in cases of reported problems.

CLINICAL JUDGMENT GUIDE: The NCLEX-RN® test plan includes nursing care that is ruled by legal requirements as well as The Joint Commission, Medicare & Medicaid Services, Centers for Disease Control and Prevention, and Occupational Safety and Health Administration rules and regulations. The nurse must be knowledgeable about these standards.

53. 1. **The nurse should "offer self" to the significant other. Ignoring the needs of the significant other at this time makes the significant other feel that the nurse does not care, and wonder "if the nurse does not care for me, then did the nurse provide adequate care to my loved one?" This action is critical to assist in the grieving process.**
    2. The UAP can gather the deceased client's belongings.
    3. The UAP can perform postmortem care.
    4. The representative of the organ donation team will make this request. Organ banks think specially trained individuals should discuss organ donation with the significant others.

CLINICAL JUDGMENT GUIDE: The NCLEX-RN® addresses questions concerned with end-of-life care, which is included in the Psychosocial Integrity section of the test plan. If unsure of the correct option, an option addressing an individual is best.

54. 1. Warfarin (Coumadin) is an oral, not IV, medication.
    2. The therapeutic PTT results should be 1.5 to 2 times the control, or 51 to 68 seconds. The client's value of 53 is within the therapeutic range. The nurse should continue the heparin drip as is.
    3. The International Normalized Ratio (INR) is not up to the therapeutic range yet, so warfarin (Coumadin) should be administered.
    4. These laboratory values do not provide any information about acetylsalicylic acid (aspirin) administration. Still, the nurse should ask the HCP whether aspirin (an antiplatelet) should be discontinued because the client is receiving two anticoagulants—heparin and warfarin.

CLINICAL JUDGMENT GUIDE: This is an alternate type of question included in the NCLEX-RN® test plan. The test taker must be able to read an EHR, know about laboratory data, and able to make appropriate decisions about the nurse's most appropriate action.

55. 1. A Rapid Response Team (RRT) is called when the nurse assesses a client with a deteriorating condition. The purpose of an RRT is to intervene to prevent a code. In the scenario described, the situation has not progressed to an arrest. The nurse should call an RRT, but administering oxygen is the first intervention.
    2. **The first action is to increase the client's oxygen to 100%.**
    3. The nurse could check the ABG results, but the client is in distress, and the nurse should implement an intervention to relieve the distress.
    4. A fast-acting inhaler should be used, but not until after the oxygen has been increased and an RRT called.

CLINICAL JUDGMENT GUIDE: The nurse should remember: If a client is in distress and the nurse can do something to relieve the distress, that should be done first, before assessment. The test taker should select an option that helps the client's condition directly.

56. 1. The client may eventually need to be transferred to a facility that accepts long-term ventilator-dependent clients, but the nurse would not anticipate it at this time.
    2. The client on a ventilator will have blood gases ordered more often than daily.
    3. The question stem does not indicate that the client is ready to be removed from the ventilator.
    4. **A client intubated for 10 to 14 days and still requiring mechanical ventilation should have a surgically placed tracheostomy to prevent permanent vocal cord damage.**

CLINICAL JUDGMENT GUIDE: The nurse must know about expected medical treatment for the client. This question is knowledge-based.

57. 1. The child's skin will normally taste salty, but this is not the priority intervention to teach.
    2. The parents should be asked about the client's stools during an assessment because the consistency of the stool evaluates the effectiveness of the pancreatic enzymes. This is not the priority intervention because the child must take the enzymes before monitoring the consistency of the stool.
    3. **Cystic fibrosis is a genetic condition that results in blockage of the pancreatic ducts. The child needs pancreatic enzymes to be administered with every meal and snack, so the enzymes will be available when the food reaches the small intestine.**
    4. Cystic fibrosis is one of the few diseases that requires salt replacement, but salt replacement is not more important than taking the pancreatic enzymes.

CLINICAL JUDGMENT GUIDE: The nurse must know about expected medical treatment for the client. This is a knowledge-based question.

58. 1. The UAP should be sensitive to the client's preferences and not insist that the client miss the program.
    2. The UAP should arrange an acceptable time for the client, and the UAP can return to complete the task at the agreed-on time.
    3. **This is the best instruction for the nurse to give to the UAP.**
    4. The bath has not been refused. The client does not want the program interrupted.

CLINICAL JUDGMENT GUIDE: Delegation means the nurse is responsible for the UAP's actions and performance. The nurse must guide the UAP.

59. 1. Effective group process involves all members of the group.
    2. Unanimous decisions may indicate groupthink, which can be a problem in a group process.

3. Effective group process involves all members of the group, not just two.
4. Not allowing deviation from the agenda is an autocratic style and limits the creativity and involvement of the group.

CLINICAL JUDGMENT GUIDE: There will be management questions on the NCLEX-RN®. There is often no test-taking strategy; the nurse must be knowledgeable about management issues.

60. 1. The ventilator should be checked to determine which alarm is sounding. This is the first step in assessing the client's problem.
    2. The nurse should assess the ventilator and the client and then notify the respiratory therapist, if needed.
    3. The client should be assessed, but the ventilator may require only a simple adjustment to fix the problem and turn off the alarm. This is one instance in which the nurse should assess the machine before assessing the client because the machine is breathing for the client.
    4. The client should be manually ventilated if the nurse cannot determine the cause of the ventilator alarm.

CLINICAL JUDGMENT GUIDE: The nurse must determine whether the client is in distress. Remember: If in distress, do not assess. The nurse must intervene to help the client. In most situations, the nurse should not select equipment over the client's body; however, when the equipment is breathing for the client, assess the equipment first.

61. 1. Acute respiratory distress syndrome is diagnosed when the client has an arterial blood gas of lower than 50% while receiving oxygen at 10 L/min. The nurse should prepare for the client to be intubated.
    2. The nurse should intervene while the client is breathing by calling the HCP and assisting in the intubation and setup of the mechanical ventilator. If the client has an arrest before this can be arranged, the client would be ventilated with a bag/mask device.
    3. If the nurse does not intervene immediately, an arrest situation will occur, at which time a Code Blue would be called and CPR started.
    4. If the client does not have a patent IV, the nurse should start one, but not before preparing for intubation.

CLINICAL JUDGMENT GUIDE: The nurse must know about expected medical treatment for the client. This is a knowledge-based question.

62. 1. These blood gases indicate respiratory acidosis that could be caused by ineffective cough, with resulting air trapping. The nurse should encourage the client to turn, cough, and deep breathe.
    2. The Pao_2 level is within normal limits, 80 to 100 mm Hg. Administering oxygen is not the first intervention.
    3. The nurse knows the ABG oxygen level, which is an accurate test. The pulse oximeter only provides an approximate level.
    4. This is not the first intervention. The nurse can intervene to treat the client before notifying the HCP.

CLINICAL JUDGMENT GUIDE: The nurse must know about expected medical treatment for the client. This is a knowledge-based question.

63. 1. The nurse should first prevent circulatory collapse by starting two IV lines and initiating normal saline or Ringer's lactate solution. The crossmatch may be needed if the shock is caused by hemorrhage.
    2. The client is exhibiting symptoms of shock. The nurse should start IV lines to prevent the client from progressing to circulatory collapse.
    3. All clients have a history taken and physical examination performed as part of the admission process to the ED, but this is not the first intervention.
    4. Checking the client's medication allergies is essential, but it is not the first intervention for a client exhibiting signs of shock.

CLINICAL JUDGMENT GUIDE: The nurse should remember: if a client is in distress and the nurse can do something to relieve the distress, that should be done first before assessment. The test taker should select an option that helps the client's condition directly.

64. Correct answers are 3 and 5.
    1. This client is nearing discharge status. Postoperative clients are progressed rapidly. A medical-surgical nurse could take care of this client.
    2. Chest tubes are frequently cared for on a medical-surgical unit; the medical-surgical nurse can care for this client.
    3. This client's status is uncertain. The ICU nurse would be an appropriate assignment for this client because the client will be transferred to the ICU soon.
    4. A medical-surgical nurse can care for this client.
    5. The ICU nurse should care for this client, requiring titration of multiple medications simultaneously.

CLINICAL JUDGMENT GUIDE: The charge nurse must decide which clients need a higher level of expertise to make this decision. Those clients requiring a higher level of expertise should be assigned to the nurse with the greatest knowledge in certain areas. This is an alternate type of question included in the NCLEX-RN®. The nurse must be able to select all the options that answer the question.

65. 1. This position allows access to the client's back area. The chest tube for a hemothorax is positioned low and posterior to allow gravity to assist in removing fluid from the thoracic area.
    2. This is the position for giving an enema.
    3. This is the position used to assist with a lumbar puncture.
    4. This is a resting position; it is not preparing for a chest tube placement.

CLINICAL JUDGMENT GUIDE: The nurse must know basic anatomy and physiology to answer this question. "Hemo" means blood, and "thorax" refers to the thoracic cavity. Blood is in the area where the lung needs to expand. Blood is heavier than air, so the client should be positioned to access the area where dependent drainage will occur.

66. 1. Starting an IV line must be done before being able to initiate a piggyback medication.
    2. To treat the client with the most effective medication and not skew the results of a sputum culture, the specimen must be obtained before initiating antibiotics.
    3. New orders for IV antibiotics must be considered a priority to prevent the client from going into gram-negative sepsis, a potentially lethal situation. However, to initiate the ceftriaxone (Rocephin) antibiotic, the nurse must make sure a correct diagnosis can be made.
    4. Respiratory treatments are important, but not before starting antibiotics.

CLINICAL JUDGMENT GUIDE: To arrive at the correct priority intervention, the test taker must decide whether one option must be accomplished before initiating other options.

67. 1. Shortness of breath after ambulating is expected for a client diagnosed with COPD.
    2. Clients diagnosed with deep vein thrombosis are at risk for pulmonary embolism (PE). Anxiety is a symptom of PE. The nurse must determine whether interventions are needed for PE, a life-threatening emergency.
    3. Anyone can take a specimen to the laboratory.
    4. An empyema is an abscess in the thoracic cavity. These vital signs are expected of this client.

CLINICAL JUDGMENT GUIDE: There are rules when deciding which client to assess first: (1) Is the situation life-threatening or life-altering? (2) Is the information/data presented abnormal or unexpected? (3) Is the information expected for the disease process? Or is the problem a psychosocial one? (4) Are the data within normal limits? The test taker should choose the correct answer based on 1 first, 2 next, 3 next, and 4 last.

68. Answer: 2,160 mL intake and 925 mL output. The nurse must add both IV fluids and oral fluids to obtain the total intake for this client: 1,500 + 100 = 1,600 IV fluids. Convert oz to mL (1 oz = 30 mL) to determine oral intake: 12 oz × 30 mL = 360 mL, 6 oz × 30 mL = 180 mL, 4 oz × 30 mL = 120 mL; 360 + 180 + 120 = 660 mL oral fluids. Total intake is 1,600 + 660 = 2,260 mL. The urinary output (800 mL) plus chest drainage (125 mL) equals 925 mL for shift output.

CLINICAL JUDGMENT GUIDE: The NCLEX-RN® test plan includes dosage calculations under Pharmacological and Parenteral Therapies. This category is included under Physiological Integrity, which promotes physical health and wellness by providing care and comfort, reducing client risk potential, and managing health alterations.

69. 1. Bronchiolitis is an inflammation of the bronchioles, the small airways in the lungs. Clinical manifestations include wheezy cough, rapid breathing, cyanosis, nasal flaring, muscle retractions, and fever. Because the client is exhibiting expected signs and symptoms, this client should be assigned to the graduate nurse.
    2. Dull percussion and vocal fremitus indicate consolidation. Consolidation is fluid instead of air in the alveolar space. This situation is potentially life-threatening and should not be assigned to a new graduate.
    3. Flail chest describes a situation in which a portion of the rib cage is separated from the rest of the chest wall, usually because of severe blunt trauma, such as a serious fall or a car accident. This affected portion is unable to contribute to the expansion of the lungs.

Flail chest is a serious condition that can lead to long-term disability and even death. The charge nurse should assign this client to a more experienced nurse.

4. The client diagnosed with reactive airway disease, asthma, should be asymptomatic; therefore, when the client is wheezing, they are having an acute exacerbation and should be assigned to a more experienced nurse.

CLINICAL JUDGMENT GUIDE: When the test taker is deciding which client should be assigned to a new graduate, the most stable client should be assigned to the least experienced nurse.

70. 1. The client diagnosed with pneumonia is expected to have bilateral crackles, and an Sao₂ of 96% is stable; therefore, this client would not be assigned to the most experienced nurse.
    2. **This client is exhibiting typical signs of ARDS; therefore, the charge nurse should assign the most experienced nurse to this client.**
    3. The postoperative client diagnosed with purulent drainage could be developing an infection and should be assessed but is not a priority over a client experiencing respiratory distress.
    4. The client with a tonsillectomy is expected to have pain on the same day of surgery; any nurse should be able to care for this client.

CLINICAL JUDGMENT GUIDE: The charge nurse must decide which clients need a higher level of expertise to make this decision. Those clients requiring a higher level of expertise should be assigned to the nurse with the greatest knowledge and experience.

71. 1. The nurse should administer the prescribed antibiotic, ceftriaxone (Rocephin), as soon as possible but not before obtaining a sputum culture.
    2. The client diagnosed with pneumonia needs more than 2 L oxygen via nasal cannula, which would be appropriate for a client diagnosed with COPD.
    3. **The nurse must obtain a sputum culture before administering ceftriaxone (Rocephin) antibiotic because the culture and sensitivity will be skewed if the client receives antibiotics. This should be the first HCP order implemented.**
    4. The client diagnosed with pneumonia is not placed in respiratory isolation. This HCP order should be questioned.

CLINICAL JUDGMENT GUIDE: The test taker must be knowledgeable in expected medical treatments for the client. This is a knowledge-based question.

72. 1. **Placing the client in the orthopneic position will help the client breathe easier. The position assumed by clients diagnosed with orthopnea is one in which they are sitting propped up in bed by several pillows.**
    2. The client diagnosed with COPD must have low oxygen levels of less than 3 L/min. COPD clients breathe because of oxygen hunger and high levels of O₂ provide so much oxygen that the client loses the stimulus to breathe.
    3. The client is in distress; therefore, the nurse should not assess but do something to help the client. The nurse should not treat a machine.
    4. The nurse should implement an intervention first because the client is in distress, then notify the respiratory therapist.

CLINICAL JUDGMENT GUIDE: The test taker should apply the nursing process in questions that ask, "Which intervention should the nurse implement first?" If the client is in distress, do not assess. The nurse should do something directly to help the client's situation.

73. 1. **The LPN could care for a client 2 days postoperative; crepitus is air in the subcutaneous tissue but is not life-threatening.**
    2. The confused client is not stable; therefore, the nurse cannot assign this client to the LPN. The nurse cannot assign assessment, teaching, evaluation, or an unstable client to the LPN.
    3. The nurse cannot assign teaching; therefore, this client cannot be assigned to an LPN.
    4. The client's pulse oximeter reading is lower than 93%; therefore, this client is unstable and cannot be assigned to an LPN.

CLINICAL JUDGMENT GUIDE: The nurse should assign the LPN the clients who have the lowest level of need but for whom the task still remains in the LPN's scope of practice. The nurse cannot assign assessing, teaching, evaluating, or an unstable client to an LPN.

74. 1. The client diagnosed with active tuberculosis is usually administered rifampin, which causes urine and bodily fluids to turn orange.
    2. The postoperative client would be expected to have pain, so this client would not need immediate intervention. The client with unexpected clinical manifestations of the disease process or condition would require immediate intervention.

3. The client diagnosed with pneumothorax should not have blood in the collection chamber; the client diagnosed with a hemothorax would be expected to have bloody drainage. This client requires immediate intervention by the charge nurse.
4. A client diagnosed with bacterial pneumonia would be expected to have elevated temperature and chills; therefore, this client does not require immediate intervention.

CLINICAL JUDGMENT GUIDE: When deciding which client to assess first, the test taker should determine whether the signs or symptoms the client is exhibiting are normal or expected for the client's situation. After eliminating the expected option, the test taker should determine which situation is more life-threatening.

75. 1. Sucralfate (Carafate) coats the stomach and must be administered on an empty stomach; therefore, the nurse would not question administering this medication.
    2. The therapeutic digoxin level is 0.8 to 2.0 mg/dL; therefore, the nurse would not question administering this medication.
    3. The therapeutic PTT for the client receiving heparin is 58 to 78 seconds; therefore, the nurse would not question administering this medication.
    4. The client on an aminoglycoside antibiotic with an elevated trough level should not receive the medication. The elevation could lead to ototoxicity or nephrotoxicity; therefore, the nurse should question administering this medication.

CLINICAL JUDGMENT GUIDE: The test taker must be knowledgeable regarding medications and associated laboratory values and be able to make a decision as to the nurse's most appropriate intervention.

76. 1. The client needs oxygen to help perfuse the lungs, heart, and body; therefore, this is the first intervention the charge nurse should tell the nurse to implement.
    2. The client will need a computed tomographic angiography (CTA), but it is not the nurse's first intervention.
    3. The nurse will need to notify the client's HCP, but not before taking care of the client's body.
    4. Assessing the client is indicated but is not the first intervention in this situation. Remember: If the client is in distress, do not assess; take action to help the client.

CLINICAL JUDGMENT GUIDE: Remember: "If the client is in distress, do not assess." Situations such as those in this question require the nurse to intervene to prevent the client's status from deteriorating. Before selecting "notify the HCP" as the correct answer, the test taker must examine the other options. If any of the other options contain data that will relieve the client's distress, prevent a life-threatening situation, or provide information the HCP will need to make an informed decision, then the test taker should eliminate the "notify the HCP" option.

77. 1. The nurse should document the client's reports in the nurse's notes, but this is not the first intervention. The nurse should first assess the client.
    2. Taking slow, deep breaths will not address the client's pain of 6 on the pain scale.
    3. The nurse must first determine whether the pain is expected for the client's condition or whether the client is experiencing a complication requiring nursing or medical intervention.
    4. The nurse must check the MAR when it is determined the pain is expected and the client requires pain medication, but it is not the first intervention.

CLINICAL JUDGMENT GUIDE: The test taker must determine whether the sign or symptom is expected for the disease process. If the sign or symptom is not expected, the nurse should assess the client. This type of questions is determining if the nurse is knowledgeable regarding potential complications.

78. Correct answers are 1, 4, and 5.
    1. The client should be in a high Fowler's position to facilitate lung expansion.
    2. The system must be patent and intact to function properly, but it should be assessed more often than every shift. It should be assessed every 2 to 4 hours.
    3. The client can have bathroom privileges, and ambulation facilitates lung ventilation and expansion.
    4. The tubing should not have any dependent loops. Looping the tubing prevents direct pressure on the chest tube and keeps the tubing off the floor, addressing both a safety and an infection control issue.
    5. The collection chamber of the chest drainage system (Pleur-evac) should be marked at the end of every shift and is part of the total output for the client.

CLINICAL JUDGMENT GUIDE: This is an alternate type of question included in the NCLEX_RN®. The nurse must be able to select the options that answer the question correctly.

79. 1. The client suspected of having ARDS is not stable and should not be assigned to an LPN. A more experienced nurse should be assigned to this client.
    2. The LPN cannot administer blood; therefore, this client should not be assigned to the LPN.
    3. Jugular vein distention and hypotension are signs of a tension pneumothorax, a medical emergency, and the client should be assigned to an RN.
    4. A client scheduled for a bronchoscopy is stable and should be assigned to the LPN. This client is the most stable and least critical.

CLINICAL JUDGMENT GUIDE: The nurse should assign the LPN the clients who have the lowest level of need but for whom the task still remains in the LPN's scope of practice. The nurse cannot assign assessing, teaching, evaluating, or an unstable client to an LPN.

80. Correct answers are 1, 2, and 5.
    1. The client's acute respiratory distress is progressing to respiratory failure. The nurse needs to prepare for immediate intubation and mechanical ventilation.
    2. The client needs a high-flow oxygen delivery system to correct hypoxia.
    3. The upright or prone positions support oxygenation and lung expansion. It can be complicated to utilize the prone position if a client is too sick.
    4. Nutritional needs are essential but not a priority over respiratory support.
    5. The client should have continuous monitoring of oxygen saturation levels.

CLINICAL JUDGMENT GUIDE: This is an alternate type of question included in the NCLEX_RN®. The nurse must be able to select the options that answer the question correctly.

81. Correct answers are 2 and 3.
    1. Arterial blood gas readings are used to assess a client's oxygenation but will not confirm ET tube placement.
    2. Listening to the breath sounds in both lungs will indicate whether both lungs are being ventilated.
    3. A portable chest x-ray will be performed to confirm correct ET tube placement.
    4. Capillary refill assesses the blood flow to the periphery; it will not confirm the correct placement of the ET tube.
    5. Suctioning secretions may be necessary but does not confirm correct ET tube placement.

CLINICAL JUDGMENT GUIDE: This is an alternate type of question included in the NCLEX_RN®. The nurse must be able to select the options that answer the question correctly.

82. Correct order is 4, 3, 5, 2, 1.
    4. The nurse should premeasure the length of the suction catheter. Length is determined by using the marking on the ET tube and adding the additional space for the adapter, usually 1 to 1.5 cm.
    3. The nurse should hyperoxygenate the client before suctioning by having the client take three or four deep breaths, manually ventilating with a bag-mask device, or activating the hyperoxygenate button on the ventilator.
    5. The nurse should lubricate the catheter tip with saline solution and insert the catheter to the premeasured length.
    2. Suction should be applied only when withdrawing the catheter.
    1. The nurse should provide mouth care for the client's comfort after the procedure is complete.

CLINICAL JUDGMENT GUIDE: This is an alternate type of question included in the NCLEX-RN® test plan. The nurse must be able to perform skills in the correct order. Assessment should always be the first intervention if the client is not in distress.

83. Correct answers are 2, 3, 4, and 5.
    1. An electrolarynx is an artificial larynx. It can be successfully used for clients with a tracheostomy.
    2. Communication boards with words, pictures, and dry erase components are helpful to facilitate communication with an intubated client on a ventilator.
    3. Hand gestures are helpful to facilitate communication with an intubated client on a ventilator.
    4. Eye blinks for yes or no questions facilitate communication with an intubated client on a ventilator.
    5. Augmented and assistive communication devices, like cell phones or tablets, use icons, pictures, and words to facilitate communication.

CLINICAL JUDGMENT GUIDE: This is an alternate type of question included in the NCLEX_RN®. The nurse must be able to select the options that answer the question correctly.

84. Correct answers are 1, 2, 3, and 4.
    1. The respiratory therapist is a part of the multidisciplinary team and responsible for the ventilator.
    2. The client should be on continuous monitoring of oxygen saturation.
    3. A manual resuscitation bag should be at the bedside in case of ventilator failure.
    4. The nurse should assess the ventilator settings frequently throughout the shift.
    5. The ventilator alarms should not be silenced, but attempts should be made to decrease alarms to avoid ICU psychosis.

CLINICAL JUDGMENT GUIDE: This is an alternate type of question included in the NCLEX_RN®. The nurse must be able to select the options that answer the question correctly.

CASE STUDY ANSWERS

1. Correct answers are 1, 2, 3, 4, 5, 6, 7, 8, and 9. Rapid respirations of 32 breaths/min, low BP of 80/53 mm Hg, elevated heart rate and temperature, abnormal SpO_2 of 86% on room air, cyanosis, disorientation, diminished lung sounds with crackles in the bases, and that the client was found wandering in the hospital lobby are abnormal and should be reported to the HCP.

    Homelessness is an assumption on the part of the nurse. At this point, there is no way to confirm the client's living arrangements.

    CLINICAL JUDGMENT GUIDE: Extended multiple responses or select all that apply questions can have one to all correct answers.

2.

Finding	COVID (+)	UTI	CVA
Respirations	X		
Blood pressure	X	X	
Level of consciousness	X	X	X
Lung sounds	X		
Location client found	X	X	X
Heart rate	X	X	
Temperature	X	X	
SpO_2	X		
Cyanosis	X		
Physical appearance	X	X	

All findings listed are consistent with the hypoxia and infectious process of COVID. Blood pressure, heart rate, and fever are directly associated with a UTI and the level of consciousness (found wandering and physical appearance) is often impacted in the elderly. The only two findings supporting a CVA as a condition are the level of consciousness and location (wandering due to confusion).

3. Correct answers are 2 and 1.
Based on the client's condition, the nurse recognizes that the client is at the highest risk for

| 2. Impaired gas exchange |

and will require

| 1. Oxygen therapy |

The client's hypoxia may worsen, reducing the gas exchange of oxygen and carbon dioxide in the alveolar beds and requiring supplemental oxygen to ensure adequate oxygenation. While a risk for injury due to the level of consciousness is relevant, there is no indication that four-extremity restraints are needed. Oxygenation is an ABC answer that takes priority. Based on the client's lab values, there is no indication of bleeding.

4.

Potential Nursing Intervention	Indicated	Not Indicated
Ensure client's code status is known	X	
Instruct staff on COVID personal protective equipment	X	
Apply wrist and ankle restraints		X
Increase oxygen to 4 L via nasal cannula		X
Start remdesivir IVPB	X	
Reorient the client as needed	X	
Place the client in a high Fowler's position.	X	
Request UAP to ambulate client in hall		X
Notify the social worker that the client is homeless		X

It is essential for the nurse to find out the client's code status so it may require a second phone call to the client's next of kin. It is also important to ensure that staff caring for this client know and use droplet precautions and personal protective equipment appropriately to protect themselves and other clients. As soon as remdesivir is available, it should be started, and the client should be reoriented and placed in a high Fowler's position to lessen the work of breathing.

There is no information indicating that the client is agitated, combative, or pulling at the IV site; therefore, restraints are not indicated, especially not four extremity restraints. While the oxygen may need to be increased at some point, it was recently increased to 3 L, so it should be monitored. Finally, the client is only to get up to bedside commode with assist; walking in the hallway would further compromise oxygenation. Unless something has changed, the client is not homeless but rather living alone in an apartment.

5. Correct answers are 1, 2, 3, 6, and 7.
    1. Initiate droplet precautions
    2. Albuterol sulfate 0.83% STAT then every 6 hours via aerosol
    3. Titrate oxygen to maintain Spo_2 >93%
    4. Hydrocortisone sodium succinate 100 mg IVP every 12 hours
    5. 0.9% NaCl via IV @ 100 mL/hr
    6. Remdesevir 100 mg IV STAT ×1, then daily
    7. Acetaminophen 1,000 mg PO PRN temperature >100.5°F (38.2°C)
    8. Urinalysis
    9. Sputum culture
    10. Regular diet as tolerated
    11. Bedrest—may use bedside commode with assist

STAT orders (albuterol and remdesivir) take priority over others and, in this case, are directly related to COVID treatment and respiratory compromise. Ensuring the staff are aware of the client's condition and are practicing droplet precautions is imperative and should occur upon admission to the unit to mitigate spread. Monitoring the client's oxygenation via pulse oximetry indicates that additional oxygen liter flow is needed. Care of the acutely ill client with COVID also requires supportive, symptom-based interventions such as administering acetaminophen for fever and comfort. The other orders should be done but are not considered priority.

6.

Finding	Improved	Declined	No Change
Temperature	X		
Heart rate		X	
Respirations	X		
Blood pressure	X		
Spo_2	X		
Level of consciousness			X

Since the previous set of vital signs, the client's temperature, respiratory rate, blood pressure, and pulse oximetry have improved. The client's heart rate has declined (*note:* the rate has increased, but in relation to the condition, it has declined), and there has been no change in the client's level of consciousness.

Gastrointestinal Management

Let whoever is in charge keep this simple question in her head—NOT how can I always do the right thing myself but how can I provide for this right thing always to be done.

—Florence Nightingale

QUESTIONS

1. The nurse is caring for clients on a medical unit. Which task should the nurse implement **first**?
   1. Change the abdominal surgical dressing so a client can ambulate in the hall.
   2. Discuss the correct method of placing Montgomery straps on the client with the UAP.
   3. Assess the client calling the desk reporting nausea and vomiting.
   4. Call the extended care facility to give report on a discharged client.

2. The nurse is preparing a client for a barium study of the stomach and esophagus. Which nursing interventions should the nurse perform? **Select all that apply.**
   1. Obtain informed consent from the client for the diagnostic procedure.
   2. Discuss the need to increase oral fluid intake after the procedure.
   3. Explain to the client that they must drink a white, chalky substance.
   4. Tell the client not to eat or drink before the procedure.
   5. Instruct the client to avoid smoking 30 minutes before the procedure.

3. Which client warrants **immediate** intervention from the nurse on the medical unit?
   1. The client diagnosed with dyspepsia experiencing eructation and bloating
   2. The client diagnosed with pancreatitis having steatorrhea and pyrexia
   3. The client diagnosed with diverticulitis experiencing left lower quadrant pain and fever
   4. The client diagnosed with Crohn's disease reporting right lower abdominal pain and diarrhea

4. The RN staff nurse and the UAP are caring for clients on a medical-surgical unit. Which tasks should the RN assign to the UAP? **Select all that apply.**
   1. Instruct the UAP to feed the 69-year-old client experiencing dysphagia.
   2. Request the UAP change the linens for the 89-year-old client diagnosed with fecal incontinence.
   3. Tell the UAP to assist the 54-year-old client with a bowel management program.
   4. Ask the UAP to obtain vital signs on the 72-year-old client diagnosed with cirrhosis.
   5. Direct the UAP to apply compression stockings to the 64-year-old client recovering from abdominal surgery.

5. Which UAP behavior requires **immediate** intervention by the RN staff nurse?
   1. The UAP is refusing to feed the client diagnosed with acute diverticulitis.
   2. The UAP would not place the client prescribed bedrest on the bedside commode.
   3. The UAP placed the client with a continuous feeding tube in the supine position.
   4. The UAP placed sequential compression devices on the client on strict bedrest.

6. The nurse is concerned about the documentation for blood administration, and other staff members agree the documentation is cumbersome, needing to be revised. Which action is **most** appropriate for the nurse to implement **first**?
   1. Discuss the blood administration documentation with the chief nursing officer.
   2. Contact an individual to help design new blood transfusion documentation.
   3. Learn to adapt to the present documentation and do not take any further action.
   4. Volunteer on an ad hoc committee to research alternate documentation.

7. The charge nurse is entering healthcare provider (HCP) orders into the electronic health record (EHR) for the client to have a barium enema. In addition to the radiology department, which hospital department should be notified of the procedure?
   1. Cardiac catheterization department
   2. Dietary department
   3. Nuclear medicine department
   4. Hospital laboratory department

8. The RN charge nurse is making assignments on a medical unit. Which client should the charge nurse assign to the new graduate nurse?
   1. The client having received 3 units of packed red blood cells
   2. The client scheduled for an esophagogastroduodenoscopy (EGD) in the morning
   3. The client diagnosed with short bowel syndrome having diarrhea and a K⁺ level of 3.3 mEq/L
   4. The client just returning from surgery for a sigmoid colostomy

9. At 0830, the day shift nurse is preparing to administer medications to the NPO (nothing by mouth) client scheduled for an endoscopy.

   Client's Name: Mr. D.   **Account Number:** 123456
   Date: Today   **Allergies:** Penicillin

Medication	1901–0700	0701–1900
Digoxin 0.125 mg PO every day		0900
Furosemide 40 mg PO bid		0900
		1600
Famotidine 20 mg IVPB every 12 hours	2100 NN	
Vancomycin 850 mg IVPB every 24 hours	2100	0900
Magnesium hydroxide, simethicone, aluminum hydroxide 30 mL PO PRN for heartburn		
Signature/Initials	Night Nurse RN/NN	Day Nurse RN/DN

   Which medication should the nurse **question** administering? **Select all that apply.**
   1. Digoxin 0.125 mg PO every day
   2. Furosemide 40 mg PO twice a day
   3. 3. Famotidine 20 mg IVPB every 12 hours
   4. Vancomycin 850 mg IVPB every 24 hours
   5. Magnesium hydroxide, simethicone, aluminum hydroxide 30 mL PO PRN heartburn

10. Which client should the nurse assess **first** after receiving the p.m. shift assessment?
    1. The client diagnosed with Barrett's esophagus having dysphagia and pyrosis
    2. The client diagnosed with proctitis experiencing tenesmus and passage of mucus through the rectum
    3. The client diagnosed with liver failure having jaundice and ascites
    4. The client experiencing abdominal pain with an 8-hour urinary output of 150 mL (5.1 oz)/hr

11. The nurse is preparing to administer morning medications to clients on a medical unit. Which medication should the nurse administer **first**?
    1. Methylprednisolone to a client diagnosed with Crohn's disease
    2. Donepezil to a client diagnosed with dementia
    3. Sucralfate to a client diagnosed with ulcer disease
    4. Enoxaparin to a client on bedrest after abdominal surgery

12. The nurse has received the morning shift report on a surgical unit in a community hospital. Which client should the nurse assess **first**?
    1. The client 6 hours postoperative for small bowel resection presenting with hypoactive bowel sounds in all four quadrants
    2. The crying and upset client scheduled for an abdominal-peritoneal resection this morning
    3. The client 1 day postoperative for abdominal surgery with a rigid, hard abdomen
    4. The client 2 days postoperative for an emergency appendectomy reporting abdominal pain, rating it as an 8 on a pain scale of 1 to 10

13. The charge nurse is reviewing the morning laboratory results. Which data should the charge nurse report to the HCP via telephone?
    1. Ms. B.G., 4 hours postoperative for gastric lap banding

Client Name: B.G.
Diagnosis:
Weight in kg: 97.7

Account Number: 3674960
Height: 61 in (154.9 cm)
Weight in lb: 215

Allergies: No known drug allergies

Laboratory Report

Laboratory Test	Client Values	Reference Values
White blood cell (WBC) count	15	4.5–11.1 10^3/microL
Red blood cell (RBC) count	4.5	Male: 4.51 to 6.01 (10^6 cells/microL)
		Female: 4.01 to 5.51 (10^6 cells/microL)
Hemoglobin (Hgb)	14	Male: 14–17.3 g/dL
		Female: 11.7–15.5 g/dL
Hematocrit (Hct)	42	Male: 42%–52%
		Female: 36%–48%
Glucose	90	Fasting: less than 100 mg/dL
		Random: less than 200 mg/dL
Potassium	3.5	3.5–5.3 mEq/L or mmol/L

2. Ms. R.M., 1 day postoperative total colectomy with creation of an ileal conduit

Client Name: R.M.
Diagnosis:
Weight in kg: 61.4

Account Number: 5903856
Height: 62 in (157.5 cm)
Weight in lbs: 135

Allergies: Sulfa

Laboratory Report

Laboratory Test	Client Values	Reference Values
WBC count	10	4.5–11.1 10^3/microL
RBC count	4.0	Male: 4.51 to 6.01 (10^6 cells/microL)
		Female: 4.01 to 5.51 (10^6 cells/microL)
Hgb	12	Male: 14–17.3 g/dL
		Female: 11.7–15.5 g/dL
Hct	36	Male: 42%–52%
		Female: 36%–48%
Glucose	95	Fasting: less than 100 mg/dL
		Random: less than 200 mg/dL
Potassium	3.5	3.5–5.3 mEq/L or mmol/L

3. Mr. S.P., 4 days postoperative for gastric bypass surgery

Client Name: S.P.
Diagnosis:
Weight in kg: 61.4

Account Number: 2640832
Height: 69 in (175.3 cm)
Weight in lbs: 300

Allergies: PCN

Laboratory Report

Laboratory Test	Client Values	Reference Values
WBC count	11	4.5–11.1 10^3/microL
RBC count	4.8	Male: 4.51 to 6.01 (10^6 cells/microL)
		Female: 4.01 to 5.51 (10^6 cells/microL)
Hgb	15	Male: 14–17.3 g/dL
		Female: 11.7–15.5 g/dL
Hct	45	Male: 42%–52%
		Female: 36%–48%
Glucose	180	Fasting: less than 100 mg/dL
		Random: less than 200 mg/dL
Potassium	4.0	3.5–5.3 mEq/L or mmol/L

4. Mr. H.C., 8 hours postoperative for exploratory laparotomy

Client Name: H.C. **Account Number:** 3721147 **Allergies:** NKDA
Diagnosis: **Height:** 72 in (182.9 cm)
Weight in kg: 86.4 **Weight in lb:** 190

Laboratory Report

Laboratory Test	Client Values	Reference Values
WBC count	11	4.5–11.1 10^3/microL
RBC count	4.8	Male: 4.51 to 6.01 (10^6 cells/microL)
		Female: 4.01 to 5.51 (10^6 cells/microL)
Hgb	16	Male: 14–17.3 g/dL
		Female: 11.7–15.5 g/dL
Hct	48	Male: 42%–52%
		Female: 36%–48%
Glucose	95	Fasting: less than 100 mg/dL
		Random: less than 200 mg/dL
Potassium	4.5	3.5–5.3 mEq/L or mmol/L

14. The nurse is preparing clients for surgery. Which client has the **greatest** potential for experiencing complications?
    1. The overweight client scheduled for removal of an abdominal mass
    2. The client scheduled for a gastrectomy diagnosed with arterial hypertension
    3. The client scheduled for an open cholecystectomy and smokes two packs of cigarettes per day
    4. The client scheduled for an emergency appendectomy and using a nasal irrigation device daily

15. The nurse is performing ostomy care for a client recovering from abdominal-peritoneal resection with a permanent sigmoid colostomy. **Rank in order of performance.**
    1. Cleanse the stomal site with mild soap and water.
    2. Assess the stoma for a pink, moist appearance.
    3. Monitor the drainage in the ostomy drainage bag.
    4. Apply stoma adhesive paste to the skin around the stoma.
    5. Attach the ostomy drainage bag to the abdomen.

16. The nurse is reviewing the HCP orders for a client scheduled for emergency appendectomy and being transferred from the emergency department (ED) to the surgical unit. Which order should the nurse implement **first**?
    1. Obtain the client's informed consent.
    2. Administer 2 mg of IV morphine every 4 hours, PRN.
    3. Shave the lower right abdominal quadrant.
    4. Administer the on-call IV piggyback (IVPB) antibiotic.

17. The client 1 day postoperative abdominal surgery has an evisceration of the wound. Which intervention should the nurse implement **first**?
    1. Place sterile saline gauze on the eviscerated area.
    2. Reinforce the abdominal dressing with an ABD pad.
    3. Assess the client's abdominal bowel sounds.
    4. Place the client in the left lateral position.

18. The medical-surgical nurse has just received the a.m. shift report. Which client should the nurse assess **first**?
    1. The client diagnosed with a paralytic ileus and absent bowel sounds
    2. The client 2 days postoperative abdominal surgery with a soft, tender abdomen
    3. The client 6 hours postoperative with an abdominal wound dehiscence
    4. The client recovering from a liver transplant being transferred to the rehabilitation unit

19. The client is being prepared for a colonoscopy in the day surgery center. The RN charge nurse observes the RN primary nurse instructing the UAP to assist the client to the bathroom. Which action should the charge nurse implement?
    1. Take no action because this is appropriate delegation.
    2. Tell the UAP to obtain a bedside commode for the client.
    3. Discuss the inappropriate delegation of the nursing task.
    4. Document the situation in an adverse occurrence report.

20. The nurse is caring for clients on a surgical unit. Which client should the nurse assess **first**?
    1. The client vomiting for 2 days with arterial blood gas (ABG) values of pH 7.47, Pao$_2$ 95 mm Hg, Paco$_2$ 44 mm Hg, HCO$_3$ 30 mmol/L
    2. The client 8 hours postoperative for splenectomy reporting abdominal pain, rating it as a 9 on a pain scale of 1 to 10
    3. The client 12 hours postoperative for abdominal surgery having dark green bile draining in the nasogastric (NG) tube
    4. The client 2 days postoperative for hiatal hernia repair reporting feeling constipated

21. The UAP angrily tells the RN primary nurse, "You are the worst nurse I have ever worked with, and I really hate working with you." Which action should the RN primary nurse implement **first**?
    1. Don't respond to the comment and appraise the situation.
    2. Tell the UAP to leave the unit immediately.
    3. Report this comment and behavior to the RN charge nurse.
    4. Explain to the UAP that they cannot talk to the RN primary nurse in this manner.

22. The client is admitted to the critical care unit after a motor vehicle accident. The client asks the nurse, "Do you know if the person in the other car is all right?" The nurse knows the person died. Which statement supports the ethical principle of veracity?
    1. "I am not sure how the other person is doing."
    2. "I will try to find out how the other person is doing."
    3. "You should rest now and try not to worry about it."
    4. "I am sorry to have to tell you, but the person died."

23. The client admitted to the critical care unit tells the nurse, "I have an advance directive, and I do not want to have cardiopulmonary resuscitation." Which intervention should the nurse implement **first**?
    1. Ask the client for a copy of the advance directive so it can be entered into the EHR.
    2. Inform the HCP of the client's request as soon as possible.
    3. Determine whether the client has a durable power of attorney for healthcare.
    4. Request the hospital chaplain to come and talk to the client about this request.

24. The client is diagnosed with esophageal bleeding. Which assessment data warrant **immediate** intervention by the nurse?
    1. The client's hemoglobin/hematocrit values are 11.4 g/dL and 32%.
    2. The client's abdomen is soft to touch and nontender.
    3. The client's vital signs are T 99°F (37.2°C), AP 114 bpm, RR 18 breaths/min, BP 88/60 mm Hg.
    4. The client's NG tube has drainage resembling coffee grounds.

25. Which task should the RN staff nurse in the long-term care facility delegate to the UAP?
    1. Assist the resident into a wheelchair for meals.
    2. Assess the incontinent client's perianal area.
    3. Discuss requirements with the client for going out on a pass.
    4. Explain how to care for the client's colostomy to the family.

26. The RN primary nurse and the UAP are caring for a client on a medical unit having difficulty swallowing and incontinent of urine and feces. Which task should the RN delegate to the UAP?
    1. Check the client's gastrostomy feeding tube for patency.
    2. Place hydrocolloid wound dressing on the client's coccyx.
    3. Apply nonmedicated ointment to the client's perineum.
    4. Suction the client during feeding to prevent aspiration.

27. Which UAP behavior **warrants** intervention by the long-term care RN staff nurse?
    1. The UAP is giving the client with a gastrostomy tube a glass of water.
    2. The UAP is ambulating the client outside using a safety belt.
    3. The UAP is assisting the client with putting a jigsaw puzzle together.
    4. The UAP is giving a back rub to the client on bedrest.

28. The nurse is preparing to teach the client how to irrigate their sigmoid colostomy. Which intervention should the nurse implement **first?**
    1. Demonstrate the procedure on a model.
    2. Provide the client with written instructions.
    3. Ask the client if they have any questions.
    4. Show the client all the equipment needed.

29. The licensed practical nurse (LPN) informs the RN primary nurse that the client diagnosed with liver failure is getting more confused. Which intervention should the RN implement **first?**
    1. Assess the client's neurological status.
    2. Notify the client's HCP.
    3. Request a STAT ammonia serum level.
    4. Tell the LPN to obtain the client's vital signs.

30. The nurse is changing the client's colostomy bag. Which interventions should the nurse implement? **Rank in order of performance.**
    1. Remove the client's colostomy bag.
    2. Apply the client's new colostomy bag.
    3. Don nonsterile gloves.
    4. Assess the client's stoma site.
    5. Cleanse the area around the client's stoma.

31. Which task is **most** appropriate for the RN home healthcare nurse to delegate to the UAP?
    1. Instruct the UAP to give ginkgo biloba to the client diagnosed with Alzheimer's disease.
    2. Ask the UAP to perform tube feedings for the client with a gastrostomy tube.
    3. Request the UAP to perform the daily colostomy irrigation for the client.
    4. Tell the UAP to wash and dry the client's hair.

32. Which behavior by the UAP **warrants** intervention by the RN home health nurse?
    1. The UAP does not accept a birthday gift from the client.
    2. The UAP gives the client a vase of flowers from the UAP's garden.
    3. The UAP picked up the client's prescriptions from the pharmacy.
    4. The UAP cleaned the client's bathroom and scrubbed the commode.

33. The client, diagnosed with diverticulosis, called the home healthcare agency and told the nurse, "I am having horrible pain in my left lower stomach, and I think I have a fever." Which action should the nurse take?
    1. Recommend the client take an antacid and lie flat on the bed.
    2. Instruct one of the nurses to visit the client immediately.
    3. Tell the client to have someone drive them to the ED.
    4. Ask the client what they ate in the last 8 hours.

34. The client with a sigmoid colostomy has an excoriated area around the stoma that has not improved for more than 2 weeks. Which intervention is **most** appropriate for the home health nurse to implement?
    1. Refer the client to the wound care nurse.
    2. Notify the client's HCP.
    3. Continue to monitor the stoma site.
    4. Place hydrocolloid paste over the excoriated area.

35. The terminally ill client tells the nurse, "I just want to live to see my grandson graduate in 2 months." Which stage of grief is the client experiencing?
    1. Anger
    2. Bargaining
    3. Depression
    4. Acceptance

36. The nurse is discussing end-of-life (EOL) care with the client diagnosed with pancreatic cancer. Which statements are the goals for EOL care? **Select all that apply.**
    1. To provide comfort and supportive care during the dying process
    2. To plan and arrange the funeral for the client
    3. To improve the client's quality of life for their remaining time
    4. To help ensure a dignified death for the client and family
    5. To assist with the financial cost of the dying process

37. The terminally ill client refuses hospice services because they say it is "giving up" and prefers their family take care of them. Which is the **most** appropriate action by the nurse?
    1. Discuss the philosophy and services of hospice care with the client.
    2. Take no other action and support the client's decision.
    3. Contact the client's HCP to discuss the prognosis.
    4. Talk to the client's family members about the choice to refuse hospice.

38. The nurse is discussing end-of-life issues with a client. The nurse is explaining the document used for listing the person the client will allow to make healthcare decisions for them if they cannot. Which document is the nurse discussing with the client?
    1. Advance directive
    2. Directive to physicians
    3. Living will
    4. Durable power of attorney for healthcare

39. The significant other of the dying client diagnosed with liver cancer asks the nurse, "What is bereavement counseling?" Which statement is the nurse's **best** response?
    1. "Bereavement counseling helps the client accept the terminal illness."
    2. "It supports you and your family in transitioning to a life without your loved one."
    3. "It counsels you and your loved one during the dying process."
    4. "It is group counseling for family members with deceased loved ones."

40. The nurse is working in a digestive disease disorder clinic. Which nursing action is an example of evidence-based practice (EBP)?
    1. Turn on the tap water to help a client urinate.
    2. Use two identifiers to identify a client before a procedure.
    3. Educate a client based on current published information.
    4. Read nursing journals about the latest procedures.

41. The RN charge nurse notices an RN staff nurse recapping a needle in a client's room. Which action should the charge nurse take **first**?
    1. Tell the staff nurse not to recap the needle.
    2. Quietly ask the staff nurse to step into the hall.
    3. Reprimand the staff nurse for not following procedures.
    4. Notify the house supervisor of the staff nurse's behavior.

42. The administrative supervisor is staffing the hospital's medical-surgical units during an ice storm and has received many calls from staff members unable to get to the hospital. Which action should the supervisor implement **first**?
    1. Inform the chief nursing officer.
    2. Notify the on-duty staff to stay.
    3. Call staff members living close to the facility.
    4. Implement the emergency disaster protocol.

43. The RN clinic nurse is working in a community health clinic. Which nursing tasks should the RN clinic nurse delegate to the UAP? **Select all that apply.**
    1. Instruct the UAP to take the client's history.
    2. Request the UAP to document the client's symptoms.
    3. Ask the UAP to obtain the client's weight and height.
    4. Tell the UAP to complete the client's follow-up care.
    5. Have the UAP take the client's temperature.

44. The staff nurse is working with a colleague acting erratically, talking loudly, and being argumentative. Which action should be taken by the nurse?
    1. Ask the supervisor to come to the unit.
    2. Determine what is bothering the nurse.
    3. Suggest the nurse go home.
    4. Smell the nurse's breath for alcohol.

45. The charge nurse is making assignments on a medical-surgical unit. Which client should be assigned to the **most** experienced nurse?
    1. The client diagnosed with lower esophageal dysfunction experiencing regurgitation
    2. The client diagnosed with Barrett's esophagitis and scheduled for an endoscopy
    3. The client diagnosed with gastroesophageal reflux disease (GERD) having bilateral wheezes
    4. The client 1 day postoperative hiatal hernia repair having pain rated a 4 on a 1 to 10 pain scale

46. The client is experiencing severe diarrhea and has a serum potassium level of 3.3 mEq/L. Which intervention should the nurse implement **first**?
    1. Notify the client's HCP.
    2. Assess the client for leg cramps.
    3. Place the client on cardiac telemetry.
    4. Prepare to administer IV potassium.

47. The UAP alerts the RN charge nurse that a client is angry with their care and packing to leave the hospital. Which intervention should the RN charge nurse implement **first**?
    1. Ask the client's nurse why the client is upset.
    2. Discuss the problem with the client.
    3. Notify the HCP.
    4. Have the client sign the against medical advice (AMA) form.

48. The RN primary nurse is caring for a 14-year-old client diagnosed with bulimia. Which intervention should the RN primary nurse delegate to the UAP?
    1. Talk with the parents about setting goals for the client.
    2. Stay with the client for 15 to 20 minutes after each meal.
    3. Encourage the client to verbalize feelings of low self-esteem.
    4. List the amount of food the client consumed for the dietitian.

49. The client tells the nurse in the bariatric clinic, "I have tried to lose weight on just about every diet out there, but nothing works." Which statement is the nurse's **best** response?
    1. "Which diets and modifications have you tried?"
    2. "How much weight are you trying to lose?"
    3. "This must be difficult. Do you want to talk?"
    4. "You may need to get used to being overweight."

50. The client 2 days postoperative from a laparoscopic cholecystectomy tells the office nurse, "My right shoulder hurts so bad I can't stand it." Which statement is the nurse's **best** response?
    1. "This is a result of the carbon dioxide gas used in surgery."
    2. "Call 911 and go to the emergency department immediately."
    3. "Increase the pain medication the surgeon ordered."
    4. "You need to ambulate in the hall to walk off the gas pains."

51. The nurse is administering medications. At 1400, the client diagnosed with gastroenteritis is reporting being nauseated and has had a formed brown stool.

Client Name: T.R. **Height:** 68 in (172.7 cm) **Date:** Today	**Account Number:** 5948726 **Weight:** 202 lbs (91.6 kg)	**Allergies:** Milk **Date of Birth:** 55 years
Medication	1901–0700	0701–1900
Diphenoxylate and atropine 1 or 2 tablets after each stool up to 8 in 24 hours	0400	0900
Ondansetron 4–8 mg IVP every 4 hours PRN for nausea	0030 (4 mg)	0630 (4 mg) 1230 (4 mg)
Signature/Initials	Night Nurse RN/NN	Day Nurse RN/DN

    Which intervention should the nurse implement?
    1. Administer ondansetron 4 mg IV push (IVP).
    2. Administer diphenoxylate and atropine 2 tabs PO.
    3. Notify the client's HCP.
    4. Tell the client nothing can be given for the nausea.

52. The nurse is caring for the client hemorrhaging from a duodenal ulcer. Which **collaborative** interventions should the nurse implement? **Select all that apply.**
    1. Prepare to administer a Sengstaken-Blakemore tube.
    2. Assess the client's vital signs.
    3. Administer a proton pump inhibitor intravenously.
    4. Obtain a type and crossmatch for 4 units of blood.
    5. Monitor the client's intake and output.

53. The nurse is caring for a client diagnosed with peptic ulcer disease. Which assessment data would require the client to have an **immediate** intervention by the nurse?
    1. The client has hypoactive bowel sounds.
    2. The client's output is 480 mL (16.2 oz) for the 12-hour shift.
    3. The client has T 98.6°F (37.0°C), AP 98 bpm, RR 22 breaths/min, BP 102/78 mm Hg.
    4. The client has emesis resembling coffee grounds.

54. The nurse is caring for the client recovering from sigmoid resection 1 day postoperative. There is a large amount of bright red blood on the dressing. Which intervention should the nurse implement **first?**
    1. Assess the client's apical pulse (AP) and blood pressure (BP).
    2. Auscultate the client's bowel sounds.
    3. Notify the HCP immediately.
    4. Reinforce the dressing with a sterile gauze pad.

55. The nurse is preparing to hang a new bag of total parenteral nutrition for the client recovering from abdominal perineal resection. The bag has 2,000 mL of 50% dextrose, 10 mL of trace elements, 20 mL of multivitamins, 20 mL of potassium chloride, and 500 mL of lipids. The bag is to infuse over the next 24 hours. At what rate should the nurse set the pump? _____

56. The UAP tells the RN staff nurse the client recovering from a laparoscopic cholecystectomy is reporting abdominal pain. Which intervention should the RN implement **first?**
    1. Check the medication administration record for the client's last pain medication.
    2. Instruct the UAP to ask the client to rate their pain on a 1 to 10 pain scale.
    3. Assess the client to rule out any postoperative surgical complications.
    4. Tell the UAP to obtain the client's vital signs and pulse oximeter reading.

57. The client is 30 minutes postprocedure liver biopsy. Which action by the UAP **warrants** intervention by the RN primary nurse?
    1. The UAP offered the client a urinal to void.
    2. The UAP gave the client a glass of water.
    3. The UAP turned the client on the left side.
    4. The UAP took the client's vital signs.

58. The client diagnosed with liver failure is experiencing pruritus secondary to severe jaundice and is scratching their upper extremities. Which intervention should the RN primary nurse implement **first?**
    1. Request the UAP to assist the client in taking a hot, soapy shower.
    2. Apply an emollient to the client's upper extremities.
    3. Place mittens on both hands of the client.
    4. Administer diphenhydramine 25 mg PO to the client.

59. The client diagnosed with hepatitis asks the nurse, "Is there any herb I can take to help my liver get better?" Which statement is the nurse's **best** response?
    1. "You should ask your healthcare provider about taking herbs."
    2. "Milk thistle is an antioxidant and may improve liver function."
    3. "You should not take any medication that is not prescribed."
    4. "Why would you want to take any herbs?"

60. Which task would be **most** appropriate for the RN staff nurse on the gastrointestinal (GI) unit to delegate to the UAP?
    1. Request the UAP to draw the serum liver function test.
    2. Ask the UAP to remove the NG tube.
    3. Tell the UAP to empty the client's colostomy bag.
    4. Instruct the UAP to enter HCP orders into the EHR.

61. The client is diagnosed with gastroenteritis. Which laboratory data **warrant immediate** intervention by the nurse?
    1. A serum sodium level of 152 mEq/L
    2. ABG values of pH 7.37, Pao_2 95 mm Hg, $Paco_2$ 43 mm Hg, HCO_3 24 mmol/L
    3. A serum potassium level of 4.8 mEq/L
    4. A stool sample that is positive for fecal leukocytes

62. The nurse has received the a.m. shift report. Which client should the nurse assess **first?**
    1. The client diagnosed with peptic ulcer disease reporting acute epigastric pain
    2. The upset client diagnosed with acute gastroenteritis wanting to go home
    3. The client diagnosed with inflammatory bowel disease receiving total parenteral nutrition
    4. The uncomfortable, jaundiced, and anorexic client diagnosed with hepatitis B

63. The client recovering from abdominal surgery is reporting pain and tells the nurse, "I felt something pop in my stomach." Which intervention should the nurse implement **first?**
    1. Check the client's apical pulse and blood pressure.
    2. Determine the client's pain on a 1 to 10 pain scale.
    3. Assess the client's surgical wound site.
    4. Administer pain medication intravenously.

64. The client 2 days postoperative for abdominal surgery has a Jackson-Pratt (JP) drain. Which assessment data indicate the JP drain is functioning appropriately?
    1. The bulb is round and has 40 mL of fluid.
    2. The drainage tube is pinned to the dressing.
    3. The drainage tube insertion site is pink and has no foul drainage.
    4. The bulb has suction and is compressed.

65. The nurse is caring for the following clients on a surgical unit. Which client should the nurse assess **first?**
    1. The postoperative client, after inguinal hernia repair, with urine output of 160 mL (5.4 oz) in 4 hours
    2. The client transferred from the postanesthesia care unit (PACU) after an emergency appendectomy
    3. The client 4 hours postoperative for abdominal surgery and reporting flatulence
    4. The client being discharged 6 hours postprocedure for colonoscopy

66. The morbidly obese client is 8 hours postoperative for gastric bypass surgery. Which nursing intervention is of the **greatest priority?**
    1. Instruct the client to use the incentive spirometer.
    2. Weigh the client daily in the same clothes and at the same time.
    3. Apply sequential compression devices to the client's lower extremities.
    4. Assist the client to sit in the bedside chair.

67. The charge nurse has completed the report. Which client should be seen **first?**
    1. The client diagnosed with ulcerative colitis and five loose stools the previous shift
    2. The elderly client admitted from another facility refusing to be seen by the nurse
    3. The client diagnosed with intractable vomiting having tented skin turgor and dry mucous membranes
    4. The client diagnosed with hemorrhoids reporting bright red blood spots on the toilet tissue

68. The RN staff nurse, an LPN, and a UAP are caring for clients on a medical floor. Which nursing tasks can the RN assign or delegate? **Select all that apply.**
    1. Instruct the UAP to discontinue the client's total parenteral nutrition.
    2. Ask the UAP to give the client 30 mL of magnesium hydroxide, aluminum hydroxide for heartburn.
    3. Tell the LPN to administer a bulk laxative to the client diagnosed with constipation.
    4. Request the LPN to assess the abdomen of a client reporting pain.
    5. Have the UAP assist the 1 day postoperative cholecystectomy client to the bathroom.

69. The RN charge nurse is making assignments. Which client should be assigned to the new graduate nurse?
   1. The 39-year-old client diagnosed with GERD reporting pyrosis
   2. The elderly client with absent bowel sounds after an endoscopy this morning
   3. The middle-aged client diagnosed with GERD exhibiting bilateral wheezing
   4. The obese client 1-day postoperative for a cholecystectomy refusing to deep breathe

70. The middle-aged client diagnosed with inflammatory bowel disease has a serum potassium level of 4.4 mEq/L. Which intervention should the nurse implement **first**?
   1. Notify the HCP.
   2. Continue to monitor the client.
   3. Request telemetry for the client.
   4. Prepare to administer potassium IV.

71. The 59-year-old client was admitted to the hospital diagnosed with hemorrhaging from a duodenal ulcer. Which **independent** interventions should the RN charge nurse instruct the primary nurse to implement? **Select all that apply.**
   1. Complete the admission assessment.
   2. Evaluate the client's BP lying, sitting, and standing.
   3. Administer antibiotics intravenously.
   4. Administer blood products.
   5. Obtain a hemoglobin and hematocrit.

72. The RN charge nurse is discharging an elderly client with a new sigmoid colostomy. Which statement made by the client indicates they need **more** teaching?
   1. "If my stoma turns purple, I will notify my HCP."
   2. "I can eat the foods I used to eat when I go home."
   3. "I should wear a colostomy pouch over my stoma."
   4. "I will irrigate my colostomy weekly with 750 mL (25.4 oz) of tap water."

73. The nurse is preparing to hang a new bag of total parenteral nutrition for a 47-year-old client recovering from abdominal perineal resection. The bag has 2,000 mL of 50% dextrose, 15 mL of trace elements, 30 mL of multivitamins, 20 mL of potassium chloride, and 200 mL of lipids. The bag is to infuse over the next 24 hours. At what rate should the nurse set the pump? _____

74. The elderly client is admitted to the medical unit with a diagnosis of acute diverticulitis. Which order should the RN charge nurse **clarify** with the HCP?
   1. Insert an NG tube.
   2. Start IV D_5W at 125 mL/hr.
   3. Schedule the client for a sigmoidoscopy.
   4. Place the client on bedrest with bathroom privileges.

75. The RN charge nurse observes the UAP turning the jaundiced client to the supine position immediately after a liver biopsy. Which action should the charge nurse implement **first**?
   1. Tell the UAP to keep the client on bedrest for 2 hours.
   2. Praise the UAP for placing the client in the supine position.
   3. Instruct the UAP to place the client on their right side.
   4. Complete an incident report on the UAP's behavior.

76. One of the primary nurses tells the RN charge nurse they stuck themself in the finger with a "used" needle and then cleansed the site with soap and water. Which intervention should the charge nurse implement **first**?
   1. Notify the infection control nurse.
   2. Complete an adverse occurrence report.
   3. Request postexposure prophylaxis.
   4. Check the hepatitis status of the client.

77. Which nursing task is **most** appropriate for the RN charge nurse to delegate to the UAP?
    1. Bathe the client diagnosed with liver failure with an inflated Sengstaken-Blakemore tube.
    2. Teach the client with an abdominal incision to splint their incision when coughing.
    3. Assist the jaundiced client diagnosed with pruritus to the bathroom for a shower and a.m. care.
    4. Tell the UAP to assist the RN staff nurse performing a paracentesis on the obese client diagnosed with liver failure.

78. The charge nurse is making rounds on the unit. Which client should the charge nurse assess **first**?
    1. The client diagnosed with peptic ulcer disease receiving blood and with a hemoglobin of 10.1 g/dL and hematocrit 35%
    2. The client diagnosed with ulcerative colitis reporting 10 loose stools and a potassium level of 3.5 mEq/L
    3. The client 1-day postoperative for abdominal surgery with a hard, rigid abdomen and elevated temperature
    4. The client diagnosed with acute diverticulitis draining green bile from their NG tube

GASTROINTESTINAL CASE STUDY

(1110) A paramedic calls the ED nurse regarding a client being transported to the ED after the client's spouse called 911. The 68-year-old client reported vomiting, abdominal pain, fatigue, and weakness for the past 3 days. The client has a history of hypertension and hyperlipidemia, and was recently diagnosed with diverticulosis following a routine colonoscopy. An IV line of normal saline started in the left antecubital vein with a 20 gauge catheter and is infusing at 150 mL/hr. Estimated time of arrival (ETA) is 10 minutes. Vital signs are below.

Vital Signs	Client Values
Blood pressure	96/58 mm Hg
Heart rate	106 bpm
Respirations	20 breaths/min
Temperature	99°F (37.2°C)
SpO_2	91% on room air
Pain	7/10

(1130) The client arrives via Emergency Medical Services (EMS) and is transferred from stretcher to the ED bed. The client reports severe nausea, abdominal pain, and weakness stating, "I was sure I was going to throw up in the ambulance, but I didn't." Color is pale, skin cool, dry and intact. Lungs are clear bilaterally. Abdomen is mildly distended and firm with hyperactive bowel sounds in the left and right upper quadrants and absent bowel sounds in both lower quadrants. While completing the assessment, the client vomits a large amount of dark brown emesis. Pedal pulses faintly present ×4. The client's spouse is at the bedside and states the client's only allergy is to strawberries.

1. **Recognize cues. What matters most?** The nurse prepares to call the ED physician. Which **priority** client data should be reported to the HCP? **Select all that apply.**
   1. Respirations
   2. Blood pressure
   3. Emesis characteristics
   4. Lung sounds
   5. Arrived via EMS
   6. Pain
   7. Temperature
   8. Spo$_2$
   9. Abdomen assessment
   10. Spouse at bedside

2. **Analyze cues. What could it mean?** For each client finding, indicate whether it is consistent with the disease process of dehydration, GI bleed, or influenza. Each finding may support more than one condition.

Finding	Dehydration	GI Bleed	Influenza
Blood pressure			
Emesis characteristics			
Pain			
Abdominal assessment			
Emesis			
Spo$_2$			

(1145) The physician visits the client and orders a complete blood count (CBC), basal metabolic panel (BMP), and an abdominal x-ray STAT; oxygen to maintain oximetry readings of 93% or higher, IV of 0.9% NaCl at 150 mL/hr. Administer 2 mg morphine sulfate and 4 mg ondansetron IV ×1 now.

(1210) Oxygen via nasal cannula started at 2 L, labs drawn, and portable abdominal x-ray completed.

(1240) Diagnostic and laboratory results are posted.

Abdominal x-ray report:
Dilated small bowel with pockets of air and fluid distally.
Impression: Consider ileus or small bowel obstruction.

Laboratory Test	Client Values	Reference Values
Hemoglobin (Hgb)	12 g/dL	Men: 14–17.3 g/dL
		Women: 11.7–15.5 g/dL
Hematocrit (Hct)	35%	Men: 42%–52%
		Women: 36%–48%
WBC count	10.6	4.5 to 11.1 × 10^3/microL
Platelets	210	140 to 400 × 10^3/microL
Creatinine	0.8 mg/dL	Male: 0.61 to 1.21 mg/dL
		Female: 0.51 to 1.11 mg/dL
Glucose	116 mg/dL	Fasting: Less than 100 mg/dL
		Random: Less than 200 mg/dL
Potassium	4.7 mEq/L	0.5 to 5.3 mEq/L or mmol/L
Sodium	141 mEq/L	135 to 145 mEq/L or mmol/L
Blood urea nitrogen	21 mg/dL	8 to 21 mg/dL
		Adult over 90 years: 10 to 31 mg/dL

EHR history: History of hypertension, hyperlipidemia, and diverticulosis. Surgical history of right knee arthroplasty 8 years ago. Allergies: Strawberries. ED bed weight of 189.2 lb (86 kg).

Home medications:

Medication	Dose, Route and Frequency
Losartan/HCTZ	50/12.5 mg, PO, every a.m.
Atorvastatin	40 mg, PO, every p.m.
Centrum Silver	1 tab, PO, every a.m.
Melatonin	5 mg, PO, as needed for sleep

(1300) Repeat vital signs obtained as follows and oxygen increased to 3 L via nasal cannula.

Vital Signs	Client Values
Blood pressure	104/64 mm Hg
Heart rate	97 bpm
Respirations	19 breaths/min
Temperature	99°F (37.2°C)
SpO_2	91% on 2L oxygen
Pain	4/10

(1320) The physician sees the client, reviews the test results, and plans to admit client for suspected small bowel obstruction (SBO) and GI bleed. Client has moderate coffee-ground emesis with flecks of bright red. Client and spouse agree to the plan of care. Provider orders entered in the chart:

PROVIDER ORDERS:

Admit to medical unit—diagnosis: suspected SBO with possible GI bleed
Consult gastroenterology
Abdominal ultrasound before transfer to the floor
Titrate oxygen to maintain SpO_2 >93%
STAT NG tube to low intermittent wall suction (LIWS)
STAT promethazine 25 mg IVP ×1
Ondansetron 4 mg IVP every 8 hours PRN nausea/vomiting. Discontinue if ineffective and administer promethazine 25 mg IVP every 8 hours as needed.
Morphine sulfate 4 mg IVP every 6 hours for severe pain of ≥7/10
Acetaminophen 650 mg IV every 4 hours for mild to moderate pain ≤6/10
IV 0.9% NaCl @ 125 mL/hr
Hold home medications
Bedrest—may use bedside commode with assist
NPO—ice chips sparingly

CHAPTER 5   GASTROINTESTINAL MANAGEMENT   133

3. **Prioritize hypotheses. Where do I start?** Complete the sentence by choosing from the drop-down list of options. Based on the client's condition at this time, the nurse recognizes that the client is at the highest risk for _____

> *Select* ▼
> 1. Fluid volume overload
> 2. Infection
> 3. Fluid volume deficit

and will require _____

> *Select* ▼
> 1. IV fluids
> 2. Anticoagulants
> 3. Antibiotics

4. **Generate solutions. What can I do?** For each intervention, specify whether the intervention is **indicated** or **not indicated** for the client's care.

Potential Nursing Intervention	Indicated	Not Indicated
Instruct client to get up slowly with assistance		
Reduce IV 0.9% NaCl to 100 mL/hr		
Notify ultrasound of abdominal order		
Increase oxygen to 4 L via nasal cannula		
Place an NG tube to LIWS		
Call gastroenterology		
Request patient care tech to ambulate the client in hall		

(1500) NG tube placed with one successful attempt, placement verified per policy and connected to LIWS (low intermittent wall suction) with immediate return of 400 mL dark brown, coffee-ground with red flecks liquid.

5. **Take action. What will I do?** Which actions are appropriate for the care of this client at this time? Highlight **one correct action from each option category.**

Possible Actions
Initiate contact precautions
Initiate droplet precautions
Initiate standard precautions
Instruct on NPO status with ice chips
Instruct on clear liquid diet
Instruct on NPO status
Verify IV normal saline rate is 100 mL/hr
Verify IV normal saline rate is 125 mL/hr
Verify IV normal saline rate is 150 mL/hr

(1800) The nurse prepares to give the oncoming shift report. Client is sleepy but arouses easily and is oriented to person, place, time, and situation. Color is pale, skin warm and dry. Lungs are clear. Abdomen firm and mildly distended with hyperactive bowel sounds in upper quadrants and absent in lower quadrants. Hand grasps and pedal pushes equal but weak. Pedal pulses (+2) bilaterally. IV left antecubital #20 gauge with normal saline @ 125 mL/hr without redness, edema, or coolness. Voided but has not been up to bedside commode. Emptied 600 mL output of greenish liquid with brown flecks from NG canister; NG tube reconnected to LIWS. The client reports slight nausea, no further emesis, and abdominal pain of 2/10. Last ondansetron and morphine administered at 1710.

Vital Signs	Client Values
Blood pressure	104/64 mm Hg
Heart rate	97 bpm
Respirations	18 breaths/min
Temperature	99°F (37.2°C)
Spo_2	93% on 2 L oxygen
Pain	2/10

6. **Evaluate outcomes. Did it help?** For each assessment finding, indicate whether the client's condition has improved, declined, or no change.

Finding	Improved	Declined	No Change
Nausea			
Bowel sounds			
Pain			
Blood pressure			
Spo_2			
Character of NG output			

ANSWERS AND RATIONALES

The correct answer number and rationale are in **boldface purple type.** Rationales for why other answer options are incorrect are also given.

1. 1. This client should be seen promptly, but not before the client who reports nausea and vomiting.
   2. This intervention can take some time and should not be hastily completed because the nurse must know the task is being done correctly before delegating it to a UAP. This task should be done at a time arranged between the UAP and the nurse.
   3. **This client has experienced a physiological problem, and the nurse must assess the client and the emesis to decide on possible interventions.**
   4. The nurse should call the extended care facility after assessing the client reporting vomiting and after assessing the abdominal dressing.

   CLINICAL JUDGMENT GUIDE: The test taker should use some tool as a reference to guide the decision-making process. In this situation, Maslow's Hierarchy of Needs should be applied. Physiological needs have priority over psychosocial ones.

2. Correct answers are 1, 3, and 4.
   1. **A barium study of the upper GI system is an x-ray procedure and requires the client to sign an informed consent form.**
   2. The barium can cause constipation after the procedure; therefore, the client should increase fluid intake.
   3. **The client will have to drink a white, chalky substance that creates a lining on the inner wall of the gastrointestinal tract.**
   4. **The test is a barium study of the upper GI system and requires the client's upper GI system to be empty. This client should be NPO for at least 8 to 10 hours before the test.**
   5. The client should not smoke for several hours before the procedure, which causes secretions to build and obstruct the diagnostic image.

   CLINICAL JUDGMENT GUIDE: The nurse must be knowledgeable regarding diagnostic tests. The nurse must know preprocedure and postprocedure interventions and which ones require informed consent.

3. 1. The nurse would expect the client diagnosed with dyspepsia (upset stomach) to have eructation (belching) and bloating; therefore, this client does not warrant immediate intervention.
   2. The nurse would expect the client diagnosed with pancreatitis to have steatorrhea (fat, frothy stools) and pyrexia (fever); therefore, this client does not warrant immediate intervention.
   3. The nurse would expect the client diagnosed with diverticulitis to have left lower quadrant pain and fever; therefore, this client does not warrant immediate intervention.
   4. **The client diagnosed with Crohn's disease should be asymptomatic, so pain and diarrhea warrant intervention by the nurse. Pain could indicate a complication.**

   CLINICAL JUDGMENT GUIDE: "Warrants immediate intervention" means the nurse must determine which client is the priority to assess. The nurse would assess a client in pain if all the other options had clients with expected clinical manifestations.

4. Correct answers are 2, 3, 4, and 5.
   1. The nurse should not delegate to the UAP the task of feeding an unstable client at risk for complications during feeding because of dysphagia. This procedure requires judgment that the UAP is not expected to possess.
   2. **UAPs can change linens for incontinent clients; therefore, this task could be delegated to a UAP.**
   3. **The UAP can assist the client to the bathroom and document the results of the attempt.**
   4. **The UAP can obtain the vital signs of a stable client.**
   5. **The UAP can apply compression stockings to the client recovering from abdominal surgery.**

   CLINICAL JUDGMENT GUIDE: This is an alternate type of question included in the NCLEX-RN®. The nurse must be able to select all the options that answer the question correctly. An RN cannot delegate assessment, teaching, evaluation, medications, or an unstable client to a UAP. Tasks that cannot be delegated are nursing interventions requiring nursing judgment.

5. 1. The client diagnosed with acute diverticulitis should be NPO; therefore, the UAP should not feed this client. This action does not warrant immediate intervention.
   2. The UAP should not allow the client on bedrest to use the bedside commode; therefore, this does not warrant immediate intervention by the nurse.

3. To prevent aspiration pneumonia, the client with a continuous feeding tube should be in the Fowler's or high Fowler's position. This action requires immediate intervention by the nurse.
4. The UAP can place sequential compression devices on a client; therefore, this does not warrant immediate intervention.

CLINICAL JUDGMENT GUIDE: Delegation means the nurse is responsible for the UAP's actions and performance. The nurse must correct the UAP's performance to ensure the client is cared for safely in the hospital or the home.

6. 1. The nurse should go through the chain of command when attempting to make a change.
   2. This may be an appropriate action at some point, but this would not be implemented until after assessing the old documentation and identifying areas to be changed.
   3. The nurse should be a change agent.
   4. The staff nurse should be a part of the solution to a problem; volunteering to be on a committee of peers is the best action to effect a change.

CLINICAL JUDGMENT GUIDE: There will be management questions on the NCLEX-RN®. Concepts of Management are included under Safe and Effective Environment and the subcategory Management of Care. This question is knowledge-based.

7. 1. A barium enema is a procedure performed in the radiology department that tests the gastrointestinal system; therefore, the cardiac catheter laboratory does not need to be informed of the procedure.
   2. The client must be NPO for 8 to 10 hours before the procedure. Therefore, the dietary department should be notified to hold the meal trays.
   3. The procedure is performed using barium or Gastrografin, neither of which contains any nuclear material. The nuclear medicine department does not need to be informed of the procedure.
   4. The procedure does not involve the clinical laboratory; therefore, this department does not need to be notified.

CLINICAL JUDGMENT GUIDE: The test taker must be knowledgeable regarding the role of all multidisciplinary healthcare team members. Referrals are included under Safe and Effective Care Environment and the subcategory Management of Care.

8. 1. This client is unstable and should not be assigned to a new graduate nurse.
   2. This client is being prepared for a test in the morning and is the least acute of the clients listed. The new graduate should be assigned to this client.
   3. This client is hypokalemic secondary to diarrhea and is at risk for cardiac dysrhythmias. This client should be assigned to a more experienced nurse. Short bowel syndrome is a malabsorption disorder caused by the surgical removal of the small intestine or rarely because of the complete dysfunction of a large segment of the bowel.
   4. A client returning from surgery with a sigmoid colostomy is at risk for postoperative complications and should be assigned to a more experienced nurse.

CLINICAL JUDGMENT GUIDE: The test taker must determine the most stable client; therefore, this is an "except" question. Three clients are either unstable or have potentially life-threatening conditions.

9. Correct answers are 1, 2, and 5.
   1. The nurse should not administer PO medications such as digoxin (Lanoxin) because the client is NPO.
   2. This medication is PO; therefore, furosemide (Lasix) should not be administered until after the endoscopy.
   3. Famotidine is an IV medication, so it can be administered even though the client is NPO.
   4. Vancomycin is an IV medication, so it can be administered even though the client is NPO.
   5. Magnesium hydroxide, simethicone, aluminum hydroxide (Mylanta) is a PRN medication and it is PO; therefore, it should not be administered until after the procedure.

CLINICAL JUDGMENT GUIDE: This is an alternate type of question included in the NCLEX-RN® test plan. The test taker must be able to read a medication administration record (MAR), be knowledgeable regarding medications, and be able to decide on the nurse's most appropriate intervention.

10. 1. The client diagnosed with Barrett's esophagus is expected to have dysphagia (difficulty swallowing) and pyrosis (heartburn); therefore, this client would not be assessed first.
    2. Proctitis is an inflammation of the anus and the lining of the rectum, affecting only the last 6 inches of the rectum. Symptoms are ineffectual straining to empty the bowels (tenesmus), diarrhea, rectal bleeding, and

possible discharge, involuntary spasms and cramping during bowel movements, left-sided abdominal pain, passage of mucus through the rectum, and anorectal pain. Because the clinical manifestations are expected, this client would not be assessed first.
3. Jaundice and ascites are expected in a client diagnosed with liver failure; therefore, the nurse should not assess this client first.
4. **The client has a urinary output of less than 30 mL/hr; therefore, this client may be going into renal failure and should be assessed first.**

CLINICAL JUDGMENT GUIDE: The test taker should ask, "Is it normal or expected for the disease process?" Do not assess this client first if it is normal or expected. If more than one option is not expected or normal, the test taker should ask which client is in a more life-threatening situation, needs more assessment, or may need the nurse to notify the HCP.

11. 1. This is a routine medication with a time frame of 30 minutes before and after the scheduled time to be administered. Methylprednisolone (Solu-Medrol), a steroid, does not need to be the first medication administered.
2. Donepezil (Aricept), an acetylcholinesterase inhibitor, can be administered within a 30-minute time frame. This medication does not need to be the first medication administered.
3. **Sucralfate (Carafate), a mucosal barrier agent, must be administered before the client eats for the medication to coat the gastric mucosa. This medication should be administered first.**
4. Enoxaparin (Lovenox), an anticoagulant, can be administered within the 30-minute time frame. This medication does not need to be the first medication administered.

CLINICAL JUDGMENT GUIDE: The test taker should know priority medications, such as life-sustaining medications, insulin, and mucolytics (Carafate). These medications should be administered first by the nurse.

12. 1. A client 6 hours postoperative abdominal surgery would be expected to have decreased bowel sounds; therefore, this client would not be assessed first.
2. Surgery is scary. The crying and upset client should be assessed, but not before a potentially life-threatening surgical emergency. Psychosocial problems do not take priority over physiological problems.
3. **A hard, rigid abdomen indicates peritonitis, which is a life-threatening emergency. This client should be assessed first.**
4. The client 2 days postoperative reporting and rating pain as an 8 should be assessed, but the pain is not life-threatening and, therefore, does not take priority over the client diagnosed with probable peritonitis.

CLINICAL JUDGMENT GUIDE: When deciding which client to assess first, the nurse should determine whether the clinical manifestations the client is exhibiting are normal or expected for the client's situation. After eliminating the expected options, the test taker should determine which situation is more life-threatening.

13. 1. **Because a client undergoing an elective procedure such as gastric lap banding is usually healthy preoperatively, an elevated postoperative WBC count may indicate infection requiring notification of the HCP.**
2. The hemoglobin and hematocrit values of 142 g/dL and 36% are within normal limits for a female client; therefore, this laboratory result does not warrant intervention.
3. The glucose level is elevated but does not indicate whether this is a fasting or random sample. Many obese clients have diabetes and must be at least 50 lb (22.7 kg) overweight to have gastric bypass surgery.
4. A serum potassium level of 4.5 mEq/L is within normal limits; therefore, this does not warrant notifying the HCP.

CLINICAL JUDGMENT GUIDE: The nurse must be knowledgeable regarding normal laboratory values. The nurse must be able to determine whether a laboratory value is normal for the client's disease process or medications the client is taking, or if the HCP should be notified.

14. 1. An overweight client having abdominal surgery is not at a higher risk for postoperative complications than any other client.
2. The client's high blood pressure should be monitored closely and medications administered to decrease the hypertension, but this would not cause the client to have a higher risk for postoperative complications.
3. **The location of the incision for an open cholecystectomy, the general anesthesia needed, and a heavy smoking history make this client high risk for pulmonary complications. Most cholecystectomies are performed laparoscopically; however, an open cholecystectomy could be indicated**

for clients with suspected gallbladder cancer, cholecystobiliary fistulas, and severe cardiopulmonary disease.
4. Use of a nasal irrigation device, such as a net pot, bulb syringe, or squeeze bottle, daily does not increase the risk of postoperative complications for a client having gastric surgery.

CLINICAL JUDGMENT GUIDE: This is an "except" question, but it does not say all the options are correct "except." Only one option would cause the nurse to suspect a high risk of postoperative complications. Remember: Smoking cigarettes puts clients at risk for multiple problems, so it would be a good choice.

15. Correct order is 3, 2, 1, 4, 5.
    3. The nurse must first assess the drainage in the bag for color, consistency, and amount.
    2. After removing the bag, the nurse should assess the site to ensure circulation to the stoma. A pink, moist appearance indicates adequate circulation.
    1. The nurse should cleanse the area with mild soap and water to ensure the skin is prepared for the adhesive paste.
    4. The nurse should apply adhesive paste to the clean, dry skin.
    5. The ostomy drainage bag is attached last.

CLINICAL JUDGMENT GUIDE: This is an alternate type of question included in the NCLEX-RN® test plan. The nurse must be able to perform skills in the correct order. Obtaining informed consent and performing an assessment should always be the first interventions.

16. 1. The nurse must first obtain the operative permit, or determine whether the client has signed a permit before implementing any other orders.
    2. The client cannot give informed consent after receiving pain medication; therefore, morphine administration cannot be implemented first.
    3. The operating room staff usually performs shave preps, but the nurse would not implement this before medicating the client.
    4. The on-call IVPB is not administered until the client's operating room (OR) is prepared. The Centers for Disease Control and Prevention recommend administering the prophylactic IVPB antibiotic within 1 hour of opening the skin during a surgical procedure.

CLINICAL JUDGMENT GUIDE: The NCLEX-RN® test plan includes perioperative nursing care. The nurse must know about preoperative and postoperative care, which is generic for all clients undergoing surgery. Obtaining informed consent is a priority intervention.

17. 1. Evisceration is the removal of viscera (internal organs, especially those in the abdominal cavity). If the bowels protrude from the abdominal incision, the nurse must apply sterile saline gauze and then notify the client's surgeon.
    2. The nurse can place an ADB pad on the sterile saline gauze.
    3. The nurse can assess the bowel sounds, but not before applying sterile saline gauze.
    4. The client should be supine; the left lateral position will not affect the client's abdominal evisceration.

CLINICAL JUDGMENT GUIDE: The test taker should apply the nursing process in questions that ask, "Which intervention should the nurse implement first?" If the client is in distress, do not assess. The nurse should do something directly to help the client's situation.

18. 1. This client diagnosed with a paralytic ileus would be expected to have absent bowel sounds; therefore, this client should not be assessed first.
    2. The postoperative abdominal surgery client should have a soft, tender abdomen; therefore, this client should not be assessed first.
    3. Wound dehiscence is the premature "bursting" opening of a wound along surgical sutures and is an emergency that would require the nurse to assess this client first.
    4. This client should be prepared for transfer to the rehabilitation unit, but not before assessing a client diagnosed with a complication of surgery.

CLINICAL JUDGMENT GUIDE: The nurse must determine which client is experiencing an unexpected or abnormal situation for the surgery or condition. All the clients should be assessed and cared for, but the nurse must determine which should be assessed first.

19. 1. The primary nurse's instruction to the UAP to assist the client to the bathroom is an appropriate delegation that ensures the safety of the client. It requires no action by the charge nurse.
    2. No information in the question's stem indicates the client needs a bedside commode; therefore, this is inappropriate.

3. The UAP can assist a stable client to ambulate; therefore, this is not an inappropriate delegation.
4. An adverse occurrence report is completed whenever potential or actual harm has come to the client. Ambulating the client with assistance is not harmful.

CLINICAL JUDGMENT GUIDE: The nurse must ensure the UAP can perform any delegated nursing tasks. The nurse's responsible for evaluating the task and demonstrating or teaching the UAP how to perform it.

20. 1. The ABGs reflect metabolic alkalosis, which is expected in a client experiencing excessive vomiting; therefore, this client would not be assessed first.
    2. Pain is a priority because the nurse must determine whether this is expected postoperative pain or a complication of the surgery. This client should be assessed first.
    3. Dark green bile should be draining from the client's NG tube; therefore, this client should not be assessed first.
    4. The client reporting constipation would not be a priority over a client with surgical pain.

CLINICAL JUDGMENT GUIDE: When deciding which client to assess first, the nurse should determine whether the clinical manifestations the client is exhibiting are normal for the client's situation. After eliminating the expected option, the test taker should determine which situation is more life-threatening.

21. 1. **The nurse should first appraise the situation and not respond or return the anger. The most essential action is empathizing with the UAP and determining the behavior's provocation.**
    2. The primary nurse could tell the UAP to leave the unit, but this is responding to the anger and not the reason for the anger.
    3. The comment may need to be reported to the charge nurse, but not until the primary nurse can determine what caused the comment. The UAP may be upset about something else entirely.
    4. This response is not the first action when dealing with an angry person. This comment may cause further angry behavior by the UAP and will not diffuse the situation. The nurse is the professional person and should control the situation.

CLINICAL JUDGMENT GUIDE: There will be management questions on the NCLEX-RN®. In many instances, there is no test-taking strategy for these questions. The nurse must be knowledgeable regarding management issues and how to deal with conflict and personnel issues.

22. 1. Beneficence is the ethical principle to do good actively for the client. Because the client is in the ICU, the client is critically ill and does not need any news that will further upset them. This statement supports the ethical principle of beneficence.
    2. The statement supports beneficence, which is to do good.
    3. This statement avoids directly telling the client the other individual is dead.
    4. **This statement supports the ethical principle of veracity, which is the duty to tell the truth. This statement will probably further upset the client and cause psychological distress, which may hinder the recovery period.**

CLINICAL JUDGMENT GUIDE: The NCLEX-RN® test plan includes nursing care that addresses ethical principles including autonomy, beneficence, justice, and veracity, to name a few.

23. 1. A copy of the advance directive should be placed in the client's EHR, but it is not the nurse's first intervention.
    2. **The nurse should first inform the HCP to document the order in the client's EHR. The HCP must write the do not resuscitate (DNR) order before the client's wishes can be honored.**
    3. The person with the durable power of attorney for healthcare can make healthcare choices for the client if the client is unable to verbalize their wishes, but the first intervention is to have the HCP write a DNR order.
    4. The client has a right to make this request, and the chaplain does not need to talk to the client about the advance directive.

CLINICAL JUDGMENT GUIDE: There will be management questions on the NCLEX-RN®. Advance directives are included under Safe and Effective Environment and the subcategory Management of Care.

24. 1. The client's hemoglobin and hematocrit are not within normal limits, but remember: "Hemoglobin 9 think about transfusion time." This laboratory information does not warrant immediate intervention.
    2. A soft, nontender abdomen is expected and does not warrant immediate intervention by the nurse.

3. The client's AP is high and the BP is low, which are findings of hypovolemic shock, which warrants immediate intervention by the nurse.
4. Coffee ground drainage indicates "old blood," which would not be unexpected in the client diagnosed with esophageal bleeding.

CLINICAL JUDGMENT GUIDE: The test taker should ask, "Are the assessment data normal for the disease process?" If the data are normal for the disease process, then the nurse would not need to intervene; if they are not normal for the disease process, then this warrants intervention by the nurse.

25. 1. Getting a client up in a wheelchair for meals is an appropriate delegation to the UAP. This task does not require nursing judgment.
    2. Assessing an incontinent client's perianal area requires nursing judgment and cannot be delegated to the UAP.
    3. Discussing requirements with a client for going out on a pass should be done by the nurse responsible for completing the required documentation and providing any medication that the resident should take along.
    4. Explaining colostomy care is teaching, and the RN cannot ask the UAP to teach.

CLINICAL JUDGMENT GUIDE: The nurse cannot delegate assessment, evaluation, teaching, administering medications, or caring for an unstable client to a UAP.

26. 1. Checking the patency of a percutaneous endoscopic gastrostomy (PEG) feeding tube requires nursing judgment, and feeding the client through the tube is based on this judgment. The UAP should not be asked to perform this task.
    2. The nurse should assess the coccyx and the area where the hydrocolloid dressing (Duo-DERM) should be placed. The UAP should not be asked to perform this task.
    3. The UAP can apply nonmedicated ointment to protect the client's perineum when bathing and changing the client's incontinence pads. This will protect the client from skin breakdown.
    4. The nurse should not delegate suctioning during feeding to a UAP. This intervention indicates the client is unstable.

CLINICAL JUDGMENT GUIDE: When the test taker is deciding which option is the most appropriate task to delegate or assign, the test taker should choose the task that allows each staff member to function within their full scope of practice. Do not assign a task to a staff member that requires a higher level of expertise than that staff member has; similarly, do not assign a task to a staff member that could be assigned to a staff member with a lower level of expertise.

27. 1. The client with a gastrostomy tube cannot eat or drink oral fluids; therefore, this behavior warrants intervention by the nurse.
    2. At the long-term care center, the clients are allowed to go outside, and the UAP ambulating the client with a safety belt is appropriate behavior.
    3. Assisting the client with an activity is an appropriate behavior by the UAP in a long-term care center.
    4. Giving a back rub to a client on bedrest is a nice thing for the UAP to do for the client.

CLINICAL JUDGMENT GUIDE: The nurse must ensure the UAP can perform delegated nursing tasks. The nurse is responsible for evaluating the task, demonstrating or teaching the UAP how to perform the task, and intervening if the UAP is exhibiting an unsafe behavior.

28. 1. The nurse should demonstrate the procedure on a model, but the first intervention should be to assess and determine whether the client has any questions.
    2. The nurse should provide the client with written instructions, but the first intervention should be to assess to determine whether the client has any questions.
    3. The client cannot learn if they have questions or concerns. Therefore, the first intervention is to ask the client whether they have any questions. Before beginning to teach the client, the nurse must allay any of the client's concerns or fears.
    4. The nurse should show the client all the equipment, but the first intervention should be to assess, to determine whether the client has any questions.

CLINICAL JUDGMENT GUIDE: The nurse should always apply the nursing process when answering a question requiring the nurse to "determine which intervention to implement first." The first part of the nursing process is to assess.

29. 1. The nurse should first assess the client's neurological status to determine the client's status.
    2. The nurse may need to contact the client's HCP, but the nurse should assess the client first before contacting the HCP.

3. Increasing confusion is a symptom of hepatic encephalopathy, and checking the client's ammonia level would be appropriate, but not before assessing the client.
4. The nurse should assess the client first, before the LPN obtaining further data.

CLINICAL JUDGMENT GUIDE: Any time the nurse receives information about a client (possibly experiencing a complication) from another staff member, the nurse must assess the client. The nurse should not make decisions about the client's needs based on another staff member's information.

30. Correct order is 3, 1, 4, 5, 2.
    3. The nurse should don nonsterile gloves because of body fluid contamination.
    1. The nurse should remove the bag carefully and ensure no drainage in the bag gets on the client's skin.
    4. The nurse should ensure the stoma site is moist and pink.
    5. The area around the stoma should be cleansed with soap and water and allowed to dry thoroughly.
    2. Lastly, the nurse should apply the new colostomy bag.

CLINICAL JUDGMENT GUIDE: The nurse must rank the interventions in order of priority. This question is an alternate type included in the NCLEX-RN® test plan. Remember, Standard Precautions are always a priority.

31. 1. Even if the client is prescribed the herb ginkgo biloba by the HCP, the nurse cannot delegate any medication administration to the UAP.
    2. In some situations, the UAP may be able to perform tube feedings in the home, but the nurse should assign the least invasive procedure to the UAP.
    3. In some situations, the UAP may be able to do colostomy irrigations in the home, but the nurse should assign the least invasive procedure to the UAP.
    4. The UAP can wash and dry the client's hair, as this is the least invasive task, so this would be the most appropriate task for the nurse to delegate to the UAP.

CLINICAL JUDGMENT GUIDE: The nurse cannot delegate assessment, teaching, evaluation, medications, or an unstable client to the UAP. The nurse should always assign the least invasive task or the task that requires the least educated employee.

32. 1. The UAP cannot accept gifts or money from the client, so this would not warrant an intervention.
    2. The UAP can bring flowers to the client. This action does not violate any rules.
    3. The UAP should not take money from the client to pick up prescriptions, and the UAP is not responsible for doing errands for the client. If money or medications are missing, this could result in a difficult situation. The home health nurse should tell the UAP not to do this activity for the client.
    4. Cleaning the house is not part of the UAP's job description, but this would not warrant intervention by the home health nurse.

CLINICAL JUDGMENT GUIDE: The nurse is responsible for knowing the scope of practice for healthcare team subordinates.

33. 1. The client is having clinical manifestations of diverticulitis, which can be potentially life-threatening; therefore, the client should get medical assistance immediately.
    2. The client needs to be seen by an HCP to be prescribed antibiotics; therefore, there is no reason for a home health nurse to visit the client.
    3. The nurse must know disease processes. The client is verbalizing findings of acute diverticulitis, which requires the client to be NPO and prescribed antibiotics. The client needs to receive immediate medical attention.
    4. The client is verbalizing clinical manifestations of acute diverticulitis, which requires medical attention. It does not matter what the client has had to eat.

CLINICAL JUDGMENT GUIDE: The nurse must know the expected medical treatments for the client. This question is knowledge-based.

34. 1. According to the NCLEX-RN® test plan under management of care, the nurse should be knowledgeable regarding referrals. The wound care nurse is trained to care for a client with a colostomy and is knowledgeable in treating complications.
    2. The most appropriate intervention is to refer the client to a multidisciplinary team member with expertise in the area in which the client is having the problem. In this case, the wound care nurse has the expertise to care for the stoma site.
    3. After 2 weeks, the nurse should obtain further assistance in treating the stoma site.
    4. Hydrocolloid (Karaya) paste will not effectively treat the excoriated area; therefore, this is not an appropriate intervention.

CLINICAL JUDGMENT GUIDE: The test taker must know the role of all multidisciplinary healthcare team members and HIPAA rules and regulations. These topics are tested on the NCLEX-RN® examination.

35.
   1. Denial is the first stage of grief. Anger is the second stage of grief: "Why me? It's not fair!" The individual recognizes that denial cannot continue. Because of anger, the person is challenging to care for because of misplaced feelings of rage and envy.
   2. Bargaining: "I'll do anything for a few more years." The third stage involves hoping the individual can somehow postpone or delay death. The client's comments indicate bargaining.
   3. Depression: "I am so sad; why bother with anything?" During the fourth stage, the dying person begins to understand the certainty of death. Because of this, the individual may become silent, refuse visitors, and spend much of the time crying and grieving.
   4. Acceptance: "It's going to be okay." In this last stage, the individual begins to come to terms with their mortality or the mortality of a loved one.

CLINICAL JUDGMENT GUIDE: The nurse caring for dying clients needs to know the stages of death. Each stage of death requires the nurse to address the psychosocial needs of the client differently.

36. Correct answers are 1, 3, and 4.
   1. This statement is a goal for EOL care.
   2. These actions will need to be done during the client's dying process, but it is not a goal for EOL care.
   3. This statement is a goal for EOL care.
   4. This statement is a goal for EOL care.
   5. Addressing the financial cost of the dying process is not a goal for EOL care.

CLINICAL JUDGMENT GUIDE: This is an alternate type of question included in the NCLEX-RN®. The nurse must be able to select all the options that answer the question. The nurse must know the roles of the other areas of nursing so that the nurse can refer the client and family to the appropriate resource.

37.
   1. Some families are close-knit and often prefer to care for their family members; therefore, they would not seek hospice or palliative care. The nurse should attempt to help the client understand the philosophy, the benefits, and the help hospice can give the client and family.
   2. The nurse should attempt to help the client and family understand hospice so the client can make an informed decision.
   3. The HCP does not need to be contacted to reaffirm the client is dying.
   4. The nurse should first talk to the client and then the family.

CLINICAL JUDGMENT GUIDE: The client has a right to refuse any healthcare, but the nurse must ensure the client fully understands the focus of the care. When the client fully understands and refuses the care, the nurse must respect the client's rights.

38.
   1. "Advance directive" is a general term that describes documents that give instructions about future medical care and treatments and who should make decisions if the client cannot.
   2. A directive to HCPs is a written document specifying the client's wish to be allowed to die without heroic or extraordinary measures.
   3. "Living will" is a lay term used frequently to describe any number of documents giving instructions about future medical care and treatments.
   4. The nurse is specifically describing the "durable power of attorney for healthcare." It is a document included in an advance directive.

CLINICAL JUDGMENT GUIDE: The nurse must be aware of documents clients use when addressing end-of-life issues. This question is knowledge-based and nurses must be able to ensure the client's last requests are honored.

39.
   1. Bereavement counseling is for survivors, not clients.
   2. This answer is the definition of bereavement counseling.
   3. Bereavement counseling is for survivors, not the client.
   4. Bereavement counseling may include group counseling, but it could also be individual counseling. This answer is not the nurse's best response.

CLINICAL JUDGMENT GUIDE: The nurse must be able to explain the support provided by hospice. Losing a loved one is a considerable loss to most people, and the nurse's responsibility is to help the survivors work through the stages of grief.

40.
   1. Many nurses follow this practice, but minimal research supports this practice.
   2. This is part of The Joint Commission's Patient Safety Goals, not evidence-based practice.

3. EBP is the conscientious use of current best evidence in making decisions about nursing care. Using the "evidence," or research, to teach a client is EBP.
4. Reading the journal is a step in EBP, but EBP requires using the information in practice.

CLINICAL JUDGMENT GUIDE: The NCLEX-RN® test plan includes nursing care based on EBP. The nurse must be knowledgeable regarding nursing research.

41. 1. The charge nurse should stop the nurse from recapping the needle, but not in front of the client.
    2. **The charge nurse should not reprimand the nurse in front of the client or the client's family. The charge nurse should ask the nurse to step into the hall where the client cannot hear.**
    3. Reprimanding the nurse is not the first action.
    4. Notifying the house supervisor is not the first action.

CLINICAL JUDGMENT GUIDE: In any business, including a healthcare facility, correcting a fellow staff member's behavior should not occur in front of a customer or, in this instance, the client.

42. 1. The chief nursing officer should be informed, but this is not the first action.
    2. **The administrative supervisor's first action is to ensure the clients receive care. The supervisor cannot allow the on-duty staff to leave until replacement staff members have been arranged.**
    3. The supervisor should call any staff that can get to the hospital to staff the hospital, but this is not the first action to implement.
    4. An emergency disaster protocol may be implemented, but the first intervention is to ensure the clients have a nurse on duty.

CLINICAL JUDGMENT GUIDE: The nurse must be knowledgeable regarding emergency preparedness. Employees receive this information in employee orientation and are responsible for implementing procedures correctly. The National Council of State Boards of Nursing (NCSBN) NCLEX-RN® test plan includes questions on a safe and effective care environment.

43. Correct answers are 3 and 5.
    1. The nurse cannot delegate any task requiring nursing judgment. Taking a client's history requires knowing which questions must be asked to assess the client's problems.
    2. Documenting the client's symptoms is a nursing responsibility that the nurse must perform and cannot be delegated to the UAP.
    3. **The nurse can delegate the UAP to obtain the client's height and weight.**
    4. The client's follow-up care may require teaching, judgment, or further assessment; therefore, the nurse should not delegate this action to a UAP. When delegating to a UAP, the nurse must provide clear, concise, and specific instructions. The nurse cannot delegate teaching.
    5. **The nurse can delegate taking the client's temperature to the UAP.**

CLINICAL JUDGMENT GUIDE: This is an alternate type of question included in the NCLEX-RN®. The nurse must be able to select all the options that answer the question. An RN cannot delegate assessment, teaching, evaluation, medications, or caring for an unstable client to a UAP. Tasks that require nursing judgment cannot be delegated.

44. 1. **The actions of the colleague indicate possible drug or alcohol impairment. The staff nurse is not in a position of authority to require the potentially impaired nurse to submit to a drug test. The administrative supervisor should assess the situation and initiate the appropriate follow-up. The nurse must ensure an impaired nurse is not allowed to care for clients.**
    2. The nurse is not a counselor; a staff nurse should not attempt to confront an impaired colleague.
    3. The administrative supervisor and the charge nurse are the only staff members with the authority to send a nurse home.
    4. The nurse should not attempt to determine the cause of the behavior as this is outside the nurse's authority.

CLINICAL JUDGMENT GUIDE: There will be management questions on the NCLEX-RN®. Concepts of Management are included under Safe and Effective Environment and the subcategory Management of Care.

45. 1. Regurgitation (effortless return of food or gastric contents from the stomach into the esophagus or mouth) is a common manifestation of GERD; therefore, this client would not be assigned to the most experienced nurse.
    2. Barrett's esophagitis is a complication of GERD; new graduates can prepare a client for a diagnostic procedure.

3. This client is exhibiting findings of asthma, a complication of GERD; therefore, the client should be assigned to the most experienced nurse.
4. Pain is expected with a surgical procedure and a less experienced nurse could administer pain medication.

CLINICAL JUDGMENT GUIDE: The test taker must determine which client is the most unstable and would require the most experienced nurse, thus making this an "except" type of question. Three clients are either stable or have non–life-threatening conditions.

46. 1. The nurse should notify the HCP, but it is not the first intervention.
    2. The nurse should assess the client for leg cramps, indicating hypokalemia, but the nurse should first ensure the client's cardiac status is stable.
    3. The client is at high risk for cardiac dysrhythmias because of hypokalemia. The nurse should first assess the cardiac status and then implement other interventions. Remember Maslow's Hierarchy of Needs.
    4. The client will need IV potassium, which requires an HCP order; therefore, this intervention is not implemented first.

CLINICAL JUDGMENT GUIDE: The test taker must examine the other three options before selecting "notify the HCP" as the correct answer. If the information in any of the other options contains data that will relieve the client's distress, prevent a life-threatening situation, or provide information the HCP will need to make an informed decision, then the test taker should eliminate the "notify the HCP" option.

47. 1. The charge nurse should discuss the client's anger with the client immediately because the client is preparing to leave the hospital. After talking with the client, the charge nurse can talk with the primary nurse.
    2. This is the first action for the charge nurse. The client is preparing to leave, and a delay in going to the client's room could result in the client leaving before the situation can be resolved.
    3. The HCP should be notified, but the charge nurse should assess the situation first.
    4. The client will be asked to sign the AMA form if they insist on leaving, but the charge nurse should attempt to resolve the situation successfully first.

CLINICAL JUDGMENT GUIDE: The nurse should always apply the nursing process when answering a question requiring the nurse to "determine which intervention to implement first." The first part of the nursing process is to assess.

48. 1. Planning the client's care cannot be delegated to a UAP; the client, not the parents, should set the goals.
    2. The UAP should stay with the client for an hour after a meal. Leaving the client after 20 minutes would allow the client time to induce vomiting.
    3. This requires the nurse to utilize therapeutic conversation and nursing judgment. The nurse cannot delegate this intervention to a UAP.
    4. The UAP can document the amount of food consumed on a calorie-count form for the dietitian to evaluate.

CLINICAL JUDGMENT GUIDE: An RN cannot delegate assessment, teaching, evaluation, medications, or an unstable client to a UAP. Tasks requiring nursing judgment cannot be delegated.

49. 1. This is an assessment question and should be asked to determine whether what the client has attempted has been unsuccessful.
    2. The amount of weight loss desired is not as important as assessment of previous unsuccessful strategies.
    3. This is a therapeutic statement, but the nurse should assess the client.
    4. This statement is not helpful, and the nurse working in a bariatric clinic should know that there are many options for weight loss, including surgery.

CLINICAL JUDGMENT GUIDE: Assessment is the first step of the nursing process, and the test taker should use the nursing process or some other systematic process to assist in determining priorities.

50. 1. During a laparoscopic cholecystectomy, carbon dioxide is instilled into the client's abdomen. Postoperatively, the gas migrates to the shoulder by gravity and causes shoulder pain.
    2. The nurse should explain to the client that this is not an emergency situation.
    3. The nurse should not tell the client to increase the pain medication as this is prescribing.
    4. These pains are "gas" pains, but they are not intestinal gas pains that can be relieved by ambulation.

CLINICAL JUDGMENT GUIDE: The nurse must know the expected medical treatment for the client. This question is knowledge-based.

51. 1. The medication is ordered every 4 hours and it has been less than 4 hours since ondansetron (Zofran) was last administered. The nurse cannot administer the PRN medication.
    2. Diphenoxylate and atropine (Lomotil) is for diarrhea, and the client has a soft, brown, formed stool; therefore, the nurse would not administer this medication.
    3. The nurse should call the HCP to discuss the situation. The client is nauseated and needs something, but nothing has been ordered that has not been given.
    4. The nurse should not tell the client nothing can be done. The nurse needs to call the HCP.

    CLINICAL JUDGMENT GUIDE: The test taker must examine the other three options before selecting "notify the HCP" as the correct answer. If information in any other options contains data that will relieve the client's distress, prevent a life-threatening situation, or provide information the HCP will need to make an informed decision, then the test taker should eliminate the "notify the HCP" option.

52. Correct answers are 1, 3, and 4.
    1. The HCP must order the insertion of a Sengstaken-Blakemore tube, so this is a collaborative nursing intervention.
    2. Assessing the client's vital signs does not require an HCP order, so this is an independent nursing intervention, not a collaborative intervention.
    3. This is a collaborative intervention that the nurse should implement. It requires an order from the HCP.
    4. Obtaining laboratory data requires an HCP order, so this is a collaborative intervention.
    5. Monitoring the client's intake and output does not require an HCP order, so this is an independent nursing intervention, not a collaborative intervention.

    CLINICAL JUDGMENT GUIDE: This is an alternate type of question included in the NCLEX-RN®. The nurse must be able to select all the options that answer the question.

53. 1. Hypoactive bowel sounds are abnormal but would not warrant immediate intervention. As long as the bowels are moving, it is not an emergency.
    2. The client should have 30 mL of urine output an hour; therefore, this information is normal and does not warrant immediate intervention.
    3. These vital signs are normal and do not warrant immediate intervention.
    4. Coffee ground emesis indicates bleeding and old blood and warrants intervention by the nurse. Further assessment is needed to determine whether the client is hypovolemic and the HCP should be notified.

    CLINICAL JUDGMENT GUIDE: The test taker should ask, "Are the assessment data normal for the disease process?" If the data are normal for the disease process, then the nurse would not need to intervene; if they are abnormal for the disease process, then this warrants intervention by the nurse.

54. 1. The nurse should first determine whether the client is hypovolemic before taking any other action, as this will determine the nurse's next action.
    2. The nurse should auscultate the client's bowel sounds to determine whether they are present, but not before taking their pulse and blood pressure.
    3. The nurse should assess the situation before notifying the HCP.
    4. The nurse may need to reinforce the dressing if the dressing becomes too saturated, but this occurs only after a thorough assessment.

    CLINICAL JUDGMENT GUIDE: The test taker must examine the other three options before selecting "notify the HCP" as the correct answer. If information in any of the other options contains data that will relieve the client's distress, prevent a life-threatening situation, or provide information the HCP will need to make an informed decision, then the test taker should eliminate the "notify the HCP" option.

55. Answer: 106 gtt/min. The nurse must divide the total amount to be infused by 24 hours to determine the IV rate: 2,550 mL divided by 24 = 106.25.

    CLINICAL JUDGMENT GUIDE: The NCLEX-RN® test plan includes dosage calculations under Pharmacological and Parenteral Therapies. This category is included under Physiological Integrity, which promotes physical health and wellness by providing care and comfort, reducing client risk potential, and managing health alterations.

56. 1. The nurse must check the medication administration record (MAR) to determine the last time the client received any pain medication, but not before assessing the client first. Remember: Assessment is the first step of the nursing process.

2. The nurse must assess the client's pain, not the UAP. The nurse cannot delegate assessment.
3. The first part of the nursing process is assessment. The nurse must first assess the client's pain to determine whether the pain indicates a complication requiring medical intervention, or if this is routine postoperative pain, which is expected.
4. The nurse should not delegate obtaining the vital signs of a potentially unstable client. The nurse must assess the client.

CLINICAL JUDGMENT GUIDE: Any time the nurse receives information about a client possibly experiencing a complication from another staff member, the nurse must assess the client. The nurse should not make decisions about the client's needs based on another staff member's information.

57. 1. The client should stay on their right side for at least 2 hours postprocedure, so giving the client a urinal to void in is appropriate and does not warrant intervention.
    2. The client is not NPO after the procedure, so giving the client water is appropriate and does not warrant intervention.
    3. Direct pressure is applied to the site, and then the client is placed on their right side to maintain site pressure for at least 2 hours. Turning the client to the left side warrants intervention by the nurse so the client will not hemorrhage.
    4. The UAP can take the vital signs for the stable client; therefore, this action would not warrant intervention.

CLINICAL JUDGMENT GUIDE: Delegation means the nurse is responsible for the UAP's actions and performance. The nurse must correct the UAP's performance to ensure the client is cared for safely in the hospital or the home.

58. 1. Hot water increases pruritus, and soap will cause dry skin, which increases pruritus; therefore, the nurse should discuss this with the UAP.
    2. This will help prevent dry skin, which will help decrease pruritus, but this is not the first intervention. The nurse should first directly protect the client's skin.
    3. Mittens will help prevent the client from scratching the skin and causing skin breakdown, which is a priority for the client diagnosed with liver failure. The client has decreased vitamin K, which will lead to bleeding. The client is also immunosuppressed, which will lead to infection.
    4. Diphenhydramine (Benadryl) will help decrease the pruritus, but it will take at least 30 minutes to work. Protecting the client's skin integrity is the priority.

CLINICAL JUDGMENT GUIDE: The nurse should remember that if a client is in distress and the nurse can do something to relieve the distress, then it should be done first, before assessment. The test taker should select an option that helps the client's condition directly.

59. 1. This statement passes the responsibility of answering the question on to another and is not the best option. The nurse should answer the client's question.
    2. Milk thistle has an active ingredient, silymarin, used to treat liver disease for over 2,000 years. It is both an antioxidant and anti-inflammatory and may improve liver function. This response gives the client factual information.
    3. The nurse should not discourage complementary therapies.
    4. This statement is judgmental, and the nurse should encourage the client to ask questions.

CLINICAL JUDGMENT GUIDE: The nurse must know about complementary alternative medicine, which includes herbs used to treat medical conditions.

60. 1. The laboratory technician draws serum blood studies, not the UAP.
    2. The nurse should not request the UAP to remove the NG tube. The NG tube is invasive, and judgment is required to remove it.
    3. The UAP can empty feces from a colostomy bag; this is not changing the bag, just emptying the feces.
    4. The UAP cannot enter HCP orders into the EHR. The UAP assists the nurse with direct client care.

CLINICAL JUDGMENT GUIDE: An RN cannot delegate assessment, teaching, evaluation, medications, or an unstable client to a UAP. Tasks that cannot be delegated are nursing interventions requiring nursing judgment. The test taker must be knowledgeable regarding the roles of all multidisciplinary healthcare team members.

61. 1. The normal serum sodium level is 135 to 145 mEq/L; this sodium level is elevated, indicating the client is dehydrated, which warrants intervention by the nurse.
    2. These are normal arterial blood gas results; therefore, the nurse would not need to intervene.

3. The normal serum potassium level is 3.5 to 5.3 mEq/L; therefore, this laboratory information does not warrant intervention by the nurse.
4. A stool specimen showing fecal leukocytes would support the diagnosis of gastroenteritis and does not warrant immediate intervention by the nurse.

CLINICAL JUDGMENT GUIDE: The nurse must know normal laboratory values and be able to determine whether a laboratory value is expected for the client's disease process or medications they are taking.

62. 1. Pain should be assessed, even if it is expected for the client's diagnosis, if the other clients are stable.
    2. The nurse needs to talk to this client, but should assess the client with pain first.
    3. The client diagnosed with inflammatory bowel disease receiving total parenteral nutrition is stable and would not be assessed first.
    4. The client diagnosed with hepatitis B would be expected to be jaundiced and anorexic, so this client would not be assessed first.

CLINICAL JUDGMENT GUIDE: The test taker should use some tool as a reference to guide in the decision-making process. In this situation, Maslow's Hierarchy of Needs should be applied. Physiological needs have priority over psychosocial ones.

63. 1. The nurse should assess the client for hypovolemia, but the first intervention is to assess the client's surgical wound to determine whether wound dehiscence has occurred.
    2. The nurse should determine the client's pain, but not before determining the cause of the pain.
    3. Assessing the surgical incision is the first intervention because this may indicate the client has wound dehiscence.
    4. The nurse should not administer pain medication without assessing for potential complications first.

CLINICAL JUDGMENT GUIDE: Assessment is the first step of the nursing process, and the test taker should use the nursing process or some other systematic process to assist in determining priorities.

64. 1. The Jackson-Pratt (JP) drain bulb should be depressed, which indicates suction is applied. In this case, the drain must be emptied and suction reapplied to function appropriately.
    2. The tube should be pinned to the dressing to prevent the client drain from accidentally being pulled out of the insertion site, but this does not indicate the drain is functioning appropriately.
    3. The insertion site should be pink and without any signs of infection, which include drainage, warmth, and redness, but it does not indicate the drain is functioning appropriately.
    4. **The Jackson-Pratt (JP) drain should be sunken in or depressed, indicating that suction is being applied, which indicates the drain is functioning appropriately.**

CLINICAL JUDGMENT GUIDE: The NCLEX-RN® includes Safe Use of Equipment as a subcategory under Safety and Infection Control, which addresses content on protecting clients, family or significant others, and healthcare personnel from health and environmental hazards.

65. 1. The client should urinate 30 mL/hr, so 160 mL in 4 hours is appropriate; the nurse should not assess this client first.
    2. **This client was just transferred from the PACU; therefore, the nurse should assess this client first to perform a baseline assessment and ensure the client is stable.**
    3. Flatulence, "gas," indicates the bowels are working, which is normal for a client with abdominal surgery, so this client should not be seen first.
    4. The client being discharged would be stable and not a priority for the nurse.

CLINICAL JUDGMENT GUIDE: The test taker must determine which clinical manifestation is expected for the surgical procedure. Clients being transferred from more intensive nursing areas to less intensive areas should be assessed upon arrival to the unit.

66. 1. **The client who is morbidly obese will have a large abdomen that prevents the lungs from expanding, which predisposes the client to respiratory complications. Having the client use an incentive spirometer will help prevent respiratory complications.**
    2. The client may be weighed daily, but this is not a priority over respiratory complications.
    3. Preventing deep vein thrombosis is an important intervention, but oxygenation is a priority.
    4. The nurse should get the client out of bed as soon as possible to help prevent deep vein thrombosis, but this is not a priority over oxygenation.

CLINICAL JUDGMENT GUIDE: The test taker should use some tool as a reference to guide in the decision-making process. In this situation, Maslow's

Hierarchy of Needs should be applied. Oxygenation is a priority.

67. 1. The client diagnosed with ulcerative colitis can have 10 to 12 loose stools a day; therefore, this client should not be seen first.
    2. This client should be assessed, but is not a priority over a client diagnosed with a physiological problem.
    3. This client has findings of dehydration. The client should remain hydrated even when they are vomiting.
    4. Bright red spots on toilet tissue is not normal, but it is expected for a client diagnosed with hemorrhoids.

CLINICAL JUDGMENT GUIDE: The test taker must determine which sign or symptom is not expected for the disease process. If the sign or symptom is not likely, then the nurse should assess that client first. This type of question determines whether the nurse is knowledgeable about the clinical manifestations of various disease processes.

68. Correct answers are 3 and 5.
    1. Total parenteral nutrition is an intravenous medication; the nurse cannot delegate medication administration to the UAP.
    2. The nurse cannot delegate medication administration to the UAP.
    3. The LPN can administer medications to a client.
    4. The RN cannot delegate a potentially unstable client assessment to the LPN.
    5. The UAP can assist the stable postoperative client to the bathroom.

CLINICAL JUDGMENT GUIDE: The nurse cannot assign assessment, teaching, evaluation, or an unstable client to an LPN. The nurse cannot delegate assessment, teaching, evaluation, medications, or an unstable client to the UAP.

69. 1. Pyrosis is heartburn and is expected in a client diagnosed with GERD. The new graduate can care for this client and administer an antacid.
    2. An endoscopy is a diagnostic test, and the client should have bowel sounds; therefore, if the client has no bowel sounds, this is an unexpected complication requiring a more experienced nurse.
    3. This client is exhibiting symptoms of asthma, a complication of GERD; therefore, the client should be assigned to the more experienced nurse.
    4. An obese postoperative cholecystectomy client, because of the pain, refusing to deep breathe is at risk of developing pneumonia. This client should have a more experienced nurse to ensure the client takes deep breaths.

CLINICAL JUDGMENT GUIDE: When the nurse is deciding which client should be assigned to the new graduate nurse, the nurse should assign the least critical client and most stable until the graduate nurse has more experience.

70. 1. The HCP would not need to be notified because the potassium level is within the normal limits of 3.5 to 5.5 mEq/L.
    2. The client's potassium level is within normal limits, so the nurse should continue to monitor the client. The normal level is 3.5 to 5.3 mEq/L or mmol/L.
    3. Hypokalemia can lead to cardiac dysrhythmias, but the client's potassium level is within normal limits.
    4. The client will need potassium to correct the hypokalemia, but the client's potassium level is within normal limits.

CLINICAL JUDGMENT GUIDE: The nurse must be knowledgeable regarding normal laboratory values and be able to determine if the laboratory value is normal for the client's disease process or medications the client is taking, or the HCP should be notified.

71. Correct answers are 1 and 2.
    1. An admission assessment is an independent intervention that the nurse should implement.
    2. Evaluating blood pressure is an independent intervention the nurse should implement. If the client can, BPs should be taken lying down, sitting, and standing to assess for orthostatic hypotension.
    3. This is a collaborative intervention that the nurse should implement. It requires an order from the HCP.
    4. Administering blood products is collaborative, requiring an order from the HCP.
    5. The HCP must order any laboratory work, so this is not an independent nursing intervention.

CLINICAL JUDGMENT GUIDE: This is an alternate type of question included in the NCLEX-RN®. The nurse must be able to select all the options that answer the question.

72. 1. A purple stoma indicates necrosis and requires immediate intervention, so the client should notify the HCP; therefore, the client understands the teaching.
    2. The client should be on a regular diet, and the colostomy will have been working for

several days before discharge. The client's statement indicates an understanding of the teaching.
3. The client should wear a colostomy pouch over the stoma so it will collect the feces coming from the stoma.
4. A sigmoid colostomy must be irrigated daily so the client will have a bowel movement daily. This statement indicates the client needs more teaching.

CLINICAL JUDGMENT GUIDE: The test taker must know which sign or symptom is not expected for a procedure or disease process and be able to evaluate if teaching was effective.

73. Answer: 94 mL/hr. First determine the total amount to be infused during 24 hours to determine the IV rate. 2000 + 15 + 30 + 20 + 200 = 2265 mL. Divide by 24 hours = 94 mL/hr.

CLINICAL JUDGMENT GUIDE: The NCLEX-RN® test plan includes dosage calculations under Pharmacological and Parenteral Therapies. This category is included under Physiological Integrity, which promotes physical health and wellness by providing care and comfort, reducing client risk potential, and managing health alterations.

74. 1. The client will have an NG tube because the client will be NPO, which will decompress the bowel and help remove hydrochloric acid.
2. Preventing dehydration is a priority for the NPO client.
3. The charge nurse should question a sigmoidoscopy. Invasive tests are not conducted during an acute exacerbation of diverticulosis.
4. The client is in severe pain and should be on bedrest, which will help rest the bowel.

CLINICAL JUDGMENT GUIDE: The nurse should be knowledgeable of disease process and their management to identify expected and contraindicated HCP orders.

75. 1. The client should be on bedrest for 2 hours, but must be on the right side to prevent hemorrhaging.
2. The client must be on the right side for 2 hours to prevent hemorrhaging.
3. The client should be placed on the right side, the same side as the liver, to prevent hemorrhaging after the liver biopsy.
4. An incident report may need to be completed, but not before taking care of the client by placing the client on their right side.

CLINICAL JUDGMENT GUIDE: The nurse is responsible for the UAP's actions. The nurse must correct the UAP's performance to ensure the client is cared for safely in the hospital.

76. 1. The nurse must notify the infection control nurse as soon as possible to start treatment if needed, but this is not the first intervention.
2. The charge nurse must first have the nurse complete the adverse occurrence report, so there is written documentation concerning the situation. Then, the charge nurse should notify the infection control nurse. They will arrange for postexposure prophylaxis and determine whether the client has hepatitis.
3. Postexposure prophylaxis may be needed, but this is not the first action.
4. The infection control nurse will check the status of the client the needle was used on before the nurse stuck themself.

CLINICAL JUDGMENT GUIDE: There will be management questions on the NCLEX-RN®. Adverse occurrence reports are included under the subcategory of Management of Care.

77. 1. The client with an inflated Sengstaken-Blakemore tube has acute esophageal varices bleeding and is unstable; therefore, this nursing task cannot be delegated.
2. The nurse cannot delegate assessment, teaching, evaluation, medications, or an unstable client to the UAP.
3. The client diagnosed with pruritus (itching) is stable and the UAP can assist with showering and a.m. care; therefore, this task can be delegated by the charge nurse.
4. The nurse cannot perform a paracentesis; only an HCP can perform this procedure. Therefore, the UAP cannot assist the nurse.

CLINICAL JUDGMENT GUIDE: The nurse cannot delegate assessment, evaluation, teaching, administering medications, or the care of an unstable client to a UAP.

78. 1. This client's hemoglobin and hematocrit are low, but the client is receiving blood; therefore, this client is stable and does not need to be assessed first.
2. The client diagnosed with ulcerative colitis would be expected to have 10 loose stools, and the potassium level is within normal limits; therefore, this client does not need to be assessed first.

3. A hard, rigid abdomen and elevated temperature is indicative of peritonitis, which is an acute postoperative complication of abdominal surgery and requires immediate intervention. The charge nurse should assess this client first.
4. Green bile draining from the NG tube is expected and does not require assessment by the charge nurse.

CLINICAL JUDGMENT GUIDE: The test taker should ask, "Is it normal or expected for the disease process or situation?" If it is normal or expected, then do not asses this client first. If more than one option is not expected or normal, then the test taker should ask which client is in a more life-threatening situation, needs more assessment, or may need the nurse to notify the HCP.

CASE STUDY ANSWERS

1. Correct answers are 2, 3, 6, 8, and 9.
   The client's blood pressure and oxygen levels (SpO_2) should be reported as they are both lower than expected. The emesis characteristics, along with the pain and abdominal assessment findings (mildly distended, firm, and bowel sounds) are abnormal and should be reported.
   The remaining findings are not a priority at this time.

2. Findings are associated with potential conditions.

Finding	Dehydration	GI Bleed	Influenza
Blood pressure	X	X	
Emesis characteristics		X	
Pain		X	
Abdominal assessment		X	
Emesis		X	
SpO_2	X	X	X

All findings listed are consistent with the blood loss due to some GI condition. The blood pressure and SpO_2 relate to both dehydration and a potential GI bleed due to loss of circulating blood volume. The only potential indicator of influenza is SpO_2 but because the client's lungs were clear and temperature is just mildly elevated, the possibility of a GI bleed is more appropriate.

3. Correct answers are 3 and 1.
   Based on the client's condition, the nurse recognizes that the client is at the highest risk for

   | 3. Fluid volume deficit |

   and will require

   | 1. IV fluids |

   The client's hemodynamic stability is compromised as a result of GI bleeding and dehydration. Both of these conditions cause a lower circulating blood volume (ABC answers most often take priority). Based on the client's lab values, there is no indication of infection that would require antibiotics.

4. Correct (indicated) and incorrect (not indicated) interventions are below.

Potential Nursing Intervention	Indicated	Not Indicated
Instruct client to get up slowly with help	X	
Reduce IV 0.9% NaCl to 100 mL/hr		X
Notify ultrasound for abdominal order	X	
Increase oxygen to 4 L via nasal cannula		X
Place an NG tube to LIWS	X	
Call gastroenterology	X	
Request patient care tech to ambulate client in hall		X

It is important to instruct the client to get up slowly and only with assistance due to the potential for orthostatic hypotension. An NG tube should be placed and the department that conducts ultrasounds and the gastroenterologist on call should be notified of the orders.

The most recent IV normal saline rate ordered is 125 mL/hr. The supplemental oxygen currently at 3 L via nasal cannula is maintaining oxygenation based on the latest pulse oximetry reading and the client is ordered bedrest, getting up with assistance only to the bedside commode.

5. The correct actions have been highlighted.

Possible Actions
Initiate contact precautions
Initiate droplet precautions
Initiate standard precautions
Instruct on clear liquid diet
Instruct on NPO status
Instruct on NPO status with ice chips
Verify IV normal saline rate is 100 mL/hr
Verify IV normal saline rate is 125 mL/hr
Verify IV normal saline rate is 150 mL/hr

6. Evaluation of findings is indicated below.

Finding	Improved	Declined	No Change
Nausea	X		
Bowel sounds			X
Pain	X		
Blood pressure			X
SpO_2	X		
Character of NG output	X		

The client's nausea, pain, oxygenation, and the description of the NG liquid output have all improved. None of the findings indicate decline, and the client's blood pressure and bowel sounds have remained unchanged.

Renal and Genitourinary Management

You are the people who are shaping a better world. One of the secrets of inner peace is the practice of compassion.

—Dalai Lama

QUESTIONS

1. The nurse is caring for the following clients on a medical unit. Which client should the nurse assess **first**?
   1. The client diagnosed with acute glomerulonephritis experiencing oliguria and periorbital edema
   2. The client diagnosed with benign prostatic hypertrophy (BPH) oozing blood from their IV site
   3. The client diagnosed with renal calculi reporting flank pain rated as a 5 on a 1 to 10 scale
   4. The client diagnosed with nephrotic syndrome having proteinuria and hypoalbuminemia

2. The nurse is inserting an indwelling catheter into a male elderly client. Which intervention should the nurse implement **first**?
   1. Ask the client if he has any prostate problems.
   2. Determine whether the client has a povidone-iodine allergy.
   3. Lubricate the end of the indwelling catheter.
   4. Ensure urine is obtained in the indwelling catheter.

3. The nurse is preparing to administer IV narcotic medication to the client diagnosed with renal calculi and reporting pain rated as 8 on a 1 to 10 pain scale. The client's vital signs are populated in the chart.

Vital Signs	Client Values
Blood pressure	132/79 mm Hg
Heart rate	90 bpm
Respirations	24 breaths/min
Temperature	98.6°F (37°C)
Spo$_2$	98% (room air)

Which intervention should the nurse implement **first**?
1. Clamp the IV tubing proximal to the port of medication administration.
2. Administer the narcotic medication slowly over 2 minutes.
3. Check the medication administration record (MAR) against the hospital identification band.
4. Determine whether the client's IV site is patent.

4. The nurse is administering medications to clients on a surgical unit. Which medication should the nurse administer **first**?
   1. Morphine IV infusion to the client 8 hours postoperative reporting pain, rating it as a 7 on a 1 to 10 pain scale
   2. Vancomycin intravenous piggyback (IVPB) to the client diagnosed with an infected abdominal wound
   3. Pantoprazole IVPB to the client at risk for developing a stress ulcer
   4. Furosemide intravenous push (IVP) to the client after surgical débridement of their right lower limb

5. The RN staff nurse and unlicensed assistive personnel (UAP) are caring for clients on a surgical unit. Which action by the UAP warrants **immediate** intervention?
   1. The UAP empties the indwelling catheter bag for the client recovering from transurethral resection of the prostate (TURP).
   2. The UAP assists a client to ambulate in the hall after an IV narcotic analgesic 30 minutes ago.
   3. The UAP provides apple juice to the client with a nephrectomy and just advanced to a clear liquid diet.
   4. The UAP applies moisture barrier cream to the elderly client diagnosed with urinary incontinence and an excoriated perianal area.

6. The RN charge nurse is making shift assignments to the surgical staff, which consists of two RNs, two licensed practical nurses (LPNs), and two UAP. Which assignment would be **most** appropriate for the RN charge nurse to make?
   1. Instruct the RN staff nurse to administer all PRN medications.
   2. Instruct the UAP to clean the recently vacated room.
   3. Assign the LPN to change the client's ileal conduit bag.
   4. Request the LPN to complete the admission for a new client.

7. The charge nurse is making assignments in the day surgery center. Which client should be assigned to the **most** experienced nurse?
   1. The 24-year-old client being prepared for discharge after a circumcision
   2. The client scheduled for a cystectomy now crying and upset about the surgery
   3. The client diagnosed with kidney cancer receiving 2 units of blood
   4. The client diagnosed with end-stage renal disease and with an arteriovenous fistula created

8. The nurse is completing the admission assessment on the client scheduled for cystectomy with creation of an ileal conduit. The client tells the nurse, "I am taking saw palmetto for my enlarged prostate." Which intervention should the nurse implement **first**?
   1. Notify the client's healthcare provider (HCP) to order the herbal supplement.
   2. Ask the client why they are taking an herb for their enlarged prostate.
   3. Consult with the pharmacist to determine any potential drug interactions.
   4. Look up saw palmetto in the *Physicians' Desk Reference* (PDR).

9. The client is upset because the HCP diagnosed them with syphilis. The client asks the nurse, "This is so embarrassing. Do you have to tell anyone about this?" Which statement is the nurse's **best** response?
   1. "Syphilis must be reported to the Public Health Department and your sexual partners."
   2. "According to HIPAA, I cannot report this to anyone without your permission."
   3. "You really should tell your sexual partners so they can be treated for syphilis."
   4. "I realize you are embarrassed. Would you want to talk about the situation?"

10. The RN primary nurse is caring for clients in the renal unit. Which task is **most** appropriate for the RN to delegate to the UAP?
    1. Instruct the UAP to calculate the clients' urinary intake and output.
    2. Request the UAP to double-check a unit of blood being administered.
    3. Tell the UAP to change the surgical dressing on the client with a kidney transplant.
    4. Ask the UAP to transfer the client from the renal unit to the intensive care unit (ICU).

11. The nurse is caring for clients on a renal unit and making assignments for the day shift. Which client should the nurse assess **first?**
    1. The client diagnosed with interstitial cystitis and urinary urgency reporting pain in the bladder
    2. The client diagnosed with acute post-streptococcal glomerulonephritis and hematuria with a smoky appearance
    3. The client diagnosed with Goodpasture syndrome, anemia, and renal failure with a pallor appearance
    4. The client diagnosed with nephrolithiasis and hematuria reporting pain, rating it as a 9 on a 1 to 10 pain scale

12. Which action by the LPN requires intervention by the critical care RN charge nurse?
    1. The LPN has the trough drawn after hanging the aminoglycoside.
    2. The LPN changes out a "sharps" container over the fill line.
    3. The LPN asks another nurse to observe the wastage of a narcotic.
    4. The LPN inserts an indwelling urinary catheter into the client.

13. The UAP informs the RN primary nurse that the client's urine output has bright red blood. Which intervention should the RN implement **first?**
    1. Instruct the UAP to take a urine specimen to the laboratory.
    2. Document the findings in the client's electronic health record (EHR) nursing notes.
    3. Assess the client's urine specimen and complete a renal assessment.
    4. Ask the UAP to take the client's vital signs.

14. The RN charge nurse is making client assignments. Which client should the charge nurse assign to the graduate nurse who has just finished orientation?
    1. The client with a cystectomy and the creation of an ileal conduit
    2. The client on continuous hemodialysis and awaiting a kidney transplant
    3. The client diagnosed with renal trauma secondary to a motor vehicle accident
    4. The client diagnosed with an eviscerated wound after abdominal surgery

15. The ICU charge nurse is notified of a bus accident with multiple injuries and victims are being brought to the emergency department (ED). The hospital is implementing a disaster policy. Which action should the nurse take **first?**
    1. Determine which clients could be discharged home immediately.
    2. Call any off-duty nurses to notify them to come into work.
    3. Assess staffing to determine which staff could be sent to the ED.
    4. Request all visitors to leave the hospital as soon as possible.

16. The 18-year-old client diagnosed with renal trauma is admitted to the critical care unit after a serious motor vehicle accident resulting from driving under the influence. The parent comes to the unit and starts yelling at their child about "driving drunk." Which action should the nurse implement?
    1. Allow the parent to continue talking to their child.
    2. Notify the hospital security to remove the parent.
    3. Escort the parent to a private area and talk to them.
    4. Tell the parent they must be quiet in order to stay.

17. The nurse is caring for a client diagnosed with benign prostatic hypertrophy. The client has undergone transurethral resection of the prostate (TURP) and is reporting bladder spasms. Which intervention should the nurse implement **first?**
    1. Administer an antispasmodic medication for bladder spasms.
    2. Calculate the client's urinary output.
    3. Palpate the client's abdomen for bladder distention.
    4. Assess the client's three-way urinary catheter for patency.

18. The nurse is caring for clients on a surgical unit. Which client should the nurse assess **first** after shift report?
    1. The client diagnosed with polycystic kidney disease with a blood pressure (BP) of 170/100 mm Hg
    2. The client diagnosed with bladder cancer and gross painless hematuria
    3. The client diagnosed with renal calculi reporting passing a stone
    4. The client diagnosed with acute pyelonephritis, with nausea and vomiting, and is dehydrated

19. The elderly client diagnosed with Alport syndrome asks the clinic nurse, "What should I do so I won't get sick this winter?" Which statements should the nurse include in the teaching? **Select all that apply.**
    1. "You should not be around any crowds during the winter months."
    2. "It is recommended you get a flu vaccine yearly."
    3. "You need to eat well-balanced meals each day."
    4. "Dress warmly when it is colder than 40°F (4.4°C) outside."
    5. "Wash your hands frequently throughout the day."

20. The elderly client tells the nurse, "I have vaginal dryness and it hurts when my partner and I make love." Which **priority** intervention should the nurse discuss with the client?
    1. Tell the client to discuss hormone replacement therapy with their HCP.
    2. Encourage the client to refrain from having sexual intercourse.
    3. Recommend the client use a vaginal lubricant before intercourse.
    4. Explain to the client that vaginal dryness is not uncommon in older adults.

21. The elderly client diagnosed with osteoporosis is prescribed alendronate. Which intervention is the **priority** when administering this medication?
    1. Administer the medication first thing in the morning.
    2. Ask the client whether they have a history of peptic ulcer disease.
    3. Encourage the client to walk for at least 30 minutes daily.
    4. Have the client remain upright for 30 minutes after administering the medication.

22. Which nursing task should the RN staff nurse on the renal unit assign to the LPN?
    1. Insert an indwelling urinary catheter for the client before surgery.
    2. Turn and reposition the client every 2 hours.
    3. Measure and record the urine in the bedside commode.
    4. Feed the client who choked on food during the client's last meal.

23. The nurse on a medical unit just received the evening shift report. Which client should the nurse assess **first**?
    1. The client diagnosed with renal vein thrombosis, with a heparin drip infusion, and a PTT of 92 seconds
    2. The client on peritoneal dialysis with clear dialysate draining from the abdomen
    3. The client on hemodialysis with an audible bruit in a right upper arm fistula
    4. The client diagnosed with cystitis reporting burning on urination

24. Which intervention should the nurse implement **first** when assisting the client diagnosed with a flaccid bladder to urinate?
    1. Perform the Credé's maneuver on the client.
    2. Perform intermittent catheterization on the client.
    3. Place the client on the bedside commode.
    4. Ask the client to drink a full glass of water.

25. The nurse is caring for clients in a family practice clinic. Which client should the nurse assess **first**?
    1. The client diagnosed with chronic pyelonephritis reporting costovertebral tenderness
    2. The client having burning and pain with urination
    3. The client diagnosed with urethritis reporting dysuria, urgency, and frequent urination
    4. The client with hesitancy, terminal dribbling, and intermittency

26. The RN clinic nurse and UAP are working in a family practice clinic. Which task should the RN delegate to the UAP?
    1. Give the client sample medications for a urinary tract infection (UTI).
    2. Show the client how to use a self-monitoring blood glucometer.
    3. Answer the telephone triage line and take messages from clients.
    4. Take the client's vital signs as part of a scheduled physical examination.

27. Which task is **most** appropriate for the RN staff nurse on the renal unit to delegate to the UAP?
    1. Escort the client diagnosed with acute pyelonephritis to radiology for a CT scan.
    2. Obtain a sterile urine specimen from the client to evaluate for urinary tract infection.
    3. Hang the bag of D_5W for the client diagnosed with post-streptococcal glomerulonephritis.
    4. Provide discharge instructions to the client diagnosed with nephrotic syndrome.

28. Which task should the employee health RN delegate to the UAP?
    1. Request the UAP read the PPD result administered to the client 72 hours ago.
    2. Ask the UAP to obtain a urine specimen from the client having drug screening.
    3. Tell the UAP to apply an ice pack to the client with a sprained right ankle after a fall.
    4. Instruct the UAP to complete an incident report for the RN with a "dirty needlestick."

29. The RN clinic nurse manager in the medical-surgical outpatient clinic is making assignments. Which task is **most** appropriate to delegate or assign to a UAP or LPN?
    1. Ask the LPN to administer the flu vaccine to the client.
    2. Tell the UAP to call the pharmacist to refill a prescription.
    3. Request the LPN to obtain the height and weight of the client.
    4. Instruct the UAP to empty the trashcans in the clients' rooms.

30. Which behavior **warrants** intervention by the RN clinical manager in the medical-surgical outpatient clinic?
    1. The UAP is discussing a client's condition in the waiting room.
    2. The LPN is talking to a client over the phone about laboratory tests.
    3. The RN is triaging phone messages during their lunch break.
    4. The UAP is taking vital signs for the client being placed in a room.

31. The UAP in the school nurse's office is listening to a student express fear about telling her parents she is pregnant. Which action should the RN school nurse implement?
    1. Tell the UAP they cannot talk to the student.
    2. Call the student's parents and report their daughter is pregnant.
    3. Do not take any action and allow the UAP to listen to the student.
    4. Ask the UAP to leave and continue to talk to the student.

32. The RN clinic nurse observes an LPN discussing an IV pyelogram, a diagnostic test, with a client in the waiting room of the outpatient clinic. Which action should the RN implement?
    1. Praise the LPN for discussing the diagnostic test with the client.
    2. The RN should tell the LPN to meet in the office area for a chat.
    3. Go to the waiting room and tell the LPN not to discuss this there.
    4. Inform the HCP that the LPN was talking to the client in the waiting room.

33. The charge nurse in a large outpatient clinic notices that the staff members are arguing and irritable, and the atmosphere has been very tense for the past week. Which action should the charge nurse take?
    1. Wait for another week to see whether the situation resolves itself.
    2. Write a memo telling all staff members to stop arguing.
    3. Schedule a meeting with the staff to discuss the situation.
    4. Tell the staff to stop arguing, or they will be terminated.

34. The employee health nurse is obtaining a urine specimen for a pre-employment drug screen. Which action should the nurse implement **first**?
    1. Obtain informed consent for the procedure.
    2. Maintain the chain of custody for the specimen.
    3. Allow the client to go to any bathroom in the clinic.
    4. Take and record the client's tympanic temperature.

35. The client comes to the clinic reporting pain and burning when urinating. Which action should the nurse implement **first**?
    1. Assess and document the client's vital signs.
    2. Determine whether the client has seen any blood in their urine.
    3. Request the client to give a midstream urine specimen.
    4. Ask the client whether they wipe front to back after a bowel movement.

36. The nurse is working at the emergency health clinic in a disaster shelter. Which intervention is the **priority** when initially assessing the client?
    1. Find out how long the client will be in the shelter.
    2. Determine whether the client has their routine medications.
    3. Document the client's health history in writing.
    4. Assess the client's vital signs, height, and weight.

37. The HCP orders an IV pyelogram for the 27-year-old client diagnosed with possible renal calculi. The client is diagnosed with schizophrenia and is delusional. Which action should the clinic nurse implement?
    1. Ask the client whether they are allergic to yeast.
    2. Request the client to sign a permit for the procedure.
    3. Obtain informed consent from the client's significant other.
    4. Discuss the local hospital's day surgery procedure with the client.

38. The home health aide tells the RN home health nurse that one of the older clients takes saw palmetto daily. Which statement is the RN's **best** response?
    1. "Herbal supplements are dangerous, and I will talk to the client about them."
    2. "Saw palmetto is used to treat benign prostatic hypertrophy. Let him take it."
    3. "I will notify the client's healthcare provider as soon as possible."
    4. "Many clients use herbal supplements. They have a right to take it."

39. The home health aide caring for the postoperative kidney transplant client asks the RN home health nurse, "Why is the physical therapist visiting the client?" Which statement is the home health RN's **best** response?
    1. "The physical therapist will evaluate the client's swallowing difficulty."
    2. "The physical therapist will assist the client with fine motor coordination."
    3. "The physical therapist will assist with caregiver concerns and making referrals."
    4. "The physical therapist will work with the client on strengthening and endurance."

40. The home health nurse is admitting a client diagnosed with end-stage renal disease, refusing hemodialysis. The client is ready to die but verbalizes having so many regrets in their life. Which intervention would be **most** appropriate for the nurse?
    1. Contact the agency chaplain to talk to the client.
    2. Call their church pastor and discuss the client's concerns.
    3. Ask the client if they want to pray with the nurse.
    4. Determine if the client has an advance directive.

41. The nurse is preparing to change a dressing on a client diagnosed with end-stage renal disease. The nurse notes the client's spouse silently holding the client's hand and praying. Which action should the nurse implement **first**?
    1. Continue to prepare for the dressing change in the room.
    2. Call the chaplain to help the client and spouse pray.
    3. Quietly leave the room and return later for the dressing change.
    4. Ask the spouse if they want the nurse to join the prayer.

42. The unit manager of the renal unit is evaluating the staff nurse. Which data should be included in the nurse's yearly evaluation? **Select all that apply.**
    1. The fact that the nurse clocked in late to work twice in the last year
    2. The client's complaint stating the nurse did not answer a call light during a code
    3. The number of times the nurse switched shifts with another nurse
    4. The appropriateness of the nurse's written documentation in the EHR
    5. The nurse's membership in the American Nephrology Nurses Association

43. The hospice nurse is providing follow-up care with the family member of a client who recently died from chronic renal disease. Which intervention is the **priority**?
    1. Attend the client's funeral service or visitation.
    2. Check on the family member 1 to 2 months after the client's death.
    3. Make sure the arrangements are what the client wants.
    4. Help the family member dispose of the client's belongings immediately.

44. The nurse is attempting to start an IV line in a dehydrated elderly client. After two unsuccessful attempts, which interventions should the nurse implement? **Select all that apply.**
    1. Keep trying to get a patent IV access.
    2. Ask the HCP to order oral fluid replacement.
    3. Ask a second nurse to attempt to start the IV line.
    4. Place cold packs on the client's arms for comfort.
    5. Obtain the portable vein finder device to assist the IV start.

45. The client diagnosed with chronic kidney disease (CKD) has a left forearm graft and is assigned to the RN primary nurse and UAP. Which action by the UAP requires **immediate** intervention by the RN?
    1. The UAP avoids using soap while bathing the client.
    2. The UAP takes the BP on the client's left arm.
    3. The UAP tells the client they should not eat chips.
    4. The UAP measures a scant amount of urine in the bedside commode.

46. The nurse is on the day shift in a long-term care facility.

Client Name: Mr. D.D. Height: 65 in (165.1 cm) Date of Birth: 78 years old	Account Number: 245869 Weight in lb: 165 Date: Today	Allergies: NKDA Weight in kg: 75
Medication	0701–1900	1901–0700
Digoxin 0.125 mg PO daily	0900	
Furosemide 40 mg PO daily	0900	
Potassium 20 mEq PO daily	0900 1800	
Biscacodyl 5 mg PO daily	0900	
Signature/Initials	Day Nurse RN/DN	Night Nurse RN/NN

    Which medication should the nurse **question** administering to the elderly client diagnosed with chronic pyelonephritis and heart failure?
    1. Digoxin
    2. Furosemide
    3. Potassium
    4. Bisacodyl

47. The elderly client diagnosed with heart failure is scheduled to receive a unit of packed red blood cells (PRBCs). The PRBCs are prepared in 350 mL of solution. At what rate should the nurse set the pump? _____

48. Which interventions should the RN staff nurse delegate to the UAP when caring for the client 2 days postoperative open nephrectomy? **Select all that apply.**
    1. Explain the procedure for using the patient-controlled analgesia (PCA) pump.
    2. Check the client's flank surgical dressing for drainage.
    3. Take and record the client's vital signs and pulse oximeter reading.
    4. Empty the client's indwelling catheter bag at the end of the shift.
    5. Assist the client to ambulate in the hallway three to four times a day.

49. After an open nephrectomy, the client has an apical pulse (AP) of 118 bpm and BP of 88/58 mm Hg. Which intervention should the nurse implement **first**?
    1. Obtain the client's pulse oximeter reading.
    2. Check the client's last hemoglobin and hematocrit.
    3. Notify the client's surgeon immediately.
    4. Monitor the client's urine output.

50. The 88-year-old client is reporting urinary frequency and dribbling. Which nursing interventions should be implemented? **Rank in order of performance.**
    1. Have the UAP make rounds on the client every 2 hours.
    2. Give the client perineal pads to place inside their underwear.
    3. Place an absorbent pad on the client's bed.
    4. Put a bedside commode at the client's bedside.
    5. Instruct the client in providing a clean-catch urine specimen.

51. The nurse in the dialysis center is initiating the morning dialysis run. Which client should the nurse assess **first?**
    1. The client with a hemoglobin of 9.0 mg/dL and hematocrit of 26%
    2. The client without a palpable thrill or auscultated bruit
    3. The client reporting a 3.6 kg (7.9 lb) weight gain and refusing dialysis
    4. The client on peritoneal dialysis reporting a hard, rigid abdomen

52. The client diagnosed with chronic kidney disease received their initial dose of erythropoietin 1 week ago. Which data **warrants** the nurse to notify the HCP?
    1. The client has a pulse oximeter reading of 95%.
    2. The client has a platelet count of 155,000/microL.
    3. The client has a blood pressure reading of 184/102 mm Hg.
    4. The client has a tympanic temperature of 99.8°F (37.7°C).

53. The client diagnosed with chronic kidney disease is placed on a fluid restriction of 1,500 mL (50.7 oz) per day. On the 7 a.m. to 7 p.m. shift the client drank an 8-oz cup of coffee, 8 oz of juice, 16 oz of tea, and 8 oz of water with medications. What amount of fluid can the 7 p.m. to 7 a.m. nurse give to the client? _____

54. The client receiving dialysis is reporting feeling dizzy and lightheaded. Which **priority** intervention should the nurse implement?
    1. Place the client in the reverse Trendelenburg position.
    2. Decrease the volume of blood being removed from the client.
    3. Administer a bolus of 300 mL of 0.9% saline solution to the client.
    4. Notify the HCP as soon as possible.

55. The client is NPO (nothing by mouth) and receiving total parenteral nutrition (TPN) via a subclavian line. Which precautions should the nurse implement? **Select all that apply.**
    1. Place the client's TPN on a gravity IV line.
    2. Monitor the client's blood glucose every 24 hours.
    3. Weigh the client daily, first thing in the morning.
    4. Change the client's IV tubing with every TPN bag administered.
    5. Monitor the client's intake and output every shift.

56. The client has received IV solutions for 3 days through a 20-gauge IV catheter placed in the left cephalic vein. On morning rounds the nurse notes the IV site is tender to palpation, edematous, and a red streak has formed. Which interventions should the nurse implement? **Rank in order of performance.**
    1. Start a new IV line in the right hand.
    2. Discontinue the IV line.
    3. Complete an incident report.
    4. Place a warm washcloth over the questionable IV site.
    5. Document the situation in the client's EHR.

57. The RN staff nurse and UAP are caring for a group of clients. Which nursing intervention should the RN perform?
    1. Measure the client's output from the indwelling catheter.
    2. Record the client's intake and output on the I&O sheet.
    3. Instruct the client on appropriate fluid restrictions.
    4. Provide water for a client diagnosed with acute pyelonephritis.

58. The nurse emptied 2,340 mL (79.1 oz) from the drainage bag of a continuous irrigation for the client recovering from a transurethral resection of the prostate (TURP). The amount of irrigation in the hanging bag was 3,000 mL (101.4 oz) at the beginning of the shift. There was 1,550 mL (52.4 oz) left in the bag 8 hours later. What is the correct urine output at the end of the 8 hours? _____

59. The client is 1-day postoperative TURP. Which action by the UAP **warrants** intervention by the RN staff nurse?
    1. The UAP increased the client's irrigation fluid to clear clots from the tubing.
    2. The UAP elevated the client's scrotum on a towel roll for support.
    3. The UAP emptied the client's indwelling urinary catheter bag.
    4. The UAP brought ice water to the client's bedside.

60. The client diagnosed with renal calculi is admitted to the medical unit. Which intervention should the nurse implement **first**?
    1. Request the client to urinate in a urinal.
    2. Assess the client's pain.
    3. Increase the client's oral fluid intake.
    4. Strain the client's urine.

61. The female client diagnosed with renal calculi is scheduled for a STAT kidney, ureter, bladder (KUB) study. Which statement by the client **warrants** intervention by the nurse?
    1. "I am allergic to shellfish and iodine."
    2. "I just had my lunch tray and ate all of it."
    3. "I have not had my period for 3 months."
    4. "I am having pain in my lower back."

62. The client diagnosed with renal calculi is scheduled for a 24-hour urine specimen collection. Which interventions should the nurse implement? **Select all that apply.**
    1. Keep the client NPO during the time the urine is being collected.
    2. Instruct the client to urinate, and include this urine when starting collection.
    3. Place the client's urine in an appropriate specimen container for 24 hours.
    4. Insert an indwelling catheter in the client after having the client empty their bladder.
    5. Post signs on the client's door alerting staff to save all the client's urine output.

63. The client diagnosed with renal calculi is 1-hour postprocedure lithotripsy. Which task is **most** appropriate for the RN primary nurse to delegate to the UAP?
    1. Tell the UAP to check the amount, color, and consistency of the client's urine output.
    2. Request the UAP to transcribe the client's HCP orders.
    3. Instruct the UAP to strain the client's urine and place any sediment in a sterile container.
    4. Ask the UAP to take the client's postprocedural vital signs.

64. The client had surgery to remove a kidney stone. Which laboratory assessment data **warrants** intervention by the nurse?
    1. A serum potassium level of 5.2 mEq/L
    2. A urinalysis showing blood in the urine
    3. A creatinine level of 1.0 mg/dL
    4. A white blood cell (WBC) count of 9.5×10^3/microL

65. Which intervention should the nurse implement **first** for the client diagnosed with urinary incontinence?
    1. Palpate the bladder after an incontinent episode.
    2. Administer oxybutynin.
    3. Ensure the client does not sit or lie in the urine.
    4. Instruct the client to go to the bathroom every 2 hours.

66. The nurse is caring for an elderly client with an indwelling catheter. Which data **warrant** notifying the HCP?
    1. Vital signs are T 98°F (36.7°C), AP 90 bpm, RR 16 breaths/min, BP 142/88 mm Hg.
    2. The client has had a change in mental status.
    3. The client's urine is cloudy with sediment.
    4. The client has no discomfort or pain.

67. The RN primary nurse is observing the UAP provide care for a client with an indwelling catheter. Which action by the UAP warrants **immediate** intervention by the RN?
    1. The UAP does not secure the tubing to the client's leg.
    2. The UAP wears gloves when providing catheter care to the client.
    3. The UAP positions the collection bag on the side of the client's bed.
    4. The UAP cares for the client's catheter after washing their hands.

68. The RN and the UAP are caring for clients on the unit. Which nursing task would be **most** appropriate for the RN to delegate to the UAP?
    1. Assist the radiology technician with a portable chest x-ray on an obese client.
    2. Evaluate the elderly client's 8-hour intake and output.
    3. Perform in and out catheterization on an adolescent client for a sterile urine specimen.
    4. Administer a cation-exchange resin enema on a 51-year-old client.

69. The RN is preparing to perform hemodialysis on a depressed middle age client diagnosed with end-stage renal disease (ESRD). Which data warrant **immediate** intervention from the RN?
    1. A hemoglobin of 9.8 mg/dL and hematocrit of 30%
    2. Inability to palpate a thrill or auscultate a bruit
    3. The client reporting being exhausted and unable to sleep
    4. No urine output in the past 12 hours

70. The client diagnosed with renal cell carcinoma is 1-day postoperative cystectomy and has a nasogastric tube in place. The client's IV is running at 150 mL/hr via an IV pump. Which data should the RN report to the HCP?
    1. The client's peripheral IV access is infiltrated.
    2. The client has hypoactive bowel sounds.
    3. The client has crackles bilaterally in the lower lobes.
    4. The client has 2+ bilateral pedal pulses.

71. The elderly client is diagnosed with chronic glomerulonephritis. Which lab value indicates the condition has worsened?
    1. The blood urea nitrogen (BUN) is 18 mg/dL.
    2. The creatinine level is 1.0 mg/dL.
    3. The glomerular filtration rate (GFR) is 60 mL/min.
    4. The 24-hour creatinine clearance is 113 mL/min.

72. The UAP emptied 3,000 mL (101.4 oz) from the drainage bag of a continuous bladder irrigation (CBI) for a 75-year-old client recovering from a TURP. The amount of irrigation in the bag hanging was 4,000 mL (135.3 oz) at the beginning of the shift. There was 2,000 mL (67.6 oz) left in the bag at 0700. What is the corrected urine volume output for the shift? _____

73. The elderly client returned from surgery after having a TURP and has P 96 bpm, R 20 breaths/min, BP 110/70 mm Hg, and light pink urine draining in the indwelling urinary catheter bag. Which interventions should the RN implement? **Select all that apply.**
    1. Assess the urine in the continuous irrigation drainage bag.
    2. Increase the irrigation fluid in the continuous irrigation catheter.
    3. Lower the head of the bed while raising the foot of the bed (Trendelenburg).
    4. Contact the surgeon to give an update on the client's condition.
    5. Monitor the client's postoperative hematocrit and hemoglobin.

74. The charge nurse is making rounds on clients in the renal unit. Which client should the charge nurse assess **first?**
    1. The depressed client diagnosed with end-stage renal disease on hemodialysis and with a palpable thrill
    2. The young client diagnosed with acute glomerulonephritis having hematuria and proteinuria
    3. The elderly client diagnosed with bladder cancer having bright red painless urination
    4. The malnourished client with an ileal conduit and no drainage in the drainage bag

75. The RN staff nurse and the LPN are caring for clients on the renal unit. Which intervention should the RN assign to the LPN?
    1. Teach the elderly client about home care of the suprapubic catheter.
    2. Monitor the obese postoperative client with a WBC count of 22 x 10 3/microL.
    3. Administer antineoplastic medications to the client diagnosed with bladder cancer.
    4. Administer a narcotic analgesic to the client diagnosed with renal calculi.

RENAL AND GENITOURINARY CASE STUDY

(0950) The nurse in a pediatrician's/HCP's office sees a 3-year old male client. While holding the client the mother describes a loss of appetite for the last 2 days, and this morning the child was lethargic, thirsty, and vomited. The client is tearful, flushed, irritable, and diaphoretic. Initial assessment findings including vital signs are shared with the HCP. The HCP requests a STAT urinalysis—straight catheterization if needed—to be done in the office.

Vital Signs	Client Values
Blood pressure	94/52 mm Hg
Heart rate	136 bpm
Respirations	30 breaths/min
Temperature	103.8°F (39.9°C)
SpO$_2$	95% on room air

(1025) The nurse asks the client's mother if she thinks the client can urinate into the specimen container. She states "he was almost potty trained but I put a diaper on him to come here"; diaper is dry. She asks the client if he can void but the client is lethargic and sleepy. The nurse instructs the mother on the procedure to straight cath for a urine sample; she agrees and asks if she can stay in the room. With the assistance of two nurses and the client's mother, a straight catheterization is performed, with 100 mL of dark cloudy urine obtained and given to the onsite lab. Emotional support is provided to both client and mother. Client is offered a hydration-replacement frozen treat but refuses.

(1045) Urinalysis results reported to HCP:

Urinalysis	Results
Color	Dark amber
Clarity	Cloudy
RBCs	6
WBCs	10–12
Nitrates	Present
Specific gravity	1.038

(1110) The nurse returns with the HCP who recommends the client be admitted to the local children's hospital for fluid replacement and treatment of a urinary tract infection (UTI). The mother is tearful but agrees with the plan and requests to go home and contact the client's father and they will both take the client within the next hour. The HCP advises the mother to have the emergency department (ED) HCP call the office for direct admit orders. The mother verbalizes understanding and agreement.

(1225) The nurse in the ED receives the client accompanied by both parents. The ED HCP contacts the pediatrician and obtains the following admission orders:

PROVIDER ORDERS:

Admit to medical unit: UTI, dehydration
IV 0.9% NaCl @ 50 mL/hr
Ampicillin 50 mg/kg/day in equally divided doses every 8 hours IV
Complete blood count (CBC) and basal metabolic panel (BMP) daily
Acetaminophen 120 mg every 6 hours PO PRN temperature >100.5°F (38.2°C)
Regular diet as tolerated—encourage PO fluids
Up with assist

(1240) Report called to unit nurse and client transported to medical unit for admission.

(1300) Admission assessment completed and IV started in left forearm #26 gauge—client tearful but cooperative. Parents at bedside. Client is lethargic and flushed with cool skin, and diaphoresis. Vital signs shown below. Client bed weight = 35 kg.

Vital Signs	Client Values
Blood pressure	92/54 mm Hg
Heart rate	140 bpm
Respirations	30 breaths/min
Temperature	103.8°F (39.9°C)
SpO_2	96% on room air

1. **Recognize cues. What matters most?** The nurse prepares to call the ED physician. Select the two highest-priority client assessments the nurse needs before administering medication(s).
   1. 24-hour intake
   2. Allergies
   3. Number of wet diapers/voids
   4. Weight
   5. Height
   6. Favorite cartoon
   7. Type of toys preferred

2. **Analyze cues. What could it mean?** For each client finding, indicate whether it is consistent with the disease process of UTI, dehydration, or shock. Each finding may support more than one condition.

Finding	UTI	Dehydration	Shock
Pallor			
Lethargy			
Vomiting			
Diaphoresis			
Irritability			
Temperature			
Thirst			
Urine specific gravity			
Urinary output			

(1400) Topical numbing cream applied predraw per facility protocol. Sample for CBC and BMP drawn with one successful attempt from client's right antecubital vein. Client tolerated procedure fair. Parents at bedside providing emotional support and encouragement to take PO fluids/popsicles.

(1500) Laboratory results posted to the EHR.

Laboratory Test	Client Values	Reference Values (3–6 years)
Hemoglobin (Hgb)	15 g/dL	11.5–14.5 g/dL
Hematocrit (Hct)	38%	34%–40%
White blood cell (WBC)	17×10^3/microL	5 to 14.5×10^3/microL
Platelets	160	150 to 450×10^3/microL
Creatinine	0.48 mg/dL	0.21 to 0.49 mg/dL
Glucose	208 mg/dL	70-110 mg/dL
Potassium	5.0 mEq/L	3.5-5.5 mEq/L or mmol/L
Sodium	141 mEq/L	135 to 145 mEq/L or mmol/L
Blood urea nitrogen (BUN)	25 mg/dL	5 to 25 mg/dL

3. **Prioritize hypotheses. Where do I start?** Complete the sentence by choosing from the drop-down list of options. Based on the client's condition at this time, the nurse recognizes that the client is at the highest risk for _____

   > Select
   > 1. Injury (falls)
   > 2. Cardiac arrest
   > 3. Urosepsis

   and will require _____

   > Select
   > 1. Telemetry monitoring
   > 2. Antibiotics
   > 3. Bedrest

4. **Generate solutions. What can I do?** For each intervention, specify whether the intervention is **indicated** or **not indicated** for the client's care.

Potential Nursing Intervention	Indicated	Not Indicated
Maintain IV 0.9% NaCLl at 50 mL/hr		
Review the "rooming in" policy with the parents		
Discourage play with other toddlers in common area		
Confirm ampicillin dosage calculation		
Reorient the client as needed		
Administer ampicillin		
Administer acetaminophen		
Encourage PO fluid intake		
Instruct parents to keep track of client's output		

5. **Take action. What will I do?** Which **four** admission orders should the nurse consider priority actions? **Select all that apply.**
   1. Maintain IV 0.9% NaCl at 50 mL/hr.
   2. Review the "rooming in" policy with the parents.
   3. Discourage play with other toddlers in common area.
   4. Confirm ampicillin dosage calculation.
   5. Administer ampicillin.
   6. Administer acetaminophen.
   7. Encourage PO fluid intake.
   8. Instruct parents to keep track of client's output.

(1835) The nurse conducts a reassessment in preparation for shift change. Client is awake watching cartoons with the mother. Skin is pale and cool, lungs clear and abdomen soft with bowel sounds ×4 quadrants. IV infusing in left forearm without redness, edema, or coolness. Client does not respond when asked about pain; the parent states "I don't think so" when asked. Intake = IV 225 mL, PO 150 mL; output = no bowel movement, 1 wet diaper. Vital signs shown below.

Vital Signs	Client Values
Blood pressure	94/56 mm Hg
Heart rate	138 bpm
Respirations	28 breaths/min
Temperature	102.6°F (39.2°C)
SpO_2	96% on room air

6. **Evaluate outcomes. Did it help?** For each assessment finding, indicate whether the client's condition has improved, declined, or no change.

Finding	Improved	Declined	No Change
Blood pressure			
Heart rate			
Respirations			
Temperature			
SpO_2			
Level of consciousness			

ANSWERS AND RATIONALES

The correct answer number and rationale are in **bold-face purple type.** Rationales for why other answer options are incorrect are also given.

1. 1. The nurse would expect the client diagnosed with acute glomerulonephritis to have oliguria and periorbital edema. Acute glomerulonephritis is a disorder of the glomeruli (glomerulonephritis) or small blood vessels in the kidneys.
   2. **The nurse would not expect the client diagnosed with BPH to have oozing blood from the IV site. This may indicate disseminated intravascular coagulation (DIC), which is a potentially life-threatening complication and requires immediate intervention.**
   3. The nurse would expect the client diagnosed with renal calculi to have pain, but a level 5 indicates the pain is under control; therefore, this client does not need to be seen first.
   4. The nurse would expect the client diagnosed with nephrotic syndrome to have proteinuria (protein in the urine) and hypoalbuminemia (decreased protein in the blood). Nephrotic syndrome is a nonspecific disorder in which the kidneys are damaged, causing them to leak large amounts of protein into the urine.

   CLINICAL JUDGMENT GUIDE: The nurse must determine which sign or symptom is not expected for the disease process. If the sign or symptom is not expected, or if it is an emergency situation, the nurse should assess the client first. This question determines whether the nurse knows the clinical manifestations of various disease processes.

2. 1. This is an appropriate question, but even clients diagnosed with prostate problems can have an indwelling catheter if inserted carefully.
   2. **Povidone-iodine (Betadine) is included in the indwelling catheter kit. Therefore, the nurse's first intervention is to check for allergies to determine whether another cleaning agent must be used.**
   3. This is appropriate but not the first intervention.
   4. Urine should be obtained in the catheter, but it is not the first intervention.

   CLINICAL JUDGMENT GUIDE: When the question asks, "Which intervention should be implemented first?" it means all the options are things a nurse could do, but only one should be done first. The nurse should use the nursing process and remember: If the client is in distress, do not assess; if the client is not in distress, the nurse should assess.

3. 1. The nurse should clamp the tubing to ensure the medication goes directly into the client and not retrograde up the tubing, but it is not the first administration.
   2. The medication should be administered over 2 minutes, but it is not the first intervention.
   3. The nurse should always ensure the medication is being administered to the correct client, but the nurse should first make sure the route of administration is safe.
   4. **Ensuring the site is patent is the first intervention because even if it is the correct client, the medication should not be administered if the IV site is infiltrated.**

   CLINICAL JUDGMENT GUIDE: When the question asks, "Which intervention should be implemented first?" it means all the options are things a nurse could implement, but only one should be implemented first. The nurse should use the nursing process and remember: If the client is in distress, do not assess; if the client is not in distress, the nurse should assess.

4. 1. **The client in pain is the priority. None of the other clients have a life-threatening condition. Pain is considered the fifth vital sign.**
   2. Routine antibiotics are not a priority over a client with postoperative pain.
   3. The risk for a stress ulcer is a potential, not an actual, problem, and proton-pump inhibitors are administered routinely to help prevent stress ulcers.
   4. The loop diuretic is a routine medication prescribed for a medical comorbid condition, not for surgical débridement.

   CLINICAL JUDGMENT GUIDE: When the nurse is making a decision about prioritizing medication administration, client comfort takes priority over regularly scheduled medications.

5. 1. The UAP can empty an indwelling catheter drainage bag because this does not require judgment.
   2. **The client who received a narcotic analgesic 30 minutes ago is at risk of falling because of the effects of the medication; therefore, the UAP should not ambulate this client. The nurse should intervene.**
   3. The UAP can provide juice to the client; apple juice is part of the client's liquid diet.
   4. Moisture barrier cream is not a medication; therefore, the UAP can apply such creams to an intact perianal area.

CLINICAL JUDGMENT GUIDE: The nurse cannot delegate assessment, evaluation, teaching, administration of medications, or an unstable client to a UAP.

6. 1. The LPN can administer routine and some PRN medications; assigning the LPN to administer all PRN medications is inappropriate.
   2. The housekeeping department, not the UAP, is assigned to clean recently vacated rooms.
   3. It is within an LPN's scope of practice to change an ileal conduit drainage bag; therefore, this would be the most appropriate assignment for the LPN.
   4. The nurse would be the most appropriate staff member to complete the admission assessment.

CLINICAL JUDGMENT GUIDE: When the nurse is deciding which option is the most appropriate task to delegate or assign, the nurse should choose the task that allows each staff member to function within their scope of practice. Remember, the nurse cannot delegate assessment, teaching, evaluation, medications, or an unstable client to the UAP and cannot assign assessment, teaching, evaluation, or an unstable client to the LPN.

7. 1. The most experienced nurse should be assigned to the client requiring teaching before discharge. Postoperative complications can occur, so the client must know when to call the HCP and how to take care of the surgical site.
   2. A less experienced nurse can talk to the crying and upset client. The most experienced nurse should care for a client requiring more knowledge.
   3. A less experienced nurse can administer and monitor a blood transfusion to the client.
   4. Although the creation of an arteriovenous fistula requires assessment and teaching from the most experienced nurse, this client is not being discharged home at this time.

CLINICAL JUDGMENT GUIDE: The nurse must determine which client is the most unstable or requires extensive teaching. This client requires the most experienced nurse, thus making this type of question an "except" question. Three clients are either stable or have non-life-threatening conditions.

8. 1. If the HCP deems that the client can continue to take the herbal supplement, then an order must be written; however, this is not the first intervention.
   2. The nurse could ask for clarification of the reason he is taking the herbal supplement, but this is not the first intervention. Many clients use herbal supplements for a variety of healthcare needs.
   3. The nurse should first consult with the pharmacist to determine whether the client is taking medications that could interact with the saw palmetto.
   4. The PDR is available to research medications, not herbal supplements.

CLINICAL JUDGMENT GUIDE: According to the NCSBN NCLEX-RN® test plan, collaboration with interdisciplinary team members is part of the management of care. The nurse must be knowledgeable regarding interventions when administering medications to clients undergoing surgery, such as the client should not receive any PO medications, the client should not receive any medications that could increase bleeding, or determining whether the client is taking any complementary alternative medications, such as herbs.

9. 1. HIPAA does not apply in some situations, including the reporting of sexually transmitted diseases to the Public Health Department. The Public Health Department will attempt to notify any sexual partners the client reports.
   2. This is a false statement. HIPAA does not apply in certain situations, and the nurse must know about HIPAA guidelines.
   3. The client should notify her sexual partners so they can be treated; however, in response to the client asking, "Does anyone have to know?" the nurse's best response is to provide facts.
   4. This is a therapeutic response to encourage the client to verbalize feelings, but the nurse should provide factual information in this situation.

CLINICAL JUDGMENT GUIDE: There will be management questions on the NCLEX-RN®. There is often no test-taking strategy for these questions; the nurse must be knowledgeable of management issues. The Health Insurance Portability and Accountability Act (HIPAA) was passed into law in 1996 to standardize the exchange of information between HCPs and to ensure patient record confidentiality.

10. 1. The UAP can calculate client intake and output. The UAP cannot evaluate the numbers to determine whether the treatment is effective but can obtain the numbers.

2. Two nurses must double-check a unit of blood before infusing the blood; therefore, this task cannot be delegated.
3. The surgeon or the nurse must change the surgical dressing for a kidney transplant. This task cannot be delegated to personnel with a lower level of expertise.
4. The UAP cannot transfer the unstable client from the renal unit to the intensive care unit.

CLINICAL JUDGMENT GUIDE: An RN cannot delegate assessment, teaching, evaluation, medications, or an unstable client to a UAP. Tasks requiring nursing judgment cannot be delegated.

11. 1. Interstitial cystitis is a chronic, painful inflammatory disease of the bladder characterized by urgency or frequency and pain in the bladder or pelvis. Because the clinical manifestations are expected, the nurse would not assess this client first.
    2. The clinical manifestations of acute post-streptococcal glomerulonephritis are varied, including generalized body edema, hypertension, oliguria, hematuria with a smoky or rusty appearance, and proteinuria. Because the clinical manifestations are expected, the nurse would not assess this client first.
    3. Goodpasture syndrome is a rare autoimmune disease seen primarily in young male smokers characterized by hematuria, weakness, pallor, anemia, and renal failure. Because the clinical manifestations are expected, the nurse would not assess this client first.
    4. **Nephrolithiasis (kidney stones) is characterized by pain and hematuria, but the nurse must assess the pain to determine whether a complication has occurred or it is the expected routine pain. Pain is the shared priority of these four clients.**

CLINICAL JUDGMENT GUIDE: The nurse can use Maslow's Hierarchy of Needs to determine which client to assess first. Pain is a physiological need.

12. 1. **The trough should be drawn before administering the aminoglycoside antibiotic, vancomycin. This requires intervention by the critical care charge nurse.**
    2. The LPN should change out a "sharps" container that is full; if not changed, this constitutes an OSHA violation.
    3. The LPN must have a narcotic wastage observed by another nurse.
    4. The LPN can insert an indwelling urinary catheter in their scope of practice.

CLINICAL JUDGMENT GUIDE: The nurse must know the scope of practice for the LPN. The nurse must know the correct medication administration procedure for the client and OSHA (Occupational Safety and Health Administration) standards.

13. 1. The UAP can take a specimen to the laboratory, but this is not the first intervention.
    2. The findings should be documented in the nurse's notes, but it is not the first intervention.
    3. **The nurse must first assess the UAP's findings and the client before taking any further action.**
    4. The UAP can take the client's vital signs, but it is not the first intervention for the nurse.

CLINICAL JUDGMENT GUIDE: A rule of thumb when answering test questions is this: If anyone gives the nurse information about a client, the nurse's first intervention is to assess the client. The nurse should always make decisions based on their assessment of the client.

14. 1. **Although cystectomy is a major surgical procedure, it has a predictable course, and no complications were identified. After removing the bladder, the client must have an ileal conduit. This is expected with this type of surgery and the new graduate nurse could be assigned this client.**
    2. A client on continuous hemodialysis would require a nurse trained in this area of nursing; therefore, this client should be assigned to a more experienced nurse.
    3. Renal trauma is unpredictable and requires continuous assessment. A more experienced nurse should be assigned to this client.
    4. An eviscerated wound indicates the client's incision has opened and the bowels are out of the abdomen. This client is critically ill and should not be assigned to an inexperienced nurse.

CLINICAL JUDGMENT GUIDE: When the test taker is deciding which client should be assigned to a new graduate, the most stable client should be assigned to the least experienced nurse.

15. 1. The charge nurse should have as many available beds as possible for clients requiring transfer to the unit. The charge nurse should send a nurse to the ED and then assess the bed situation.
    2. This may need to be done, but it is not the first intervention, and the charge nurse could assign this to a staff member who is not providing direct client care.

3. Most disaster policies require one nurse to be sent immediately from each area; therefore, this intervention should be implemented first. The charge nurse must determine which staff nurse would be most helpful in the ED without compromising the staffing in the ICU.
4. The charge nurse should not request anyone to leave the hospital. This is not typical protocol for a disaster.

CLINICAL JUDGMENT GUIDE: The nurse must be knowledgeable regarding emergency preparedness. Employees receive this information in employee orientation and are responsible for implementing procedures correctly. The NCSBN NCLEX-RN® test plan includes questions on a safe and effective care environment.

16. 1. The nurse must diffuse the situation and remove the parent from the client's room because a seriously ill client does not need to be yelled at.
    2. Hospital security does not need to be called unless the parent refuses to leave the client's room in the critical care unit.
    3. The nurse should remove the parent from the room and allow them to vent feelings about the injury their child sustained while under the influence.
    4. The nurse should remove the parent because they are upset and let them vent. Telling the parent they must be quiet is condescending. When someone is upset, telling the person to be quiet is not helpful.

CLINICAL JUDGMENT GUIDE: The NCLEX-RN® test plan includes Therapeutic Communication as a subcategory in Psychosocial Integrity. The nurse should allow clients and families to vent their feelings.

17. 1. The nurse may need to administer an antispasmodic medication, but not before assessment of the client. Bladder spasms in a client after a TURP are usually caused by clots remaining in the bladder. A three-way indwelling catheter that is working correctly will flush the clots from the bladder.
    2. The nurse should calculate the client's urine output, but that is not the first intervention and will not address the client's pain.
    3. The nurse could palpate the client's bladder for distention, but this will not help decrease the client's pain.
    4. The three-way indwelling catheter is placed during surgery to keep blood clots from remaining in the bladder and causing bladder spasms and increasing bleeding. The nurse should first assess the drainage system to ensure it has not become obstructed by a clot.

CLINICAL JUDGMENT GUIDE: The test taker should use a systematic guide when deciding on a priority intervention. The nursing process is an excellent tool for the test taker to use in this question. Assessment is the first step of the nursing process.

18. 1. The client diagnosed with polycystic kidney disease, the most common life-threatening genetic disease in the world, is expected to have hypertension along with hematuria and a feeling of heaviness in the back, side, or abdomen. The nurse should not assess this client first because the clinical manifestations are expected.
    2. The clinical manifestation of bladder cancer is painless gross hematuria; therefore, the nurse would not assess this client first.
    3. The nurse should check to determine whether the client has passed a stone, but this is a desired outcome and could wait until the client with an emergency has been assessed and appropriate interventions initiated.
    4. The client diagnosed with acute pyelonephritis, an inflammation of the renal parenchyma and collecting system, is not expected to get dehydrated; therefore, this client should be assessed first.

CLINICAL JUDGMENT GUIDE: The test taker must read all the options to determine whether an option contains a life-threatening situation. If an option contains expected information or values within normal limits, that client does not have priority.

19. Correct answers are 2, 3, 4, and 5.
    1. Avoiding all crowds may help the elderly client avoid getting a cold or the flu, but it is not usually possible and can be detrimental mentally and physically to the client.
    2. The yearly flu shot helps prevent getting sick during the winter months, because the flu can cause serious illness and even death in the elderly. Alport syndrome is also known as hereditary nephritis.
    3. Eating a well-balanced diet is essential to maintain health and support a healthy immune system.
    4. Dressing appropriately in winter is important as poor circulation can cause distress and impact immunity in older adults.
    5. Frequent hand washing can help avoid illness and prevent spreading germs to others.

CLINICAL JUDGMENT GUIDE: This is an alternate type of question included in the NCLEX-RN®. The nurse must select all the options that answer the question correctly. The nurse must be able to teach health promotion to clients. Immunizations are a priority for children and older adults.

20. 1. Hormone replacement therapy may be needed, but not because of vaginal dryness. The client should discuss this with her HCP, but it does not address the client's statement.
    2. Many elderly people are sexually active and sexual activity should be encouraged, not discouraged, by the nurse.
    3. Vaginal lubricant will help with the vaginal dryness and help decrease pain during sexual intercourse.
    4. Vaginal dryness is common in the elderly, but the nurse should discuss ways to address the dryness, not explain that it is normal.

CLINICAL JUDGMENT GUIDE: When the question asks for the priority intervention, it means one or more of the options could be something a nurse might discuss with the client. The test taker should select the option that directly answers the client's statement.

21. 1. The bisphosphonate medication alendronate (Fosamax) should be administered in the morning on an empty stomach to increase absorption, but it is not a priority over the client's sitting up for 30 minutes. The client should remain upright for at least 30 minutes to prevent regurgitation into the esophagus and esophageal erosion.
    2. The client diagnosed with peptic ulcer disease may be more at risk for esophageal erosion, but the HCP should have assessed this before prescribing this medication for the client.
    3. The client diagnosed with osteoporosis should be encouraged to walk to increase bone density, but this is not pertinent when administering the medication.
    4. The bisphosphonate medication alendronate (Fosamax) should be administered on an empty stomach with a full glass of water to promote absorption of the medication. The client should remain upright for at least 30 minutes to prevent regurgitation into the esophagus and esophageal erosion.

CLINICAL JUDGMENT GUIDE: The nurse must be aware of interventions that must be implemented when administering medications. The nurse must know which interventions will help prevent untoward complications when administering medications.

22. 1. The LPN is qualified to perform a sterile procedure, such as inserting an indwelling catheter before surgery. This is an appropriate assignment.
    2. Turning and repositioning a client can be delegated to a UAP.
    3. Emptying a client's bedside commode and recording the amount of urine can be delegated to a UAP.
    4. The nurse should feed the client who choked during their last meal to assess the client's ability to swallow. This client is unstable and cannot be assigned or delegated.

CLINICAL JUDGMENT GUIDE: The nurse cannot delegate or assign assessment, teaching, evaluation, or an unstable client to an LPN. The LPN can transcribe HCP orders, call HCPs to obtain orders, and perform sterile procedures.

23. 1. The therapeutic PTT level of a client on heparin should be 1.5 to 2 times the normal PTT of 39 seconds. The therapeutic levels in this case are 58 and 78 seconds. With a PTT of 92 seconds, the client is at risk for bleeding, and the heparin drip should be held. The nurse should assess this client first.
    2. The client on peritoneal dialysis should have clear dialysate so this client does not have to be assessed first.
    3. The client on hemodialysis should have an audible bruit over the fistula, which indicates the fistula is patent.
    4. Cystitis is inflammation of the urinary bladder, and burning on urination is an expected symptom.

CLINICAL JUDGMENT GUIDE: The test taker must determine whether any assessment data are normal or abnormal for the client's diagnosis. If the data are abnormal, then this client should be seen first.

24. 1. Credé's maneuver is used to express urine by pressing the hand on the bladder, especially a paralyzed bladder. It is a noninvasive procedure and should be implemented first before catheterization, which is an invasive procedure.
    2. Intermittent catheterization is an invasive procedure that may lead to possible infection when done every 3 to 4 hours.

3. The nurse could place the client on the bedside commode, which is used for clients diagnosed with uninhibited bladder patterns.
4. Drinking water before attempting to urinate will not help the client.

CLINICAL JUDGMENT GUIDE: If the nurse is undecided between an invasive and a noninvasive procedure, the nurse should select the noninvasive procedure first.

25. 1. The client diagnosed with pyelonephritis typically presents with costovertebral tenderness over the affected side; therefore, this is expected, and the nurse would not assess this client first.
    2. This client likely has a urinary tract infection, which requires a midstream urinalysis. Of these four clients, this client should be seen first to have the test ordered.
    3. The client diagnosed with urethritis would present with these symptoms; therefore, the clinic nurse would not need to see this client first.
    4. Hesitancy, terminal dribbling, and intermittency are clinical manifestations of BPH, which may require surgery; therefore, this client should not be seen before a client diagnosed with a possible urinary tract infection.

CLINICAL JUDGMENT GUIDE: When deciding which client to assess first, the test taker should determine whether the clinical manifestations the client is exhibiting are normal for the client's situation. After eliminating the expected options, the test taker should determine which situation can be cured and which is more life-threatening.

26. 1. The nurse should not delegate medication administration, including giving the client boxes of sample medications, to a UAP.
    2. Showing the client how to use a glucometer is teaching the client, and the nurse cannot delegate teaching.
    3. Triaging calls requires nursing judgment; this responsibility cannot be delegated to the UAP.
    4. The UAP is trained to take the vital signs of a stable client. This task can be safely delegated by the nurse.

CLINICAL JUDGMENT GUIDE: The nurse cannot delegate assessment, evaluation, teaching, administration of medications, or care of an unstable client to a UAP.

27. 1. The UAP can escort a stable client to the radiology department; therefore, this is the most appropriate task to delegate to the UAP.
    2. The UAP cannot obtain a sterile specimen; therefore, this task cannot be delegated.
    3. The UAP cannot hang IV bags because they are medications, and medication administration cannot be delegated to a UAP.
    4. Discharge instructions are teaching, and teaching cannot be delegated to a UAP.

CLINICAL JUDGMENT GUIDE: An RN cannot delegate assessment, teaching, evaluation, medications, or an unstable client to a UAP. Tasks that cannot be delegated are nursing interventions requiring nursing judgment.

28. 1. The UAP cannot administer medication or evaluate the effectiveness of medication; therefore, this task cannot be delegated.
    2. This legal issue should not be delegated to the UAP.
    3. The UAP can apply ice to the right ankle because the client is stable.
    4. The nurse should complete the incident report, not the UAP.

CLINICAL JUDGMENT GUIDE: The nurse cannot delegate assessment, teaching, evaluation, medications, or an unstable client to the UAP. Remember, most forms should be completed by the individual the form is about, not by someone unaware of the situation.

29. 1. The LPN can administer medication to the client; therefore, this assignment is appropriate.
    2. The UAP cannot call in prescription refills to the pharmacist.
    3. The LPN can obtain the weight and height of a client, but the UAP can do this task, so it is more appropriate to delegate it to the UAP.
    4. The UAP can empty the trashcans, but the custodian or housekeeper would be a more appropriate delegation of this task.

CLINICAL JUDGMENT GUIDE: The nurse cannot delegate assessment, teaching, evaluation, medications, or an unstable client to the UAP. The nurse cannot assign assessment, teaching, evaluation, or an unstable client to the LPN. Remember to delegate or assign the task to the least educated person capable of doing the task safely.

30. 1. The UAP is violating HIPAA rules concerning confidentiality, so the clinical manager should intervene.
    2. The LPN can talk to the client over the phone about laboratory tests so this does not warrant intervention.
    3. The RN can triage phone messages, so this does not warrant intervention.
    4. The UAP can take the vital signs on a stable client. Clients in an outpatient clinic are considered stable unless otherwise specified.

    CLINICAL JUDGMENT GUIDE: The nurse is responsible for the actions and behavior of UAPs and LPNs working in the unit. The nurse must correct behavior as needed.

31. 1. The UAP is a healthcare team member and should be able to listen to a student's concerns.
    2. The nurse cannot violate the student's rights, even in the school nurse setting.
    3. The nurse should allow the UAP to continue to talk to the student, and then the nurse can speak to the student.
    4. The UAP has established a relationship with the student and should be allowed to talk to the student. If the student wanted to speak to the school nurse, they would have done so.

    CLINICAL JUDGMENT GUIDE: The nurse is responsible for the actions and behavior of UAPs in any healthcare setting. The nurse should know when to intervene and when not to intervene.

32. 1. This is a breach of confidentiality. The LPN should not discuss the client's health problem in the waiting room where everyone can hear.
    2. The nurse should remove the LPN from the situation without embarrassing the LPN. Asking the LPN to come to the office area is the appropriate action for the nurse to take. The LPN's action is a violation of HIPAA.
    3. The nurse should not correct the LPN's behavior in front of the client as this is embarrassing to both the LPN and the client.
    4. The nurse does not have to report this to the HCP. The nurse can talk to the LPN concerning this breach of confidentiality.

    CLINICAL JUDGMENT GUIDE: The nurse is responsible for knowing and complying with local, state, and federal standards of care. The LPN's discussion of a confidential matter in a public area violates HIPAA.

33. 1. The charge nurse must address this situation because it has been happening for over a week.
    2. Writing a memo does nothing to discover the cause of the tense atmosphere.
    3. The charge nurse should call a meeting and attempt to determine what is causing the staff's behavior and the tense atmosphere. The charge nurse could then problem-solve, with the goal of having a more relaxed atmosphere in which to work.
    4. This is threatening, which is not an appropriate way to resolve a staff problem.

    CLINICAL JUDGMENT GUIDE: In any business, including a healthcare facility, arguing should not occur among staff of any level where the customers—in this case, the clients—can hear it or see it. The nurse should address the situation directly with the staff members.

34. 1. Obtaining a urine sample is not an invasive procedure and does not require informed consent.
    2. The urine specimen must adhere to a chain of custody so the client cannot dispute the results.
    3. The bathroom for drug testing should not have access to water via a sink so the client cannot dilute the urine specimen.
    4. The tympanic temperature is taken in the client's ear and is not required for a urine drug sample.

    CLINICAL JUDGMENT GUIDE: There are management questions on the NCLEX-RN®. In many instances, there is no test-taking strategy for these questions. The nurse must be knowledgeable regarding management issues and know what must comply with local, state, and federal requirements.

35. 1. Any client seen in the clinic should have the vital signs taken, but given the clinical manifestations of the client, the nurse should first obtain a urinalysis.
    2. The nurse should determine whether there has been blood in the urine, but it is not the nurse's first intervention. The HCP needs a urinalysis to confirm the probable diagnosis.
    3. The client is verbalizing the classic clinical manifestations of a urinary tract infection, but it must be confirmed with a urinalysis. The nurse should first obtain the specimen so the results will be available when the HCP sees the client.

4. The nurse should always teach the client, and asking this question is appropriate, but it is not the clinic nurse's first intervention.

CLINICAL JUDGMENT GUIDE: The client's clinical manifestations often provide the nurse with the most likely problem, and the nurse should confirm the condition with a laboratory test, if possible. Clinic and ED nurses obtain tests so the HCP will have the results when seen.

36. 1. The nurse may need to know how long the client will be in the shelter, but this is not a priority during the initial client assessment.
    2. During a disaster, the priority is determining whether the client has routine medications to take while in the shelter. If clients have life-sustaining medications, then obtaining the medications becomes a priority. Remember, psychiatric medications are life-sustaining.
    3. The client's health history is important, but no matter what the history is, if the client does not have life-sustaining medications, the client will end up in the hospital.
    4. The client should be assessed, but unless the client has verbalized a specific symptom in this situation, assessment of vital signs, height, and weight is not a priority.

CLINICAL JUDGMENT GUIDE: The nurse must be knowledgeable regarding emergency preparedness. The NCSBN NCLEX-RN® test plan includes questions on a safe and effective care environment.

37. 1. The nurse should ask whether the client is allergic to iodine or shellfish.
    2. An incompetent client cannot sign the consent form. Because the client is diagnosed with schizophrenia, asking them to sign a permit form is not an appropriate intervention.
    3. An incompetent client is not autonomous and cannot give or withhold consent—for example, individuals who are cognitively impaired, mentally ill, neurologically incapacitated, or under the influence of mind-altering drugs. This client is diagnosed with schizophrenia, a mental illness, and is delusional; therefore, the client's significant other must consent to the procedure.
    4. This procedure is performed in the radiology department, not in a day surgery department.

CLINICAL JUDGMENT GUIDE: The NCLEX-RN® test plan includes questions on nursing care ruled by legal requirements. The nurse must be knowledgeable regarding these issues.

38. 1. Some herbal supplements can interact with prescribed medications and become dangerous, but saw palmetto is not one of them.
    2. The herbal supplement, saw palmetto, is recommended by many urologists and used to treat BPH; therefore, this is the most appropriate statement.
    3. The nurse should notify the client's HCP, but the best response is to support the client's use of saw palmetto for BPH.
    4. This is a true statement, but the nurse should address the client taking the saw palmetto, not make a general statement.

CLINICAL JUDGMENT GUIDE: The NCLEX-RN® tests complementary alternative medicine (CAM), so the nurse must be familiar with the common herbs used to treat disease processes.

39. 1. This is the speech therapist's role, a home care team member.
    2. This is the occupational therapist's role, a member of the home care team.
    3. This is the social worker's role, a member of the home care team.
    4. This is the physical therapist's role, a member of the home care team.

CLINICAL JUDGMENT GUIDE: The home health nurse must know the roles of the home care team members. The home health nurse must be able to make appropriate referrals.

40. 1. The NCSBN NCLEX-RN® test plan includes referrals under Management of Care. The client is in spiritual distress. The chaplain is a member of the team to address spiritual needs.
    2. The nurse should not discuss the client's concerns with the client's pastor. The nurse should contact the agency chaplain; then, if needed, the agency chaplain could talk to the client's pastor.
    3. This is crossing professional boundaries. The nurse should not impose their religious beliefs on the client. If the client asks the nurse to pray, then the nurse could—but the nurse should not ask the client to pray.
    4. The client is verbalizing thoughts about dying, not asking questions about living wills. This would not be an appropriate intervention.

CLINICAL JUDGMENT GUIDE: The test taker must know the roles of all members of the multidisciplinary healthcare team.

41. 1. This is a private moment between the client and spouse; the nurse should not impose on the situation.
    2. The client and spouse did not ask for help; the nurse should not assume help is needed.
    3. **This is a private moment and should be respected by the nurse. The nurse should allow the client and spouse quiet time together.**
    4. This is a private moment between the client and spouse; the nurse should not impose on the situation.

CLINICAL JUDGMENT GUIDE: The nurse must be aware of spiritual needs and help to support the client's needs whenever possible.

42. Correct answers are 4 and 5.
    1. Clocking in late twice in a year is not a pattern of behavior.
    2. The nurse involved in a code could not leave the code to answer a call light.
    3. The nurse has covered themself, or may be changing to cover someone else. This action assumes responsibility for the client's care on the unit and does not require a mention in the evaluation unless the nurse changes at the request of management.
    4. **The nurse's care is being evaluated, including the nurse's documentation. The completeness of documentation should be included in the evaluation.**
    5. **The nurse's membership in the American Nephrology Nurses Association helps the nurse remain up to date on current trends impacting the care provided. This information should be included in the evaluation.**

CLINICAL JUDGMENT GUIDE: This is an alternate type of question included in the NCLEX-RN®. The nurse must select all the options that answer the question correctly. There will be management questions on the NCLEX-RN®. There is often no test-taking strategy for these questions.

43. 1. This is a nice gesture, but the priority is to provide support when the family and friends have returned to their own lives.
    2. **The family and friends will have returned to their own lives 1 to 2 months after a family member has died, so this is when the next of kin needs support from the hospice nurse. Hospice will follow up with the significant other for up to 13 months.**
    3. This is the family's responsibility, not the hospice nurse's.
    4. This is not the nurse's responsibility and should be discouraged for a short period. In the immediate grieving period, the significant other may get rid of possessions they wish had been kept later.

CLINICAL JUDGMENT GUIDE: The test taker must know the roles of all multidisciplinary healthcare team members. This knowledge will be tested on the NCLEX-RN® examination.

44. Correct answers are 3 and 5.
    1. The nurse should not continue to attempt IV access if another nurse is available and can insert the IV line successfully.
    2. The client needs IV replacement at this time.
    3. **After two attempts, the nurse should arrange for a second nurse to attempt the placement.**
    4. Cold packs would cause the circulatory system to contract and make it more difficult to start an IV line. Hot packs dilate the blood vessels.
    5. **With a portable vein finder device, infrared light is absorbed by hemoglobin in the blood, making the veins appear darker in contrast to the surrounding tissue, facilitating IV starts.**

CLINICAL JUDGMENT GUIDE: The nurse must be able to perform skills safely. The nurse should not continue to inflict pain on the client after attempting invasive procedures more than twice.

45. 1. The UAP should not use soap when bathing a client diagnosed with CKD. Soap will dry the skin, and the client diagnosed with CKD has altered skin integrity.
    2. **The nurse should stop the UAP from using the arm with the graft. Pressure on the graft could occlude the graft.**
    3. The UAP can tell the client not to eat contraband food. This statement is not teaching.
    4. This is an appropriate action for the UAP; the nurse would not need to intervene.

CLINICAL JUDGMENT GUIDE: "Delegation" means that the nurse is responsible for the UAP's actions and performance. The nurse must correct the UAP's performance to ensure the client is cared for safely in the hospital or the home.

46. 1. Digoxin (Lanoxin) is frequently ordered for elderly clients with a history of heart failure. The nurse should take an apical heart rate and hold the medication if the apical pulse is lower than 60 bpm. This is a maintenance dose of the medication.

2. Furosemide (Lasix), a loop diuretic, is frequently prescribed for clients with a history of heart failure. The nurse should determine whether the client is having muscle cramping, which is a sign of potassium deficiency. The nurse would not question administering this medication without an indication of potassium deficiency.
3. Potassium (K Dur) is given to prevent potassium depletion when administering a diuretic.
4. Bisacodyl (Dulcolax) is a stimulant laxative. Overuse of stimulant laxatives can cause laxative dependency and colon obstruction. The nurse should contact the HCP and arrange a bulk laxative if the client requires a daily one.

CLINICAL JUDGMENT GUIDE: This is an alternate type of question included in the NCLEX-RN® test plan. The test taker must be able to read a medication administration record (MAR), be knowledgeable regarding medications, and make an appropriate decision as to the nurse's most appropriate intervention.

47. Answer: 88 mL/hr (350 divided by 4 hours = 87.5 mL/hr).
    The client is diagnosed with heart failure, which indicates the client is at high risk for fluid volume overload when administering any type of fluids. Blood must be administered within 4 hours.

CLINICAL JUDGMENT GUIDE: The NCLEX-RN® test plan includes dosage calculations under Pharmacological and Parenteral Therapies. This category is included under Physiological Integrity, which promotes physical health and wellness by providing care and comfort, reducing client risk potential, and managing health alterations.

48. Correct answers are 3, 4, and 5.
    1. Teaching is the nurse's responsibility and cannot be delegated to a UAP.
    2. The word "check" indicates a step in the assessment process, and the nurse cannot delegate assessment to a UAP.
    3. The client is 2 days postoperative, and vital signs should be stable so the UAP can take vital signs. The nurse must ensure the UAP knows when to immediately notify them of vital signs outside the guidelines the nurse provides to the UAP.
    4. This action does not require judging, assessing, teaching, or evaluating on the part of the UAP so this task can be delegated.
    5. A client 2 days postoperative should be ambulating frequently. The UAP can perform this task.

CLINICAL JUDGMENT GUIDE: This is an alternate type of question included in the NCLEX-RN®. The nurse must be able to select options that answer the question correctly.

49. 1. The nurse could obtain the client's pulse oximeter reading, but this client is hemorrhaging, and the surgeon should be notified immediately.
    2. Checking the client's last Hgb and Hct could be done, but this client's AP and BP are indicating hemorrhaging; therefore, the first intervention is to notify the client's surgeon.
    3. The client's apical pulse and blood pressure indicate that the client is hemorrhaging; therefore, the nurse should first notify the client's surgeon.
    4. The nurse could monitor the client's urine output, but it will not help the client's hemorrhaging; therefore, this is not the nurse's first intervention.

CLINICAL JUDGMENT GUIDE: The test taker must read all the options carefully before choosing "Notify the HCP." If any options provide information the HCP needs to know to make a decision, the test taker should choose that option. If the HCP does not need any additional information to make a decision and the nurse suspects the condition is severe or life-threatening, the priority intervention is to call the HCP.

50. Correct order is 4, 5, 2, 3, 1.
    4. Safety should be the primary concern of the nurse. A bedside commode will provide the client with an option that is easier to get to than walking to the bathroom and prevent the client from slipping on urine that may be dribbled.
    5. The nurse needs to obtain a urine culture to initiate antibiotic therapy.
    2. This will help the client stay dry and not soil clothes and allow some independence in ambulation in the room and hallways.
    3. This will protect the bed and the client from soiling.
    1. Providing frequent assistance with toileting will prevent the client from having incontinence.

CLINICAL JUDGMENT GUIDE: This is an alternate type of question included in the NCLEX-RN® test plan. The nurse must be able to implement interventions in the correct order.

51.
1. These laboratory findings are low but would not require a blood transfusion. These laboratory findings are often expected in an anemic client secondary to chronic kidney disease.
2. This client's dialysis access is compromised and should be assessed, but this is not life-threatening.
3. This client should be seen, but not before a potentially life-threatening situation.
4. **The client on peritoneal dialysis with a hard, rigid abdomen has a potentially life-threatening complication; this client should be assessed first and then sent to the hospital.**

CLINICAL JUDGMENT GUIDE: The test taker must determine whether any assessment data are normal or abnormal for the client's diagnosis. If the data are abnormal, then this client should be seen first. If the data are normal, then a client diagnosed with a physiological problem is the client the nurse should assess first.

52.
1. This pulse oximeter reading is above 93%; therefore, this information does not warrant notifying the HCP.
2. The client's platelet count is within normal limits; therefore, this information does not warrant notifying the HCP.
3. **After the initial administration of erythropoietin, a biological response modifier, the client's antihypertensive medications may need to be adjusted. Therefore, this elevated blood pressure warrants notifying the HCP. Erythropoietin therapy is contraindicated for clients diagnosed with uncontrollable hypertension.**
4. The client's tympanic temperature is within normal limits; therefore, this does not warrant notifying the HCP.

CLINICAL JUDGMENT GUIDE: The test taker should select the potentially life-threatening option or a complaint requiring the medication to be adjusted or discontinued. The nurse should notify the HCP if the medication is causing an adverse effect, not an expected side effect.

53. Answer: 300 mL.

The nurse must add up how many milliliters of fluid the client drank on the 7 a.m. to 7 p.m. shift, then subtract that number from 1,500 mL to determine how much fluid the client can receive on the 7 p.m. to 7 a.m. shift. One ounce is equal to 30 mL. The client drank 40 oz (8 + 8 + 16 + 8) of fluid, or 1,200 mL (40 × 30) of fluid. Therefore, the client can have 300 mL (1,500 − 1,200) of fluid on the 7 p.m. to 7 a.m. shift.

CLINICAL JUDGMENT GUIDE: The NCLEX-RN® test plan includes dosage calculations under Pharmacological and Parenteral Therapies. This category is included under Physiological Integrity, which promotes physical health and wellness by providing care and comfort, reducing client risk potential, and managing health alterations.

54.
1. The reverse Trendelenburg position has the nurse elevating the client's chair, which will not help the client's dizziness and lightheadedness.
2. Decreasing the volume of blood being removed is an appropriate intervention, but it will not help the client's dizziness and lightheadedness as fast as infusing normal saline.
3. **Normal saline infusion increases the volume in the bloodstream, decreasing the client's lightheadedness and dizziness.**
4. Hypotension is expected in clients receiving dialysis; therefore, the HCP does not need to be notified.

CLINICAL JUDGMENT GUIDE: When the question asks, "Which intervention should be implemented first?" it means all the options are things a nurse could implement, but only one should be implemented first. The nurse should use the nursing process and remember: If the client is in distress, do not assess; if the client is not in distress, the nurse should assess.

55. Correct answers are 3, 4, and 5.
1. TPN is a hypertonic solution with enough calories, proteins, lipids, electrolytes, and trace elements to sustain life. It is administered via a pump to prevent a too-rapid infusion. It should not be administered without a pump or via a gravity IV line.
2. TPN contains 50% dextrose solution; therefore, the client is monitored to ensure the pancreas adapts to high glucose levels. The glucose level is checked every 6 hours, not every 24 hours.
3. **The client is weighed daily in the same clothes and at the same time to monitor for fluid overload and evaluate daily weight.**
4. **The IV tubing is changed with every bag because the high glucose level can cause bacterial growth.**
5. **Intake and output are monitored to observe for fluid balance.**

CLINICAL JUDGMENT GUIDE: This is an alternate type of question included in the NCLEX-RN®. The nurse must select all the options that answer the question correctly.

56. Correct order is 2, 1, 4, 5, 3.
    2. The client has signs of phlebitis, and the IV line must be removed to prevent further complications.
    1. A new IV line will be started in the right hand after the left IV line is discontinued.
    4. A warm washcloth on an IV site sometimes comforts the client. If done, it should be placed for 20 minutes four times a day.
    5. All pertinent situations should be documented in the client's EHR.
    3. Depending on the healthcare facility, this may or may not be done, but client care comes before documentation.

CLINICAL JUDGMENT GUIDE: This is an alternate type of question included in the NCLEX-RN® test plan. The nurse must be able to perform skills in the correct order. Documentation is completed after direct client care.

57. 1. A UAP can empty the catheter and measure the amount.
    2. The UAP can record intake and output on the I&O sheet.
    3. The nurse cannot delegate teaching to the UAP.
    4. The client has a disease, but the UAP is only asked to take water to the client.

CLINICAL JUDGMENT GUIDE: This is an "except" question. The nurse could determine which task is appropriate to delegate to the UAP; three options would be appropriate to delegate. The nurse should implement tasks that are not appropriate for delegating. Remember, the nurse cannot delegate assessment, teaching, evaluation, medications, or an unstable client to the UAP.

58. Answer: 890 mL. First, determine the amount of irrigation fluid: 3,000 − 1,550 = 1,450 mL of irrigation fluid. Then, subtract 1,450 irrigation fluid from the drainage of 2,340 mL to determine the urine output: 2,340 − 1,450 = 890 mL of urine output.

CLINICAL JUDGMENT GUIDE: The NCLEX-RN® test plan includes dosage calculations under Pharmacological and Parenteral Therapies. This category is included under Physiological Integrity, which promotes physical health and wellness by providing care and comfort, reducing client risk potential, and managing health alterations.

59. 1. The UAP cannot increase the irrigation fluid because this requires assessment and judgment. This behavior warrants intervention by the nurse.
    2. Elevating the scrotum on a towel for support is an intervention a UAP can implement. It does not require judgment, and the client is stable; therefore, action does not warrant intervention by the nurse.
    3. The UAP can empty catheter bags because this does not require any judgment. This action does not warrant intervention by the nurse.
    4. The UAP can bring ice water to the client's bedside because the client is not NPO.

CLINICAL JUDGMENT GUIDE: "Delegation" means the nurse is responsible for the UAP's actions and performance. The nurse must correct the UAP's performance to ensure the client is cared for safely in the hospital or the home.

60. 1. The client should use a urinal so the nurse can strain the urine before placing it in the commode.
    2. Assessment is the first part of the nursing process and is always the priority. The intensity of the renal colic pain can be so intense it can cause a vasovagal response, with resulting hypotension and syncope.
    3. Increased fluid increases urinary output, which will facilitate the movement of the renal stone through the ureter and help decrease pain, but it is not the first intervention.
    4. The nurse should strain the client's urine to determine whether the renal calculi have been passed via the urine.

CLINICAL JUDGMENT GUIDE: When the question asks, "Which intervention should be implemented first?" it means that all the options are things a nurse could implement, but only one should be implemented first. The nurse should use the nursing process and remember: If the client is in distress, do not assess; if the client is not in distress, the nurse should assess.

61. 1. A KUB study is an x-ray and does not include administering any contrast dye.
    2. Food, fluids, and ordered medication are not restricted before a KUB study.
    3. An x-ray should not be completed on a possibly pregnant client. The x-rays could harm the fetus.

4. The client diagnosed with renal calculi is expected to have pain, depending on where the calculi are located, but this statement would not warrant intervention for the KUB study.

CLINICAL JUDGMENT GUIDE: This question asks the nurse to identify which statement warrants intervention, indicating three options are appropriate for the disease process or disorder but one is incorrect. This is an "except" question, but it does not say all the options are correct "except."

62. Correct answers are 3 and 5.
    1. The HCP may order certain foods and medications when obtaining a 24-hour urine collection to evaluate for calcium oxalate or uric acid, but the client will not be NPO.
    2. When the collection begins, the client should completely empty their bladder and discard that urine. The first urine specimen is not included.
    3. **All urine for 24 hours should be saved and put in a container with a preservative, refrigerated, or put on ice, as indicated. Not following specific instructions will result in an inaccurate test result.**
    4. The urine is obtained in some type of urine collection device such as a bedpan, bedside commode, or commode hat. The client is not catheterized.
    5. **Posting signs will help ensure that all the urine is saved during the 24-hour period. If urine is discarded, the test may result in inaccurate information or the need to start the test again.**

CLINICAL JUDGMENT GUIDE: This is an alternate type of question included in the NCLEX-RN®. The nurse must be able to select all the options that answer the question correctly. There are no partially correct answers.

63. 1. The urine must be assessed for bleeding and cloudiness. Initially, the urine is bright red, but the color soon diminishes, and cloudiness may indicate an infection. This assessment should not be delegated to a UAP.
    2. The UAP cannot transcribe an HCP's orders.
    3. **The UAP can strain the client's urine. This task does not require judgment or evaluation. Any sediment should be placed in a sterile container and sent to the laboratory for analysis.**
    4. The kidney is highly vascular. Hemorrhaging and the resulting shock are potential complications of lithotripsy, so the nurse should not delegate vital signs postprocedure.

CLINICAL JUDGMENT GUIDE: The nurse cannot delegate assessment, teaching, evaluation, medications, or an unstable client to a UAP. Tasks that cannot be delegated are nursing interventions requiring nursing judgment.

64. 1. This potassium level is within normal limits, 3.5 to 5.5 mEq/L.
    2. **Hematuria is not uncommon after the removal of a kidney stone, but causes further assessment by the nurse. It may indicate hemorrhaging, which is life-threatening.**
    3. A creatinine level of 1 mg/dL is normal for a male or a female client.
    4. This WBC count is within the normal limits of 4.5 to 11.1 10^3/microL.

CLINICAL JUDGMENT GUIDE: The nurse must be knowledgeable regarding normal laboratory values and be able to determine whether the laboratory value is expected for the client's disease process or for medications the client is taking.

65. 1. **The nurse should assess first to determine the etiology of the incontinence before the treatment plan can be formulated. By palpating the bladder after voiding, the nurse can determine whether the incontinence resulted from overdistention of the bladder.**
    2. Medications—for instance, anticholinergic agents such as oxybutynin—can cause adverse effects. Nonpharmacological methods of treatment are preferred before medications are administered.
    3. The nurse should ensure the client does not have skin breakdown secondary to urinary incontinence, but the first intervention is assessment.
    4. The nurse should instruct the client to use the bathroom every 2 hours and attempt to urinate, which may decrease the number of incontinent episodes.

CLINICAL JUDGMENT GUIDE: When the question asks, "Which intervention should be implemented first?" it means that all the options are things a nurse could implement, but only one should be implemented first. The nurse should use the nursing process and remember: If the client is in distress, do not assess; if the client is not in distress, the nurse should assess.

66. 1. These vital signs are within normal limits and would not require further investigation.
    2. When an elderly client's mental status changes, the nurse should notify the HCP because it is not normal or expected. This

could indicate a urinary tract infection secondary to an indwelling catheter. Elderly clients often do not present with classic clinical manifestations of infection.

3. The client's urine should be clear and light yellow, but cloudy urine with sediment is not life-threatening. The nurse would not need to notify the client's HCP.
4. The client should have no discomfort and pain; this would not warrant further investigation.

CLINICAL JUDGMENT GUIDE: When the question asks, "Which data set warrants notifying the HCP?" it is an "except" question. Three data sets are expected with the client's disease process or condition, whereas one is not expected and warrants notifying the HCP.

67. 1. The client's catheter should be secured on the leg to prevent manipulation, increasing the urinary tract infection risk. This warrants immediate intervention by the nurse.
2. The UAP must adhere to Standard Precautions when providing care to the client; therefore, this doesn't warrant immediate intervention by the nurse.
3. The drainage bag should be kept below the bladder level to prevent urine reflux into the renal system; therefore, this does not warrant intervention by the nurse.
4. Hand hygiene is essential before and after handling any portion of the drainage system; therefore, this does not warrant intervention by the nurse.

CLINICAL JUDGMENT GUIDE: When the question asks, "Which intervention warrants immediate intervention?" it is an "except" question. Three of the interventions indicate that the UAP understands the appropriate care for the client, and one indicates that the UAP does not understand the appropriate care.

68. 1. The UAP can assist the radiology technician with the portable chest x-ray. The RN cannot delegate assessment, teaching, evaluation, medications, or an unstable client. If the UAP is pregnant, then the nurse should not delegate this task.
2. The UAP can obtain the client's intake and output, but the nurse must evaluate the data to determine whether interventions are needed or effective.
3. In some units, UAPs can perform urinary catheterization, but the nurse should delegate the least invasive task of the four options.
4. This is a medication enema, and the UAP cannot administer medications. Also, the client must be unstable and have an excessively high serum potassium level for this to be ordered.

CLINICAL JUDGMENT GUIDE: The nurse cannot delegate assessment, evaluation, teaching, administration of medications, or care of an unstable client to a UAP.

69. 1. The laboratory findings are low but would not require a blood transfusion. These laboratory findings are often expected in an anemic client secondary to ESRD.
2. The dialysis access is compromised; therefore, this client warrants intervention by the RN because the hemodialysis cannot be performed.
3. It is common for a client undergoing dialysis to be exhausted and sleep through the treatment; therefore, this does not warrant intervention.
4. The client in end-stage renal disease would not have urinary output; therefore, this does not warrant intervention from the RN.

CLINICAL JUDGMENT GUIDE: The nurse must determine which sign or symptom is not expected for the disease process. If the sign or symptom is not expected, or if it is an emergency situation, the nurse should assess the client first. This question determines whether the nurse knows the clinical manifestations of various disease processes.

70. 1. The RN can restart the client's IV access without notifying the HCP.
2. Hypoactive bowel sounds may be abnormal, but airway problems take priority over gastrointestinal distress. Remember Maslow's Hierarchy of Needs.
3. The client may be developing pneumonia or acute respiratory distress syndrome, which are surgical complications; therefore, the RN should notify the HCP.
4. A 2+ pedal pulse is expected data; therefore, the RN does not need to notify the HCP.

CLINICAL JUDGMENT GUIDE: When the question asks, "Which data set warrants notifying the HCP?" it is an "except" question. Three data sets are expected with the client's disease process or condition, whereas one is not expected and warrants notifying the HCP.

71. 1. Normal blood urea nitrogen levels are 8 to 21 mg/dL or 10 to 31 mg/dL for clients older than age 90 years.

2. Normal creatinine levels are 0.61 to 1.21 mg/dL for male clients and 0.51 to 1.04 mg/dL for female clients.
3. GFR is approximately 120 mL/min. If the GFR is decreased to 60 mL/min, the kidneys are functioning at about one-half filtration capacity.
4. Normal creatinine clearance is 85 to 125 mL/min for males and 75 to 115 mL/min for females.

CLINICAL JUDGMENT GUIDE: The nurse must be knowledgeable regarding normal laboratory values and determine whether the laboratory value is expected for the client's disease process or for medications the client is taking.

72. Answer: 1,000 mL. First, determine the amount of irrigation fluid: 4,000 – 2,000 = 2,000 mL of irrigation fluid. Then, subtract 2,000 of irrigation fluid from the drainage of 3,000 to determine the urine output: 3,000 – 2,000 = 1,000 mL of urine output.

CLINICAL JUDGMENT GUIDE: The NCLEX-RN® test plan includes dosage calculations under Pharmacological and Parenteral Therapies. This category is included under Physiological Integrity, which promotes physical health and wellness by providing care and comfort, reducing client risk potential, and managing health alterations.

73. Correct answers are 1 and 5.
    1. **The client is stable, but the RN should assess the drainage. The drainage should be light pink for a client recovering from a TURP.**
    2. The client is stable; therefore, the RN should not increase the irrigation fluid unless the drainage is dark red.
    3. If the client is hypovolemic, the head of the bed should be lowered, and the foot should be elevated to protect the brain. This client is stable.
    4. The surgeon must be notified if the client is unstable or experiencing a complication of surgery. This client is stable; therefore, the RN should not notify the surgeon.
    5. **The RN should monitor the client's laboratory values for bleeding or infection.**

CLINICAL JUDGMENT GUIDE: This is an alternate type of question included in the NCLEX-RN®. The nurse must select all the options that answer the question correctly.

74. 1. The client with a palpable thrill is stable; therefore, the charge nurse would not need to see this client first.
    2. The client diagnosed with acute glomerulonephritis is expected to have hematuria and proteinuria; therefore, the charge nurse should not assess this client first.
    3. The sign of bladder cancer is painless hematuria; therefore, the charge nurse would not need to see this client first.
    4. **An ileal conduit is a procedure that diverts urine from the bladder and provides an alternate cutaneous pathway for urine to exit the body. Urinary output should always be at least 30 mL/hr. This client should be assessed to make sure that the stents placed in the ureters have not become dislodged, or to ensure that edema of the ureters is not occurring.**

CLINICAL JUDGMENT GUIDE: The test taker must determine whether any assessment data are normal or abnormal for the client's diagnosis. If the data are abnormal, then this client should be seen first.

75. 1. Teaching cannot be assigned to an LPN, no matter how knowledgeable the LPN.
    2. This client has the laboratory symptoms of an infection; therefore, the RN cannot assign an unstable client to the LPN.
    3. Antineoplastic medication can only be administered by a qualified registered nurse.
    4. **The LPN can administer narcotic analgesics to a client; therefore, this would be an appropriate assignment.**

CLINICAL JUDGMENT GUIDE: The nurse cannot delegate assessment, teaching, evaluation, or an unstable client to the LPN.

CASE STUDY ANSWERS

1. **Correct answers are 2 and 4.**
   While the remaining answer choices would be "nice to know," the client's allergies and weight are needed to ensure dose verification and safe administration.

2. Findings associated with the conditions are indicated below.

Finding	UTI	Dehydration	Shock
Pallor			X
Lethargy	X	X	X
Vomiting	X		
Diaphoresis	X		
Irritability		X	X
Temperature	X		
Thirst	X	X	X
Urine specific gravity	X	X	
Urinary output	X	X	X

Findings are indicative of the marked conditions. While the client is being admitted for a UTI and dehydration, the nurse also needs to be familiar with signs of early, compensatory, shock so that condition changes are recognized and managed.

3. **Correct answers are 3 and 2.**
   Based on the client's condition, the nurse recognizes that the client is at the highest risk for

3. Urosepsis

   and will require

2. Antibiotics

   The client's urinary tract infection and dehydration may continue to worsen and lead to urosepsis. Initiating the antibiotics as soon as possible is the priority at this point. There is no evidence of a risk for cardiac arrest or an injury from a fall. The parents are currently at the bedside and can be instructed to let the nurse know if they are not going to be directly with the client.

4. Correct indicated and not indicated interventions are marked below.

Potential Nursing Intervention	Indicated	Not Indicated
Maintain IV 0.9% NaCl at 50 mL/hr	X	
Review the "rooming in" policy with the parents	X	
Discourage play with other toddlers in common area		X
Confirm ampicillin dosage calculation	X	
Reorient the client as needed	X	
Administer ampicillin	X	
Administer acetaminophen	X	
Encourage PO fluid intake	X	
Instruct parents to keep track of client's output	X	

From a physical perspective, maintaining both IV and PO fluid intake, as well as output is important to restore hemodynamics and hydration. Since the ampicillin was ordered for dosage based on weight, the nurse should confirm the dose when it is received from the pharmacy. Ampicillin and acetaminophen should be given as soon as possible. Finally, while physical interventions most often take priority over psychosocial actions, when caring for young children, the nurse is also caring for the parents. Reviewing the policy allowing parent(s) to room in with the client provides reassurance.

Since the client is noninfectious, the toddler/parents can socialize with other toddlers/parents depending on how the client feels.

5. Correct answers are 1, 4, 5, 6.
   1. Maintain IV 0.9% NaCl at 50 mL/hr.
   2. Review the "rooming in" policy with the parents.
   3. Encourage play with other toddlers in common area.
   4. Confirm ampicillin dosage calculation.
   5. Administer ampicillin.
   6. Administer acetaminophen.
   7. Encourage PO fluid intake.
   8. Instruct parents to keep track of client's output.

The client's physical needs take priority, especially those that are one of the ABCs. IV fluids are circulatory, the ampicillin is needed to treat infection, and the acetaminophen will lower fever. While encouraging PO fluid intake is also circulatory, pay attention to the number of priority interventions in the question; IV fluids will replace circulatory volume faster than oral fluids.

6. Answers are indicated below.

Finding	Improved	Declined	No Change
Blood pressure			X
Heart rate			X
Respirations			X
Temperature	X		
SpO$_2$			X
Level of consciousness	X		

Both temperature and level of consciousness have improved since admission. No findings indicate a decline in condition, and although there are subtle differences in the other vital signs, they all remain within the normal range, indicating no change.

Neurological Management 7

Let us never consider ourselves finished nurses . . . we must be learning all our lives.

—Florence Nightingale

QUESTIONS

1. The charge nurse has received laboratory data for clients in the medical department. Which client would require intervention by the charge nurse?
   1. The client diagnosed with a stroke with platelet levels of 250×10^3/microL
   2. The client diagnosed with a seizure disorder and a valproic acid level of 75 mcg/mL
   3. The client diagnosed with multiple sclerosis on prednisone with a glucose level of 208 mg/dL
   4. The client receiving phenytoin with serum levels of 24 mcg/dL

2. The nurse is administering medications for clients on a neurological unit. Which medication should the nurse administer **first**?
   1. Pain medication to a client reporting headaches rated an 8 on a 1 to 10 pain scale
   2. Steroids to the client experiencing an acute exacerbation of multiple sclerosis
   3. An anticholinesterase medication to a client diagnosed with myasthenia gravis
   4. Antacid to a client diagnosed with pyrosis calling several times over the intercom

3. The nurse has just received the shift report. Which client should the nurse assess **first**?
   1. The client diagnosed with Guillain-Barré syndrome and ascending paralysis to the knees
   2. The client diagnosed with a C6 spinal cord injury (SCI) and autonomic dysreflexia
   3. The client diagnosed with Parkinson's disease experiencing a "pill-rolling" tremor
   4. The client diagnosed with Huntington's disease with writhing, twisting face movements

4. The RN primary nurse and unlicensed assistive personnel (UAP) are caring for a client diagnosed with right-sided paralysis. Which action by the UAP **requires** the RN to intervene?
   1. The UAP places the gait belt around the client's waist before ambulating.
   2. The UAP places the client on the abdomen with the client's head to the side.
   3. The UAP places their hand under the client's right axilla to help the client move up in bed.
   4. The UAP praises the client for performing activities of daily living (ADLs) independently.

5. The charge nurse is making client assignments for a neurological medical floor. Which client should be assigned to the **most** experienced nurse?
   1. The elderly client experiencing a stroke-in-evolution
   2. The client diagnosed with a transient ischemic attack 48 hours ago
   3. The client diagnosed with Guillain-Barré syndrome reporting leg pain
   4. The client diagnosed with Alzheimer's disease wandering in the halls

6. The client diagnosed with a cerebrovascular accident (CVA) has residual right-sided hemiparesis and difficulty swallowing but is scheduled for discharge. Which referral is **most** appropriate for the case manager to make at this time?
   1. Inpatient rehabilitation unit
   2. Home healthcare agency
   3. Long-term care facility
   4. Outpatient therapy center

7. The RN primary nurse and licensed practical nurse (LPN) are caring for a client diagnosed with a stroke. Which intervention should the RN assign to the LPN?
   1. Feed the client being allowed to eat for the first time.
   2. Administer the client's anticoagulant subcutaneously.
   3. Check the client's neurological signs and limb movement.
   4. Teach the client to turn their head and tuck the chin to swallow.

8. The RN staff nurse is caring for a client diagnosed with Alzheimer's disease. Which nursing tasks can the RN staff nurse delegate to the UAP? **Select all that apply.**
   1. Check the client's skin under the restraints.
   2. Administer the client's antipsychotic medication.
   3. Perform the client's morning hygiene care.
   4. Ambulate the client to the bathroom.
   5. Obtain the client's routine vital signs.

9. The RN primary nurse on the surgical unit is working with a UAP. Which task is **most** appropriate for the RN to delegate to the UAP?
   1. Change the abdominal dressing for a 2 days postoperative client.
   2. Check the client's IV insertion site on their right arm.
   3. Monitor vital signs on a client returning from surgery.
   4. Escort a discharged client to the client's vehicle.

10. Which client diagnosed with an SCI should the charge nurse assess **first** after receiving the change-of-shift report?
    1. The client diagnosed with a C6 SCI reporting dyspnea symptoms with a respiratory rate of 12 breaths/min
    2. The client diagnosed with an L4 SCI frightened about being transferred to the rehabilitation unit
    3. The client diagnosed with an L2 SCI reporting a headache and suddenly feeling very hot
    4. The client diagnosed with a C4 SCI on a ventilator with a pulse oximeter reading of 98%

11. The client diagnosed with a C6 SCI comes to the emergency department reporting a throbbing headache and has a BP of 200/120 mm Hg. Which intervention should the nurse implement **first**?
    1. Place the client on a telemetry unit.
    2. Complete a neurological assessment.
    3. Insert an indwelling urinary catheter.
    4. Request a STAT CT scan of their head.

12. The RN intensive care unit (ICU) nurse and UAP are caring for a client diagnosed with right-sided paralysis secondary to a CVA. Which action by the UAP **requires** the RN to intervene?
    1. The UAP performs passive range-of-motion (ROM) exercises for the client.
    2. The UAP places the client on their abdomen with the head to the side.
    3. The UAP uses a lift sheet when moving the client up in bed.
    4. The UAP praises the client for attempting to feed themself.

13. The critical care RN charge nurse is making client assignments for the shift. Which client should the charge nurse assign to the graduate nurse just completing orientation?
    1. The dying client diagnosed with amyotrophic lateral sclerosis on a ventilator while their family is at the bedside.
    2. The client diagnosed with a closed head injury and increasing intracranial pressure receiving IV mannitol.
    3. The client diagnosed with a C5 SCI experiencing spinal shock and on dopamine.
    4. The client diagnosed with a seizure disorder experiencing status epilepticus for the past 24 hours.

14. The critical care nurse is caring for a client diagnosed with a head injury secondary to a motorcycle accident. On morning rounds the client is responsive to painful stimuli and assumes decorticate posturing. Two hours later, which data would warrant **immediate** intervention by the nurse?
    1. The client has purposeful movement when the nurse rubs their sternum.
    2. The client extends their upper and lower extremities in response to painful stimuli.
    3. The client aimlessly thrashes in their bed when a noxious stimulus is applied.
    4. The client is able to squeeze the nurse's hand on a verbal request.

15. The RN charge nurse is making rounds and notices the sharps container in the client's room is above the fill line. Which action should the charge nurse implement?
    1. Complete an adverse occurrence report.
    2. Discuss the situation with the primary nurse.
    3. Instruct the UAP to change the sharps container.
    4. Notify the infection control nurse immediately.

16. The spouse of a client diagnosed with a brain tumor tells the nurse, "I don't know how I will make it if something happens to my partner. I love them so much." Which statement is **most** appropriate for the nurse?
    1. "I will call the chaplain to come and talk to you."
    2. "Do you have any family support to be with you?"
    3. "You don't know how you will make it if something happens."
    4. "Do not worry, everything will be all right. You are a strong person."

17. To which collaborative healthcare team member should the RN critical care nurse refer the client diagnosed with myasthenia gravis (MG) in the late stages?
    1. Occupational therapist
    2. Physical therapist
    3. Social worker
    4. Speech therapist

18. The nurse caring for a client is accidentally stuck with the stylet used to start an IV infusion. Which actions should the nurse implement next? **Rank in order of performance.**
    1. Have the laboratory draw the client's and the nurse's blood.
    2. Notify the charge nurse and follow hospital protocol.
    3. Contact the infection control nurse to start postexposure prophylactic medication.
    4. Follow up with the employee health nurse to have laboratory work drawn.
    5. Flush the skin with water and attempt to get the area to bleed.

19. The nurse is caring for clients in a long-term care facility. Which client should the nurse assess **first** after receiving the morning report?
    1. The client diagnosed with Parkinson's disease starting to hallucinate during the night
    2. The client diagnosed with congestive heart failure and 3+ pitting edema of both feet
    3. The client diagnosed with Alzheimer's disease found wandering in the hall at 0200
    4. The client diagnosed with terminal cancer weighing 8 pounds less than 4 weeks ago

20. The nurse in a long-term care facility is administering medications to a client group. Which medication should the nurse administer **first**?
    1. Acetylsalicylic acid to a client diagnosed with cerebrovascular disease
    2. Neostigmine to a client diagnosed with myasthenia gravis
    3. Cephalexin to a client diagnosed with an acute urinary tract infection
    4. Acyclovir to a client diagnosed with Bell's palsy

21. The nurse in a long-term care facility is developing a plan of care for a client diagnosed with end-stage Alzheimer's disease. Which client problem is **priority** for this client?
    1. Inability to do ADLs
    2. Increased risk for injury
    3. Potential for constipation
    4. Ineffective family coping

22. The clinic nurse is providing discharge instructions to an elderly client diagnosed with cataracts. Which interventions are important for the nurse to implement? **Select all that apply.**
    1. Teach the client to increase the light in the home.
    2. Encourage the client to wear dark glasses outside.
    3. Discuss the need to have the cataracts removed.
    4. Ask the family to avoid rearranging the furniture in the home.
    5. Provide instructions with visual aids or large print.

23. A spouse tells the clinic nurse that their partner has been fine but is now confused, doesn't know where they are, and is acting unusual. Which intervention should the nurse implement **first**?
    1. Perform a neurological assessment.
    2. Notify the client's healthcare provider (HCP).
    3. Ask the spouse to explain more about the client's behavior.
    4. Determine when the client last had something to eat.

24. The RN charge nurse observes the client's RN primary nurse telling the UAP to feed an elderly client diagnosed with a CVA. Which question should the charge nurse ask the client's nurse?
    1. "How does the client swallow the medications?"
    2. "Did you complete your head-to-toe assessment?"
    3. "Does the client have some thickener in the room?"
    4. "Why would you delegate feeding to a UAP?"

25. The client diagnosed with a CVA is confined to a wheelchair for most of their waking hours. Which intervention is **priority** for the nurse to implement?
    1. Encourage the client to move their buttocks every 2 hours.
    2. Order a high-protein diet to prevent skin breakdown.
    3. Get a pressure-relieving cushion to place in their wheelchair.
    4. Refer the client to physical therapy for transfer teaching.

26. As the nurse enters the room of a newly admitted client, the client experiences a tonic-clonic seizure. Which actions should the nurse implement? **Select all that apply.**
    1. Identify the first area that began seizing.
    2. Note the time the client's seizure began.
    3. Begin to pad the client's bed rails.
    4. Provide the client with privacy during the seizure.
    5. Immediately insert an oral airway.

27. The RN rehabilitation unit nurse tells the UAP to assist the client recovering from Guillain-Barré syndrome with a.m. care. Which action by the UAP warrants **immediate** intervention?
    1. The UAP closes the client's door and cubicle curtain.
    2. The UAP massages the client's back with lotion.
    3. The UAP checks the temperature of the bathing water.
    4. The UAP puts the side rails up when bathing the client.

28. The client diagnosed with a right-sided CVA or stroke is admitted to the rehabilitation unit. Which interventions should be included in the nursing care plan? **Select all that apply.**
    1. Position the client to prevent shoulder adduction.
    2. Refer the client to occupational therapy daily.
    3. Encourage the client to move the affected side.
    4. Perform quadriceps exercises five times a day.
    5. Instruct the client to hold their fingers in a fist.

29. The nurse is the **first** person on a motor vehicle accident scene. The driver is unconscious. Which action should the nurse implement **first**?
    1. Stabilize the driver's cervical spine.
    2. Do not move the client from the accident.
    3. Ensure the driver has a patent airway.
    4. Control any external bleeding.

30. The clinic nurse is making assignments for the large family practice clinic. Which task should be assigned to a staff nurse now 4 months pregnant?
    1. Have the staff nurse answer the telephone calls from clients.
    2. Instruct the staff nurse to work in the radiology department.
    3. Tell the staff nurse to work in the front desk triage area.
    4. Assign the staff nurse to work in the oncology clinic.

31. Which task is **most** appropriate for the RN clinic nurse to delegate to the UAP?
    1. Request that the UAP ride in the ambulance with a client.
    2. Ask the UAP to escort the client in a wheelchair to their car.
    3. Instruct the UAP to show the client how to use crutches.
    4. Tell the UAP to call the pharmacy to refill a prescription.

32. The employee health nurse is caring for an employee describing low back pain radiating down both their legs after falling from a ladder. Which intervention should the nurse implement **first**?
    1. Refer the client to an HCP for further evaluation.
    2. Complete the workers' compensation documentation.
    3. Investigate the cause of the fall off the ladder.
    4. Notify the employee's supervisor of the incident.

33. The employee health nurse is caring for an employee describing right knee pain after tripping. There is no visible injury, and the client has a normal neurovascular assessment. Which intervention should the nurse implement?
   1. Request the employee to return to work.
   2. Obtain a urine specimen for a drug screen.
   3. Send the client to the emergency department.
   4. Place a sequential compression device on their leg.

34. The rural emergency department nurse is triaging victims at a disaster site. The victims are tagged using a color code system. Which client should be evacuated first? **Rank in order of priority.**
   1. The alert client diagnosed with a sucking chest wound assigned a red tag
   2. The inconsolable crying client assigned a green tag and unable to answer questions
   3. The client assigned a yellow tag with a hard and tender abdomen to the touch
   4. The client assigned a black tag with full-thickness burns over 60% of their body
   5. The client assigned a white tag with no injuries and is comforting the victims

35. The home health nurse enters the home of an 80-year-old client recovering from a CVA, or stroke, 2 months ago. The client is reporting a severe headache. Which intervention should the nurse implement **first?**
   1. Determine what medication the client has taken.
   2. Assess the client's pain on a pain scale of 1 to 10.
   3. Ask whether the client has any acetaminophen.
   4. Tell the client to sit down and take their blood pressure.

36. A client is suspected of having bacterial meningitis, and the nurse is assisting the HCP with a lumbar puncture. Which intervention should the nurse implement **first?**
   1. Have the client lie in the lateral recumbent position.
   2. Tell the client to empty their bladder.
   3. Encourage the client to complete an advance directive.
   4. Keep the client NPO before the procedure.

37. The home health nurse is scheduling daily visits. Which client should the nurse visit **first?**
   1. The client diagnosed with an L4 SCI describing a severe, pounding headache
   2. The depressed client diagnosed with amyotrophic lateral sclerosis (ALS) wanting to die
   3. The client diagnosed with Parkinson's disease walking with a short, shuffling gait
   4. The client diagnosed with a C5 SCI reporting redness and drainage at the halo vest sites

38. The clinic nurse is triaging client telephone calls. Which client should the nurse call **first?**
   1. The client diagnosed with AIDS developing Kaposi's sarcoma
   2. The client diagnosed with dementia having difficulty dressing themself
   3. The client diagnosed with trigeminal neuralgia having lightning-like shock to the cheeks
   4. The client with vomiting and abdominal cramping pain, and a friend with botulism

39. The home health nurse is caring for a 22-year-old client diagnosed with an L5 SCI 2 months ago. The client says, "I will never be happy again. I can't walk or drive, and I had to quit college." Which intervention should the nurse implement **first?**
   1. Allow the client to express their feelings of powerlessness.
   2. Refer the client to the home healthcare agency social worker.
   3. Recommend contacting the American Spinal Cord Association.
   4. Ask the client whether they have any friends to visit.

40. The client diagnosed with transient ischemic attack (TIA) being admitted is reporting a headache. The client is allergic to morphine, iodine, and codeine. Which HCP order should the nurse **question**?
    1. Schedule the client for a CT scan with contrast in the a.m.
    2. Administer acetaminophen 650 mg PO for headache.
    3. Take the client's vital signs per protocol.
    4. Provide the client with a low-fat, low-cholesterol diet.

41. The home health nurse is admitting a client diagnosed with myasthenia gravis. The client tells the nurse, "Even with my medication, I get exhausted when I do anything." Which intervention should the nurse implement?
    1. Talk to the client's spouse about helping around the house more.
    2. Contact the home health occupational therapist to discuss the client's concerns.
    3. Allow the client to verbalize their feelings of being exhausted.
    4. Recommend the client make an appointment with their HCP.

42. The nurse is caring for clients in the emergency department. Which client should the nurse assess **first**?
    1. The client diagnosed with an epidural hematoma
    2. The client diagnosed with a seizure and in a postictal state
    3. The client diagnosed with encephalitis with a headache
    4. The client diagnosed with multiple sclerosis with scanning speech

43. The nurse in the neurological clinic is triaging phone calls. Which client should the nurse contact **first**?
    1. The client diagnosed with a tension headache reporting nausea and vomiting
    2. The client diagnosed with a migraine headache reporting bilateral throbbing pain
    3. The client diagnosed with a cluster headache reporting unilateral sharp pain
    4. The client diagnosed with hypertension reporting pressure-type pain in the back of the head

44. A client sustained a severe head injury; their spouse is concerned about what to do if the client has a seizure when they go home. Which statement indicates the spouse understands the **most** important action to take if the client has a seizure?
    1. "I should check to see if my partner urinates on themself."
    2. "I will move the furniture out of their way."
    3. "I will call 911 as soon as their seizure begins."
    4. "I will make sure my spouse rests after the seizure is over."

45. The multidisciplinary team is meeting to discuss a client diagnosed with right-sided weakness and a stage 2 pressure injury over the sacral area that is **not** healing. Which **priority** intervention should the client's home health nurse recommend?
    1. Recommend the client get a hospital bed with a trapeze bar.
    2. Recommend a home health aide provide the client care 7 days a week.
    3. Recommend the client be transferred to a skilled nursing unit.
    4. Recommend a referral to the home healthcare agency wound care nurse.

46. The home health aide informs the RN home health nurse the client diagnosed with multiple sclerosis having problems transferring from their bed to their chair is now having problems getting into the shower. Which intervention should the RN implement?
    1. Ask the home health aide whether the bathroom has grab bars.
    2. Assess the client's ability to transfer in the home.
    3. Instruct the home health aide to give the client a bed bath.
    4. Contact the agency physical therapist about the situation.

47. The nurse is teaching the client diagnosed with tension-type headaches. Which statement indicates the client needs **more** teaching?
    1. "I will do some type of exercise every day."
    2. "I am going to practice yoga techniques when I get a headache."
    3. "Cold packs to the back of my neck will help relieve my headache."
    4. "Foods containing amines like cheese and chocolate can cause headaches."

48. The client in a multiple vehicle crash dies in the emergency department. Which **priority** intervention should the emergency department nurse implement when addressing the needs of the client's family?
    1. Ask if the client wanted to be an organ donor.
    2. Give the family the client's personal belongings.
    3. Escort the family to a private room to grieve.
    4. Determine which funeral home should be contacted.

49. A 22-year-old client diagnosed with a traumatic brain injury after a motor vehicle accident is placed on a ventilator. The neurologist explained to the family that the client has **no** brain function. Which referral is appropriate at this time?
    1. Local funeral director
    2. Hospice agency
    3. Home health nurse
    4. Organ procurement organization

50. The nurse is caring for clients in an ophthalmology clinic. Which client **warrants** intervention by the nurse?
    1. The client diagnosed with cataracts reporting decreased vision and abnormal color perception
    2. The client diagnosed with a retinal detachment reporting a painless loss of peripheral vision
    3. The client diagnosed with an external hordeolum reporting a reddened tender area under their eye
    4. The client diagnosed with primary open-angle glaucoma reporting excruciating eye pain

51. The nurse is at the park and observes a person falling and a stick impaled in their right eye. Which intervention should the nurse implement **first**?
    1. Tell someone to call 911 immediately.
    2. Stabilize the stick in the accident victim's eye.
    3. Apply direct pressure to the right eye.
    4. Use a nontoxic liquid and irrigate the eye.

52. The RN staff nurse and UAP are caring for a minimally responsive client diagnosed with multiple sclerosis weighing more than 400 pounds (181.4 kg). Which action is **priority** when moving the client in the bed?
    1. Obtain a lifting device made for heavy clients.
    2. Do not attempt to move the client because of the weight.
    3. Get another UAP to help move the client in the bed.
    4. Tell the family that the client must assist in moving in the bed.

53. The terminally ill client diagnosed with amyotrophic lateral sclerosis (ALS), also known as Lou Gehrig's disease, has a DNR (do not resuscitate) order. The client is reporting "pain all over." The nurse notes the client has shallow breathing and P 67 bpm, R 8 breaths/min, BP 104/62 mm Hg. Which intervention should the nurse implement?
    1. Administer the narcotic pain medication IV push (IVP).
    2. Turn and reposition the client for comfort.
    3. Refuse to administer pain medication.
    4. Notify the HCP of the client's vital signs.

54. The nurse in a rehabilitation facility is evaluating the progress of a recovering client diagnosed with a C6–C7 SCI. Which outcome indicates the client is **improving?**
    1. The client can maneuver the automatic wheelchair into the hallway.
    2. The client states they will be able to return to work in a few weeks.
    3. The client uses eye blinks to communicate yes and no responses.
    4. The client's spouse built a wheelchair ramp onto their house.

55. The nurse is triaging phone calls in a neurosensory clinic. Which client should the nurse contact **first?**
    1. The client diagnosed with Ménière's disease reporting vertigo and tinnitus
    2. The client diagnosed with otitis media with effusion feeling fullness in their ear
    3. The client diagnosed with external otitis reporting serosanguineous drainage and otalgia
    4. The client diagnosed with otosclerosis reporting bilateral hearing loss

56. A client comes to the emergency department reporting bleach splashed in their eyes. Which intervention should the nurse implement **first?**
    1. Cover both their eyes with sterile patches.
    2. Assess the client's visual acuity.
    3. Irrigate their eyes with a sterile solution.
    4. Elevate the head of their bed 45 degrees.

57. The 24-year-old client diagnosed with a traumatic brain injury is transferring to a rehabilitation unit. Which HCP order should the nurse **question?**
    1. Physical therapy for lower extremity strength daily
    2. Occupational therapy to work on cognitive functioning twice a day
    3. A soft diet with mechanically ground meats and thickening agent in fluids
    4. Methylprednisolone IVP every 6 hours

58. The rehabilitation nurse is planning the discharge of a 68-year-old client with residual speech and balance deficits diagnosed with a subarachnoid hemorrhage. Which referral should the nurse initiate at this time?
    1. Hospice organization
    2. Speech therapist
    3. Physical therapist
    4. Home health agency

59. The client is postoperative right eye enucleation. Which statement indicates the client needs **more** discharge teaching?
    1. "It will be approximately 2 weeks before I can get a prosthetic eye."
    2. "I can show you how I insert the conformer in the socket in case it falls out."
    3. "I should insert eye drops into the lower conjunctiva of my eye."
    4. "If I develop a fever, I should call my HCP."

60. The nurse is caring for a client newly diagnosed with multiple sclerosis. Which referral is appropriate at this time?
    1. Social worker to apply for disability
    2. Dietitian for a nutritional consult
    3. Psychological counselor for therapy
    4. Chaplain to discuss spiritual issues

61. The RN staff nurse, LPN, and UAP have been assigned to care for clients on a neurology unit. Which nursing task is **most** appropriate to assign to the LPN?
    1. Administer adrenocorticotropic hormone to the client diagnosed with multiple sclerosis.
    2. Take the vital signs for the client experiencing status epilepticus.
    3. Assist the client diagnosed with Parkinson's disease ambulating to the bathroom.
    4. Assess the newly admitted client diagnosed with pneumonia and restless legs syndrome.

62. The nurse is administering medications on a neurological unit. Which medication should the nurse administer **first?**
    1. The osmotic diuretic to the client diagnosed with a closed head injury
    2. The morning medications to the client scheduled for physical therapy
    3. The narcotic pain medication to a client diagnosed with increased intracranial pressure
    4. Gabapentin to the client diagnosed with restless legs syndrome

63. The RN charge nurse observes the new graduate nurse delegating tasks to the UAP. The UAP appears to be ignoring the graduate nurse. Which action should the charge nurse implement **first?**
    1. Wait and observe how the graduate nurse handles the situation.
    2. Tell the UAP to get busy and complete the assigned tasks.
    3. Discuss asserting authority techniques with the new graduate.
    4. Informally counsel the UAP about their response to the new nurse.

64. The nurse on the day shift of a rehabilitation unit reviews the following medication administration record (MAR).

Client Name: D. F. **Height:** 69 in (175.3 cm) **Date of Birth:** 05/07/1955	**Account Number:** 9251645 **Weight in lb:** 178 **Date:** Today	**Allergies:** Penicillin **Weight in kg:** 80.9
Medication	1901–0700	0701–1900
Levothyroxine 0.75 mcg PO daily		
Morphine sulfate 30 mg PO bid		
Fleets enema per rectum daily		
Metformin 850 mg PO bid		
Signature/Initials	Night Nurse RN/NN	Day Nurse RN/DN

    Which medication should the nurse administer **first?**
    1. Levothyroxine
    2. Morphine sulfate
    3. Fleets enema
    4. Metformin

65. The recovering client in the rehabilitation unit after a motor vehicle accident has been prescribed 50 mg of baclofen per dose orally for muscle spasms. Baclofen comes in 10-mg, 20-mg, and 75-mg tablets. How many tablets should the nurse administer and in which quantity? _____

66. The 19-year-old client diagnosed with a traumatic brain injury is recovering in the rehabilitation unit. Which intervention should the RN staff nurse delegate to the UAP? **Select all that apply.**
    1. Make safety rounds hourly.
    2. Refer the client to a college and career counselor.
    3. Assist the client with meals.
    4. Clamp and unclamp the indwelling catheter every 2 hours.
    5. Discuss discharge placement with the parents.

67. The 69-year-old client diagnosed with a right CVA is in the rehabilitation unit and diagnosed with left-sided weakness. Where should the nurse place the quad cane when assisting the client to ambulate?

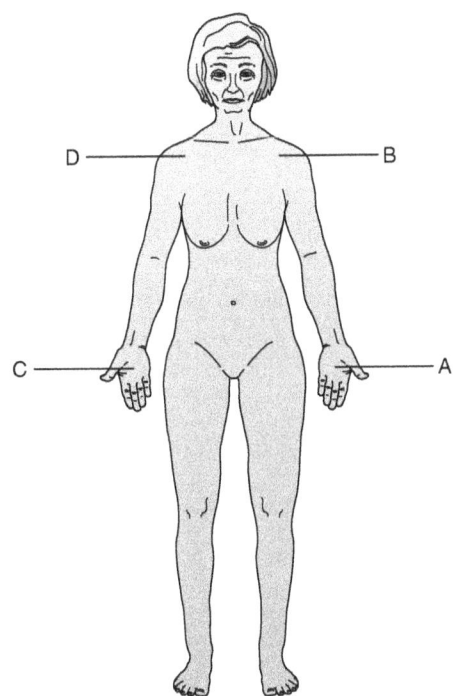

   1. A
   2. B
   3. C
   4. D

68. The client is in the emergency department after a fall that resulted in a closed head injury. The admitting nurse notes the client responds by opening their eyes and pushing the nurse's arm away when painful stimuli is applied but does **not** respond verbally.

Glasgow Coma Scale Appropriate Stimulus Response Score

Eye-Opening		
*Approach to bedside	Spontaneous response	4
*Verbal command	Opens eyes to name on command	3
*Pain	Lack of opening of eyes to previous stimuli but opens to pain	2
	Lack of opening of eyes to any stimulus	1
	Untestable	0
Best Verbal Response		
Verbal questioning with maximum arousal	Oriented to person, place, time, and events	5
	Confusion, conversant but disoriented	4
	Disorganized use of words	3
	Incomprehensible words, groaning	2
	Lack of sound even with painful stimuli	1
	Untestable	0
Best Motor Response		
Verbal command	Follows verbal command	6
Pain (pressure on proximal nail bed)	Localizes pain, attempts to remove offending stimulus	5
	Flexion withdrawal of arm in response to pain without abnormal posturing	4
	Abnormal flexion, flexing of arm at elbow and pronation, making a fist	3
	Abnormal extension, extension of arm at elbow with adduction, and internal rotation of arm at shoulder	2
	Lack of response	1
	Untestable	0

Which rating on the Glasgow Coma Scale should be documented by the nurse?
1. Client scored a 12 on the Glasgow Coma Scale.
2. Client scored a 10 on the Glasgow Coma Scale.
3. Client scored an 8 on the Glasgow Coma Scale.
4. Client scored a 6 on the Glasgow Coma Scale.

69. The day shift RN staff nurse and the UAP are caring for an elderly client diagnosed with a right-sided CVA and hemiparalysis. Which action by the UAP **requires** the RN to intervene?
    1. The UAP places the call light on the client's left side.
    2. The UAP assists the client in eating their breakfast meal.
    3. The UAP uses the draw sheet to move the client up in bed.
    4. The UAP places a small pillow under the client's left shoulder.

70. The 45-year-old hypertensive client diagnosed with a right-sided CVA is reporting a severe headache. Which intervention should the nurse implement **first**?
    1. Administer acetaminophen.
    2. Prepare for a STAT computed tomography (CT) scan.
    3. Notify the client's HCP.
    4. Assess the client's neurological status.

71. The nurse is caring for clients in the neurological ICU. Which client should the nurse assess **first**?
    1. The client diagnosed with a C6 SCI reporting dyspnea with crackles in their lungs
    2. The young adult client diagnosed with Guillain-Barré syndrome reporting ascending paralysis
    3. The client diagnosed with traumatic brain injury and a Glasgow Coma Scale score of 6
    4. The obese client diagnosed with a CVA and expressive aphasia

72. The ICU unit is very busy. The charge nurse is reviewing the HCP's admission orders for an elderly client diagnosed with a closed head injury. Which medication order should the charge nurse **question**?
    1. A subcutaneous anticoagulant
    2. An IV osmotic diuretic
    3. An IV anticonvulsant
    4. An IV proton-pump inhibitor

73. The nurse is caring for a quadriplegic client diagnosed with a C6 SCI 2 years ago admitted for stage IV pressure injuries in the coccyx area. The client is reporting a severe headache and their BP is 190/110 mm Hg. Which intervention should the nurse implement **first**?
    1. Insert a urinary catheter into the client.
    2. Complete a neurological assessment.
    3. Put the client in the Trendelenburg position.
    4. Palpate the client's bladder.

74. The charge nurse is making rounds and enters the room of a pediatric client having a tonic-clonic seizure. Which **priority** intervention should the charge nurse implement?
    1. Place the client on their side.
    2. Call the Rapid Response Team.
    3. Determine whether the client is incontinent of urine.
    4. Provide the client with privacy during the seizure.

75. The UAP is attempting to put an oral airway in the mouth of a client having a tonic-clonic seizure. Which intervention should the RN charge nurse take **first**?
    1. Complete an adverse occurrence report.
    2. Instruct the UAP to stop inserting the oral airway.
    3. Assist the UAP to insert the oral airway.
    4. Note the time of the seizure and observe the seizure.

76. The charge nurse is teaching the graduate nurse the correct procedure for assisting the HCP with a lumbar puncture to rule out meningitis on a young adult. Which interventions should the charge nurse discuss with the graduate nurse? **Select all that apply.**
    1. Obtain an informed consent from the client or spouse.
    2. Determine whether the client is allergic to iodine or shellfish.
    3. Place the client supine with the foot of the bed elevated.
    4. Instruct the client to relax and breathe normally.
    5. Explain to the client what to expect during the procedure.

77. The charge nurse is making shift assignments. Which client should be assigned to the **most** experienced nurse?
    1. The malnourished client diagnosed with bacterial meningitis experiencing photophobia
    2. The paraplegic client diagnosed with an L4 SCI and spastic muscle spasms of the lower extremities
    3. The elderly client diagnosed with Parkinson's disease with a mask-like face with pill rolling
    4. The client diagnosed with amyotrophic lateral sclerosis (ALS) having respiratory distress.

78. The nurse is caring for clients in a neurological ICU. Which client should be assessed **first?**
    1. The client recovering from an motor vehicle accident diagnosed with increased intracranial pressure and with a Glasgow Coma Scale score that went from 11 to 14
    2. The quadriplegic client diagnosed with a C6 SCI, bradycardia, hypotension, and hyperreflexia
    3. The client diagnosed with a brainstem herniation and their big toe moving toward the top surface of their foot while the other toes fan out after the sole has been firmly stroked
    4. The 20-year-old client diagnosed with West Nile virus reporting generalized body aches with a temperature of 101.2°F (38.4°C)

NEUROLOGICAL CASE STUDY

(1700) A 62-year-old woman with a history of hypertension and hyperlipidemia arrives at the emergency department (ED) with the report of a sudden, severe headache described as "the worst headache of my life." She reports associated nausea and vomiting, and upon arrival, appears diaphoretic and agitated.

(1715) Upon assessment the triage nurse find that the client is alert and oriented to person, place, and time, but she exhibits decreased verbal fluency and right-sided facial droop. Skin is intact, warm, and clammy. Lungs are clear to auscultation. Bowel sounds are active in all four quadrants. The client's left pupil measures 7 mm; her right pupil measures 3 mm. Grip strength is equal bilaterally, but arm and leg coordination is mildly impaired on the right side. Client reports a pain level of 10/10. She reports taking 500 mg of ibuprofen (Motrin) 30 minutes prior to arrival without relief. Vital signs are as follows:

Vital Signs	Client Values
Blood pressure	180/110 mm Hg
Heart rate	120 bpm
Respirations	18 breaths/min
Temperature	98.9°F (37.2°C)
Spo₂	98% (room air)

The nurse takes a complete medical history and reviews the patient's medications and places them in the electronic health record (EHR).

EHR history. Past medical history of hypertension, hyperlipidemia, allergies: shellfish and sulfonamides.

ED bed weight of 185 lb (84.1 kg). Allergies: Shellfish and sulfonamides.

Medication List	
Medication	Time Taken
Multivitamin PO daily	Before breakfast
Metoprolol 28 mg PO daily	Before breakfast
Aspirin 81 mg PO daily	Before breakfast
Lovastatin 60 mg PO	At bedtime
Motrin 500 mg PO	PRN for pain

1. **Recognize cues. What matters most?** The nurse prepares to call the ED physician. Which **priority** client data should be reported to the HCP? **Select all that apply.**
   1. Blood pressure 180/110 mm Hg
   2. Decreased verbal fluency and right-sided facial droop
   3. Lung sounds
   4. History of hypertension and hyperlipidemia
   5. Heart rate of 120 bpm
   6. Temperature of 98.9°F (37.2°C)
   7. Spo₂ 98% on room air
   8. Headache pain 10/10
   9. Pupil sizes
   10. Respirations 18 breaths/min

2. **Analyze cues. What could it mean?** What at-risk issues should the nurse be concerned for the client developing? **Select three answers.**
   1. Ineffective tissue perfusion
   2. Sepsis
   3. Anxiety
   4. Decreased skin integrity
   5. Seizures

(1745) The physician visits the client and orders a complete blood count (CBC), basal metabolic panel (BMP), and a coagulation panel to be done STAT, followed by a head CT with contrast. The physician orders are populated in the chart.

PROVIDER ORDERS:

CBC, BMP, coagulation panel STAT
0.9% NaCl via IV at 50 mL/hr
Head CT with contrast
Lumbar puncture
Morphine 15 mg IV every 4 hours PRN for pain
Phenytoin 100 mg IV every 8 hours

(1830) Diagnostic and laboratory results are posted:

Laboratory Test	Client Values	Reference Values
Hemoglobin (Hgb)	7.8 g/dL	Male: 14–17.3 g/dL
		Female: 11.7–15.5 g/dL
Hematocrit (Hct)	34%	Male: 42%–52%
		Female: 36%–48%
White blood cell (WBC) count	**9.8**	4.5 to 11.1 × 103/microL
Platelets	153	140 to 400 × 103/microL
Creatinine	1.6 mg/dL	Male: 0.61 to 1.21 mg/dL
		Female: 0.51 to 1.11 mg/dL
Glucose	124 mg/dL	Fasting: Less than 100 mg/dL
		Random: Less than 200 mg/dL
Potassium	4.2 mEq/L	3.5 to 5.3 mEq/L or mmol/L
Sodium	144 mEq/L	135 to 145 mEq/L or mmol/L
Blood urea nitrogen	20 mg/dL	8 to 21 mg/dL
		Adult over 90 years: 10 to 31 mg/dL
Prothrombin time	13 seconds	11 to 13.5 seconds
Partial thromboplastin time	35 seconds	25 to 37 seconds

3. **Prioritize hypotheses. Where do I start?** Complete the sentence by choosing from the drop-down list of options. Based on the client's condition at the time, the nurse recognizes that the client is at the **highest** risk for

and will require

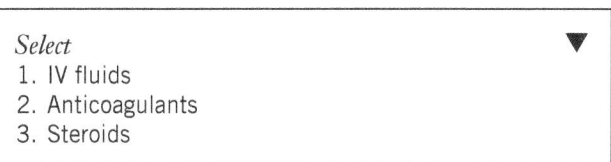

(1930) CT scan of the head reveals an aneurysm at the bifurcation of the internal carotid artery and a small amount of blood in the subarachnoid space. Lumbar puncture shows the presence of blood in the cerebrospinal fluid (CSF).

4. **Generate solutions. What can I do?** For each intervention, specify whether the intervention is **indicated** or **not indicated** for the client's care.

Potential Nursing Intervention	Indicated	Not Indicated
Begin oral fluids		
Prepare patient for surgery		
Apply wrist restraints		
Start oxygen at 2 L via nasal cannula		
Apply antiembolism stockings		
Reorient the client as needed		
Place the client in a high Fowler's position.		

5. **Take action. What will I do?** The patient is admitted to the ICU following aneurysm coiling. Which admission orders should the nurse consider a **priority** action? **Select all that apply.**
   1. Seizure precautions
   2. Vital signs every 4 hours
   3. Complete bedrest
   4. Routine measurement of intake and output
   5. Diet as tolerated
   6. CBC and BMP in a.m.

(0400) Client awakens when her name is called. She is oriented to person, place, and time. Skin is warm, dry, and pale. The client's left pupil measures 5 mm; her right pupil measures 3 mm. Hand grasps are equal bilaterally. Lung sounds are clear. Abdomen is soft with bowel sounds present ×4. Oxygen given at 2 L via nasal cannula. Client states she is having pain at surgical site; pain level is 4 out of 10. Vital signs are listed here:

Vital Signs	Client Values
Blood pressure	140/72 mm Hg
Heart rate	96 bpm
Respirations	18 breaths/min
Temperature	98.5°F (36.9°C)
Spo₂	99% (2 L)

6. **Evaluate outcomes. Did it help?** For each assessment finding, indicate whether the client's condition has **improved**, **declined**, or **no change**.

Finding	Improved	Declined	No Change
Temperature			
Heart rate			
Respirations			
Blood pressure			
Pain			
Spo₂			
Level of consciousness/ Neurological status			

One week later the client is being ready for discharge. The client is oriented ×4 and denies pain. Skin is pink, warm, and dry. PERRLA. Both pupils measure 3 mm. Hand grasps are equal bilaterally. Gait is steady. Lung sounds are clear. Abdomen is soft with bowel sounds present ×4. The suture line is well approximated and without signs of infection.

Vital Signs	Client Values
Blood pressure	130/72 mm Hg
Heart rate	80 bpm
Respirations	20 breaths/min
Temperature	98.6 °F (37.0°C)
Spo₂	100% room air
Pain	0/10

ANSWERS AND RATIONALES

The correct answer number and rationale are in **bold-face purple type.** Rationales for why other answer options are incorrect are also given.

1. 1. The serum platelet level is within the normal range of 140 to 400 × 10³/microL; therefore, this client does not warrant intervention by the charge nurse.
   2. A therapeutic valproic acid (Depakote) level is 50 to 125 mcg/mL; therefore, this laboratory result does not warrant action by the nurse.
   3. Steroids, such as prednisone, elevate a client's blood glucose level; therefore, this does not warrant intervention by the nurse.
   4. **The therapeutic range for the anticonvulsant phenytoin (Dilantin) is 10–20 mcg/mL. This client's higher level warrants intervention because the serum level is above the therapeutic range.**

   CLINICAL JUDGMENT GUIDE: The nurse must know normal laboratory values and be able to determine whether the laboratory value is expected for the client's disease process or the medications the client is taking.

2. 1. A pain medication is important to administer in a timely manner, but giving this medication is not a priority over administering a medication on time to prevent respiratory complications.
   2. A steroid medication is not a priority over a client experiencing respiratory difficulty. Steroids must be given to prevent adrenal sufficiency, but they do not have to be administered first.
   3. **Anticholinesterase medications administered for myasthenia gravis must be administered on time to preserve muscle functioning, especially the functioning of the upper respiratory tract muscles. This is the priority medication.**
   4. Clients calling for medications should be attended to, but this client would not receive an antacid for heartburn before the client diagnosed with myasthenia gravis or the client in pain.

   CLINICAL JUDGMENT GUIDE: The nurse must be aware of the expected actions of medications and use that information to prioritize which clients should receive their medications first.

3. 1. The nurse would expect the client diagnosed with Guillain-Barré syndrome to have ascending paralysis, and the problem has just reached the knees, so the nurse should not need to assess this client first.
   2. **The client diagnosed with a C6 SCI is expected to have autonomic dysreflexia, but it is an emergency situation; therefore, the nurse should assess this client first.**
   3. "Pill rolling," a hand tremor wherein the thumb and forefinger appear to move in a rotary fashion as if rolling a pill, is an expected clinical manifestation of Parkinson's; therefore, the nurse would not assess this client first.
   4. The client diagnosed with Huntington's disease has chorea, which includes abnormal and excessive involuntary movements; therefore, this client would not be assessed first.

   CLINICAL JUDGMENT GUIDE: The nurse must determine which sign or symptom is not expected for the disease process. If the sign or symptom is unexpected or it is an emergency situation, then the nurse should assess the client first. This type of question determines whether the nurse knows signs or symptoms of various disease processes.

4. 1. Placing a gait belt on a client before ambulating is appropriate for safety and would not require the nurse to intervene.
   2. Placing the client in a prone position helps promote hyperextension of the hip joints, which is essential for normal gait and helps prevent knee and hip flexion contractures; therefore, this would not require the nurse to intervene.
   3. **This action is inappropriate and would require intervention by the nurse because pulling on a flaccid shoulder joint could cause shoulder dislocation; the client should be pulled up by placing the arm underneath the client's back or using a lift sheet.**
   4. The client should be encouraged and praised for attempting to independently perform activities like combing hair or brushing teeth.

   CLINICAL JUDGMENT GUIDE: The nurse must ensure the UAP can perform any delegated tasks. It is the nurse's responsibility to demonstrate to or teach the UAP how to perform a task and evaluate the results.

5. 1. With an evolving stroke, the client experiences a worsening of signs or symptoms over several minutes to hours; thus, the client is at risk of dying and should be cared for by the most experienced nurse.
   2. A transient ischemic attack, by definition, lasts fewer than 24 hours; thus, this client should be stable now.
   3. Pain is expected in clients diagnosed with Guillain-Barré syndrome; symptoms typically occur on the lower half of the body, which wouldn't affect the airway. Therefore, a less experienced nurse could care for this client.
   4. The charge nurse could assign this client to a UAP.

   CLINICAL JUDGMENT GUIDE: When the nurse makes client assignments, the most critical and unstable client should be assigned to the most experienced nurse.

6. 1. This client should be referred to an inpatient rehabilitation facility for intensive therapy before deciding on long-term placement (home with home healthcare or a long-term care facility). The initial rehabilitation a client receives can set the tone for all further recuperation. This is the appropriate referral at this time.
   2. A home healthcare agency may be needed when the client returns home, but the most appropriate referral is to a rehabilitation center where intensive therapy can occur.
   3. A long-term care facility may be needed at some point, but the client should be allowed to regain as much lost ability as possible.
   4. The outpatient center would be utilized when the client is ready for discharge from the inpatient center.

   CLINICAL JUDGMENT GUIDE: The nurse must know the roles of all members of the multidisciplinary healthcare team, as well as HIPAA (Health Insurance Portability and Accountability Act) rules and regulations. These will be tested on the NCLEX-RN® examination.

7. 1. The nurse should be the first one to feed the client in order for the nurse to evaluate the client's ability to swallow and not aspirate.
   2. The LPN could administer routine parenteral medications. This is the best task to assign to the LPN.
   3. This involves assessing the client; therefore, the nurse should not delegate this assignment to the LPN.
   4. Teaching is the responsibility of the RN.

   CLINICAL JUDGMENT GUIDE: The nurse cannot assign assessment, teaching, evaluation, or an unstable client to an LPN.

8. Correct answers are 3, 4, and 5.
   1. Checking the client's skin involves assessment; therefore, the nurse cannot delegate this assignment to the UAP.
   2. The nurse cannot delegate medication administration to a UAP.
   3. The UAP can perform routine hygiene care. The nurse must then make the time to assess the client's skin.
   4. The UAP can ambulate a client to the bathroom.
   5. The UAP can take routine vital signs.

   CLINICAL JUDGMENT GUIDE: This type of alternate question is included in the NCLEX-RN® examination. The nurse must be able to select all the options that answer the question correctly.

9. 1. The UAP cannot change abdominal dressings because the incision must be assessed for healing.
   2. The UAP cannot check the client's IV site. Remember, "check" is assessment.
   3. The nurse must monitor the vital signs of a client who recently returned from surgery to determine whether the client is stable; the UAP can take vital signs and report results to the nurse.
   4. The UAP can escort the client to the vehicle after discharge.

   CLINICAL JUDGMENT GUIDE: A nurse cannot delegate assessment, teaching, evaluation, medications, or an unstable client to a UAP. Tasks that require nursing judgment cannot be delegated.

10. 1. This client diagnosed with dyspnea and a respiration rate of 12 has signs and symptoms of a respiratory complication and should be assessed first because ascending paralysis at the C6 level could cause the client to stop breathing.
    2. This is a psychosocial need and should be addressed, but it is not a priority over a physiological problem.
    3. A client diagnosed with a lower SCI would not be at risk for autonomic dysreflexia; therefore, a report of headache and feeling hot would not be a priority over an airway problem.

4. The client with a pulse oximeter reading greater than 93% is receiving adequate oxygenation.

CLINICAL JUDGMENT GUIDE: When deciding which client to assess first, the test taker should determine whether the signs and symptoms the client exhibits are normal or expected for the situation. After eliminating the expected options, the test taker should determine which situation is more life-threatening.

11. 1. The client is experiencing autonomic dysreflexia, a complication of SCI above the T6, and the most common cause is a full bladder. Placing the client on telemetry is not the nurse's first intervention.
    2. Completing a neurological assessment is an intervention a nurse could implement, but it should not be the first for a client experiencing autonomic dysreflexia.
    3. **Autonomic dysreflexia is a life-threatening condition and can be considered a medical emergency requiring immediate attention. The nurse should not assess but should intervene, and the most common cause is a full bladder.**
    4. A head CT scan would be appropriate if the elevated BP was secondary to a CVA, not because of a complication of an SCI.

CLINICAL JUDGMENT GUIDE: When the test question asks the test taker to determine which intervention should be implemented first, it means that all the options are something a nurse could implement. The test taker should apply the nursing process: If the client is in distress then do not assess; the nurse should do something to help the client.

12. 1. It would be appropriate for the UAP to perform ROM exercises to help prevent contractures; therefore, this action would not require the nurse to intervene.
    2. **This is not an appropriate intervention because the client is at risk for increased intracranial pressure; therefore, the client should not be placed on their stomach. The prone position helps promote hyperextension of the hip joints, which is essential for normal gait and helps prevent knee and hip flexion contractures, and is done in rehabilitation.**
    3. The client should be pulled up in bed by placing the arm underneath the back or using a lift sheet; therefore, the nurse would not need to intervene.
    4. The client should be encouraged and praised for attempting to perform any activities independently, such as combing hair, brushing teeth, or feeding themselves. The nurse would not need to intervene.

CLINICAL JUDGMENT GUIDE: The nurse must ensure the UAP can perform any delegated tasks. It is the nurse's responsibility to demonstrate to or teach the UAP how to perform the task, and then the nurse will evaluate the task.

13. 1. **The less experienced nurse could care for the client on a ventilator and console the family as needed.**
    2. A client diagnosed with increased intracranial pressure requires a more experienced critical care nurse.
    3. This client is unstable and requires a more experienced critical care nurse.
    4. Status epilepticus is a state of continuous seizure activity and is the most serious complication of epilepsy, a neurological emergency. This client should be assigned to a more experienced nurse.

CLINICAL JUDGMENT GUIDE: The graduate nurse should be assigned the most stable client. The more critical clients should be assigned to the more experienced nurses.

14. 1. Purposeful movement following painful stimuli would indicate an improvement in the client's condition and would not warrant intervention by the nurse.
    2. **Extension of the upper and lower extremities is assuming a decerebrate posture, which indicates the client's intracranial pressure is increasing. This would warrant immediate intervention by the nurse.**
    3. Aimless thrashing would indicate an improvement in the client's condition and would not warrant intervention by the nurse.
    4. If the client can follow simple commands, then the client's condition is improving and would not warrant intervention by the nurse.

CLINICAL JUDGMENT GUIDE: The test taker should ask, "Are the assessment data normal?" for the disease process. If the data are normal for the disease process, then the nurse would not need to intervene; if they are not normal for the disease process, then this warrants intervention.

15. 1. An adverse occurrence report is completed for incidents occurring to clients.

2. The nurse should talk to the primary nurse, but the sharps container should be changed immediately.
3. The UAP can change a sharps container. This must be done because a sharps container above the fill line violates Occupational Safety and Health Administration (OSHA) rules and can result in a financial fine.
4. The infection control nurse does not need to be notified of this situation.

CLINICAL JUDGMENT GUIDE: The nurse is responsible for knowing and complying with local, state, and federal standards of care.

16. 1. The nurse should address the client's comment and not shift the responsibility to someone else.
    2. The nurse should address the client's statement and not attempt to problem-solve at this point.
    3. The nurse is reflecting the client's comments, which will encourage the client to vent their feelings. This is the most appropriate response.
    4. This is false reassurance and an inappropriate response to the client's statement.

CLINICAL JUDGMENT GUIDE: The NCLEX-RN® test plan includes Therapeutic Communication as a subcategory of Psychosocial Integrity. The nurse should allow clients and family to express feelings.

17. 1. The occupational therapist addresses assisting the client with ADLs, but with MG the client will have no problems with ADLs if the client takes the medication correctly 30 minutes before performing ADLs.
    2. A physical therapist addresses transfer and movement issues with the client, but this would not be a priority in the critical care unit.
    3. The social worker assists the client with discharge or financial issues, but this would not be appropriate for the client in the critical care unit.
    4. Speech therapists address swallowing problems, and clients diagnosed with MG are dysphagic and are at risk for aspiration; the speech therapist can help match food consistency to the client's ability to swallow and thus help enhance client safety. This referral would be appropriate in the critical care unit.

CLINICAL JUDGMENT GUIDE: The NCLEX-RN® integrates the nursing process throughout the Client Needs categories and subcategories. The nursing process is a scientific, clinical reasoning approach to client care, including assessment, analysis, planning, implementation, and evaluation. The nurse will be responsible for identifying nursing diagnoses for clients.

18. Correct order is 5, 2, 1, 3, 4.
    5. The nurse should flush the area with soap and water and attempt to get the site to bleed.
    2. The nurse should notify the charge nurse immediately after cleaning the area to avoid any treatment delays and initiate hospital protocol.
    1. The laboratory should draw the client's and the nurse's baseline laboratory blood work.
    3. If applicable, postexposure prophylaxis should be started within 4 hours of the stick.
    4. Follow-up with the employee health nurse is done at 3 months and 6 months.

CLINICAL JUDGMENT GUIDE: The NCLEX-RN® test plan includes nursing care that is ruled by legal requirements as well as The Joint Commission, Centers for Medicare & Medicaid Services, the Centers for Disease Control and Prevention, and OSHA rules and regulations. The nurse must know these standards.

19. 1. The client diagnosed with Parkinson's disease and beginning to hallucinate may be experiencing an adverse reaction to one of the medications used to treat the disease. The nurse should assess this client first.
    2. Peripheral edema is expected in a client diagnosed with heart failure. This client does not need to be assessed first.
    3. Wandering and lack of sleep are expected in a client diagnosed with Alzheimer's disease. This client does not need to be assessed first.
    4. Weight loss in a client diagnosed with terminal cancer is expected. Before intervening, the nurse should review the client's intake, food preferences, and pain control. Weight loss does not occur in minutes to hours, and this client's needs do not merit assessment before the client diagnosed with a new problem.

CLINICAL JUDGMENT GUIDE: The nurse should determine whether a new problem is occurring or whether the problem is expected for the disease process. If the symptom is expected for the disease process and is not life-threatening, then that client does not have priority.

20. 1. A daily acetylsalicylic acid (aspirin) tablet is not a priority medication. This medication can be administered 30 minutes before or 30 minutes after the scheduled time.
    2. Neostigmine (Prostigmin) promotes muscle function in clients diagnosed with myasthenia gravis. This medication should always be administered on time to prevent loss of muscle tone, especially the upper respiratory tract muscles. This is the priority medication to administer at this time.
    3. Cephalexin (Keflex), an oral antibiotic, can be administered within 30 minutes before or after the scheduled time frame.
    4. Acyclovir (Zovirax) alone or in combination with prednisone may be used to treat Bell's palsy, but this is not a priority medication.

    CLINICAL JUDGMENT GUIDE: When deciding on priority medications, the test taker must first know the expected response of the client. If the expected response prevents or treats an emergency, that medication becomes the priority medication to administer.

21. 1. Clients diagnosed with Alzheimer's disease may have problems completing ADLs, but this is not the client's priority problem.
    2. Safety is the highest priority for clients diagnosed with end-stage Alzheimer's disease because the client is unaware of their surroundings and can easily wander from an area of safety.
    3. The client in end-stage disease may have an increased risk for constipation, but this is not a priority over the safety of the client.
    4. The client's family is often distraught over seeing their loved one deteriorate because of Alzheimer's, but it is not a priority over the safety of the client.

    CLINICAL JUDGMENT GUIDE: The test taker can use Maslow's Hierarchy of Needs to determine the correct answer. On the pyramid of needs, beginning at the bottom, physiological needs have priority, followed by safety.

22. Correct answers are 1, 2, 4, and 5.
    1. Cataracts cause less light to be filtered through an opaque lens to the retina. The client should have as much light as possible in the home to prevent falls.
    2. Dark glasses protect the eyes from the sun's rays when outside, as they do for anyone, so they should be encouraged in this client.
    3. This is the responsibility of the HCP, not the nurse.
    4. The furniture in the client's house should not be moved. The client will be less likely to fall or stumble if the furniture remains in its usual position.
    5. Discharge instructions should be provided with visual aids or large print, allowing the client to review the materials with less difficulty.

    CLINICAL JUDGMENT GUIDE: This question requires the test taker to use knowledge of the disease process and Maslow's Hierarchy of Needs. Cataracts cause opacity of the eye lens. The test taker should address nursing interventions that promote client safety and independence.

23. 1. The nurse should assess the client's neurological status first. It is not normal for an older person to have behavioral changes so they should be assessed.
    2. The nurse may need to notify the HCP, but not before completing a neurological assessment.
    3. The nurse should assess the client before further interviewing the client's wife.
    4. The nurse could determine the last time the client ate because the confusion could be caused by hypoglycemia, but the first intervention is to complete a neurological assessment.

    CLINICAL JUDGMENT GUIDE: Any time the nurse receives information about a client experiencing a possible complication, the nurse must assess the client.

24. 1. This question will determine whether the nurse has assessed the client's swallowing ability. The nurse cannot delegate unstable clients, and a client newly diagnosed with a CVA may be unstable and have difficulty swallowing.
    2. This question does not address the client's ability to swallow.
    3. Thickener (Thick-It) might be needed if the client has difficulty swallowing, but the charge nurse has not established that the client has swallowing difficulty.
    4. A UAP can feed stable clients, and the task does not require nursing judgment.

    CLINICAL JUDGMENT GUIDE: The nurse cannot delegate assessment, evaluation, teaching, administering medications, or caring for an unstable client to a UAP.

25. 1. The client should be encouraged to move the buttocks to increase blood circulation to the area, but a wheelchair cushion used every time the client is in the wheelchair will help prevent pressure injuries.
    2. A high-protein diet will assist with maintaining a positive nitrogen balance that will support wound healing, but it will not prevent pressure from causing skin breakdown.
    3. All clients in a wheelchair for extended periods should have a wheelchair cushion that relieves pressure to prevent skin breakdown.
    4. The more the client can move from the wheelchair to a chair to the bed, the more it will help decrease the possibility of a pressure injury, but a wheelchair cushion helps relieve pressure continuously.

    CLINICAL JUDGMENT GUIDE: The nurse must know the expected medical treatment for the client. This question is a knowledge-based, or comprehension, question.

26. Correct answers are 1, 2, and 4.
    1. Identifying the first area that began seizing will provide information and clues as to the origin of the seizure in the brain.
    2. The nurse should look at their watch and time the seizure.
    3. The client's bed rails should be padded, but this intervention should not be performed when a client begins to have a seizure. The nurse should protect the client and assess the seizure. The seizure may be over by the time the nurse can pad the side rails.
    4. The client should be protected from onlookers as much as possible.
    5. The nurse should never attempt to insert anything into a client's mouth during a seizure. Doing so can cause injury to the client's mouth or obstruction of the client's airway.

    CLINICAL JUDGMENT GUIDE: This is an alternate type of question included in the NCLEX-RN® examination. The nurse must be able to select all the correct options.

27. 1. Closing the door and cubicle curtain protects the client's privacy and would not warrant immediate intervention from the nurse.
    2. Providing a back massage is a comfort action and would not warrant intervention by the nurse.
    3. Checking the temperature of the bathwater prevents scalding the client with water that is too hot or making the client uncomfortable with water that is too cold. This action would not warrant immediate intervention.
    4. The client is recovering from a potentially debilitating disease, and in the rehabilitation unit, the client should be out of bed as much as possible. Bathing the client in bed would warrant intervention by the nurse.

    CLINICAL JUDGMENT GUIDE: Delegation means the nurse is responsible for the UAP's actions and performance. The nurse must correct the UAP's performance to ensure the client is cared for safely in the hospital, the rehabilitation unit, or the home.

28. Correct answers are 1, 2, 3, and 4.
    1. Placing a small pillow under the shoulder will prevent the shoulder from adducting toward the chest and developing a contracture.
    2. The client should be referred to occupational therapy for assistance with performing activities of daily living (ADLs).
    3. The client should not ignore the paralyzed side, and the nurse must encourage the client to move it as much as possible; a written schedule may assist the client in exercising.
    4. These exercises should be done at least five times a day for 10 minutes to help strengthen the muscles used for walking.
    5. The fingers should be positioned to be barely flexed, to prevent contracture.

    CLINICAL JUDGMENT GUIDE: This is an alternate type of question included in the NCLEX-RN®. The nurse must be able to select all the options that answer the question correctly.

29. 1. The nurse should stabilize the client's cervical spine to help prevent an SCI, or the client's spine can sustain irreparable damage during movement.
    2. The nurse should not move the driver unless the driver is in danger such as the car on fire or in water.
    3. The nurse should first ensure a patent airway. According to Maslow's Hierarchy of Needs, the airway is always the priority.
    4. The nurse should control external bleeding, but the first intervention is the airway.

    CLINICAL JUDGMENT GUIDE: The test taker should use some tool as a reference to guide the decision-making process. In this situation, Maslow's Hierarchy of Needs should be applied.

30. 1. This would be the most appropriate assignment because the nurse would not be exposed to contagious diseases or dangerous radiological procedures.
    2. The pregnant nurse should not be exposed to x-rays, which could endanger the fetus.
    3. Working in the front desk triage area would expose the pregnant nurse to any contagious or infectious disease. This is not an appropriate assignment.
    4. The oncology clinic will have clients receiving chemotherapeutic agents that may endanger the fetus; this would not be the most appropriate assignment. Even if the nurse is not administering the medication, the most appropriate assignment is to assign the nurse to an area that poses no danger to the fetus.

CLINICAL JUDGMENT GUIDE: Pregnant nurses can refuse and should not be assigned duties that could harm the fetus. Most medications and many diagnostic tests and treatments can harm the fetus.

31. 1. If the client must be transferred from the clinic to the hospital, then the client is unstable and should not be assigned to a UAP.
    2. The client is stable because they are being sent home; therefore, the UAP could safely complete this task.
    3. Showing the client how to walk with crutches is teaching, and the nurse cannot delegate teaching to the UAP.
    4. The UAP should not be calling a pharmacy because this is not within the scope of practice of unlicensed personnel. The HCP is responsible for completing this task.

CLINICAL JUDGMENT GUIDE: A nurse cannot delegate assessment, teaching, evaluation, medications, or an unstable client to a UAP. Tasks that cannot be delegated are nursing interventions requiring nursing judgment.

32. 1. The nurse should first care for the client and refer the client to an HCP for possible x-rays, pain medication, and further treatment. The employee health nurse's responsibility is to ensure the employee is safe to work, and this client is not.
    2. This information should be completed because workers' compensation insurance must cover any injury on the job to cover all costs for the client. Documentation is never a priority over caring for the client.
    3. The employee health nurse should determine whether there are unsafe areas in the workplace or whether the employee was negligent, but this is not the nurse's first intervention.
    4. The employee's supervisor does need to be notified, but this is not the nurse's first intervention. The safety of the client is always first.

CLINICAL JUDGMENT GUIDE: When the question asks which intervention should be implemented first, it means all the options are something a nurse could implement, but only one should be implemented first. The test taker should use the nursing process to determine the appropriate action: If the client is in distress, do not assess; if the client is not in distress, then the nurse should assess.

33. 1. If a client is reporting pain, the nurse should not ask the client to return to work. If nothing else, the client should be allowed to stay in the clinic until the pain subsides.
    2. The employee must submit to a urine drug screen any time an injury occurs. This is standard practice by many employers to help determine whether the employee was under the influence during the accident. Workers' compensation will not be responsible if the employee is under the influence of alcohol or drugs.
    3. A referral to the emergency department is not warranted because there are no visible injuries and the neurovascular assessment is normal. The employee health nurse could send the employee home with further instructions. None of the symptoms warrant the employee needing an x-ray.
    4. A sequential compression device is used to help prevent deep vein thrombosis for clients on bedrest. This is not an appropriate intervention.

CLINICAL JUDGMENT GUIDE: The NCLEX-RN® test plan includes nursing care that is ruled by legal requirements as well as The Joint Commission, Centers for Medicare & Medicaid Services, Centers for Disease Control and Prevention, and OSHA rules and regulations. The nurse must be knowledgeable of these standards.

34. Correct order is 1, 3, 2, 4, 5.
    1. An alert client diagnosed with a sucking chest wound and categorized as red should be evacuated first. A red tag means the injury is life-threatening but survivable with minimal intervention. These clients can deteriorate rapidly without treatment.

3. A client with a hard and tender abdomen and categorized as a yellow should be evacuated second. A yellow tag means the injury is significant and requires medical care but is currently stable.
2. An inconsolable client who is unable to answer questions and is categorized as green should be evacuated third. A green tag means the injury is minor, and treatment can be delayed hours to days. These clients should be moved away from the main triage area. Clients diagnosed with behavioral and psychological problems are included in this category.
4. This client categorized as black should be evacuated fourth. A black tag means the injury is extensive and chances of survival are unlikely even with definitive care. Clients should receive comfort measures and be separated from other casualties, but not abandoned.
5. The client categorized as white does not need to be evacuated until last. A white tag means no care is required.

CLINICAL JUDGMENT GUIDE: The NCLEX-RN® test plan includes questions on disaster management. The nurse must be aware of triaging clients, nursing care, procedures, and protocols during disasters.

35. 1. The nurse should determine what medication the client has taken, but the nurse should first attempt to determine whether the headache is secondary to high blood pressure.
2. No matter the client's number on the pain scale in the home setting, the nurse must attempt to determine the cause. One way to determine the cause or eliminate a possible cause is to take the client's blood pressure.
3. If the client's blood pressure is not elevated, the client could take the non-narcotic analgesic acetaminophen (Tylenol). Still, if the client's blood pressure is elevated, the acetaminophen will not help.
4. The number 1 risk factor for a CVA is arterial hypertension. Because the client has a history of CVA and is reporting a severe headache, which is a symptom of hypertension, the nurse should first take the client's blood pressure. If it is elevated, the client must be taken to the emergency department. In the home setting, asking about the pain scale would not affect the care the nurse provides.

CLINICAL JUDGMENT GUIDE: When the question asks which intervention should be implemented first, it means that all the options are something a nurse could implement, but only one should be implemented first. The test taker should use the nursing process to determine the appropriate action: If the client is in distress, do not assess; if the client is not in distress, then the nurse should assess.

36. 1. The nurse should assist the client in lying in the "C" position with the back as near as possible to the edge of the bed, but it is not the first intervention.
2. The first intervention is to empty the client's bladder before the procedure.
3. All clients should have an advance directive, but it is not mandated by law, and clients can decide not to have one.
4. The client does not have to be NPO for this procedure.

CLINICAL JUDGMENT GUIDE: The nurse must know about normal diagnostic tests and pre- and post-procedure interventions. The nurse must be able to determine whether the client can have the diagnostic procedure and provide postprocedure care to ensure the client is safe.

37. 1. A severe, pounding headache would be the priority for a client diagnosed with a T6 or above SCI because it could be autonomic dysreflexia, but not in a client diagnosed with a lower-level lesion.
2. The client's psychosocial need is not a priority over clients diagnosed with physiological problems. This client does not need to be visited first.
3. The client diagnosed with Parkinson's disease is expected to have a short, shuffling gait; therefore, this client does not need to be seen first.
4. The client is reporting an infection at the insertion sites into the bone, which can lead to osteomyelitis. This client is exhibiting a potentially life-threatening condition and should be seen first.

CLINICAL JUDGMENT GUIDE: When deciding which client to assess first, the test taker should determine whether the signs or symptoms the client is exhibiting are normal or expected for the situation. After eliminating the expected option, the test taker should determine which situation is more life-threatening.

38. 1. A client diagnosed with AIDS would be expected to have Kaposi's sarcoma; therefore, this client would not need to be visited first.

2. A client diagnosed with dementia would be expected to have difficulty dressing; therefore, this client would not need to be visited first.
3. The classic feature of trigeminal neuralgia is excruciating pain described as a burning, knife-like, or lightning-like shock in the lips, upper or lower gums, cheek, forehead, or side of the nose. The nurse would not return this call first because the client is experiencing the normal signs and symptoms of the disease process.
4. Botulism is the most serious type of food poisoning, and the client is exhibiting signs and symptoms of it; therefore, the nurse should return this phone call first.

CLINICAL JUDGMENT GUIDE: When deciding which client to assess first, the nurse should determine whether the clinical manifestations the client is exhibiting are normal or expected for the situation. After eliminating the expected options, the test taker should determine which situation is more dangerous for the client.

39. 1. Therapeutic communication addresses the client's feelings and attempts to allow the client to verbalize feelings. The client is still grieving over their loss, and the nurse should let them vent those feelings.
2. The social worker may be able to help the client with driving and going back to college, but this is not the nurse's first intervention.
3. The American Spinal Cord Association is an excellent resource for clients diagnosed with spinal cord injuries. However, the client is still grieving, and the nurse should allow the client to express their feelings.
4. Attempting to help identify a support system for the client is an appropriate intervention, but the first intervention is to allow the client to vent their feelings.

CLINICAL JUDGMENT GUIDE: The NCLEX-RN® test plan includes Therapeutic Communication as a subcategory of Psychosocial Integrity. The nurse should allow clients and family to vent their feelings.

40. 1. The client is allergic to iodine; therefore, the client cannot have the CT scan with contrast agent because it is iodine. The nurse should question this HCP order.
2. The client is not allergic to acetaminophen; therefore, this order should not be questioned.
3. The client should have vital signs taken; therefore, this order should not be questioned.
4. A low-fat, low-cholesterol diet would be appropriate for this client.

CLINICAL JUDGMENT GUIDE: When the question stem asks the nurse to determine which HCP order to question, the test taker should realize this is an "except" question. Three of the options are appropriate for the HCP to prescribe, and one is not appropriate for the client's disease process or procedure.

41. 1. The client has a chronic illness. The nurse should empower the client to deal with their disease process, not put more responsibility on the spouse.
2. The occupational therapist could assist the client in identifying ways to save energy when performing ADLs. Myasthenia gravis is a neurological condition that causes skeletal muscle weakness.
3. The home health nurse should realize that exhaustion is a symptom of the client's disease process and should utilize any member of the home healthcare team who is able to help the client. Allowing the client to verbalize their feelings about exhaustion is an appropriate therapeutic intervention, but this client needs specific advice on handling it.
4. If the client is taking their medication, the client does not need to be referred to their HCP. Myasthenia gravis is a chronic illness; muscle weakness is the primary symptom.

CLINICAL JUDGMENT GUIDE: The test taker must know the roles of all members of the multidisciplinary healthcare team as well as HIPAA rules and regulations. These are tested on the NCLEX-RN® examination.

42. 1. An epidural hematoma results from bleeding between the dura and the inner surface of the skull and is a medical emergency. This client should be seen first.
2. Postictal state is the client's sleepy state after a seizure. This client is stable; therefore, this client does not have to be assessed first.
3. The client diagnosed with encephalitis may have a fever, headache, nausea, and vomiting. The client needs to be assessed, but not before a head injury with active arterial bleeding.
4. The client diagnosed with multiple sclerosis is expected to have scanning speech; therefore, the nurse should not assess this client first.

CLINICAL JUDGMENT GUIDE: The test taker should use some tool as a reference to guide the decision-making process. In this situation, Maslow's Hierarchy of Needs should be applied.

43. 1. The tension headache does not involve nausea or vomiting but may involve photophobia or phonophobia. The nurse should return this phone call first because the nausea and vomiting are not expected.
    2. The migraine headache is a recurring headache characterized by unilateral or bilateral throbbing pain; therefore, this client should not be contacted first.
    3. The pain of cluster headaches is sharp and stabbing on one side of the head, often near the eye. It is not similar to the pulsing pain of a migraine headache. This client does not need to be contacted first.
    4. This is the typical type of pain clients diagnosed with hypertension experience; therefore, this client does not need to be contacted first.

CLINICAL JUDGMENT GUIDE: The test taker must determine which sign or symptom is not expected for the disease process. If the sign or symptom is not expected, then the nurse should assess the client first. This type of question determines whether the nurse knows about clinical manifestations of various disease processes.

44. 1. The spouse should check to determine whether the client is incontinent of urine, but the client's safety is the priority.
    2. **The most important action the spouse can take if the client has a seizure is to ensure the client does not get injured during the seizure. Moving all the furniture out of the way will help ensure the client's safety.**
    3. Seizures are not life-threatening. If the spouse calls 911, the ambulance will probably arrive after the client's seizure has ended. Seizures lasting longer than 4 to 5 minutes warrant calling 911.
    4. The client should be allowed to rest after the seizure when they are in the postictal state, but it is not the most important action to take. The safety of the client during the seizure is the priority.

CLINICAL JUDGMENT GUIDE: The nurse must know the expected medical treatment for the client's condition. Safety is the priority for the client, especially when the client is at home.

45. 1. The client may benefit from a hospital bed, but this is not the priority intervention to address the client's nonhealing pressure injury.
    2. Home healthcare agencies do not provide care 7 days a week. Even if the client could have an aide 7 days a week, it is not the priority intervention to address the client's nonhealing pressure injury.
    3. The client does not need to be transferred to a skilled nursing unit. The wound care nurse should first attempt to heal the pressure injury in the home.
    4. **The wound care nurse's primary role is to address nonhealing pressure injuries. This referral is the priority intervention.**

CLINICAL JUDGMENT GUIDE: The test taker must know the roles of all members of the multidisciplinary healthcare team as well as HIPAA rules and regulations. These are tested on the NCLEX-RN® examination.

46. 1. Grab bars address safety issues, but the client is having transfer difficulty, which requires the help of the physical therapist.
    2. In most situations, the nurse should assess the client before taking action, but the home health aide has the ability and knowledge to determine whether the client is having problems getting out of bed and into the shower. The nurse should allow the physical therapist to assess the client's transfer ability.
    3. The goal of home health nursing is to keep the client as independent as possible, and having the client receive a bed bath increases the client's dependency on the home health aide.
    4. **The physical therapist is the healthcare team member responsible for helping the client diagnosed with mobility issues.**

CLINICAL JUDGMENT GUIDE: The test taker must know the roles of all members of the multidisciplinary healthcare team, as well as HIPAA rules and regulations. These are tested on the NCLEX-RN® examination.

47. 1. Daily exercise, relaxation periods, and socializing are encouraged because each can help decrease the occurrence of headaches. This statement indicates the client understands the teaching.
    2. Alternative ways of handling a headache's pain include relaxation, meditation, yoga, and self-hypnosis. This statement indicates the client understands the teaching.
    3. **Massage and moist hot packs to the neck and head can help a client diagnosed with**

tension-type headaches. This statement indicates the client needs more teaching.
4. Foods containing amines (cheese, chocolate), nitrites (hot dogs), vinegar, onions, caffeine, and alcohol (especially red wine) can trigger a headache. The statement indicates the client understands the teaching.

CLINICAL JUDGMENT GUIDE: This question asks the nurse to identify which statement indicates the client understands the teaching, indicating that three options are appropriate, but one is incorrect. This is an "except" question, even though it does not say all the options are correct "except."

48. 1. Most organ procurement organizations prefer to ask the family if the client wishes to be an organ or tissue donor. The priority intervention for the nurse is to address the family's grieving.
2. The nurse should give the client's belongings to the family, but the priority intervention is to address the family's grieving.
3. **The nurse's priority intervention should be to address the family's grieving process.**
4. The client's body will have to be sent to a funeral home, but it is not the nurse's priority intervention.

CLINICAL JUDGMENT GUIDE: The nurse must address all areas of the client's death, but the priority intervention is to address the client's family. Helping the client's family initially after the death with the grieving process should be the nurse's priority.

49. 1. The family should designate a funeral home. The nurse does not make this referral.
2. Hospice is for dying clients, but this client is considered brain dead.
3. A home health nurse cannot help this client or family.
4. **A 22-year-old client, after experiencing a traumatic brain death, could be a good candidate for organ donation. Most organ procurement organizations prefer to be the ones to approach the family. This is the best referral.**

CLINICAL JUDGMENT GUIDE: The NCLEX-RN® test plan includes nursing care that is ruled by legal requirements as well as The Joint Commission, Centers for Medicare & Medicaid Services, Centers for Disease Control and Prevention, and OSHA rules and regulations. The nurse must be knowledgeable of these standards.

50. 1. The client diagnosed with cataracts is expected to have decreased vision and abnormal color perception and will need surgery, but it is elective surgery. Therefore, this client does not warrant intervention.
2. Loss of peripheral vision is an expected symptom of a retinal detachment and should be seen because the client needs surgery; without surgery, the condition could lead to blindness. But this does not warrant intervention over the client having pain.
3. A hordeolum is a "sty," an infection of the sebaceous glands in the lid margin. It is not an emergency and is treated with warm, moist compresses to the eye four times a day.
4. **The client diagnosed with primary open-angle glaucoma reports no symptom of pain or pressure, so a client reporting eye pain warrants intervention by the nurse.**

CLINICAL JUDGMENT GUIDE: The test taker must determine which sign or symptom is not expected for the disease process. If the sign or symptom is unexpected, the nurse should assess the client first. This type of question determines whether the nurse is knowledgeable about clinical manifestations of various disease processes.

51. 1. Someone should call 911 because the client needs to go to the emergency department, but the nurse should first take care of the client.
2. **The nurse should first stabilize the foreign object to help prevent further damage. The stick should not be removed because it will cause more damage and possibly enucleate the eye.**
3. The nurse should not apply direct pressure to the eye. The nurse should stabilize the foreign object and not apply pressure, which could cause further damage.
4. The eye should be irrigated for a chemical exposure, not an impaled object.

CLINICAL JUDGMENT GUIDE: The nurse should remember that if a client is in distress and the nurse can do something to relieve the distress, that action should be done first before assessment. The nurse should select an intervention that directly helps the client's condition or prevents further damage.

52. 1. The nurse and the UAP should protect themselves from injury by obtaining a lifting device before attempting to move the client.
2. The nurse and the UAP should provide the best care possible, including turning the client every 2 hours.

3. One other person may not be enough to turn or move the client adequately without injuring the staff.
4. The client is not responsive enough to assist in movement.

CLINICAL JUDGMENT GUIDE: The NCLEX-RN® test plan includes nursing care that is ruled by legal requirements as well as The Joint Commission, Centers for Medicare & Medicaid Services, Centers for Disease Control and Prevention, and OSHA rules and regulations. The nurse must be know these standards.

53. 1. The nurse should administer the IVP narcotic pain medication even if the client has shallow breathing, with respirations of 8 breaths/min. A nurse should never administer medication with the intent of hastening the client's death, but medicating a dying client to achieve a peaceful death is an appropriate intervention.
2. Repositioning the client would not be effective for "pain all over."
3. It is cruel to refuse to administer pain medication to a dying client. The vital signs are decreased, but the client has signed a DNR and should be supported in a peaceful death.
4. The HCP has all the orders needed in place. There is no reason to notify the HCP.

CLINICAL JUDGMENT GUIDE: The NCLEX-RN® addresses questions concerned with end-of-life care, which is included in the Psychosocial Integrity section of the test plan. If unsure of the correct option, an intervention addressing an individual is better.

54. 1. The client's ability to maneuver a wheelchair indicates that the client has progressed in therapy.
2. This statement indicates the client is in denial about the prognosis of the injury.
3. Eye blinks may be used for communication with a client with a higher-level injury.
4. The building of a wheelchair ramp indicates the spouse is preparing for the client's return home, not that the client is progressing in therapy.

CLINICAL JUDGMENT GUIDE: The NCLEX-RN® integrates the nursing process throughout the Client Needs categories and subcategories. The nursing process is a scientific, clinical reasoning approach to client care, including assessment, analysis, planning, implementation, and evaluation. The nurse will be responsible for determining whether or not goals are being met.

55. 1. Ménière's disease, an excessive accumulation of endolymph in the membranous labyrinth, is characterized by episodic vertigo, tinnitus, fluctuating sensorineural hearing loss, and aural fullness. This client does not need to be contacted first.
2. Otitis media with effusion is an inflammation of the middle ear in which a collection of fluid is present in the middle ear space, resulting in a feeling of fullness of the ear and decreased hearing. Since this is expected, the nurse does not need to contact this client first.
3. This client needs to be contacted so culture and sensitivity (C&S) tests and mild analgesics can be prescribed. The ear canal has to be cleaned, and antibiotic eardrops must be administered to the ear. Otalgia is ear pain. This client should be contacted for treatment.
4. Otosclerosis is an autosomal disease, the fixation of the footplate of the stapes of the oval window, and results in conductive hearing loss; therefore, this client does not need to be contacted first.

CLINICAL JUDGMENT GUIDE: The test taker must determine which sign or symptom is not expected for the disease process. If the sign or symptom is unexpected, the nurse should assess the client first. This question determines whether the nurse knows about clinical manifestations of various disease processes.

56. 1. The nurse must irrigate the eyes, not patch the eyes.
2. The client is in distress, and the nurse needs to flush the client's eyes, not assess the visual acuity.
3. For chemical injuries, the nurse should begin ocular irrigation with sterile, pH-balanced, physiological solution.
4. The nurse should elevate the head of the bed, but it is not the nurse's first intervention.

CLINICAL JUDGMENT GUIDE: The nurse should remember that if a client is in distress and the nurse can do something to relieve the distress, it should be done first, before assessment. The nurse should select an option that directly helps the client's condition.

57. 1. The client admitted to a rehabilitation unit is expected to participate in therapy for at least 3 hours daily. The nurse would not question this order.
2. The client admitted to a rehabilitation unit is expected to participate in therapy for at least 3 hours daily. The nurse would not question this order.

CHAPTER 7 NEUROLOGICAL MANAGEMENT 217

3. Clients diagnosed with neurological deficits may have trouble swallowing. The nurse would not question this order.
4. A client in a rehabilitation unit for a brain injury should not require IV medications. The nurse should question this order.

CLINICAL JUDGMENT GUIDE: When the stem asks the nurse to determine which HCP order to question, the test taker must realize this is an "except" question. Three options are appropriate for the HCP to prescribe, and one is not appropriate for the client's disease process or procedure.

58. 1. A hospice organization is designed for terminally ill clients. The client is not terminally ill.
    2. The speech therapist helps clients regain speech and swallowing abilities. This therapy should have occurred while the client was in the rehab facility.
    3. The physical therapist assists the client with gait and muscle strengthening. This therapy should have occurred while the client was in the rehab facility.
    4. **The client is being discharged. The nurse should plan for continuity of care by arranging for a home health agency to follow the client at home.**

CLINICAL JUDGMENT GUIDE: The test taker must know the roles of all members of the multidisciplinary healthcare team, as well as HIPAA rules and regulations. The NCLEX-RN® examination tests this information.

59. 1. It will take approximately 6 weeks for the wound to heal sufficiently before being fitted for a prosthetic eye.
    2. The nurse should ensure the client can insert the conformer in the eye socket, and the client should be able to demonstrate this to the nurse. The client does not need more teaching.
    3. Eye drops must be placed in the lower conjunctiva; therefore, the client does not need more discharge teaching.
    4. The client is at risk for infection and should call the HCP if an elevation in temperature occurs. The client does not need more discharge teaching.

CLINICAL JUDGMENT GUIDE: This question asks the nurse to identify which statement supports the notion that the client needs more teaching, indicating three statements are appropriate for the disease process or disorder, but one is incorrect. This question is an "except" question even though it does not say all the options are correct "except."

60. 1. The client may be able to maintain the ability to work for several years before needing to apply for disability. The stem does not suggest the client is disabled.
    2. The client is newly diagnosed; nutrition would not be a problem now.
    3. **The client should be referred to a psychological counselor to develop skills for coping with long-term chronic illness.**
    4. The chaplain may need to see the client, but the stem did not indicate the client was having a problem with spiritual distress.

CLINICAL JUDGMENT GUIDE: The test taker must know the roles of all members of the multidisciplinary healthcare team, as well as HIPAA rules and regulations. The NCLEX-RN® examination will test this information.

61. 1. The LPN can administer medications to clients; therefore, this task is appropriate for the nurse to assign to the LPN.
    2. The client experiencing status epilepticus is an unstable client, and the nurse should not assign this task to the LPN.
    3. **The UAP could assist the client to the bathroom. Remember to assign and delegate tasks based on staff members' education and job description.**
    4. The nurse cannot assign the assessment to the LPN.

CLINICAL JUDGMENT GUIDE: When the test taker decides which option is the most appropriate task to delegate or assign, the test taker should choose the task that allows each staff member to function within their full scope of practice. Do not assign a task to a staff member that falls outside the staff member's or volunteer's expertise. Remember: The nurse cannot delegate assessment, teaching, evaluation, or the care of an unstable client to the LPN.

62. 1. **The client diagnosed with a closed head injury is at risk for increased intracranial pressure, and the osmotic diuretic is a priority medication.**
    2. The nurse should administer the medications to the client before leaving the unit, but the client diagnosed with a physiological, potentially life-threatening complication is a priority.
    3. Before administering a narcotic, the nurse must first assess the client to make sure that administering the medication is not going to mask symptoms.
    4. The anticonvulsant gabapentin (Neurontin) is a routine medication that can be administered

30 minutes before or after the scheduled time. This is not a priority medication.

CLINICAL JUDGMENT GUIDE: The test taker should know which medications are priority, such as those indicated in life-threatening situations. These must be administered first.

63. 1. The charge nurse will not always be available to intercede for the new graduate. The charge nurse should wait and see whether the new graduate can handle the situation before intervening.
    2. The charge nurse should wait, allowing the new graduate to deal with the UAP.
    3. The charge nurse should wait, allowing the new graduate to deal with the UAP.
    4. The charge nurse should wait, allowing the new graduate to deal with the UAP.

CLINICAL JUDGMENT GUIDE: Management questions will be on the NCLEX-RN®. There is often no test-taking strategy; the nurse must be knowledgeable of management issues.

64. 1. Levothyroxine (Synthroid) is a daily medication.
    2. Morphine sulfate (MS Contin) is a narcotic analgesic in sustained-release form. Clients experiencing pain are unlikely to be able to participate fully in the treatment program. The client should be medicated to ensure compliance with the treatment regimen.
    3. The Fleets enema is utilized daily to assist the client in regaining control of their bowels. This should be administered sometime during the evening hours because administering it during the day would interfere with other therapies, such as physical or occupational therapy. Most therapy is performed during the daytime hours.
    4. Metformin (Glucophage) should be administered with meals to prevent nausea and could be the second medication administered.

CLINICAL JUDGMENT GUIDE: This is an alternate type of question included in the NCLEX-RN® test plan. The test taker must be able to read an MAR, be knowledgeable of medications, and make a decision as to the nurse's most appropriate intervention.

65. Answer: Two 20-mg tablets and one 10-mg tablet.
    20 + 20 + 10 = 50 mg
    The nurse cannot split a 75-mg tablet into two-thirds, so the client must receive multiple tablets.

CLINICAL JUDGMENT GUIDE: This is an alternate type of question included in the NCLEX-RN®. The nurse must know how to solve math questions.

66. Correct answers are 1, 3, and 4.
    1. The UAP can make hourly rounds on the client, taking the client to the bathroom, giving the client a drink of water, checking to ensure the client is not climbing out of bed, and so on.
    2. This is the responsibility of the registered nurse or the social worker.
    3. This client is in rehab and should be stable so the UAP can set up the tray or feed the client.
    4. The UAP can clamp and unclamp an indwelling catheter in a rehab area. This is a noninvasive skill that can be taught to the UAP. It does not require judgment.
    5. This is the responsibility of the registered nurse or the social worker.

CLINICAL JUDGMENT GUIDE: This is an alternate type of question included in the NCLEX-RN®. The nurse must be able to select all the options that answer the question correctly.

67. 1. The left hand is weak and cannot be depended on to hold a cane.
    2. The shoulder is not appropriate for a cane.
    3. The right hand is the strongest hand because right-sided CVA damages the left side of the body; therefore, the right hand should be the one holding the cane.
    4. The shoulder is not appropriate for a cane.

CLINICAL JUDGMENT GUIDE: This is an alternate type of question on the NCLEX-RN® called "hot spot," which asks the nurse to identify the area with the computer arrow.

68. 1. The client scored much lower than 12 on the Glasgow Coma Scale.
    2. The client has a lower score than 10 on the scale.
    3. The client received 2 points for lack of opening of eyes to previous stimuli but opens to pain; the client received 1 point for lack of sound even with painful stimuli; and the client received 5 points for localizing pain and attempts to remove offending stimulus. This is a total of 8 points.
    4. The client has a higher score than 6.

CLINICAL JUDGMENT GUIDE: This is an alternate type of question included in the NCLEX-RN® test plan. The test taker must be able to read an EHR, assess the client, and decide on the nurse's most appropriate action.

69. 1. The client diagnosed with a right-sided CVA has left-sided paralysis, so placing the call light on the left side is inappropriate. The client would not be able to use the call light because the left side is paralyzed; the nurse should intervene.
   2. The UAP should assist the client with meals because the client cannot use the left arm.
   3. Using a draw sheet is an appropriate way to move the client up in bed.
   4. Placing a small pillow under the shoulder will prevent the shoulder from adducting toward the chest and developing a contracture, so this action does not require the nurse to intervene.

CLINICAL JUDGMENT GUIDE: The nurse is responsible for evaluating the care provided by the UAP and correcting their performance as needed.

70. 1. The client may need acetaminophen, a non-opioid analgesic, for the pain but the nurse should first assess the client to determine whether this is a headache or whether the client has an evolving CVA, which would require notifying the HCP.
   2. The client may need a CT scan but that cannot be determined until the nurse assesses the client to determine whether the headache is indicative of an evolving stroke.
   3. The nurse must assess the client to obtain data that will be needed when notifying the HCP; therefore, this is not the nurse's first intervention.
   4. **The nurse must first assess the client to determine whether the client's neurological status is deteriorating, which requires notifying the HCP; or if the headache is expected, then it would require an analgesic.**

CLINICAL JUDGMENT GUIDE: Assessment is the first step of the nursing process. The nurse should assess to determine more information about the headache and identify whether the client is deteriorating.

71. 1. The client may be developing pneumonia and needs to be assessed but not before a client with a Glasgow Coma Scale of 6, which is life-threatening.
   2. Ascending paralysis is a symptom of Guillain-Barré syndrome; therefore, the nurse would not need to assess this client first.
   3. **A 15 on the Glasgow Coma Scale indicates the client is neurologically intact, and a 6 indicates the client is not neurologically intact; therefore, the nurse should see this client first.**
   4. The nurse should expect a client diagnosed with a CVA (stroke) to have some sequelae of the problem, including the inability to speak.

CLINICAL JUDGMENT GUIDE: When deciding which client to assess first, the test taker should determine whether the signs and symptoms the client exhibits are expected for the situation. After eliminating the expected options, the test taker should determine which situation is more life-threatening.

72. 1. **This medication could possibly cause bleeding; therefore, this medication should be questioned by the charge nurse.**
   2. An osmotic diuretic is the medication of choice used to treat increased intracranial pressure, which can occur with a closed head injury.
   3. Any client diagnosed with a head injury will be on prophylactic anticonvulsants to prevent seizure activity, so the nurse would not question this order.
   4. Clients in the ICU are administered proton-pump inhibitors to help prevent stress ulcers; therefore, the nurse would not question this order.

CLINICAL JUDGMENT GUIDE: When the stem asks the nurse to determine which HCP order to question, the test taker must realize this is an "except" question. Three options are appropriate for the HCP to prescribe, and one is not.

73. 1. If the client's bladder is full, the nurse needs to insert a urinary catheter, which will relieve the headache. The client may be experiencing autonomic dysreflexia, but the nurse will need to palpate the bladder first.
   2. The client is in distress; therefore, the nurse should not assess the client first.
   3. The client should be put in the Trendelenburg position for hypovolemia, not for autonomic dysreflexia.
   4. **The nurse should first palpate the client's bladder to determine whether the client is experiencing autonomic dysreflexia, which is what the nurse should consider first with the client's clinical manifestations.**

CLINICAL JUDGMENT GUIDE: The nurse must know the clinical manifestations of severe complications of disease processes and assess the client accordingly.

74. 1. The charge nurse's priority intervention is placing the client on the side to maintain a patent airway.
    2. The Rapid Response Team is called when the client is alive, but the nurse thinks the client is in a potentially life-threatening situation. This is a possible intervention, but it is not a priority as the nurse walks into the room.
    3. The nurse should determine whether the client is incontinent of urine or stool and assess the client's seizure for the type of activity. Still, it is not a priority over maintaining a patent airway.
    4. The client should have privacy, but maintaining a patent airway is the priority.

    CLINICAL JUDGMENT GUIDE: When deciding which intervention should be a priority, the test taker should determine which intervention would address the most life-threatening complication.

75. 1. An occurrence report may need to be completed, but it is not the nurse's first intervention.
    2. The charge nurse's first intervention is to stop the UAP from inserting the oral airway. Once the seizure has started, there should be no attempts to insert anything in the mouth. If the client experiences an aura before the seizure, an oral airway could be inserted, but not once the seizure has started.
    3. Nothing should be inserted into the client's mouth once a seizure has started.
    4. The nurse should observe the time the seizure started and the seizure activity, but this is not the first intervention.

    CLINICAL JUDGMENT GUIDE: The nurse must know the immediate care of a client experiencing a seizure and stop the UAP from performing a potentially harmful intervention.

76. Correct answers are 1, 4, and 5.
    1. Informed consent is required for an invasive procedure, such as a lumbar puncture.
    2. A lumbar puncture does not insert dye into the client; therefore, this is inappropriate.
    3. The client should be in the side-lying position with the back arched. This position increases the space between the vertebrae, which allows the HCP to enter the spinal column more easily.
    4. The client is encouraged to relax and breathe normally; the client should feel some pressure in the back, but there should be no pain.
    5. The nurse should always explain to the client what happens before and during a procedure.

    CLINICAL JUDGMENT GUIDE: This type of alternate question is included in the NCLEX-RN® examination. The nurse must be able to select all the options that answer the question correctly.

77. 1. The client diagnosed with bacterial meningitis would be expected to have photophobia, so the most experienced nurse would not need to be assigned to this client.
    2. The client diagnosed with an L4 SCI could have spastic muscle spasms, which are not a complication; therefore, a less experienced nurse could care for this client.
    3. A less experienced nurse would be assigned the client diagnosed with Parkinson's disease because these symptoms are expected for this client.
    4. The client diagnosed with ALS has deteriorating respiratory distress, which is expected. Still, with these four clients the most experienced nurse should be assigned to the client diagnosed with respiratory distress. Maslow's Hierarchy of Needs identifies airway as a priority.

    CLINICAL JUDGMENT GUIDE: The most unstable client should be assigned to the most experienced nurse.

78. 1. A Glasgow Coma Scale score of 15 indicates intact neurological status, so an increase from 11 to 14 is good and the nurse would not need to see this client first.
    2. These clinical manifestations indicate spinal shock; therefore, this client should be assessed first, and appropriate medications should be administered.
    3. This is a positive Babinski sign, which is expected in a client diagnosed with a brainstem herniation, so this client would not need to be assessed first.
    4. These are expected clinical manifestations of West Nile virus; therefore, the nurse would not need to assess this client first.

    CLINICAL JUDGMENT GUIDE: When deciding which client to assess first, the test taker should determine whether the signs and symptoms the client exhibits are expected for the situation. After eliminating the expected options, the test taker should determine which situation is more life-threatening.

CASE STUDY ANSWERS

1. Correct answers are 1, 2, 4, 5, 8, and 9.
   1. Blood pressure 180/110 mm Hg is higher than expected.
   2. Decreased verbal fluency and right-sided facial droop
   3. Lung sounds
   4. History of hypertension and hyperlipidemia are pertinent to the client's clinical findings.
   5. Heart rate of 120 bpm indicates tachycardia.
   6. Temperature of 98.9°F (37.2°C)
   7. Spo$_2$ 98% on room air
   8. Headache pain 10/10: "the worst headache of my life"
   9. Pupil sizes are not equal.
   10. Respirations 18 breaths/min

   CLINICAL JUDGMENT GUIDE: The test taker should examine each answer option individually. Alternative question formats, such as this extended multiple response or select all that apply question, can have one to all correct answers.

2. Correct answers are 1, 3, and 5.
   1. The client is experiencing a sudden and severe headache, a BP of 180/110 mm Hg, and neurological changes. These findings place the client at risk for decreased tissue perfusion to the brain.
   2. No assessment information indicates this client is at risk for sepsis.
   3. The client is experiencing a sudden, severe headache described as "the worst headache of my life." The client is also diaphoretic and agitated and has decreased verbal fluency and facial droop. These findings align with the patient being at risk for anxiety.
   4. No assessment information indicates this client is at risk for decreased skin integrity.
   5. The client's neurological changes, such as decreased verbal fluency, facial droop, change in pupil size, and a sudden and severe headache align with decreased tissue perfusion to the brain, which puts the client at risk for seizure activity.

3. Correct answers are 2 and 3.
   Based on the client's condition, the nurse recognizes that the client is at the highest risk for

   | 2. Anaphylaxis |

   and will require

   | 3. Steroids |

   The physician has ordered the patient to have a CT scan with contrast. The patient is allergic to shellfish. Premedication with a steroid may be used to prevent an anaphylactic reaction to the contrast dye.

4. Correct answers are marked.

Potential Nursing Intervention	Indicated	Not Indicated
Begin oral fluids		X
Prepare the client for surgery	X	
Apply wrist restraints		X
Start oxygen at 2 L via nasal cannula		X
Apply antiembolism stockings	X	
Reorient the client as needed	X	
Place the client in high Fowler's position.		X

   1. The nurse should not start fluids as the client is being prepared for surgery and needs to be NPO.
   2. The nurse should prepare the client for surgery.
   3. No information in the case study indicates the client is agitated, combative, or pulling at their IV site; therefore, wrist restraints are not indicated.
   4. The client's SpO2 is 98% on room air so oxygen is not needed.
   5. Clients should be reoriented to person, place, and time as needed.
   6. Clients with brain aneurysms should be placed in semi-Fowler's position not high Fowler's.

5. Correct answers are 1, 2, 3.
   1. The client has had trauma to the brain, putting them at risk for seizures. Seizure precautions are a priority nursing intervention.
   2. Vital signs every 4 hours are a priority to allow the nurse to observe subtle changes in the client's condition.
   3. Complete bedrest is important to prevent increased intracranial pressure.
   4. Routine intake and output are not a priority for this client.
   5. A meal tray can be ordered if the client is hungry, but it is not a priority.
   6. Scheduling routine blood work is not a priority for this client.

6. Correct answers are marked.

Finding	Improved	Declined	No Change
Temperature	X		
Heart rate	X		
Respirations			X
Blood pressure	X		
Pain	X		
Spo_2		X	
Level of consciousness/ Neurological status		X	

The client's Spo_2 is higher than on admission, but the patient is now on 2 L of oxygen by nasal cannula. This finding indicates that the client's condition has declined. The client was alert and oriented ×4 on admission. The client is now oriented ×3 and only awakens when her name is called. This finding indicates that the client's condition has declined. The client's respiratory rate is unchanged from admission. The remaining findings indicate an improvement in the client's condition.

Endocrine Management

Intuition will tell the thinking mind where to look next.

—John Salk

QUESTIONS

1. After receiving the shift report, the 7:00 p.m. to 7:00 a.m. nurse is reviewing the medication administration record (MAR) of the client diagnosed with type 2 diabetes.

Client's Name: M.P. **Height:** 70 in (177.8 cm)	**Account Number:** 1234567 **Weight:** 265 lb (120.2 kg)	**Allergies:** NKDA **Date:** Today
Medication	1901–0700	0701–1900
Regular insulin by bedside glucose (BG) measurement subcutaneously before meals and at bedtime		
Lower than 60 mg/dL notify HCP <150 mg/dL 0 units 151–200 mg/dL 2 units		0730 DN BG 420 mg/dL 0 units
201–250 mg/dL 4 units 251–300 mg/dL 6 units		1130 DN BG 245 mg/dL 4 units
301–350 mg/dL 8 units 351–400 mg/dL 10 units Greater than 400 mg/dL notify HCP		1630 DN BG 398 mg/dL 10 units
Insulin isophane 48 units SQ BID		0730 DN 1630 DN
Signature/Initials	Night Nurse RN/NN	Day Nurse RN/DN

   Which intervention should the nurse implement?
   1. Make sure the client receives a snack at bedtime.
   2. Check the client's blood glucose level immediately.
   3. Have the unlicensed assistive personnel (UAP) give the client orange juice.
   4. Teach the client about the symptoms of diabetic ketoacidosis (DKA).

2. Which task is **most** appropriate for the RN staff nurse to delegate to the UAP?
   1. Request the UAP to take the diabetic client's evening snack to the client.
   2. Ask the UAP to silence the client's PCA pump alarm.
   3. Tell the UAP to witness the client's advance directive.
   4. Ask the UAP to show the client how to take the client's radial pulse.

3. Which task is **most** appropriate for the RN charge nurse to assign to the licensed practical nurse (LPN)?
   1. Tell the LPN to change the client's subclavian dressing.
   2. Request the LPN to obtain the client's daily weight.
   3. Assign the LPN to care for the client in myxedema coma.
   4. Ask the LPN to complete discharge teaching to the client.

4. The new graduate nurse on the endocrine unit is having difficulty completing the workload on time. Which suggestion could the RN preceptor make to help the new graduate become **more** organized?
   1. Suggest the new nurse take a break whenever the nurse feels overwhelmed with tasks.
   2. Tell the new nurse to start the shift with a work organization sheet for the assigned clients.
   3. Instruct the new nurse to take five deep breaths at the beginning of the shift and then begin.
   4. Review each day's assignments for the new nurse and organize the work for the new nurse.

5. The rehabilitation nurse is caring for a client diagnosed with type 2 diabetes and is 1 week postoperative for left carotid endarterectomy. The client's 11:30 a.m. bedside glucometer reading is 408 mg/dL.

Client's Name: P. S. **Height:** 69 in (175.3 cm)	**Account Number:** 1234569 **Weight:** 165 lb (74.8 kg)	**Allergies:** NKDA **Date:** Today
Medication	1901–0700	0701–1900
Regular insulin by bedside glucose subcu ac & hs		
Lower than 60 mg/dL notify HCP		0730 DN
<150 mg/dL 0 units		BG 142 mg/dL
		0 units
151–200 mg/dL 2 units		
201–250 mg/dL 4 units		
251–300 mg/dL 6 units		
301–350 mg/dL 8 units		
351–400 mg/dL 10 units		
Greater than 400 mg/dL notify HCP		
Signature/Initials	Night Nurse RN/ NN	Day Nurse RN/DN

Based on the MAR, which intervention should the nurse implement **first**?
1. Notify the healthcare provider (HCP).
2. Administer 10 units regular insulin.
3. Notify the laboratory to draw a serum glucose level.
4. Recheck the bedside glucometer reading.

6. The RN charge nurse on the endocrine surgical unit is making assignments. Which task should be delegated or assigned to the team members?
   1. Request the LPN assess the hypoglycemic client.
   2. Ask the UAP to assist in feeding the client with an adrenalectomy diagnosed with a paralytic ileus.
   3. Instruct the UAP to insert a nasogastric tube into the client recovering from a thyroidectomy.
   4. Tell the LPN to perform an intermittent urinary catheterization for the client diagnosed with acromegaly.

7. Which task is **most** appropriate for the RN staff nurse to delegate or assign when caring for clients on a surgical unit?
   1. Instruct the LPN to feed the client 1-day postoperative unilateral thyroidectomy.
   2. Ask another nurse to administer an IV push (IVP) pain medication to a postoperative client in severe pain.
   3. Request the UAP check the client with vital signs of AP 112 bpm, RR 26 breaths/min, BP 92/58 mm Hg.
   4. Instruct the LPN to obtain the pretransfusion assessment on a postoperative client.

8. The client diagnosed with Addison's disease is being prepared for emergency surgery and is asking to complete an advance directive. Which type of advance directive should the nurse recommend the client complete at this time?
   1. Power of attorney
   2. Living will
   3. Do not resuscitate (DNR) order
   4. Durable power of attorney for healthcare

9. The nurse is caring for clients in the postanesthesia care unit (PACU). Which client requires **immediate** intervention by the PACU nurse?
   1. The client with a bilateral adrenalectomy and exhibiting masseter rigidity
   2. The client with a subtotal thyroidectomy and has not urinated since surgery
   3. The client with general anesthesia and is sleepy but arouses easily to verbal stimuli
   4. The client with a pituitary tumor removed and with hypoactive bowel sounds

10. The RN charge nurse on a busy 20-bed endocrinology unit must send one staff member to the nursery. Which staff member is **most** appropriate to send to the nursery?
    1. The nurse with 4 years of experience working on the endocrinology unit
    2. The graduate nurse on the endocrinology unit for 6 months
    3. The LPN having worked in a newborn nursery at another facility
    4. The UAP with parenting experience for six small children

11. The nurse is working in an endocrinology unit. Which client warrants **immediate** intervention by the nurse?
    1. The client diagnosed with acromegaly presenting with club-like fingertips and large feet
    2. The client diagnosed with syndrome of inappropriate antidiuretic hormone secretion (SIADH) with decreased urine output
    3. The client diagnosed with Cushing's syndrome, with truncal obesity and thin, fragile skin
    4. The client diagnosed with pheochromocytoma reporting a severe pounding headache and chest pain

12. The night nurse enters the client's room and finds the client crying. The client asks the nurse, "Am I dying? I think something is terribly wrong with me, but no one is telling me." The nurse knows the client has pancreatic cancer and has less than 6 months to live. Which response is an example of the ethical principle of veracity?
    1. "You are concerned no one is telling you something is wrong."
    2. "Your diagnosis is pancreatic cancer."
    3. "If you feel something is wrong, you should speak with your doctor in the morning."
    4. "What makes you think something is wrong and you are dying?"

13. The critical care nurse just received the a.m. shift report on a client diagnosed with heart failure and pre-existing type 2 diabetes.

    Client's Name: A. R. **Account Number:** 1234560 **Allergies:** Penicillin
    Height: 67 in (170.2 cm) **Weight:** 148 lb (67.1 kg) **Date:** Today

Medication	1901–0700	0701–1900
Metformin 100 mg PO twice a day	2000	0800
70/30 insulin 24 units subcutaneous		0730
Digoxin 0.125 mg IVP daily		0800
Ceftriaxone 100 mg IVPB	0700	
Signature/Initials	Night Nurse RN/NN	Day Nurse RN/DN

    After reviewing the client's MAR, which medication should the nurse administer **first**?
    1. Metformin 100 mg PO
    2. Digoxin 0.125 mg IVP
    3. Ceftriaxone 100 mg IV piggyback (IVPB)
    4. 70/30 insulin subcutaneous

14. Which client should the charge nurse on a medical unit assign to the nurse 5 months pregnant?
    1. The client completing chemotherapy treatment and immunosuppressed
    2. The client diagnosed with postoperative hyperparathyroidism and shingles (herpes zoster)
    3. The client diagnosed with hyperthyroidism receiving radioactive iodine I-131
    4. The client diagnosed with AIDS and a cytomegalovirus infection

15. The client, diagnosed with hypothyroidism and myxedema coma, is admitted to the critical care unit. Which assessment data warrant **immediate** intervention by the nurse?
    1. The client's blood glucose level is 74 mg/dL.
    2. The client's vital signs are T 96.2°F (35.7 °C); AP 54 bpm; RR 12 breaths/min; and BP 90/58 mm Hg.
    3. The client's arterial blood gas (ABG) values are pH 7.33; Pao_2 78 mm Hg; $Paco_2$ 48 mm Hg; HCO_3 25 mmol/L.
    4. The client is lethargic and sleeps all the time.

16. The nurse is preparing to administer morning medications. Which medication should the nurse administer **first**?
    1. The levothyroxine to a client diagnosed with hypothyroidism
    2. The insulin isophane to a client diagnosed with type 2 diabetes
    3. The prednisone to a client diagnosed with Addison's disease
    4. The tiotropium inhaler to a client diagnosed with chronic asthma

17. The nurse is working on an endocrinology unit. Which client should the nurse assess **first**?
    1. The client diagnosed with diabetes insipidus having polyuria and polydipsia
    2. The client 1-day postoperative thyroidectomy presenting with neck edema
    3. The client diagnosed with hypoparathyroidism reporting painful muscle cramps and irritability
    4. The client diagnosed with Addison's disease experiencing weakness, fatigue, and anorexia

18. The client is admitted to the endocrinology unit newly diagnosed with an acute exacerbation of central diabetes insipidus (DI). Which intervention is the **priority** nursing intervention?
    1. Obtain the client's baseline weight.
    2. Administer desmopressin acetate intranasally.
    3. Administer IV hypotonic saline.
    4. Monitor the client's intake and output.

19. The UAP takes the vital signs of the client recovering from a thyroidectomy. The client's vital signs are populated in the chart.

Vital Signs	Client Values
Blood pressure	164/88 mm Hg
Pulse	128 bpm
Respirations	26 breaths/min
Temperature	104°F (40°C)

    Which intervention should the nurse implement **first**?
    1. Prepare to administer propranolol.
    2. Notify the HCP immediately.
    3. Assess the client's vital signs and surgical dressing.
    4. Administer acetaminophen orally (PO) STAT.

20. The UAP tells the RN primary nurse that a client is crying and upset after learning their spouse has just died. Which intervention should the nurse implement?
    1. Tell the UAP to go and sit with the client.
    2. Make a referral for the chaplain to see the client.
    3. Ask the HCP to prescribe a mild sedative.
    4. Leave the client alone in the room to grieve.

21. At 1000, the client diagnosed with type 1 diabetes is reporting being jittery, having a headache, and feeling dizzy. Which intervention should the nurse implement **first**?
    1. Give the client glucose tablets.
    2. Provide the client with the lunch meal.
    3. Request the laboratory to draw a serum glucose level.
    4. Determine the last time the client received insulin.

22. An elderly client diagnosed with thyroid cancer frequently makes statements that are inappropriate for the situation and is not oriented to place, time, or date. The HCP has ordered a magnetic resonance imaging (MRI) scan of the client's brain. Which intervention should the nurse implement?
    1. Administer a mild sedative to prevent claustrophobia.
    2. Order a vest restraint for use by the client during the MRI.
    3. Make sure the client does not have a pacemaker.
    4. Ask a family member to stay with the client while the test is performed.

23. An elderly client is admitted from the long-term care facility diagnosed with hyperglycemic hyperosmolar nonketotic coma. The client does not have any family or friends present. Which resource(s) should the admission nurse use to obtain client information?
    1. Having the nurse wait until a significant other can be contacted
    2. The verbal report from the ambulance workers and STAT laboratory work
    3. The transfer form from the nursing home and old hospital records
    4. The HCP's telephone orders about the care needed

24. The nurse administering medications to clients on a medical unit discovers the wrong medication was administered to a client, Ms. Jones. Ms. Jones replied she was Ms. Smith when the nurse asked her name from the MAR. Which step in medication administration did the nurse violate when administering the medication?
    1. Asking the client to repeat their name
    2. Verifying the client's armband with the MAR
    3. Checking the medication against the MAR
    4. Documenting the medication on the MAR

25. The female client diagnosed with type 2 diabetes and a urinary tract infection (UTI) describes frequent UTIs. Which interventions should the nurse implement? **Select all that apply.**
    1. Encourage the client to empty their bladder regularly and completely.
    2. Instruct the client to drink 8 ounces of cranberry or lingonberry juice daily.
    3. Explain the importance of taking oral hypoglycemic medications.
    4. Discuss the importance of taking all their prescribed antibiotics.
    5. Teach the client to measure their urine output with each voiding.

26. Which laboratory data should the nurse monitor for the client receiving IV methylprednisolone?
    1. Potassium level
    2. Sodium level
    3. Liver enzymes
    4. Glucose level

27. The nurse is working in an outpatient clinic triaging phone calls. Which client **warrants** notifying the HCP?
    1. The client diagnosed with type 2 diabetes receiving hemodialysis and weighing 6 pounds more since the last dialysis treatment
    2. The client diagnosed with type 1 diabetes and early-stage chronic renal disease reporting having to go to the bathroom several times at night
    3. The client diagnosed with SIADH feeling very upset because no one has returned the previous phone call
    4. The client diagnosed with type 1 diabetes and with a kidney transplant reporting decreased urine output with flu-like symptoms

28. Which client should the endocrinology nurse assess **first** after receiving the shift report?
    1. The 1-day postoperative transsphenoidal hypophysectomy client with clear drainage from the nose
    2. The client diagnosed with Graves' disease presenting with exophthalmos and bruits over the thyroid gland
    3. The client diagnosed with hyperparathyroidism reporting weakness, loss of appetite, and constipation
    4. The client diagnosed with Addison's disease and orthostatic hypotension reporting nausea and vomiting

29. Which client is the **priority** to be assigned to a case manager in the outpatient clinic so that care can be achieved?
    1. The client diagnosed with renal calculi and 2 weeks post–lithotripsy procedure
    2. The client diagnosed with type 2 diabetes and coronary artery disease (CAD)
    3. The client diagnosed with hypothyroidism receiving radiation treatment
    4. The client diagnosed with Addison's disease and on corticosteroid therapy

30. Which client is **most** appropriate for the parish nurse to care for?
    1. The post-gestational diabetic client with newborn triplets and is a single parent
    2. The Catholic client confined to their home because of severe arthritis
    3. The obese client diagnosed with Cushing's syndrome requesting help with losing weight
    4. The client diagnosed with chronic renal disease being cared for in the home by the spouse

31. Which task should the RN ambulatory care nurse delegate to the UAP?
    1. Ask the UAP to remove the trash from the room of the client diagnosed with hyperthyroidism and receiving radioactive iodine treatment.
    2. Instruct the UAP to escort the client asking to smoke a cigar outside.
    3. Request the UAP to check the surgical dressing on the client with an ileal conduit.
    4. Tell the UAP to take the glucometer reading on the client about to go to surgery.

32. The nurse is hanging 1,000 mL of IV fluids to run for 8 hours. The IV tubing is a microdrip. At how many gtt/min should the IV rate be set? _____

33. The clinic nurse is caring for clients using complementary alternative medicine (CAM). Which intervention is an example of CAM? **Select all that apply.**
    1. The client diagnosed with hypothyroidism taking *Centella asiatica*
    2. The client diagnosed with type 2 diabetes taking cinnamon daily
    3. The client diagnosed with coronary artery disease taking daily low-dose aspirin
    4. The client using acupuncture to help quit smoking cigarettes
    5. The client using hypnosis to improve memory function

34. Which statement is an example of community-oriented, population-focused nursing?
    1. The nurse cares for an elderly client in the community recovering from a kidney transplant.
    2. The nurse develops an educational program for clients in the local area diagnosed with type 2 diabetes.
    3. The nurse refers a client diagnosed with Cushing's syndrome to the registered dietitian.
    4. The nurse provides pamphlets to the client diagnosed with chronic renal disease.

35. Which **priority** intervention should the nurse implement when teaching about glucometer testing for a client diagnosed with type 2 diabetes?
    1. Instruct the client to keep a written record of their glucometer readings.
    2. Recommend the client check the glucometer reading in the morning.
    3. Have the client demonstrate correctly performing their blood sugar test.
    4. Teach the client how to dispose of the lancets and strips appropriately.

36. Which client would **most** benefit from acupressure, a traditional Chinese medicine considered CAM?
    1. The client diagnosed with thyroid cancer with chemotherapy-induced nausea
    2. The client diagnosed with type 2 diabetes and chronic renal disease
    3. The postpartum client diagnosed with Sheehan syndrome
    4. The client diagnosed with arterial hypertension

37. The home health RN director of nurses hears a nurse and the occupational therapist loudly disagreeing about the care of a newly admitted client while they are sitting in an area that is accessible to anyone coming into the office. Which action should the director of nurses implement **first**?
    1. Ask the staff members to move the argument to another room.
    2. Request both individuals to come into the director's office.
    3. Call the secretary with instructions for the staff to quit arguing.
    4. Tell the staff members that arguing is not allowed in the office.

38. Which client should the nurse on the endocrinology unit assess **first**?
    1. The client diagnosed with hypothyroidism with vital signs of T 94.2°F (34.6°C), AP 48 bpm, RR 14 breaths/min, BP 90/68 mm Hg
    2. The client diagnosed with hypoparathyroidism demonstrating a positive Chvostek's sign
    3. The client 1-day postoperative thyroidectomy reporting hoarseness
    4. The client diagnosed with diabetes insipidus drinking large amounts of water

39. Which activities are examples of home healthcare nurse responsibilities when caring for clients diagnosed with endocrine disorders? **Select all that apply.**
    1. Complete nutritional counseling and teaching for a client on a high-fiber diet.
    2. Discuss preoperative teaching for the client having a total right hip replacement.
    3. Manage oxygen therapy for a client diagnosed with chronic obstructive pulmonary disease (COPD).
    4. Teach the client and family about administration and side effects of medications.
    5. Draw blood for studies related to monitoring disease processes and therapy.

40. The UAP just took the blood pressure of a client recovering from a thyroidectomy. The UAP tells the RN primary nurse that the client's hand turned into a claw when the blood pressure was taken. Which intervention should the nurse implement **first**?
    1. Prepare to administer IV calcium gluconate.
    2. Assess the client for clinical manifestations of hypoparathyroidism.
    3. Request the UAP to elevate the client's head of the bed.
    4. Notify the client's HCP immediately.

41. The client diagnosed with type 2 diabetes and chronic renal disease asks the nurse, "How can I qualify for home healthcare when I go home?" Which statement is the nurse's **best** response?
    1. "You must need constant skilled care by the nurse."
    2. "You must have a family member living with you."
    3. "You must be homebound to receive home healthcare."
    4. "You must be referred by the hospital social worker."

42. The nurse is providing CAM therapy by teaching the client diagnosed with hyperthyroidism to focus attention, increase self-awareness, and increase concentration on an object. Which type of mind-body intervention is the nurse teaching?
    1. Meditation
    2. Imagery
    3. Aromatherapy
    4. Acupressure

43. Which **priority** intervention should the nurse implement for the client diagnosed with SIADH?
    1. Maintain the prescribed daily fluid restriction.
    2. Position the client's head of bed with no more than 10 degrees of elevation.
    3. Turn and reposition the client every 2 hours while on bedrest.
    4. Provide frequent oral hygiene every 2 hours for the client.

44. The home health agency chief nursing officer (CNO) is making assignments for the nurses. Which client should be assigned to the new graduate nurse having just completed orientation?
    1. The client diagnosed with Cushing's syndrome experiencing dyspnea and confusion
    2. The client who does not have the money to get prescriptions filled
    3. The client diagnosed with full-thickness burns on the arm needing a dressing change
    4. The client diagnosed with diabetic neuropathy reporting pain

45. The RN staff nurse on the endocrinology unit is caring for clients, assisted by a UAP. Which task is **most** appropriate to delegate to the UAP?
    1. Feed the client 1-day postoperative transsphenoidal hypophysectomy.
    2. Obtain a urine specimen from the client diagnosed with diabetes insipidus.
    3. Take the vital signs for the client diagnosed with myxedema coma.
    4. Assess the pulse oximeter reading of the client diagnosed with an addisonian crisis.

46. The clinical nurse manager on the endocrine unit overhears the staff nurses arguing and upset about how the charge nurse is assigning clients. Which statement indicates a democratic leadership style by the clinical nurse manager?
    1. "My charge nurse makes the assignments, and I support how they do them."
    2. "As long as there are no concerns from the clients, I will not interfere."
    3. "I appreciate you telling me about the situation, and I will handle it."
    4. "I will schedule a meeting, and we will all sit down and discuss the situation."

47. The UAP tells the RN staff nurse the terminally ill client diagnosed with thyroid cancer is having deep-rapid breathing but then doesn't breathe for about a minute. Which intervention should the nurse implement **first**?
    1. Explain the client is having Cheyne-Stokes respirations.
    2. Notify the hospital chaplain to come to the client's room.
    3. Go to the client's room immediately and assess the client.
    4. Inform the client's family that the client's death is near.

48. Which interventions should the RN primary nurse implement for the client diagnosed with hyperthyroidism? **Select all that apply.**
    1. Establish a supportive and trusting relationship to help the client cope.
    2. Assist with exercises involving large muscle groups.
    3. Instruct the UAP to apply multiple blankets to the bed.
    4. Explain that the caregiver should not leave the client alone.
    5. Place the client in a cool room away from high-traffic areas.

49. Which statement by the client experiencing exophthalmos indicates the client needs **more** teaching by the endocrinology nurse?
    1. "I will use artificial tears to moisten my eyes."
    2. "I need to wear dark glasses to prevent irritation."
    3. "I should not move my eyes unless absolutely necessary."
    4. "I should lightly tape my eyes shut when I sleep."

50. Which action by the UAP **warrants** intervention by the RN primary nurse caring for the client on hemodialysis diagnosed with type 2 diabetes and chronic renal disease?
    1. The UAP times the client's activities to help conserve energy.
    2. The UAP applies a lubricant to the lips and oral mucous membranes.
    3. The UAP ties a sheet around the client sitting in the chair.
    4. The UAP uses a fan to facilitate movement of cool air.

51. The RN nurse supervisor in the home health office is assigning tasks for the day. Which task is **most** appropriate for the nurse supervisor to assign to the LPN?
    1. Tell the LPN to complete the admission assessment for the client diagnosed with Cushing's disease.
    2. Request the LPN to evaluate the client's response to the new pain medication regimen.
    3. Request the LPN to perform wound care for the client diagnosed with a stage 4 pressure injury.
    4. Instruct the LPN to visit the stable client diagnosed with type 2 diabetes needing a hospital bed.

52. The charge nurse is reviewing the morning laboratory results for the clients. Which laboratory results **require** notifying the client's HCP?
    1. The client diagnosed with hypoparathyroidism and a decreased serum calcium level
    2. The client diagnosed with Cushing's disease and a decreased urine cortisol level
    3. The client diagnosed with diabetes insipidus and a low urine specific gravity
    4. The client diagnosed with hyperthyroidism and an increased thyroid-stimulating hormone (TSH) level

53. The nurse on the medical unit is preparing to administer 0900 medications. Which medication should the nurse **question** administering?
    1. Levothyroxine to the client diagnosed with hypothyroidism
    2. Metformin to the client diagnosed with type 2 diabetes after a CT scan with dye
    3. Insulin (human recombinant) to the no longer NPO client diagnosed with type 1 diabetes
    4. Prednisone to a client diagnosed with Addison's disease

54. The RN staff nurse and UAP are caring for clients on an endocrinology unit. Which tasks should the RN delegate to the UAP? **Select all that apply.**
    1. Ambulate the client recovering from a unilateral adrenalectomy.
    2. Change the linens for the diaphoretic client diagnosed with acute thyrotoxicosis.
    3. Bring ice-cold water to the client diagnosed with diabetes insipidus.
    4. Take the vital signs of a client just returning from the PACU.
    5. Deliver the lunch tray to the client receiving regular insulin on a sliding scale.

55. The unit manager of an endocrinology unit is over budget for the year and must transfer one staff member to another unit. Which option is the **best** action for the unit manager to take before deciding which staff member to transfer?
    1. Assess each staff member's abilities.
    2. Choose the last staff member hired.
    3. Ask for input from the staff members.
    4. Request the transfer documentation form.

56. The overhead page has just announced a Code Red, an actual fire, on a unit two floors below the unit where the RN staff nurse is working. Which action should the nurse implement **first**?
    1. Turn off the oxygen supply to the rooms.
    2. Evacuate the clients to a lower floor.
    3. Close all of the doors to the clients' rooms.
    4. Make a list of clients to discharge.

57. The nurse is preparing to administer medications for clients on a medical unit. The client diagnosed with hypothyroidism is describing being hot all the time, feeling palpitations, and being jittery. Which intervention should the nurse implement **first**?
    1. Check the client's serum thyroid levels.
    2. Assess the client for diarrhea.
    3. Document the findings in the (EHR).
    4. Hold the client's thyroid medication.

58. The nurse is administering medications on an endocrinology unit. Which medication should the nurse **question** administering?
    1. The propylthiouracil to the client diagnosed with hyperthyroidism
    2. The desmopressin acetate to the client diagnosed with diabetes insipidus
    3. The somatropin to the client diagnosed with hypopituitarism
    4. The propranolol to the client diagnosed with hypothyroidism

59. The hospice nurse caring for a client diagnosed with diabetes mellitus type 2 observes the client eating a bowl of ice cream. Which intervention should the nurse implement **first?**
    1. Allow the client to enjoy the ice cream.
    2. Check the client's blood glucose.
    3. Remind the client not to eat ice cream.
    4. Suggest the client eat low-fat sweets.

60. The RN staff nurse is caring for the client 1-day postoperative transsphenoidal hypophysectomy. Which action by the UAP **warrants** intervention by the nurse?
    1. The UAP places the client with the head of the bed (HOB) 30 degrees elevated.
    2. The UAP tells the client not to cough vigorously.
    3. The UAP is helping the client splint the incision.
    4. The UAP is taking the client's vital signs.

61. The charge nurse of a surgical unit has been notified of an external disaster with multiple casualties. Which client should the charge nurse request to be discharged from the hospital to make room for clients from the disaster?
    1. The client scheduled for a bilateral adrenalectomy in the morning and preoperative teaching has not been started
    2. The client recovering from a total abdominal hysterectomy 2 days ago and their PCA machine has been discontinued
    3. The client postoperative bilateral thyroidectomy with a hemoglobin of 7 mg/dL and a hematocrit of 22.1%
    4. The client diagnosed with type 2 diabetes recovering from a kidney transplant experiencing fever and pain at the surgical site

62. Which client's laboratory data should cause the charge nurse to notify the HCP?
    1. The potassium level of 3.6 mEq/L in a client diagnosed with heart failure taking furosemide
    2. The partial thromboplastin time (PTT) of 78 seconds in the client diagnosed with pulmonary embolism receiving IV heparin
    3. The blood urea nitrogen (BUN) of 84 mg/dL in a client diagnosed with end-stage renal disease (ESRD) and peripheral edema
    4. The blood glucose level of 543 mg/dL in a client diagnosed with uncontrolled diabetes mellitus type 1

63. Which nursing intervention is the **priority** for the intensive care unit (ICU) nurse to implement when caring for a client diagnosed with diabetic ketoacidosis (DKA)?
    1. Assess for a fruity breath odor.
    2. Check blood glucose levels ac and hs.
    3. Monitor the client's pulse oximeter readings.
    4. Maintain the regular insulin IV rate on an infusion pump.

64. The client diagnosed with type 2 diabetes mellitus has a hemoglobin A1C of 11 mg/dL. Which intervention should the nurse implement **first?**
    1. Check the client's current blood glucose level.
    2. Assess the client for neuropathy and retinopathy.
    3. Teach the client about the effects of uncontrolled hyperglycemia.
    4. Monitor the client's BUN and creatinine levels.

65. The nurse in a primary healthcare clinic is reviewing laboratory data. Which laboratory data should the nurse report to the HCP **first?**
    1. The male client seen for an annual physical examination

    ### Laboratory Report

Laboratory Test	Client Values	Reference Values
White blood cell (WBC) count	16.3	4.5 to 11.1 × 10^3/microL
Red blood cell (RBC) count	4.6	Male: 4.51 to 6.01 × 10^6 cells/microL Female: 4.01 to 5.51 × 10^6 cells/microL
Hemoglobin (Hgb)	13.3	Male: 14 to 17.3 g/dL Female: 11.7 to 15.5 g/dL
Hematocrit (Hct)	42	Male: 42% to 52% Female: 36% to 48%
Platelets	149	150 to 450 × 10^3/microL

    2. The female client reporting a runny nose and cough

    ### Laboratory Report

Laboratory Test	Client Values	Reference Values
White blood cell (WBC) count	5.3	4.5 to 11.1 × 10^3/microL
Red blood cell (RBC) count	4.2	Male: 4.51 to 6.01 × 10^6 cells/microL Female: 4.01 to 5.51 × 10^6 cells/microL
Hemoglobin (Hgb)	12	Male: 14 to 17.3 g/dL Female: 11.7 to 15.5 g/dL
Hematocrit (Hct)	36.9	Male: 42% to 52% Female: 36% to 48%
Platelets	150	150 to 450 × 10^3 mm

    3. The female client receiving an influenza vaccination

    ### Laboratory Report

Laboratory Test	Client Values	Reference Values
Glucose	125	Fasting: Less than 100 mg/dL Random: Less than 200 mg/dL
Potassium	4.9	3.5 to 5.3 mEq/L or mmol/L
Sodium	140	135 to 145 mEq/L or mmol/L

    4. The male client reporting insomnia and work stress

    ### Laboratory Report

Laboratory Test	Client Values	Reference Values
Glucose	100	Fasting: Less than 100 mg/dL Random: Less than 200 mg/dL
Potassium	5.1	3.5 to 5.3 mEq/L or mmol/L
Sodium	136	135 to 145 mEq/L or mmol/L

66. The client diagnosed with type 1 diabetes is receiving regular insulin by sliding scale. The client's glucometer reading is 249 mg/dL. The order reads blood glucose level:
    Less than 150 mg/dL 0 units
    151–200 mg/dL 5 units
    201–250 mg/dL 8 units
    251–300 mg/dL 12 units
    More than 301 mg/dL Contact HCP
    How much insulin should the nurse administer to the client? _____

67. The RN clinic nurse in the outpatient clinic is working with a UAP. Which tasks are **most** appropriate for the nurse to delegate to the UAP? **Select all that apply.**
    1. Put the client in the examination room and take the vital signs.
    2. Weigh the client and document the weight in the client's EHR.
    3. Prepare the examination room for the next client.
    4. Discuss the prescriptions prescribed by the HCP.
    5. Call the pharmacy to authorize a refill on a client's prescription.

68. The nurse in an outpatient clinic is triaging telephone calls. **Rank in order of priority.**
    1. The call from a spouse stating their client started on the prescribed antidepressant and will not wake up
    2. The call from a client stating the medication that was prescribed for their type 2 diabetes mellitus is too expensive
    3. The client diagnosed with hypothyroidism reporting feeling hot, having hand tremors, and diarrhea
    4. The call from the pharmacist requesting authorization to change a medication from a brand name to a generic drug
    5. The call from the client having not received results after an MRI scan 2 days ago

69. The 24-year-old client diagnosed with type 1 diabetes mellitus is reporting nausea and vomiting. Which interventions should the nurse implement? **Select all that apply.**
    1. Ask the client about the number of vomiting episodes.
    2. Determine the client's blood glucose level.
    3. Find out what medications the client has taken for the nausea.
    4. Tell the client to drink diet sodas to avoid dehydrating.
    5. Make sure the client does not take insulin during the illness.

70. The 19-year-old client, newly diagnosed with type 1 diabetes mellitus, asks the nurse about "sick day rules." Which instructions should the nurse include in the teaching? **Select all that apply.**
    1. Tell the client to monitor their urine ketones when sick.
    2. Instruct the client to go immediately to the ED when feeling sick.
    3. Teach the client to take over-the-counter medications that are sugar-free.
    4. Have the client call the HCP if showing ketones in the urine.
    5. Discuss trying to intake carbohydrates equal to usual caloric intake.

71. The nurse is caring for an obese client reporting to the ED with nausea and vomiting. The client is diagnosed with DKA and admitted to the ICU. Which interventions should the ICU nurse implement at this time? **Select all that apply.**
    1. Assess the client for dehydration and electrolyte imbalance.
    2. Perform bedside glucose monitoring hourly.
    3. Initiate an IV drip of normal saline and regular insulin.
    4. Perform oral care.
    5. Monitor potassium and sodium levels frequently.

72. The RN ICU nurse and the UAP are caring for an elderly client diagnosed with DKA. The UAP is performing foot care on the client. Which action by the UAP **requires** the nurse to intervene?
    1. The UAP cleans the feet with warm water and soap.
    2. The UAP thoroughly dries the feet, patting gently.
    3. The UAP applies lotion to the feet between the toes.
    4. The UAP places cotton socks on the client's feet.

73. The young adult client diagnosed with type 1 diabetes recovered from DKA and is being discharged from the hospital. The nurse is preparing the discharge information. Which information should the nurse include in the discharge instructions? **Select all that apply.**
    1. Discuss "sick day rules" with the client.
    2. Review self-monitoring of blood glucose.
    3. Instruct the client to perform an inspection of their feet daily.
    4. Encourage weight loss.
    5. Instruct the client to have regular eye examinations.

74. The 22-year-old client newly diagnosed with type 1 diabetes is being discharged from the hospital after recovering from DKA. Which referral should the nurse initiate at this time?
    1. Referral to the physical therapist
    2. Referral to a hospice organization
    3. Referral to a diabetes educator
    4. Referral to a fitness trainer

75. The client diagnosed with type 1 diabetes asks the nurse, "What are the benefits of continuous glucose monitoring (CGM)?" Which statement is the nurse's **best** response?
    1. "You will never have to perform a fingerstick blood glucose check again."
    2. "The CGM system is much cheaper than performing fingerstick checks."
    3. "The CGM system automatically adjusts your insulin dosage to the blood sugar results."
    4. "You will be able to see the trends in your blood glucose levels."

76. The nurse is teaching the client with an insulin pump. Which statement indicates the client **needs more** teaching?
    1. "When I sleep, I will clip my insulin pump to my pajamas."
    2. "My insulin pump will help stabilize my blood sugar levels."
    3. "I will need to monitor my blood glucose frequently."
    4. "I can perform any exercise wearing my insulin pump."

77. The obese client diagnosed with lipohypertrophy uses an insulin pump to control blood sugar. The client asks the nurse, "How can I prevent lipohypertrophy?" Which **priority** intervention should the nurse discuss with the client?
    1. "Rotate the catheter insertion site frequently."
    2. "Wash your hands before adjusting your insulin pump."
    3. "Avoid insertion of the catheter in the inner thigh."
    4. "Take all oral antibiotics as prescribed."

78. The nurse is performing a triple preparation procedure for insertion of an insulin pump catheter into a diabetic client. Which interventions should the nurse implement? **Rank in order of performance.**
    1. Apply an antiseptic and adhesive wipe to the area and let dry.
    2. Insert the infusion catheter set in a continuous motion.
    3. Wash the insertion area with antibacterial soap and let dry.
    4. Wash hands and don nonsterile gloves.
    5. Cleanse the area with an antibacterial solution and let dry.

ENDOCRINE CASE STUDY

(1750) The nurse in the ED receives a call from the Emergency Medical Services (EMS) regarding a 46-year-old client being transported after he "passed out while coaching his son's baseball game." The client's spouse reported that the client has been weak, shaky, fatigued, and "fighting a stomach bug" with vomiting. The client was feeling better today and decided to coach the game. The client has no significant medical history, although he had similar symptoms a few weeks ago that resolved without issue. Client is lethargic and oriented to person and place only. An IV line of normal saline (NS) was started in the right antecubital (AC) vein with a 20-gauge catheter and is infusing at 150 mL/hr. The client's spouse will come to the hospital when they get child care for their three children.

Vital Signs	Client Values
Blood pressure	88/50 mm Hg
Heart rate	124 bpm
Respirations	18 breaths/min
Temperature	100.6°F (38.1°C)
Spo$_2$	96% on room air
Pain	Denies

(1820) The client arrives via EMS and is transferred from the stretcher to the bed. Color is pale, skin cool and diaphoretic. Lungs are clear bilaterally. Abdomen is soft with bowel sounds in all four quadrants. Pedal pulses present ×4 with no edema. Client states, "I don't know what happened. I was tired and remember getting dizzy, but then I don't remember anything until I was in the ambulance." IV infusing to the right AC vein with no edema or coolness, NS at 150 mL/hr. The client states, "I don't think so," when asked if he has any allergies.

1. **Recognize cues. What matters most?** The nurse prepares to call the ED physician. Which **priority** client data should be reported to the HCP? **Select all that apply.**
   1. Respirations
   2. Blood pressure
   3. Syncope
   4. Vertigo
   5. Weakness
   6. Diaphoresis
   7. Temperature
   8. Heart rate
   9. Abdomen assessment

(1830) The ED physician visits the client and orders a complete blood count (CBC), basal metabolic panel (BMP), and urinalysis STAT, increasing the flow rate of the IV infusion to 200 mL/hr × 2 L. The nurse draws the STAT labs and instructs the client about needing a urine sample. While awaiting lab results, the nurse obtains additional information from the client's spouse, who just arrived in the ED.

Past History: Mild hypertension, right rotator cuff repair (7 years ago), and pneumonia "last winter"

The spouse confirmed the client has no known allergies.

ED bed weight: 215.6 lb (98 kg)

Home Medications: None

(1910) Diagnostic and laboratory results are received.

Laboratory Test	Client Values	Reference Values
Hemoglobin (Hgb)	10	Male: 14–17.3 g/dL Female: 11.7–15.5 g/dL
Hematocrit (Hct)	28	Male: 42%–52% Female: 36%–48%
White blood cell (WBC) count	12.8	4.5 to 11.1 × 10^3/microL
Platelets	165	140 to 400 × 10^3/microL
Creatinine	0.8	Male: 0.61 to 1.21 mg/dL Female: 0.51 to 1.11 mg/dL
Glucose	82	Fasting: Less than 100 mg/dL Random: Less than 200 mg/dL
Potassium	3.1	3.5 to 5 mEq/L or mmol/L
Sodium	125	135 to 145 mEq/L or mmol/L
Blood urea nitrogen	27	8 to 21 mg/dL Adult over 90 years: 10 to 31 mg/dL

2. **Analyze cues. What could it mean?** For each client finding, indicate whether it is consistent with the listed disease process(es). Each finding may support more than one condition.

Finding	Dehydration	Addison's Disease	Diabetes Mellitus
Hypotension			
Anemia			
Hypoglycemia			
Hyponatremia			
Fatigue			
Weakness			
Vertigo			
Increased BUN level			

(2100) The physician sees the client, reviews the laboratory results, and orders admission to the medical intensive care unit (MICU) for suspected new-onset Addison's disease. The client and spouse verbalize understanding and agree to plan. Provider orders are populated in the chart.

PROVIDER ORDERS:

Admit to MICU: suspected new-onset Addison's disease
Consult Endocrinology
STAT electrocardiogram, then continuous telemetry
Adrenocorticotropic hormone (ACTH) stimulation test tomorrow in a.m.
CBC and BMP every morning
Ensure urinalysis has been obtained; straight cath ×1 if needed
IV 0.9% NaCl @ 150 mL/hr
Ondansetron 4 mg IVP every 8 hours as needed for nausea/vomiting
Diet: regular, encourage PO fluids and salt intake
Activity as tolerated
Vital signs: orthostatic vital signs every morning, then routine

3. **Prioritize hypotheses. Where do I start?** Complete the sentence by choosing from the drop-down list of options. Based on the client's condition at this time, the nurse recognizes that the client is at the highest risk for _____

> *Select* ▼
> 1. Decreased cardiac output
> 2. Infection
> 3. Fluid volume overload

and will require _____

> *Select* ▼
> 1. Diuretics
> 2. IV fluids
> 3. Antibiotics

(2130) Client is transferred from the ED to MICU. The MICU nurse assesses the client, reviews the ED notes and transfer orders, and establishes the initial plan of care.

4. **Generate solutions. What can I do?** For each intervention, specify whether the intervention is **indicated** or **not indicated** for the client's care.

Potential Nursing Intervention	Indicated	Not Indicated
Instruct client to get up slowly with assistance		
Reduce IV 0.9% NaCl to 100 mL/hr		
Provide teaching on ACTH suppression test		
Ensure continuous telemetry		
Instruct on the need for a urine sample		
Call Endocrinology consult		
Encourage oral fluid intake		

(2145) The endocrinology resident visits the client and orders hydrocortisone 100 mg IVP STAT, then hydrocortisone 200 mg IV over 24 hours. The client continues to state he does not feel the need to urinate.

5. **Take action. What will I do?** Which actions are appropriate for the care of this client at this time? **Drag and drop one correct action from the options listed in the left column into the right column.**

Possible Actions	Correct Actions
Reinforce the need for a urine sample	
Straight cath ×1 and send urine to lab	
Place an indwelling urinary catheter	
Instruct on oral fluid restriction	
Encourage oral fluids	
Instruct on NPO status	
Administer IVP 100 mg hydrocortisone	
Administer IVP 200 mg hydrocortisone	
Initiate a second IV site	

(Day 3 of hospitalization; 0900) The client has been diagnosed with Addison's disease, stabilized, and the nurse has provided discharge instructions.

6. **Evaluate outcomes. Does the client understand the teaching?** For each client statement, indicate whether the teaching regarding the new diagnosis of Addison's disease has or has not been effective.

Client Statement	Teaching Effective	Teaching Not Effective
"I will take the prednisone for 7 days."		
"I should check my blood pressure once a week."		
"I should drink at least 64 ounces of water every day."		
"I should restrict my daily intake of sodium."		
"I should order a medical alert bracelet and wear it all the time."		

ANSWERS AND RATIONALES

The correct answer number and rationale are in **bold-face purple type.** Rationales for why other answer options are incorrect are also given.

1. 1. **The client received intermediate-acting insulin at 1630 plus the sliding-scale insulin dose to lower the client's blood glucose level. This client should receive a bedtime snack to make sure the client does not experience a hypoglycemic reaction during the night. Intermediate insulin generally peaks 6 to 8 hours after administration, 2230 to 0030 for this client.**
   2. The nurse should check the client's blood glucose at 2100 hours, not at the current time.
   3. Nothing indicates the client needs an intervention for hypoglycemia at this time.
   4. The client diagnosed with type 2 diabetes would experience hyperglycemic hyperosmolar nonketotic coma (HHNC) syndrome, not DKA.

   CLINICAL JUDGMENT GUIDE: This is an alternate type of question included in the NCLEX-RN® test plan. The test taker must be able to read an MAR, be knowledgeable of medications, and be able to decide on the nurse's most appropriate intervention.

2. 1. **The UAP can take food to the client because this is not a medication and the client is stable.**
   2. The RN staff nurse should not have the UAP silence the alarm on the client's PCA pump. The nurse should assess the client and the pump to determine the reason for the PCA alarm.
   3. No hospital employees should witness the client's advance directive.
   4. The RN cannot delegate teaching to the UAP.

   CLINICAL JUDGMENT GUIDE: The nurse should not delegate assessment, teaching, evaluation, medications, or an unstable client to the UAP.

3. 1. **The LPN can change sterile dressings according to their scope of practice.**
   2. The UAP can obtain the client's weight; therefore, it should not be assigned to the LPN.
   3. The client in myxedema coma is not stable and should be assigned to the RN, not the LPN.
   4. Teaching should not be assigned to the LPN, only to the RN.

   CLINICAL JUDGMENT GUIDE: The RN should not assign assessment, teaching, evaluation, or the care of an unstable client to an LPN. If any task can be assigned to a UAP, it should not be assigned to an LPN.

4. 1. The new graduate cannot take a break when overwhelmed because the work may never get done. The new graduate should schedule breaks throughout the shift, not when they want to take them.
   2. **The preceptor should recommend that the new graduate use some tool to organize the work so important tasks, such as medication administration and taking vital signs, are not missed.**
   3. Encouraging the new graduate to calm down (five deep breaths) before beginning work is good, but it will not help the new graduate with time management.
   4. The new graduate must find the best way to organize. Doing the organizing for the new graduate will not help.

   CLINICAL JUDGMENT GUIDE: There will be management questions on the NCLEX-RN®. Concepts of Management are included under the category Safe and Effective Care Environment and the subcategory Management of Care.

5. 1. The HCP should be notified when the laboratory verifies the glucose level.
   2. The sliding scale indicates a blood glucose level of 351 to 400 mg/dL requires 10 units of regular insulin. There is no insulin dosage administered for 408 mg/dL.
   3. This should be done, but not until the nurse rechecks the blood glucose level at the bedside.
   4. **The nurse should first recheck the blood glucose level at the bedside before taking any further action.**

   CLINICAL JUDGMENT GUIDE: The test taker needs to read all options carefully before choosing the option that says, "Notify the HCP." If any of the options will provide information the HCP needs to know to make a decision, the test taker should choose that option. Assessment is the first step in the nursing process.

6. 1. **The LPN is not licensed to assess the hypoglycemic client, nor should the RN assign or delegate an unstable client. This client is unstable and requires the RN's assessment skills.**

2. The client diagnosed with a paralytic ileus is NPO and should not have any food.
3. The UAP does not have the skill or training to insert a nasogastric tube.
4. The LPN can perform a sterile procedure, such as completing an intermittent urinary catheterization.

CLINICAL JUDGMENT GUIDE: The test taker must know which tasks should be delegated or assigned to the UAP and LPN, and the RN must also know which interventions are appropriate for the client's condition.

7. 1. This would be an inappropriate assignment because the UAP, not the LPN, could feed this stable client.
   2. The RN could request that another nurse administer pain medication to relieve the client's immediate pain.
   3. This client's vital signs indicate that the client is unstable; therefore, the RN should check on this client and not delegate the assessment to a UAP.
   4. The client who requires a blood transfusion is unstable. The RN should complete the pretransfusion assessment. The RN, not the LPN, assesses.

CLINICAL JUDGMENT GUIDE: The RN cannot delegate assessment, teaching, evaluation, medications, or an unstable client to a UAP. The RN cannot assign assessment, teaching, evaluation, or an unstable client to an LPN. The nurse can assign a task to another nurse.

8. 1. A power of attorney is a legal document authorizing an individual to conduct business for the client. The nurse should not recommend this type of document for a healthcare situation.
   2. The living will usually requests the client refuse life-sustaining treatment. General anesthesia requires the client to be intubated and placed on a ventilator; therefore, the client's request to deny this type of life-sustaining effort will not be honored in the operating room. The nurse should not recommend this type of advance directive.
   3. A DNR order must be written in the client's EHR by the HCP and may reflect the client's wishes, but it is not an advance directive.
   4. This document would be most appropriate for the nurse to recommend because it names an individual to be responsible if the client cannot make healthcare decisions for themself.

CLINICAL JUDGMENT GUIDE: Questions on advance directives are included in the NCLEX-RN®. This content is included under the category Safe and Effective Care Environment and the subcategory Management of Care.

9. 1. Masseter rigidity is a sign of malignant hyperthermia, which is a life-threatening complication of surgery. The client will also exhibit tachycardia, hypotension, decreased cardiac output, and oliguria. It is a rare muscle disorder chemically induced by anesthesia.
   2. The client was NPO after midnight and during surgery; therefore, not urinating since surgery warrants no immediate intervention.
   3. The client receiving general anesthesia is expected to be sleepy after surgery and easy to arouse; therefore, this client warrants no immediate intervention.
   4. As long as the client has bowel sounds after surgery, hypoactive or hyperactive, then this client warrants no immediate intervention.

CLINICAL JUDGMENT GUIDE: When deciding which client to assess first, the test taker should determine whether the clinical manifestations the client is exhibiting are normal or expected for the client's situation. After eliminating the expected option, the test taker should determine which situation is more life-threatening.

10. 1. The nurse with 4 years' experience on the unit should not be sent because the nurse's expertise is needed on the unit.
    2. Although knowledgeable of the endocrinology unit with 6 months of experience, the graduate nurse would not be sent because of a lack of experience in the maternal-child area.
    3. The LPN with maternal-child area experience would be most helpful to the nursery.
    4. The charge nurse should not make assignments based on a staff member's personal life.

CLINICAL JUDGMENT GUIDE: There will be management questions on the NCLEX-RN®. Charge nurse responsibilities are included under the category Safe and Effective Care Environment.

11. 1. Acromegaly, an excessive secretion of growth hormone, results in overgrowth of the bones and soft tissues. Clubbed fingertips and large feet are expected; therefore, this client doesn't warrant intervention.
    2. The client diagnosed with SIADH, because of sustained secretion of antidiuretic hormone (ADH), would be expected to have a low

urinary output. This client warrants no intervention by the nurse.

3. The client diagnosed with Cushing's syndrome would have truncal obesity and thin, fragile skin; therefore, this client warrants no intervention by the nurse. Cushing's syndrome is caused by excess secretion of glucocorticoids by the adrenal gland.
4. **The client diagnosed with pheochromocytoma, a tumor of the adrenal medulla that produces excessive catecholamine, is expected to have a severe pounding headache and chest pain. Still, of these four clients, this client has pain, which is a priority. This client warrants intervention by the nurse.**

CLINICAL JUDGMENT GUIDE: The test taker should use some tool as a reference to guide the decision-making process. In this situation, Maslow's Hierarchy of Needs should be applied. Pain is a priority even if it is expected.

12. 1. This statement is a therapeutic response but does not tell the client the truth.
2. **The ethical principle of veracity is the duty to tell the truth.**
3. This statement shifts responsibility to another person, which the nurse should not do if possible.
4. This is attempting to obtain more information about the situation but is not telling the truth.

CLINICAL JUDGMENT GUIDE: The NCLEX-RN® test plan includes nursing care addressing ethical principles, including autonomy, beneficence, justice, and veracity, to name a few.

13. 1. After the a.m. shift report, the priority medication should be insulin before breakfast, not metformin (Glucophage).
2. After the a.m. shift report, the priority medication should be insulin before breakfast, not digoxin.
3. Ceftriaxone (Rocephin), an antibiotic, IVPB, is a routine, scheduled medication and should have been administered by the night nurse; there's also a 1-hour leeway when administering this medication. The nurse would have to see whether the IVPB apparatus was hanging at the client's bedside or contact the night nurse before administering this medication.
4. **Insulin is a medication that must be administered before the meal; therefore, this medication is a priority.**

CLINICAL JUDGMENT GUIDE: The test taker should know which medications are priority medications, such as life-sustaining medications and insulin, and medications that have specific requirements for effectiveness, such as mucosal barrier agents (Carafate). These medications should be administered first by the nurse.

14. 1. The pregnant nurse can care for clients receiving antineoplastic medications. The nurse should not be exposed to antineoplastic agents outside the administration bags and tubing. The pregnant nurse can care for an immunosuppressed client.
2. Shingles (herpes zoster) is a painful, blistering skin rash caused by the varicella-zoster virus, which causes chickenpox. The pregnant nurse should not be assigned this client.
3. The client receiving radioactive iodine should not be around pregnant women or young children; therefore, the pregnant nurse should not care for this client.
4. The client has cytomegalovirus, which crosses the placental barrier. Therefore, a pregnant nurse should not be assigned this client. Any client diagnosed with a communicable disease that crosses the placental barrier should not be assigned to a pregnant nurse.

CLINICAL JUDGMENT GUIDE: There will be management questions on the NCLEX-RN®. Charge nurse responsibilities are included under the category Safe and Effective Care Environment.

15. 1. This is below the normal fasting range of 100 mg/dL. Hypoglycemia is expected in a client diagnosed with myxedema; therefore, a 74 mg/dL blood glucose level would be expected.
2. The client's metabolism is slowed in myxedema coma, which would result in these vital signs.
3. These ABG values indicate respiratory acidosis (pH lower than 7.35, PaCO2 higher than 45 mm Hg) and hypoxemia (O2 lower than 80%); therefore, this client would warrant immediate intervention by the nurse. Untreated respiratory acidosis can result in death if not treated immediately.
4. Lethargy is an expected symptom in a client diagnosed with myxedema; therefore, this would not warrant immediate intervention.

CLINICAL JUDGMENT GUIDE: The nurse must know the expected medical treatment for the client. This is a knowledge-based question. The nurse must be knowledgeable of normal laboratory values and be able to determine whether the laboratory value is normal for the client's disease process or the medications the client is taking.

16. 1. Levothyroxine (Synthroid), a thyroid hormone, is a daily medication that can be administered within a 1-hour time frame (30 minutes before and 30 minutes after the dosing time).
    2. Insulin isophane (Humulin N), a pancreatic hormone, should be administered before a meal for best effects. This medication should be administered first.
    3. Prednisone, a glucocorticoid, is a routine medication and can be administered within the 1-hour time frame (30 minutes before and 30 minutes after the dosing time).
    4. Tiotropium (Spiriva) inhaler, a bronchodilator, is a routine daily medication and can be administered within the 1-hour time frame (30 minutes before and 30 minutes after the dosing time).

CLINICAL JUDGMENT GUIDE: The test taker should know priority medications, such as life-sustaining medications, insulin, and medications with specific requirements for effectiveness, such as mucosal barrier agents (Carafate). These medications should be administered first by the nurse.

17. 1. The client diagnosed with diabetes insipidus, a deficiency in the production of the ADH, will have increased thirst and urination. The nurse should not assess this client first.
    2. **The nurse should assess the client with a thyroidectomy for hemorrhaging every 2 hours. Neck edema, irregular breathing, and frequent swelling are signs of hemorrhaging; therefore, the nurse should assess this client first.**
    3. The client diagnosed with hypofunction of the parathyroid gland is expected to have muscle cramps and irritability; therefore, the nurse should not assess this client first. Bleeding and loss of airway are the priority over an expected symptom of the disease process, which is not as immediately life-threatening.
    4. Addison's disease, hypofunction of the adrenal gland, causes the client weakness, fatigue, and anorexia. These signs or symptoms are expected; therefore, the nurse should not assess this client first.

CLINICAL JUDGMENT GUIDE: The test taker must determine which sign or symptom is expected for the disease process. If the sign or symptom is not likely, the nurse should assess the client first. This question determines whether the nurse knows the clinical manifestations of various disease processes.

18. 1. The nurse should obtain the client's baseline weight, but it is not the priority intervention over restoring the client's circulatory status.
    2. Desmopressin acetate (DDAVP), an analog of the ADH, is the hormone replacement of choice for central DI. It is not the first intervention because restoring circulatory volume is the priority.
    3. In acute DI, hypotonic saline is administered intravenously and is titrated to replace urinary output. Restoring circulatory volume is the priority intervention. Remember Maslow's Hierarchy of Needs; physiological needs are the priority.
    4. Monitoring the client's intake and output is an appropriate nursing intervention but not a priority over restoring circulatory volume.

CLINICAL JUDGMENT GUIDE: All options are plausible in questions that ask the test taker to identify a priority intervention. The test taker must identify the most important intervention.

19. 1. The beta-adrenergic blocker propranolol (Inderal) treats thyrotoxicosis, a thyroid storm, but it is not the nurse's first intervention.
    2. The nurse should notify the HCP of this rare condition, thyrotoxic crisis, but the nurse should first assess the client before calling the HCP.
    3. **Because the UAP gave the RN this information, the nurse must assess the client before taking further action.**
    4. The nurse should administer acetaminophen (Tylenol) PO STAT to help decrease the fever, but the RN should first assess the client because the UAP gave the nurse the information.

CLINICAL JUDGMENT GUIDE: Any time a nurse receives information from another staff member about a client possibly experiencing a complication, the RN must assess the client. A nurse should not decide about the client's needs based on another staff member's information.

20. 1. The UAP cannot sit for an extended time with a grieving client.
    2. A chaplain is a spiritual adviser who can stay with the client until a family member or the client's spiritual adviser can come to the hospital to be with the client.
    3. The client should not be sedated. Grieving is a natural process that must be worked through. Sedating the client will delay the

grieving process. The nurse should allow the client to vent their feelings to foster the grieving process, not numb the client.
4. The client may request to be left alone, but the nurse should first refer the client for spiritual support and not assume the client wants to be left alone. Most clients feel the need for someone's presence.

CLINICAL JUDGMENT GUIDE: The test taker must know the roles of all multidisciplinary healthcare team members, as well as HIPAA (Health Insurance Portability and Accountability Act) rules and regulations. These will be tested on the NCLEX-RN® examination.

21. 1. The client is exhibiting hypoglycemia; therefore, the nurse should treat the client's symptoms with a simple carbohydrate, such as glucose tablets. This is the first intervention.
    2. The nurse should provide the client with complex carbohydrates so another episode of hypoglycemia will not occur.
    3. The nurse could obtain a glucometer reading at the bedside, but having the laboratory draw a serum blood glucose level should not be the nurse's first intervention.
    4. The nurse should determine the last time the client received insulin, but it is not the first intervention. Remember: The nurse should not assess if the client is in distress.

CLINICAL JUDGMENT GUIDE: When the question asks which intervention should be implemented first, it means all the options are something a nurse could implement, but only one should be implemented first. The test taker should use the nursing process to determine the appropriate response: If the client is in distress, do not assess; if the client is not in distress, then the nurse should assess.

22. 1. The client has not reported claustrophobia. The client has some neurological abnormality.
    2. A vest restraint will not keep the client's head still during the MRI.
    3. The nurse should ensure that the client has no medical device implanted that could react with the magnetic field created by the MRI scanner. An implanted electronic device, such as a pacematker, could prevent the client from having an MRI, depending on the age of the pacemaker and the material with which it was made.
    4. Family members are requested to stay outside the area where the MRI is performed.

CLINICAL JUDGMENT GUIDE: The nurse must know about normal diagnostic tests pre- and postprocedure interventions, be able to determine whether the client can have the diagnostic procedure, and provide postprocedure care to ensure the client is safe.

23. 1. The nurse needs as much information as possible to provide client care. The client may or may not have a significant other to be contacted. This is not the best way to get information about the client.
    2. The ambulance workers will only be able to give a cursory report based on the limited information provided to them. This is not the best place to get information about the client.
    3. The nursing home should send a transfer form with the client that details current medications, diagnoses, and hygiene needs. Previous hospital records will include a history, physical examination, and discharge summary. These records are the best place to start to glean information regarding the client.
    4. The HCP orders may contain a current diagnosis but will not include any information about the client's medical history. This is not the best place to get information about the client.

CLINICAL JUDGMENT GUIDE: Assessment is the first step of the nursing process, and the test taker should use the nursing process or some other systematic process to assist in determining priorities. The nurse should access documentation that has objective data about the client's condition.

24. 1. The nurse asked the client their name, and the client replied that they were a different person.
    2. The step the nurse did not take was to verify the client's armband against the MAR. Checking the identification band against the MAR would have prevented the error.
    3. This step was not overlooked.
    4. This step was not missed.

CLINICAL JUDGMENT GUIDE: The NCLEX-RN® test plan includes the category Medication Administration under Physiological Integrity: Pharmacological and Parenteral Therapies. This is a knowledge-based question.

25. Correct answers are 1, 2, 3, and 4.
    1. Health promotion activities that help prevent UTIs include emptying the bladder; bacteria can grow in stagnated urine in the bladder, and emptying the bladder will help prevent this.

2. Enzymes found in cranberries inhibit attachment of urinary pathogens (especially E. coli) to the bladder epithelium. Daily cranberry juice helps prevent UTIs.
3. Women diagnosed with diabetes are two to three times more likely to have bacteria in their bladders than women without diabetes. Taking hypoglycemic medication is important to maintain appropriate blood sugar levels.
4. Antibiotic therapy is a priority intervention for the client diagnosed with a UTI.
5. Measuring urine output will not prevent the development of UTIs.

CLINICAL JUDGMENT GUIDE: This is an alternate type of question included in the NCLEX-RN® examination. The nurse must be able to select all the options that answer the question correctly.

26. 1. Steroids do not affect the client's potassium level.
2. Glucocorticoids do not affect the client's sodium level.
3. Steroids do not affect the client's liver enzymes.
4. Methylprednisolone (Solu-Medrol), a glucocorticoid steroid, is excreted as glucocorticoids from the adrenal gland and is responsible for insulin resistance by the cells, which may cause hyperglycemia; therefore, the nurse should monitor the glucose level.

CLINICAL JUDGMENT GUIDE: The nurse must know laboratory values affected by medication and be able to determine whether the laboratory value is normal for the client's disease process or the medications the client is taking.

27. 1. A 6-pound weight gain between dialysis treatments is expected; therefore, the nurse would not need to notify the client's HCP.
2. In the early stage of renal insufficiency, polyuria results from the inability of the kidneys to concentrate urine, which most often happens at night (nocturia). The nurse would not notify the client's HCP.
3. The nurse should call this client, but psychosocial problems do not take priority over physiological, potentially life-threatening problems.
4. These are signs of an acute transplant rejection, which is potentially a life-threatening problem; therefore, the nurse should notify the HCP about this client.

CLINICAL JUDGMENT GUIDE: The nurse should ask, "Are the assessment data normal?" for the disease process. If they are normal for the disease process, then the nurse would not need to intervene; if they are not normal for the disease process, then this warrants intervention.

28. 1. This client should be seen first because clear nasal drainage could be cerebrospinal fluid (CSF), which is a potentially life-threatening complication from surgery. The nurse needs to determine whether the drainage has glucose. If it does, it is CSF, and the surgeon needs to be notified.
2. The client diagnosed with Graves' disease has exophthalmos (protruding eyes) and bruits (swishing sound) over the thyroid gland, so the nurse would not assess this client first.
3. The client diagnosed with hyperparathyroidism is expected to have weakness, loss of appetite, and constipation; therefore, the nurse would not assess this client first.
4. The client diagnosed with Addison's disease is expected to have orthostatic hypotension, nausea, and vomiting; therefore, the nurse would not assess this client first.

CLINICAL JUDGMENT GUIDE: The test taker must determine which sign or symptom is unexpected for the disease process. If the sign or symptom is unexpected, the nurse should assess the client first. This type of question determines whether the nurse is knowledgeable of clinical manifestations of various disease processes.

29. 1. A case manager is assigned to a client diagnosed with a chronic illness; therefore, a client who was diagnosed with renal calculi and had lithotripsy would not be appropriate for a case manager.
2. It would be appropriate to assign this client to a case manager because this client has two chronic illnesses, often having multiple hospitalizations and chronic complications, and requires long-term healthcare.
3. Hypothyroidism is not a disease process resulting in multiple hospitalizations or chronic complications.
4. A client diagnosed with Addison's disease on corticosteroid therapy would not be a client referred to a case manager.

CLINICAL JUDGMENT GUIDE: Diabetes and CAD are well-known chronic disease processes and should make the test taker consider this option the correct answer. Postoperative clients, for the most part, return to their normal life, which would not require a case manager.

30. 1. This client would benefit from a home health nurse but not a parish nurse.
    2. A parish nurse is an RN with a minimum of 2 years of experience working in a faith community, addressing the health issues of its members and those in the broader community or neighborhood. Parish nursing was recognized as a specialty in 1998 by the American Nurses Association. The client is a Catholic, so that is the reason the parish nurse should care for this client.
    3. This option has no faith base; therefore, the parish nurse should not be assigned this client.
    4. The client diagnosed with chronic renal disease and the caregiver need assistance in the home, but the parish nurse does not need to offer it.

    CLINICAL JUDGMENT GUIDE: The nurse must know the roles and responsibilities of nurses working in different hospital and community areas.

31. 1. The UAP should not remove anything from the room. The nuclear medicine personnel will check the waste from the room for radioactivity before removal and, if radioactive, will arrange for disposal in a way that protects the environment.
    2. The UAP is hired to care for clients in the ambulatory care unit, not to take a client out to smoke. Clients in ambulatory care should not be smoking before or after surgery or procedures.
    3. The UAP cannot assess the client's surgical dressing.
    4. The UAP can obtain a glucometer reading on a stable client. Clients in the ambulatory care unit are stable.

    CLINICAL JUDGMENT GUIDE: The RN cannot delegate assessment, teaching, evaluation, medications, or an unstable client to the UAP.

32. **Answer: 125 gtt/min.**
    A microdrip delivers 60 gtt/mL. The formula for this dosage problem is as follows:
    1,000 mL divided by 8 = 125 mL/hr
    125 × 60 = 7,500 gtt/hr
    7,500 divided by 60 minutes = 125 gtt/min

    CLINICAL JUDGMENT GUIDE: This is an alternate type of question included in the NCLEX-RN®.

The nurse must know how to perform math calculations.

33. **Correct answers are 1, 2, 4, and 5.**
    1. Some herbal remedies commonly recommended for hypothyroid conditions include *Equisetum arvense*, *Avena sativa*, *Centella asiatica*, *Coleus forskohlii*, and *Fucus vesiculosus*. This is an example of an herbal CAM, a healing practice that does not fall within conventional medicine.
    2. Cinnamon is a popular spice and flavoring with considerable evidence of lowering blood sugar. This is an example of a CAM, a healing practice that does not fall within conventional medicine.
    3. Daily low-dose aspirin is a medically accepted practice prescribed by medical doctors. This is not an example of a CAM.
    4. This is an example of a CAM, a healing practice that does not fall within conventional medicine. Acupuncture is a type of traditional Chinese medicine.
    5. Hypnosis is used in clients for concentration and memory improvement. This is an example of a CAM.

    CLINICAL JUDGMENT GUIDE: The NCLEX-RN® tests candidates on complementary alternative medicine, so the test taker should know the types of CAMs. Many clients use these along with conventional medical interventions.

34. 1. This is an example of community-based nursing wherein nurses care for an individual client living in the community.
    2. Community-oriented, population-focused nursing practice involves the engagement of nursing in promoting and protecting the health of populations, not individuals in the community. Therefore, this is an example of community-oriented, population-focused nursing.
    3. This is an example of community-based nursing wherein nurses care for an individual client living in the community.
    4. This is an example of community-based nursing wherein nurses care for an individual client living in the community.

    CLINICAL JUDGMENT GUIDE: The test taker should note options 1, 3, and 4 all address an individual client, but option 2 is the "odd man out" and addresses a group of clients; this should cause the test taker to select this option as the correct answer.

35. 1. The client should keep a written record of the results, but this is not a priority.
    2. The glucometer readings should be done in the morning when the client has not had anything to eat, but it can be done several times daily. This is not a priority.
    3. Have the client demonstrate the skill to ensure the client can correctly perform the glucometer reading. This is the priority when teaching about glucometer tests.
    4. Proper disposal of lancets and strips with blood on them is important, but not a priority over the client demonstrating the skill.

CLINICAL JUDGMENT GUIDE: All options are plausible in questions that ask the nurse to identify a priority intervention. When teaching the client any skill, the priority intervention is having the client perform the skill in front of the nurse.

36. 1. Acupressure applies pressure along the body's energy meridian. Applying pressure on the medial forearm helps decrease the client's feeling of nausea.
    2. This client must have medical interventions and would not benefit from acupressure.
    3. Sheehan syndrome is a postpartum condition of pituitary necrosis and hypopituitarism that occurs after circulatory collapse from uterine hemorrhaging. This client would not be treated with acupressure.
    4. The client diagnosed with hypertension needs medications and would not benefit from acupressure.

CLINICAL JUDGMENT GUIDE: The NCLEX-RN® tests CAM therapies, so the nurse must be familiar with the different types of activities and therapies used for clients.

37. 1. Moving the staff members to another room will only allow the argument to continue. This is not the director's first intervention.
    2. The nursing supervisor should intervene, listen to both staff members' concerns, and attempt to help resolve the disagreement. This is the director's first intervention.
    3. The director should not ask another staff member to intervene in the argument. The director should address the professional staff about unprofessional behavior.
    4. The director should not act unprofessionally and correct the staff in front of everyone in the office. This should be done in private.

CLINICAL JUDGMENT GUIDE: In any business, including a healthcare facility, arguments or discussions of confidential information should not occur among staff of any level where the customers or other staff can hear or see it.

38. 1. These are signs of myxedema coma, characterized by subnormal temperature, hypotension, and hypoventilation. This client should be seen first by the nurse.
    2. The client diagnosed with hypoparathyroidism is expected to have a positive Chvostek's sign (twitching of the facial muscles when the facial nerve is tapped); therefore, the nurse should not assess this client first.
    3. Hoarseness is expected 3 to 4 days after surgery because of edema; therefore, the nurse should not assess this client first.
    4. The client diagnosed with diabetes insipidus has polyuria and compensates for the fluid loss by drinking great amounts of water; therefore, the nurse should not assess this client first.

CLINICAL JUDGMENT GUIDE: The test taker must determine which sign or symptom is not expected for the disease process. If the sign or symptom is unexpected, the nurse should assess the client first. This type of question determines whether the nurse is knowledgeable of clinical manifestations of various disease processes.

39. Correct answers are 1, 3, 4, and 5.
    1. Nutritional counseling and teaching is an example of an activity the home health nurse would implement in the home.
    2. Preoperative teaching is not an activity the home health nurse performs in the home. The preoperative nurse usually completes this.
    3. Managing oxygen therapy is an example of an activity the home health nurse would implement in the home.
    4. Teaching the client and family about administration and side effects of medications is an example of an activity the home health nurse would implement in the home.
    5. Drawing blood for studies related to monitoring disease processes and therapy is an example of an activity the home health nurse would implement in the home.

CLINICAL JUDGMENT GUIDE: This is an alternate type of question included in the NCLEX-RN®. The nurse must select all the options that answer the question correctly.

40. 1. The client is exhibiting Trousseau's sign indicating hypoparathyroidism and requiring treatment with IV calcium gluconate, but it is not the nurse's first intervention. The nurse must first assess the client before taking any action.
    2. **When the UAP gives information about a client to the RN, the RN must assess the client before taking action.**
    3. The client is exhibiting clinical manifestations of hypoparathyroidism, which makes this client unstable. The RN should not delegate any task to the UAP for the unstable client.
    4. The nurse will need to notify the HCP, but not before assessing the client first.

CLINICAL JUDGMENT GUIDE: Any time the RN receives information from another staff member about a client possibly experiencing a complication, the nurse must assess the client. A nurse should not make decisions about the client's needs based on another staff member's information.

41. 1. The client must need intermittent professional skilled care (such as nursing), not constant care.
    2. The client does not have to have a family member living in the home to be eligible for home healthcare.
    3. **The client must be confined to the home or require a considerable and taxing effort to leave the home for brief periods to be eligible for home healthcare.**
    4. The client can be referred directly from an HCP's office or a long-term care facility, and clients may also request home healthcare for themselves.

CLINICAL JUDGMENT GUIDE: The nurse must know the areas of nursing and how and why the client would qualify for the care. The nurse must be a resource and advocate for the client.

42. 1. This is an example of meditation.
    2. Imagery uses the client's mind to generate images to help calm the body.
    3. Aromatherapy, a biologically based therapy, involves using plants' essential oils for their beneficial effect.
    4. Acupressure is a manipulative and body-based method of applying finger and hand pressure to specific body areas.

CLINICAL JUDGMENT GUIDE: The NCLEX-RN® tests complementary alternative medicine (CAM), so the nurse must be familiar with the different types of activities and therapies used for clients.

43. 1. The priority intervention is to restrict fluids to help prevent weight gain, edema, or a serum sodium decline.
    2. This position enhances venous return to the heart and increases left atrial filling pressure, reducing ADH release, but it is not a priority over fluid restriction.
    3. The edematous skin is fragile and at risk for skin breakdown. Turning every 2 hours is a pertinent intervention, but it is not a priority over fluid retention.
    4. The client needs oral hygiene, but it is not a priority over fluid restriction.

CLINICAL JUDGMENT GUIDE: Physiological problems have the highest priority when deciding on a course of action. The nurse should use Maslow's Hierarchy of Needs; fluid and electrolyte balance is the priority.

44. 1. Dyspnea and confusion are not expected in a client diagnosed with Cushing's syndrome; therefore, this client would warrant a more experienced nurse to assess the reason for the complications.
    2. The client with financial problems should be assigned to a social worker, not a nurse.
    3. A full-thickness (third-degree) burn is the most serious and requires excellent assessment skills to determine whether complications occur. This client should be assigned to a more experienced nurse.
    4. The client diagnosed with diabetic neuropathy would be expected to have pain; therefore, this client could be assigned to a nurse new to home health nursing. The client is not exhibiting a complication or an unexpected clinical manifestation.

CLINICAL JUDGMENT GUIDE: When the test taker is deciding which client should be assigned to a new graduate, the most stable client should be assigned to the least experienced nurse.

45. 1. The client 1-day postoperative transsphenoidal hypophysectomy can feed themselves; therefore, this task should not be delegated.
    2. The UAP can obtain a urine specimen from the client. This task is not assessment, teaching, evaluation, medications, or caring for an unstable client.
    3. The client diagnosed with myxedema coma is unstable; therefore, this task cannot be delegated.
    4. The UAP cannot assess. The client diagnosed with an addisonian crisis is not stable; therefore, this task cannot be delegated.

CLINICAL JUDGMENT GUIDE: This is an "except" question. The test taker could ask which task is appropriate to delegate to the UAP; one option would be appropriate, and three would not. Remember: The RN cannot delegate assessment, teaching, evaluation, medications, or an unstable client to the UAP.

46. 1. This statement does not allow the nurses to have any input into the assignments; therefore, this is the statement of an autocratic manager. These managers use an authoritarian approach to direct the activities of others.
    2. Laissez-faire managers maintain a permissive climate with little direction or control. Allowing the assistants to have total control is laissez-faire management. Supporting the assistants in front of the charge nurse is an appropriate action, but it does not address the needs of the field nurses.
    3. This statement does not support a democratic leadership style. It is more autocratic: The director will take care of the problem.
    4. Democratic managers are people-oriented and emphasize efficient group functioning. The environment is open, and communication flows both ways. Meetings to discuss concerns illustrate a democratic leadership style.

CLINICAL JUDGMENT GUIDE: There will be management questions on the NCLEX-RN®. Concepts of Management is included under the category Safe and Effective Care Environment and the subcategory Management of Care.

47. 1. This type of breathing is called Cheyne-Stokes respirations, a pattern of breathing characterized by alternating periods of apnea and deep-rapid breathing. This is not the nurse's first intervention.
    2. The nurse should notify the chaplain, but this is not the nurse's first intervention.
    3. **The RN must first assess the client because the UAP gave the nurse the information.**
    4. The family should be contacted, but not before assessing the client.

CLINICAL JUDGMENT GUIDE: Whenever any other person gives the RN information about a client, the nurse must assess the client before taking any other action.

48. Correct answers are 1, 2, and 5.
    1. This is an intervention the nurse should establish with every client.
    2. Exercises with large muscles release nervous tension and restlessness. Tremors can interfere with small-muscle coordination.
    3. The UAP should use light coverings, not heavy coverings, because the client diagnosed with hyperthyroidism feels hot.
    4. The client diagnosed with hyperthyroidism is not terminal, and there is no reason the caregiver cannot leave the client's bedside.
    5. A calm, quiet, cool room should be provided because increased metabolism causes sleep disturbances and the feeling of being hot.

CLINICAL JUDGMENT GUIDE: The test taker will have alternate types of questions on the NCLEX-RN®. The test taker must select all the correct options for full credit.

49. 1. This statement indicates that the client understands the teaching and does not need more. The exophthalmos that occurs with the disease allows the eyes to dry out, making them uncomfortable and exposing the client to sclera damage.
    2. The client should wear dark glasses; therefore, the client understands the teaching.
    3. **To maintain flexibility, the client should exercise the intraocular muscles several times daily by turning the eyes in the complete range of motion. This statement indicates the client needs more teaching.**
    4. The client should tape the eyes shut; therefore, this client understands the teaching.

CLINICAL JUDGMENT GUIDE: This is an "except" question. Three of the comments indicate the client understands the teaching, and one suggests the client does not understand the teaching. These are occasionally found on the NCLEX-RN® and are worded in this manner. The test taker must realize that the reverse of the usual is in place. A hint: If the test taker is sure more than one option is correct, then the test taker should reread to ensure that a word or words such as "inappropriate" or "needs more teaching" have not been overlooked.

50. 1. Conserving the energy of the dying client is an appropriate intervention and warrants no intervention by the RN.
    2. Applying lubricant to the client's dry lips and mouth is an appropriate intervention and warrants no intervention by the hospice nurse.
    3. This is a form of restraint. The UAP cannot restrain the client in the home or the

acute care setting. This behavior warrants intervention by the RN.
4. This is an appropriate action to help with shortness of breath, or dyspnea. This action would not warrant intervention by the nurse.

CLINICAL JUDGMENT GUIDE: The RN must ensure the UAP can perform delegated tasks. The nurse is responsible for demonstrating or teaching the UAP how to perform the task and then evaluating it.

51. 1. The LPN cannot perform assessments on new admissions.
    2. The RN cannot assign an evaluation of the client's medical regimen to the LPN.
    3. The wound care RN should perform care for a stage 4 pressure injury, not the LPN.
    4. **The LPN can contact medical supply companies and request durable medical equipment (DME); therefore, assigning the LPN is the most appropriate task.**

CLINICAL JUDGMENT GUIDE: The RN cannot assign assessment, teaching, evaluation, or an unstable client to the LPN in the home or the acute care setting.

52. 1. The client diagnosed with hypoparathyroidism is expected to have a decreased serum calcium level; therefore, the nurse would not contact the client's HCP.
    2. The client diagnosed with Cushing's syndrome is expected to have a urine cortisol level of 50 to 100 mcg/day; therefore, the nurse would not notify the client's HCP.
    3. The client diagnosed with diabetes insipidus is expected to have a low urine specific gravity (lower than 1.005); therefore, the nurse would not notify the client's HCP.
    4. **The client diagnosed with hyperthyroidism should have a decreased TSH level; therefore, the nurse should notify the client's HCP.**

CLINICAL JUDGMENT GUIDE: The nurse must know normal laboratory values and be able to determine whether the laboratory value is normal for the client's disease process or the medications the client is taking.

53. 1. The nurse would expect to administer the hormone levothyroxine (Synthroid) to the client diagnosed with hypothyroidism.
    2. **Metformin (Glucophage) must be held 24 hours after a client has received any contrast dye because it can cause renal failure. The nurse should question this medication.**
    3. The client diagnosed with type 1 diabetes should receive their prescribed (human recombinant) insulin (Humulin N) when they are no longer NPO.
    4. The client diagnosed with Addison's disease would be receiving the steroid prednisone; therefore, the nurse would not question administering this medication.

CLINICAL JUDGMENT GUIDE: The nurse must be aware of interventions that have to be implemented before administering medications. The nurse must know what to monitor before administering medications because untoward reactions and possibly death can occur.

54. Correct answers are 1, 2, 3, and 5.
    1. The client with a unilateral adrenalectomy should be ambulated to prevent postoperative complications. This task could be delegated to the UAP.
    2. The UAP can change linens for a client. Acute thyrotoxicosis is not a life-threatening condition.
    3. The client diagnosed with DI is thirsty and craves ice water; therefore, this task can be delegated to the UAP.
    4. The client just returned from surgery and PACU and should be assessed immediately by the RN. The UAP is not qualified to identify an unstable situation.
    5. The UAP can deliver meal trays to clients receiving regular insulin on a sliding scale.

CLINICAL JUDGMENT GUIDE: The RN must ensure the UAP can perform delegated tasks. It is the nurse's responsibility to demonstrate or teach the UAP how to perform and evaluate the task.

55. 1. **The manager should assess each staff member's abilities for the unit's needs before deciding which staff member to transfer.**
    2. This may be the method used by many managers, but the best action is to evaluate the unit's needs and the staff's abilities.
    3. The unit manager often makes hard decisions without consulting the staff members. Asking for the staff members' input could cause tension; therefore, this intervention is not appropriate.
    4. This will be completed after the decision has been made and the staff member is notified.

CLINICAL JUDGMENT GUIDE: There will be management questions on the NCLEX-RN®. Concepts of Management is included under the category Safe and Effective Care Environment and subcategory Management of Care.

56. 1. On a floor not directly affected by the fire, the oxygen is turned off only at the instruction of the administrative supervisor or plant operations director.
    2. The clients are safer on the floor where they are, not in an area closer to the fire.
    3. The first action in a Code Red (actual fire) is to rescue (R) the clients in immediate danger, followed by confine (C), closing the doors. Doors in a hospital must be fire-rated to confine a blaze for an hour and a half.
    4. This could be done, but a charge nurse's responsibility is not called for at this time.

CLINICAL JUDGMENT GUIDE: The nurse must be knowledgeable of emergency preparedness. Employees receive this information in employee orientation and are responsible for implementing procedures correctly. The National Council of State Boards of Nursing (NCSBN) NCLEX-RN® test plan includes questions on promoting a Safe and Effective Care Environment.

57. 1. The nurse should check the laboratory tests to determine the thyroid levels, but this is not the first intervention.
    2. Assessing the client for diarrhea could be done, but it is more important not to worsen the problem, and, therefore, the nurse should hold the thyroid medication first.
    3. Documentation of the client's symptoms is always important, but it is not the first intervention.
    4. The client is describing symptoms of hyperthyroidism. Because the client is diagnosed with hypothyroidism, has been prescribed thyroid hormone replacement, and now has symptoms of hyperthyroidism, it can be assumed that the client now has an excess of thyroid hormone. Therefore, the nurse should hold the thyroid medication and check the client's thyroid profile.

CLINICAL JUDGMENT GUIDE: The nurse must know the expected actions of medications. The nurse must be aware of assessment data indicating whether the medication is effective or whether the medication is causing a side effect or an adverse effect.

58. 1. Propylthiouracil (PTU) blocks peripheral conversion of thyroxine (T4) to triiodothyronine (T3) and is prescribed for the client diagnosed with hyperthyroidism. The nurse would not question administering this medication.
    2. Desmopressin acetate (DDAVP) is the treatment of choice for the client diagnosed with central diabetes insipidus.
    3. Somatropin (Genotropin), a growth hormone, is the treatment of choice for clients diagnosed with hypofunction of the pituitary gland.
    4. The client diagnosed with hypothyroidism has a decreased pulse rate; therefore, the nurse should not administer a beta blocker, which could further decrease the pulse rate. The client diagnosed with thyrotoxicosis (hyperthyroidism) would receive propranolol (Inderal). The nurse should question administering this medication.

CLINICAL JUDGMENT GUIDE: The nurse must know about medications prescribed for specific conditions and disease processes. The nurse is the last person to ensure the client receives the correct medications.

59. 1. A terminally ill client should be allowed comfort measures even when the activity would typically not be encouraged or allowed. If needed, the client can receive sliding-scale insulin to cover the ice cream.
    2. The nurse could do this after the ice cream has been metabolized to determine whether an insulin injection is needed.
    3. The nurse should tell the client that food such as ice cream may be consumed in moderation and with the appropriate coverage.
    4. Low-fat sweets may be a good substitute for some foods the client may want.

CLINICAL JUDGMENT GUIDE: The NCLEX-RN® addresses questions concerned with end-of-life care. This is included in the Psychosocial Integrity section of the test plan. Supporting the client's choice is an appropriate option when working with dying clients.

60. 1. The HOB should be elevated 30 degrees because the elevation avoids pressure on the sella turcica and decreases headaches, a frequent postoperative problem.
    2. A hypophysectomy is surgery that removes the pituitary gland by making an incision in the inner aspect of the upper lip and gingiva. The client should avoid vigorous coughing, sneezing, and straining at stool.
    3. A hypophysectomy is surgery that removes the pituitary gland by making an incision in the inner aspect of the upper lip and gingiva. The sella turcica is entered through the floor of the nose and

sphenoid sinuses. There are no visual incisions, and the nose cannot be splinted.
4. The UAP can take the client's vital signs; this action would not warrant intervention by the RN.

CLINICAL JUDGMENT GUIDE: The RN must ensure the UAP can perform delegated tasks. It is the nurse's responsibility to demonstrate and teach the UAP how to perform the task, and evaluate it.

61. 1. The client needs preoperative teaching, and the charge nurse should not request a discharge for a client who has surgery in the morning.
    2. This client is stable and could be prescribed oral pain medication. The client could be discharged home and followed by home health nursing if needed. This client is the most appropriate client for the charge nurse to request to be discharged.
    3. This client is experiencing a complication of surgery and is hemorrhaging; the Hgb/Hct are very low. Therefore, this client cannot be discharged home.
    4. This client may be showing signs of acute rejection; therefore, this client cannot be discharged home.

CLINICAL JUDGMENT GUIDE: When the nurse is deciding which client should be discharged home, the most stable client should be discharged.

62. 1. This is a normal potassium level. The HCP does not need to be notified.
    2. This level is within the therapeutic range. The HCP does not need to be notified.
    3. A BUN of 84 mg/dL is an abnormal laboratory value, but it would be expected in a client diagnosed with ESRD. The HCP does not need to be notified.
    4. This is a very high blood glucose level. The client diagnosed with type 1 diabetes will be catabolizing fats at this level and is at risk for DKA coma.

CLINICAL JUDGMENT GUIDE: The nurse must be knowledgeable of normal laboratory values and be able to determine whether the laboratory value is normal for the client's disease process or the medications the client is taking.

63. 1. The client diagnosed with DKA would have fruity breath; therefore, this nursing intervention does not have priority.
    2. Glucose levels are monitored at least every hour.
    3. The pulse oximeter reading is not a priority for a client in DKA.
    4. The client will be on a regular insulin drip, which must be maintained on an IV pump device at the prescribed rate. Decreasing the client's blood glucose level is the priority nursing intervention.

CLINICAL JUDGMENT GUIDE: The nurse should remember that if a client is in distress and the nurse can do something to relieve the distress, it should be done first before assessment. The test taker should select an option that helps the client's condition directly.

64. 1. The client's hemoglobin A1C test reveals the average blood glucose for the previous 2 to 3 months. The current blood glucose level may or may not be in the desired range, but the client's diabetes with this level of hemoglobin A1C is not controlled.
    2. The nurse should assess for complications of diabetes, but this is not the first intervention. Getting the client to realize the meaning of a high hemoglobin A1C is the priority now.
    3. **The client must be taught the long-term effects of hyperglycemia. A hemoglobin A1C of 11% indicates an average blood glucose of 269 mg/dL. Over time, a level higher than 120 to 140 mg/dL can damage many body systems.**
    4. Monitoring blood work is not a priority over teaching the client about complications of diabetes when having such a high A1C.

CLINICAL JUDGMENT GUIDE: The nurse must be knowledgeable of normal laboratory values and be able to determine whether the laboratory value is normal for the client's disease process or the medications the client is taking.

65. 1. This client has an elevated WBC count, which could indicate an infection. The HCP should be made aware of this client first.
    2. These are normal laboratory values.
    3. These are normal laboratory values.
    4. These are normal laboratory values.

CLINICAL JUDGMENT GUIDE: This is an alternate type of question included in the NCLEX-RN® test plan. The test taker must be able to read an EHR, be knowledgeable of laboratory data, and make decisions concerning the nurse's most appropriate action.

66. The nurse should administer 8 units of regular insulin, a pancreatic hormone, because 249 mg/dL is between 201 and 250.

CLINICAL JUDGMENT GUIDE: A fill-in-the-blank question is an alternate type of question included in the NCLEX-RN®. The test taker must use the number keyboard to answer fill-in-the-blank questions.

67. Correct answers are 1, 2, and 3.
    1. The UAP can escort the client to the examination room and take the initial vital signs.
    2. The UAP can weigh the client and document the weight.
    3. The UAP can prepare the examination room for the next client.
    4. Discussing prescriptions is teaching, and the RN cannot delegate teaching.
    5. Calling the pharmacy requires knowledge of medications and medication administration. This task cannot be delegated to a UAP.

    CLINICAL JUDGMENT GUIDE: This is an alternate type of question included in the NCLEX-RN®. The nurse must be able to select all the options that answer the question correctly to get full credit. The RN cannot delegate assessment, teaching, evaluation, medications, or an unstable client to the UAP.

68. Correct order is 1, 3, 4, 2, 5.
    1. This client may have overdosed accidentally or on purpose. This is a physiological problem, and the nurse must determine which intervention is required next. This is a potentially life-threatening situation, so the nurse should return this phone call first.
    3. The client diagnosed with hypothyroidism is reporting signs of hyperthyroidism, indicating the client is overdosing on thyroid hormone replacement and needs to be seen in the clinic. This is a physiological problem; therefore, the nurse should call this client second.
    4. The pharmacist needs to know whether the substitution can be made to fill this prescription. This call should be returned third.
    2. The nurse needs to discuss the prescribed medication with the HCP to see whether a different, less expensive medication would work as well for the client, or whether an alternative medication program could be discussed with the client. This phone call should be returned fourth.
    5. The nurse must first determine where the breakdown in the communication of the results of the MRI occurred, then obtain the results and provide them to the HCP before returning the call. This phone call can be returned last.

    CLINICAL JUDGMENT GUIDE: This is an alternate question requiring the nurse to assess clients in order of priority. Answering requires the nurse to evaluate each client's situation and determine which are life-threatening and which are expected for the client's situation, as well as which client has a psychosocial problem.

69. Correct answers are 1, 2, 3, and 5.
    1. This is an assessment question and is needed to determine the extent of the current situation.
    2. Knowing the blood glucose level is important for the nurse to determine whether the client is at risk for DKA.
    3. This will determine what has been tried and the next step.
    4. The client should drink liquids that provide calories, such as sports drinks, and alternate with water to maintain hydration.
    5. The client will still need to take insulin. Without insulin, the client's body will begin to break down fats. A by-product of fat catabolism is acid. The buildup of acid in the body will result in DKA, which can lead to coma and death.

    CLINICAL JUDGMENT GUIDE: The nurse must be knowledgeable about expected medical treatment for the client and their symptoms.

70. Correct answers are 1, 3, 4, and 5.
    1. The client should monitor for urine ketones. The body usually does not spill ketones in the urine until after the blood glucose levels reach 240 mg/dL and above. Urine ketones indicate the client's body will begin to break down fats; ketones are the by-product of fat metabolism.
    2. The client should try to practice "sick day rules" to manage diabetes mellitus during times of illness. Clients do not need to go to the emergency department with an illness immediately.
    3. Over-the-counter (OTC) medications to control cough and nasal congestion are safe, but the client should be taught to avoid those OTC medications that contain sugar.
    4. The HCP must adjust the insulin dosage if the client is "spilling" ketones in the urine.
    5. To prevent DKA, the client must continue taking insulin. To prevent hypoglycemia, the client should attempt to ingest calories to balance the insulin. The antidote for insulin is food.

    CLINICAL JUDGMENT GUIDE: This is an alternate type of question on the NCLEX-RN® examination. The test taker must select all the correct answers.

71. Correct answers are 1, 2, 3, 4, and 5.
    1. The client should be assessed for fluid volume deficit and electrolyte imbalance. Intake and output should be strictly monitored.
    2. Bedside glucose assessments should be monitored at least hourly to evaluate the client's response to treatments.
    3. IV fluids and regular insulin are initial treatments for DKA.
    4. The client was admitted for nausea and vomiting, so oral care is an important intervention for the nurse to perform.
    5. The client in DKA loses potassium from increased urinary output, acidosis, catabolic state, and vomiting. Monitoring and replacement are essential for preventing cardiac dysrhythmias secondary to hypokalemia.

CLINICAL JUDGMENT GUIDE: The nurse must be knowledgeable about expected medical treatment for the client and their symptoms.

72. 1. The client should be cleaned with warm water and mild soap.
    2. The client's feet should be thoroughly dried by patting, not rubbing the skin.
    3. Lotion can be applied to the feet but should not be used between the toes. The moisture of the lotion can cause skin breakdown. The nurse should intervene.
    4. The client should wear cotton or wool socks, which are moisture-resistant, and avoid going barefoot.

CLINICAL JUDGMENT GUIDE: The RN must ensure the UAP can perform delegated tasks. The nurse is responsible for demonstrating or teaching the UAP how to perform the task and then evaluating it. If the UAP is performing a task incorrectly, the nurse should intervene immediately.

73. Correct answers are 1, 2, 3, and 5.
    1. The client should be taught about "sick day rules" to maintain blood sugar during illness.
    2. Regular monitoring of blood glucose should be reinforced with the client.
    3. Diabetes affects all the tissues in the body, and the feet are particularly at risk for the development of foot ulcers.
    4. Type 1 diabetes occurs in young clients who have no production of insulin from the beta cells of the pancreas. These clients are usually underweight. This teaching is not indicated.
    5. The client should have regular examinations with the diagnosis of type 1 diabetes.

CLINICAL JUDGMENT GUIDE: Teaching is a critical responsibility of the RN. Test takers should know information that should be taught to clients with common diagnoses.

74. 1. There is no indication that the client recovering from DKA needs a physical therapist.
    2. There is no indication that the client newly diagnosed with type 1 diabetes would need a referral to a hospice organization.
    3. A diabetes educator can educate and support this client with the new diagnosis. This is an appropriate referral.
    4. There is no indication that the client needs a fitness trainer.

CLINICAL JUDGMENT GUIDE: The nurse should be knowledgeable of the roles and responsibilities of all members of the multidisciplinary healthcare team and appropriate referrals.

75. 1. CGM gives glucose readings every 5 minutes; fingerstick tests are still required, but less often.
    2. The CGM system is more expensive than performing fingerstick tests.
    3. CGM is a blood glucose monitoring system only, but it can be used with an insulin pump for better blood sugar maintenance.
    4. The CGM system is designed to show real-time blood glucose measurements and trends over time, allowing for a better understanding of the client's glucose level fluctuations. CGM systems can send information and alerts directly to the client's smartphone.

CLINICAL JUDGMENT GUIDE: The nurse must be knowledgeable regarding wearable devices utilized to manage common health issues.

76. 1. The client can place the pump on the bed or attach it to their clothing or pillow. This statement indicates the client understands the teaching.
    2. An insulin pump allows the client to administer a continuous dose of insulin and bolus doses to cover meals high in carbohydrates. This helps to avoid large fluctuations in blood glucose levels. This statement indicates the client understands the teaching.
    3. The client must continue monitoring blood glucose levels to ensure the insulin pump works correctly. If the insulin pump malfunctions, the client could experience DKA. This statement indicates the client understands the teaching.

4. An insulin pump allows the client to match insulin to exercise and activities. When performing some exercise, such as swimming or contact sports, the insulin pump should be disconnected to avoid damage to the pump or injury to the client. This statement indicates the client needs more teaching.

CLINICAL JUDGMENT GUIDE: The nurse must be knowledgeable regarding wearable devices utilized to manage common health issues.

77. 1. Lipohypertrophy is an abnormal fat accumulation under the skin's surface and is most often associated with repeated injections at the same location. The priority intervention is to rotate catheter insertion sites to avoid lipohypertrophy.
    2. The client should be taught to perform frequent hand washing to prevent infection at the catheter insertion site; however, the priority intervention is to rotate insertion sites.
    3. The client should be taught to avoid inserting the insulin pump catheter in the inner thigh. The inner thigh has many nerves and blood vessels, which can cause increased discomfort and reduce insulin absorption. This is not the priority intervention to avoid lipohypertrophy.
    4. The client should be instructed to complete the prescribed course of antibiotics to treat the lipohypertrophy, but this will not prevent the reoccurrence. The priority intervention is to prevent lipohypertrophy by rotating catheter insertion sites.

CLINICAL JUDGMENT GUIDE: The nurse must be knowledgeable regarding wearable devices utilized to manage common health issues and how to teach the client ways to avoid device complications.

78. Correct order is 4, 3, 5, 1, 2.
    4. The nurse should wash their hands and don nonsterile gloves.
    3. The nurse should wash the insertion area with antibacterial soap and let it dry thoroughly.
    5. The nurse should cleanse the area with an antibacterial solution and let it dry thoroughly.
    1. The next step is to apply an antiseptic and adhesive wipe to the area.
    2. The final step is to insert the catheter in a slow, continuous motion.

CLINICAL JUDGMENT GUIDE: The nurse must be able to perform skills in the correct order. This is an alternate type of question included in the NCLEX-RN® examination.

CASE STUDY ANSWERS

1. Correct answers are 2, 3, 4, 5, 6, 7, and 8. The client's blood pressure, heart rate, and temperature should be reported as vital signs outside the normal range. The syncope, vertigo, weakness, and diaphoresis should also be reported as these indicators may help determine the underlying cause of the client's illness. The remaining findings are not a priority at this time.

2. Correct answers are marked here.

Finding	Dehydration	Addison's Disease	Diabetes Mellitus
Hypotension	X	X	
Anemia		X	X
Hypoglycemia		X	
Hyponatremia		X	
Fatigue	X	X	X
Weakness	X	X	X
Vertigo	X	X	
Increased BUN level	X	X	

All findings listed are consistent with the diagnosis of Addison's disease, with hyponatremia and hypoglycemia being some of the most prevalent due to the decrease in glucocorticoid and mineralocorticoid levels. Some of the findings are also present in clients with diabetes mellitus (anemia, fatigue, and weakness), and other more nonspecific findings are associated with dehydration (hypotension, fatigue, weakness, vertigo, and increased BUN levels).

3. Correct answers are 1 and 2.
Based on the client's condition, the nurse recognizes that the client is at the highest risk for

| 1. Decreased cardiac output |

and will require

| 2. IV fluids |

The client's hemodynamic stability is compromised owing to an inability to retain sodium and water. The low circulating blood volume puts the client at risk for decreased cardiac output, requiring IV fluids to avoid tissue and organ damage due to poor perfusion. There is no indication of infection or the need for antibiotics, and given the vital signs and electrolyte levels, the client is at risk for fluid volume *deficit* rather than *overload*; diuretics would worsen the client's condition.

4. Correct interventions are marked.

Potential Nursing Intervention	Indicated	Not Indicated
Instruct client to get up slowly with help	X	
Reduce IV 0.9% NaCl to 100 mL/hr		X
Provide teaching on ACTH suppression test	X	
Ensure continuous telemetry	X	
Instruct on the need for a urine sample	X	
Call Endocrinology consult	X	
Encourage oral fluid intake	X	

It is important to instruct the client to get up slowly and only with assistance because of the potential for orthostatic hypotension. An ACTH suppression test has been ordered for the next morning; the client has not been taught the purpose or process of this test. Continuous telemetry has been ordered and is important for ongoing monitoring due to electrolyte imbalance and hemodynamic instability. The client should be reminded about the need for a urine sample and to drink as much fluids as possible.

The most recent IV normal saline rate ordered is 150 mL/hr; reducing the rate would worsen hypotension and decrease tissue perfusion.

5. Correct answers are marked.

The client should be catheterized to obtain a urine specimen for evaluation. Oral fluids should be encouraged to counter the effects of adrenal insufficiency. 100mg of hydrocortisone is the appropriate medication to administer.

Possible Actions	Correct Actions
Reinforce the need for a urine sample	Straight cath ×1 and send urine to lab
Place an indwelling urinary catheter	
Instruct on oral fluid restriction	Encourage oral fluids
Instruct on NPO status	
Administer IVP 200 mg hydrocortisone	Administer IVP 100 mg hydrocortisone
Initiate a second IV site	

6. Correct answers are marked.

Client Statement	Teaching Effective	Teaching Not Effective
"I will take the oral hydrocortisone for 7 days."		X
"I should check my blood pressure once a month."		X
"I should drink at least 64 ounces of water everyday."	X	
"I should restrict my daily intake of sodium."		X
"I should order a medical alert bracelet and wear it all the time."	X	

The client should continue to drink 64 oz or more of water every day, which will assist in countering the effects of adrenal insufficiency. A medical alert bracelet is recommended so that caregivers and first responders are aware of the client's condition if he cannot verbalize.

The client will require lifelong mineralocorticoid and glucocorticoid replacement therapy. At least initially, the client should check their blood pressure at least daily for early detection of hypotension. Finally, the client will be encouraged to eat high-sodium foods; these will result in helping the body retain water for hemodynamic stability.

Integumentary Management 9

Believe you can and you're halfway there.

—Theodore Roosevelt

QUESTIONS

1. The client with a history of cerebrovascular accident (CVA) is admitted to the orthopedic unit diagnosed with a fractured right hip. The client is reporting bleeding when brushing their teeth. The nurse reviews the client's medication administration record (MAR).

Client's Name: P.W. **Height:** 72 in (182.9 cm)	**Account Number:** 1230456 **Weight:** 240 lb (108.9 kg)	**Allergies:** NKDA **Date:** Today
Medication	**0701–1900**	**1901–0700**
Levothyroxine 1 tablet PO daily	0900 DN	
Atenolol 50 mg PO daily	0900 DN AP 72	
Warfarin 5 mg PO	1700 DN	
Hydrocodone 5 mg/500 mg PO every 4–6 hours PRN for pain		
Signature/Initials	Day Nurse RN/DN	Night Nurse RN/DN

   Which intervention should the nurse implement **first**?
   1. Prepare to administer vitamin K.
   2. Determine whether the client is using a soft-bristle toothbrush.
   3. Check the client's apical pulse and blood pressure.
   4. Request the laboratory to draw a STAT International Normalized Ratio (INR).

2. The nurse received the a.m. shift report on the following clients. Which client should the nurse assess **first**?
   1. The client with a right total knee replacement wanting to be removed from the continuous passive motion (CPM) machine
   2. The client diagnosed with chronic low back pain crying and upset about being discharged home
   3. The client 1 week postoperative for right total hip replacement and a temperature of 100.4°F (38°C)
   4. The client diagnosed with full-thickness burns needing to be medicated before being taken to whirlpool

3. The nurse is working in an orthopedic unit. Which client should the nurse assess **first**?
   1. The client 2 weeks postoperative ORIF of the right hip reporting pain when ambulating
   2. The client 10 days postoperative for left total knee replacement refusing to use the continuous passive motion (CPM) machine
   3. The client 1 week postoperative for L3–L4 laminectomy reporting numbness and tingling of their feet
   4. The client being admitted to the rehabilitation unit from the orthopedic surgical unit after a motor vehicle accident (MVA)

4. The client is 1 week postoperative for right below-the-knee amputation secondary to arterial occlusive disease. The nurse is unable to assess a pedal pulse in the left foot. Which intervention should the nurse implement **first**?
   1. Assess for paresthesia and paralysis.
   2. Utilize the Doppler device to auscultate the pulse.
   3. Place the client's leg in the dependent position.
   4. Wrap the client's left leg in a warm blanket.

5. The nurse is preparing to administer morning (a.m.) medications to the following clients. Which medication should the nurse administer **first**?
   1. The NSAID to the client diagnosed with osteoarthritis
   2. The IV antibiotic to the client diagnosed with cellulitis
   3. The antiviral agent to the client diagnosed with herpes zoster (shingles)
   4. The antihistamine for the client diagnosed with urticaria and pruritus

6. The client tells the nurse, "I have a mole on my back that is darker and getting larger." Which intervention should the nurse implement **first**?
   1. Tell the client to use corticosteroid cream on the area.
   2. Recommend the client use SPF 15 or higher when in the sun.
   3. Instruct the client to notify their healthcare provider (HCP) immediately.
   4. Encourage the client to wear dark, woven clothing when outside.

7. The nurse is at a local playground, and the nurse's 10-year-old child falls and reports hurting their left ankle and foot. Which intervention should the nurse implement **first** at the scene of the accident?
   1. Instruct the child not to move their left leg.
   2. Elevate the left leg on two rolled towels.
   3. Apply an ice pack to the left ankle.
   4. Check the child's pedal pulse bilaterally.

8. The nurse is preparing to change a dressing on an 82-year-old client diagnosed with a stage III pressure injury. Which intervention should the nurse implement **first**?
   1. Obtain the needed equipment to perform the procedure.
   2. Remove the client's old dressing with nonsterile gloves.
   3. Explain the procedure to the client in understandable terms.
   4. Check to determine whether the client has received pain medication.

9. Which client should the charge nurse on the rehabilitation unit assess **first** after receiving the a.m. shift report?
    1. The male client who is postoperative ORIF of the right hip

Client Name: J.L.	Account Number: 1133557	Allergies: PCN
Laboratory Report		
Laboratory Test	Client Values	Reference Values
WBC	9.1	4.5 to 11.1 × 10³/microL
Hgb	8	Male: 14 to 17.3 g/dL
		Female: 11.7 to 15.5 g/dL
Hct	24	Male: 42% to 52%
		Female: 36% to 48%
Glucose	89	Fasting: Less than 100 mg/dL
		Random: Less than 200 mg/dL
Rheumatoid factor	12	Less than 14 IU/mL

    2. The female client diagnosed with rheumatoid arthritis

Client Name: M.P.	Account Number: 2299483	Allergies: NKDA
Laboratory Report		
Laboratory Test	Client Values	Reference Values
WBC	8.2	4.5 to 11.1 × 10³/microL
Hgb	14.3	Male: 14 to 17.3 g/dL
		Female: 11.7 to 15.5 g/dL
Hct	43	Male: 42% to 52%
		Female: 36% to 48%
Glucose	95	Fasting: Less than 100 mg/dL
		Random: Less than 200 mg/dL
Rheumatoid factor	20	Less than 14 IU/mL

    3. The male client diagnosed with a stage IV pressure injury

Client Name: P.G.	Account Number: 8833774	Allergies: NKDA
Laboratory Report		
Laboratory Test	Client Values	Reference Values
WBC	14	4.5 to 11.1 × 10³/microL
Hgb	14	Male: 14 to 17.3 g/dL
		Female: 11.7 to 15.5 g/dL
Hct	42	Male: 42% to 52%
		Female: 36% to 48%
Glucose	99	Fasting: Less than 100 mg/dL
		Random: Less than 200 mg/dL
Rheumatoid factor	10	Less than 14 IU/mL

4. The female client diagnosed with systemic allergies and taking a prednisone dose pack

Client Name: K.C. **Account Number:** 2255449 **Allergies:** NKDA

Laboratory Report

Laboratory Test	Client Values	Reference Values
WBC	8.5	4.5 to 11.1 × 10³/microL
Hgb	12.3	Male: 14 to 17.3 g/dL
		Female: 11.7 to 15.5 g/dL
Hct	36	Male: 42% to 52%
		Female: 36% to 48%
Glucose	189	Fasting: Less than 100 mg/dL
		Random: Less than 200 mg/dL
Rheumatoid factor	8	Less than 14 IU/mL

10. The unassisted client ambulating the orthopedic hallway fell to the floor. Which action should the nurse implement **first**?
    1. Complete an adverse occurrence report.
    2. Notify the clinical manager on the unit.
    3. Determine whether the client has any injuries.
    4. Ask why the client was in the hall alone.

11. The RN rehab nurse and the unlicensed assistive personnel (UAP) are caring for clients in a rehabilitation unit. Which nursing task is **most** appropriate for the RN to delegate to the UAP?
    1. Flush the triple-lumen lines on a central venous catheter.
    2. Demonstrate to the client how to ambulate with a walker.
    3. Assist with bowel training by escorting the client to the bathroom.
    4. Apply corticosteroid cream to the client diagnosed with allergic dermatitis.

12. The UAP tells the RN primary nurse the client with a right above-the-knee amputation has a large amount of bright red blood on the right leg residual limb. Which action should the nurse implement?
    1. Assess the client's residual limb dressing.
    2. Tell the UAP to take the client's pulse and blood pressure.
    3. Remove the dressing to assess the incision.
    4. Request the UAP to reinforce the dressing.

13. Which action by the UAP **warrants immediate** intervention by the RN staff nurse?
    1. The UAP tied the confused client to a chair with a sheet.
    2. The UAP escorted the client downstairs to smoke a cigarette.
    3. The UAP bought the client a carbonated beverage from the cafeteria.
    4. The UAP assisted the client to ambulate to the dayroom area.

14. The RN charge nurse, a licensed practical nurse (LPN), and two UAPs are caring for clients. Which action is **most** appropriate for the charge nurse to assign or delegate?
    1. Ask the UAP to apply warm compresses to the client diagnosed with tinea corporis.
    2. Request the LPN to apply antifungal cream to the client diagnosed with tinea pedis.
    3. Tell the UAP to remove the toenail of the client diagnosed with onychomycosis.
    4. Instruct the LPN to administer isotretinoin to the pregnant client.

15. The RN staff nurse in the rehabilitation unit is caring for clients along with a UAP. Which action by the UAP **warrants immediate** intervention?
    1. The UAP assists a client 1 week postoperatively in eating a regular diet.
    2. The UAP calls for assistance when taking a client to the shower.
    3. The UAP assists the client weighing 181 kg (399 lb) to the bedside commode.
    4. The UAP places the call light within reach of the client sitting in the chair.

16. The UAP in the rehabilitation unit is placing the client with a left above-the-knee amputation in the prone position. Which action should the RN rehab nurse implement?
    1. Tell the UAP to place the client on their back.
    2. Praise the UAP for positioning the client prone.
    3. Report this action verbally to the charge nurse.
    4. Explain to the UAP that the client should not be on their stomach.

17. The UAP is applying elastic compression stockings to the client. Which action by the UAP indicates to the RN primary nurse the UAP **understands** the correct procedure for applying the elastic compression stockings?
    1. The UAP applies the stockings while the client sits in a chair.
    2. The UAP cannot insert two fingers under the proximal end of the stocking.
    3. The UAP had the client elevate their legs before putting on the stockings.
    4. The UAP places the toe opening of the elastic stocking on top of the client's foot.

18. The charge nurse on the acute care rehabilitation unit is making assignments for the shift. Which client should the charge nurse assign to the **most** experienced nurse?
    1. The client diagnosed with a full-thickness burn and refusing to go to therapy
    2. The client diagnosed with osteomyelitis and having bone pain and a fever
    3. The client diagnosed with a fractured tibia and having deep, unrelenting pain
    4. The client diagnosed with low back pain radiating down the left leg

19. The busy 36-bed rehabilitation unit RN charge nurse must send one staff member to the emergency department (ED). Which staff member is the **most** appropriate person to send?
    1. The LPN working in the rehabilitation unit for 3 years
    2. The RN employed in the rehabilitation unit for 8 years
    3. The UAP completing the 4-week orientation to the rehabilitation unit
    4. The RN recently transferred to the rehabilitation unit from the medical unit

20. Which task should the RN rehabilitation nurse delegate to the UAP?
    1. Tell the UAP to show the client how to perform self-catheterization.
    2. Request the UAP to place the newly confused client in the inclusion bed.
    3. Ask the UAP to give the client 30 mL of magnesium hydroxide aluminum hydroxide.
    4. Encourage the UAP to attend the multidisciplinary team meeting.

21. The client is 8 hours postoperative spinal surgery. Which **priority** intervention should the nurse implement?
    1. Evaluate how much pain medication the client uses via the patient-controlled analgesia (PCA) pump.
    2. Logroll the client with three staff members when turning the client side to side.
    3. Assist the client to ambulate to the bathroom using an elevated commode seat.
    4. Place pillows under the thighs of each leg when the client is supine.

22. The elderly spouse of a client with a total hip replacement being discharged home tells the nurse, "I am really worried about taking my spouse home. I don't know how I can take care of them." Which intervention is **most** appropriate for the nurse?
    1. Refer the client to the home health nurse.
    2. Discuss the possibility of placing the client in a nursing home.
    3. Request the client's HCP to talk to the client's spouse.
    4. Allow the client's spouse to vent their feelings about the situation.

23. On previous occasions, the nurse has been told by their coworker not to talk about their body, then the nurse says, "You really look hot in those scrubs. You have a great-looking body." Which action should the coworker nurse implement **next**?
    1. Document the comment in writing and file a formal grievance.
    2. Tell the offending nurse this makes them feel very uncomfortable.
    3. Notify the clinical manager of the sexual harassment.
    4. Discuss the nurse's behavior with the hospital lawyer.

24. The client admitted to the rehabilitation unit because of a diagnosed debilitative state asks the nurse, "Why do I have to go to physical therapy every day?" Which statement is the nurse's **best** response?
    1. "The physical therapy will help you become **more** independent in caring for yourself."
    2. "You must have at least 3 hours of therapy daily to stay in this rehab unit."
    3. "The multidisciplinary team determined that you should be in physical therapy daily."
    4. "The physical therapist will help you with exercises to improve your muscle strength."

25. The client diagnosed with a fractured right ankle must be instructed on crutch walking. Which member of the multidisciplinary team should address this problem?
    1. The physical therapist
    2. The social worker
    3. The occupational therapist
    4. The rehabilitation physician

26. The client with bilateral amputations tells the nurse, "I was told I can't go back to my job because they do not have handicap-accessible bathrooms or ramps." Which action by the nurse is **most** helpful to the client?
    1. Discuss the situation with the multidisciplinary healthcare team.
    2. Explain the Americans with Disabilities Act (ADA) to the client.
    3. Contact the client's employer via telephone and discuss the situation.
    4. Encourage the client to hire an attorney and sue the employer.

27. Which action by the RN primary nurse would **warrant immediate** intervention by the RN charge nurse on the rehabilitation unit?
    1. The primary nurse tells the UAP to escort a client to the swimming pool.
    2. The primary nurse evaluates the client's plan of care with the family member.
    3. The primary RN asks another RN to administer an injection prepared by the primary RN.
    4. The primary nurse requests another nurse to watch their clients for 30 minutes.

28. The client in a motor vehicle accident is in critical condition diagnosed with a pelvic fracture, flail chest, bilateral arm fractures, and a left hip fracture. The client tells the nurse, "I just want to die. I can't feed myself or clean myself." Which statement is the nurse's **best** response?
    1. "I know this must be hard for you, but you can have a life."
    2. "I can see you must feel helpless; I am here to listen."
    3. "Have you thought about killing yourself?"
    4. "You are in shock; things will get better in time."

29. The nurse on the surgical unit is being sent to the neonatal intensive care unit (NICU) to work because they are short-staffed. The nurse has never worked in the NICU. Which response by the nurse supports the ethical principle of nonmaleficence?
    1. The nurse requests not to be floated to the NICU.
    2. The nurse accepts the assignment to the NICU.
    3. The nurse asks why another nurse can't go to the NICU.
    4. The nurse talks another nurse into going to the NICU.

30. The client's spouse is frustrated and tells the nurse, "Everyone is telling me something different about when my spouse will be able to go home. I don't know whom to believe." Which statement is the rehabilitation nurse's **best** response?
    1. "I can see you are frustrated. Do you want to talk about how you feel?"
    2. "I will contact the case manager and have them talk to you as soon as possible."
    3. "Do not worry. Your spouse won't go home until you and the client are both ready."
    4. "Your spouse's HCP should be able to give you that information."

31. The client with a right upper extremity amputation tells the nurse, "I do everything with my right hand, and now it is gone. I have no idea what I will do after I get discharged. How will I support my family? I will need to get a new job." Which statement is the nurse's **best** response?
    1. "With time, you will be able to do everything with your left hand."
    2. "The state rehabilitation commission will help retrain you."
    3. "You should ask the social worker about applying for disability."
    4. "You are worried about how you will be able to support your family."

32. The client tells the nurse, "I do not like my doctor, and I want another doctor." Which statement is the nurse's **best** response?
    1. "You should tell your doctor you are unhappy with their care."
    2. "Can you tell me what you don't like about your doctor's care?"
    3. "I will notify my nursing supervisor and report your concern."
    4. "I am sorry, but you must keep this doctor until you are discharged."

33. The RN staff nurse and the UAP are caring for a 74-year-old client now 3 days postoperative right total hip replacement. Which nursing task should be delegated to the UAP?
    1. Place the abductor pillow between the client's legs.
    2. Ensure the client stays on complete bedrest.
    3. Feed the client their evening meal.
    4. Check the client's right hip surgical dressing.

34. The RN staff nurse tells the UAP to assist the client who is 1 day postoperative spinal surgery with a.m. care. Which action by the UAP **warrants immediate** intervention?
    1. The UAP closes the door and cubicle curtain.
    2. The UAP requests the client to turn to their side.
    3. The UAP checks the temperature of the bathing water.
    4. The UAP puts the side rails up when bathing the client.

35. The client with a right below-the-knee amputation, also diagnosed with impetigo, is admitted to a rehabilitation unit. Which interventions should be included in the nursing care plan? **Select all that apply.**
    1. Elevate the client's right leg on two pillows.
    2. Refer the client to occupational therapy daily.
    3. Encourage the client to push the residual limb against a pillow.
    4. Use warm soap and water to remove the crusts secondary to impetigo.
    5. Ensure all staff members wear gloves when caring for clients.

36. The overhead page has issued a Code Black, indicating a tornado in the area. Which intervention should the charge nurse implement?
    1. Instruct the hospital staff to assist the clients and visitors to the cafeteria.
    2. Request the client and visitors go into the bathroom in the client's room.
    3. Have the clients and visitors remain in the hallway with the doors closed.
    4. Tell the client and visitors to remain in the client's room with the door open.

37. The client is placed in a double hip spica cast for 3 months. The client's significant other tells the nurse, "My partner said we are supposed to talk to the case manager. What is a case manager?" Which statement is the nurse's **best** response?
    1. "A case manager discusses the cost and insurance issues concerning the rehabilitation."
    2. "The case manager is responsible for the medical treatment regimen for your partner."
    3. "The case manager is a member of the team assisting your partner in finding another job."
    4. "The case manager is coordinating the rehabilitation team and keeping you informed."

38. The 28-year-old client sustained traumatic bilateral amputations secondary to a motor vehicle accident and is being discharged home to live with their spouse and 3-year-old child. Which **priority** psychosocial intervention should the rehabilitation nurse discuss with the client?
    1. Ask the client whether they have any sexual concerns that need to be discussed.
    2. Determine whether their home is safe for ambulating with prosthetic devices.
    3. Discuss the procedure for obtaining a specially equipped car.
    4. Explain the importance of getting psychological counseling.

39. The RN primary nurse overhears the UAP telling a family member of a client, "One of the clients will be going to prison because that person was charged with vehicular manslaughter. Two people in the motor vehicle accident died." Which action should the primary nurse implement **first**?
    1. Apologize to the family member for the UAP's comments.
    2. Tell the UAP that the comment is a violation of HIPAA.
    3. Allow the UAP to complete the conversation and then discuss the situation.
    4. Interrupt the conversation and tell the UAP to go to the nurse's station.

40. The clinical nurse manager verbally warned a staff nurse about being late to work on two occasions. The nurse was 35 minutes late for today's shift. Which action should the charge nurse take?
    1. Ask the staff nurse why they were late again today.
    2. Notify the human resources department in writing.
    3. Initiate the hospital policy for unacceptable behavior.
    4. Do not allow the staff nurse to work on the unit today.

41. The RN charge nurse on the rehabilitation unit is making assignments for the day shift. Which assignment would be **most** appropriate for the LPN?
    1. Have the LPN call the HCP to order a diet change.
    2. Instruct the LPN to complete the admission assessment.
    3. Ask the LPN to teach the client about a high-fiber diet.
    4. Request the LPN to obtain the intake and output for the clients.

42. The charge nurse received laboratory data on the following clients. Which client **warrants immediate** intervention by the charge nurse?
    1. The client diagnosed with chronic obstructive pulmonary disease (COPD) and arterial blood gas (ABG) values of pH 7.35; Pao_2 77 mm Hg; $Paco_2$ 57 mm Hg; HCO_3 24 mmol/L.
    2. The client diagnosed with bilateral total knee replacement and a white blood cell (WBC) count of 10,400/microL.
    3. The client receiving antibiotic therapy with a serum potassium level of 3.3 mEq/L.
    4. The client receiving total parenteral nutrition (TPN) with a glucose level of 145 mg/dL.

43. The client tells the primary nurse, "I just finished completing my living will, and I need you to witness my signature." Which action should the nurse implement?
    1. Witness the client's living will using an ink pen.
    2. Explain that the nurse cannot witness this document.
    3. Tell the client the document does not need a witness's signature.
    4. Offer to have the hospital attorney notarize the form.

44. The nurse is preparing to ambulate the client diagnosed with full-thickness burns on the lower extremities down the hall. Which **priority** intervention should the nurse implement?
    1. Place rubber-soled shoes on the client.
    2. Put a gait belt around the client's waist.
    3. Explain the procedure to the client.
    4. Provide a clear path for the client to walk.

45. The client in the rehabilitation unit tells the nurse, "I will not go to physical therapy again because it hurts so much when I do the exercises." Which statement **supports** the nurse's role as a client advocate?
    1. "You do not have to go to physical therapy if it causes pain."
    2. "I will talk to the physical therapist about the exercises that cause you pain."
    3. "Let me check and see if you can receive pain medication before therapy."
    4. "I will discuss your concerns at the next multidisciplinary team meeting."

46. The rehabilitation nurse enters the client's room and the client is talking on the phone. The client asks the nurse to speak with their spouse because they have questions. Which action should the nurse take?
    1. Explain that HIPAA regulations prevent the nurse from talking to the spouse.
    2. Tell the client it would be best for the nurse to talk to the spouse in person.
    3. Request the client's spouse to ask questions at the weekly team meeting.
    4. Honor the client's request and answer the spouse's questions on the phone.

47. The school nurse notes the child has impetigo. Which interventions should the nurse implement? **Select all that apply.**
    1. Administer an antibiotic ointment four times a day.
    2. Instruct the parents to keep the child at home until the lesions crust over.
    3. Tell the parents to use separate towels for their child.
    4. Do not remove the crusts from the skin lesions.
    5. Tell the parents to have the child wear nonlatex sterile gloves over both hands until there is no crusting.

48. Which action by the primary nurse **requires immediate** intervention by the charge nurse?
    1. The nurse is teaching the client how to use a glucometer.
    2. The nurse leaves the computer screen open to the electronic health record at the nurse's station.
    3. The nurse is discussing a client situation on the phone with the HCP.
    4. The nurse contacts the chaplain to come and talk to a client.

49. The nurse is triaging phone calls in a dermatological clinic. Which client **warrants** the nurse making an appointment **immediately?**
    1. The client reports having white spots on both of their hands.
    2. The client reports redness and itching on their hands.
    3. The client reports a cherry angioma on their right lower leg.
    4. The client reports red patches on one side of their body.

50. The client has an area on their skin the dermatologist thinks may be basal cell carcinoma. Which intervention will the nurse implement to confirm the diagnosis?
    1. Refer the client for the magnetic resonance imaging (MRI).
    2. Explain how to obtain a washing of the abnormal skin area.
    3. Prepare the client for a biopsy of the abnormal skin growth.
    4. Tell the client there is no definitive way to confirm the diagnosis.

51. The nurse is assisting the client to use a cane when ambulating. **Rank in order of performance.**
    1. Request the client to move their cane forward.
    2. Move their weaker leg one step forward.
    3. Ensure the client places the cane in their strong hand.
    4. Move their stronger leg one step forward.
    5. Apply a gait belt around the client's waist.

52. Which **priority** intervention should the nurse implement to help prevent pressure injuries in the client on strict bedrest?
    1. Provide adequate skin care for the client.
    2. Turn the client every 2 hours or more often.
    3. Ensure sufficient nutritional intake.
    4. Use pressure-relieving devices such as waterbeds.

53. Which intervention should the nurse implement **first** for the client diagnosed with a fractured femur suspected of having a fat embolism?
    1. Assess the client's bilateral breath sounds.
    2. Encourage the client to cough and deep breathe.
    3. Administer oxygen via a nasal cannula.
    4. Prepare to administer IV heparin therapy.

54. The client diagnosed with an electrical burn is brought to the ED. The entrance wound is on their right hand, and the exit wound is on their left foot. Which intervention should the nurse implement **first?**
    1. Place sterile gauze on the entrance and exit wounds.
    2. Assess the client's vital signs.
    3. Monitor the client's pulse oximetry.
    4. Place the client on cardiac telemetry.

55. The nurse is using an electric client lift to transfer the client from their bed to a stretcher. Which **priority** intervention should the nurse implement?
    1. Have two staff members assist when using the lift.
    2. Ensure the client is correctly placed in the lift before moving.
    3. Lift the client slowly off their bed when turning on the lift.
    4. Ensure the stretcher is in the correct position and locked.

56. The RN staff nurse is assessing the functional ability of a client using the Katz Index of Activities of Daily Living (ADLs). Which assessment score would require the nurse to delegate feeding, bathing, and toileting to the UAP?
    1. Katz Index of ADLs score 6
    2. Katz Index of ADLs score 4
    3. Katz Index of ADLs score 3
    4. Katz Index of ADLs score 0

57. The client has cellulitis on their right lower arm. Which intervention should the nurse implement?
    1. Place the client's right arm in the dependent position.
    2. Apply warm, moist heat to the affected area.
    3. Wash the affected area with anti-staphylococcal soap.
    4. Wrap the right arm with elastic bandages.

58. The UAP is transferring the client from their bed to the wheelchair. Which interventions should the RN primary nurse ensure the UAP implements during this procedure? **Rank in order of priority.**
    1. Assist the client to sit when the client's legs touch the edge of the chair.
    2. Place the wheelchair at an angle on the client's strong side.
    3. Assist the client to stand and put their strong hand on the wheelchair armrest.
    4. Keep the client's weight forward and pivot the client.
    5. Lock the wheelchair brakes and secure the chair position.

59. The RN charge nurse on the rehabilitation unit is assigning and delegating tasks to the UAP and the LPN. Which task is **most** appropriate for the RN to delegate or assign?
    1. Tell the UAP to elevate the client's residual limb above their heart.
    2. Instruct the LPN to give the diabetic clients their HS snacks.
    3. Request the UAP to insert an indwelling urinary catheter.
    4. Ask the LPN to assess the client diagnosed with possible herpes zoster.

60. The RN burn unit nurse is caring for a client diagnosed with a full-thickness burn over their right lower extremity. Which task should the nurse delegate to the UAP?
    1. Instruct the UAP to check the client's right dorsalis pedal pulse.
    2. Ask the UAP to cleanse the client's dentures and place them in their container.
    3. Request the UAP to perform passive range-of-motion (ROM) exercises.
    4. Tell the UAP to keep the client's right leg in the dependent position.

61. The client is admitted to the ED diagnosed with a third-degree burn over the front of both legs. Which **priority** intervention should the nurse implement?
    1. Maintain a sterile environment when caring for the client.
    2. Insert two large-bore IV access routes.
    3. Administer IV antibiotic therapy.
    4. Assess the client's pain level on a 1 to 10 pain scale.

62. The day nurse is preparing to administer medications to the client reporting lightheadedness when getting out of bed.

Client's Name: J.S.	Account Number: 1032456	Height: 72 in (182.9 cm)
Weight: 75 kg (165.3 lb)	Date: Today	

Medication	0701–1900	1901–0700
Atenolol 50 mg PO daily	0900	
Ceftriaxone 150 mg IVBP every 12 hours	0900	
Bisacodyl 2 PO PRN constipation		
Hydrocodone 5 mg/500 mg PO every 4–6 hours PRN for pain		
Signature/Initials	Day Nurse RN/DN	Night Nurse RN/DN

    Which medication should the day nurse **question** administering?
    1. Atenolol 50 mg PO
    2. Ceftriaxone 150 mg IV piggyback (IVPB)
    3. Bisacodyl 2 PO
    4. Administer all medications as ordered.

63. The nurse is discussing complementary and alternative medicine (CAM) with a client in the rehabilitation unit. Which therapies should the nurse discuss with the client? **Select all that apply.**
    1. Acupuncture
    2. Guided imagery
    3. Compression sequential devices
    4. Music therapy
    5. Muscle-strengthening exercises

64. The nurse tells the client, "I am referring you to the vocational counselor." The client asks the nurse, "Why are you making this referral?" Which statement is the nurse's **best** response?
    1. "The counselor will assist you with job placement, training, or further education."
    2. "The counselor specializes in rehabilitative medicine and will help you get better."
    3. "The counselor will help develop your fine motor skills to help perform ADLs."
    4. "The counselor will help you continue or develop hobbies or interests."

65. The nurse is assessing the client's daily schedule and habits. Which question is **most** appropriate for the nurse to ask the client?
    1. "Do you have a family member able to assist you when you go home?"
    2. "What time do you prefer bathing, and do you take a tub bath or a shower?"
    3. "Do you have insurance to help with the cost of rehabilitation?"
    4. "Are you concerned about the care you are receiving here?"

66. The nurse is administering medication to the client diagnosed with a third-degree burn on their chest area.

Client Name: A.M.	Account Number: 1432223	Allergies: NKDA
Height: 68 in (172.7 cm)	Weight in lb: 140	Weight in kg: 63.63
Date of Birth: 65 years	Date: Today	

Medication	1901–0700	0701–1900
Vancomycin IVPB 500 mg daily		
Pantoprazole 40 mg IVPB daily		
Silver sulfadiazine topical ointment to burn TID three times a day		
Morphine 2 to 5 mg IVP PRN pain		
Signature/Initials	Night Nurse RN/NN	Day Nurse RN/DN

    Which medication requires a laboratory test?
    1. Vancomycin
    2. Pantoprazole
    3. Silver sulfadiazine topical ointment
    4. Morphine

67. The home health nurse is arranging for the spouse of an elderly client diagnosed with heart failure to administer furosemide. The medication is to be administered 20 mg on Monday/Wednesday/Friday and 40 mg on Sunday/Tuesday/Thursday/Saturday. The prescription is for 40 mg scored tablets. How many tablets should the nurse teach the spouse to administer on Sundays? _____

68. The RN home health nurse has arranged for a home health aide to assist a 79-year-old client diagnosed with Alzheimer's disease. Which interventions should the nurse delegate to the home health aide? **Select all that apply.**
    1. Weigh the client once a week and document the weight on the client record.
    2. Stay with the client twice a week while the spouse goes out to run errands.
    3. Take and record the client's vital signs.
    4. Take the client to the bank and store for personal business.
    5. Listen to the client's heart sounds and notify the HCP if abnormal sounds are heard.

69. The nurse is at the local mall when a young person begins having shortness of breath, has hives on their face and arms, and is reporting itching. Which intervention should the nurse implement **first**?
    1. Tell a bystander to call 911 immediately.
    2. Ask the person if they have an epinephrine autoinjector.
    3. Check the client for a medical alert bracelet.
    4. Place a soft cushion under the client's head.

70. The home health nurse is planning to make rounds for the day and is deciding in which order to see their assigned clients. **Rank in order of priority.**
    1. The 29-year-old client diagnosed with spinal cord injury (SCI) after a MVA needing a dressing changed on a stage IV pressure area
    2. The 56-year-old client diagnosed with breast cancer needing an injection of filgrastim subcutaneously
    3. The 67-year-old client diagnosed with emphysema calling to report their sputum is a rusty color this morning
    4. The 80-year-old client diagnosed with Alzheimer's disease wandering around their house in confusion
    5. The 72-year-old client diagnosed with atrial fibrillation needing a prothrombin time performed and called to the HCP

71. The client is admitted to the burn unit after a boiling pot of hot water accidentally spilled on their lower legs. The assessment reveals blistered, mottled red skin, and both feet are edematous. Which depth of burn should the nurse document?
    1. Superficial partial thickness
    2. Deep partial thickness
    3. Full thickness
    4. First degree

72. The nurse is caring for a client diagnosed with a full-thickness burn to 65% of their body 12 hours ago. After establishing a patent airway, which nursing intervention is the **priority** for the client?
    1. Replace the client's fluids and electrolytes.
    2. Prevent the client from developing Curling's ulcers.
    3. Implement interventions to prevent infection.
    4. Prepare to assist with an escharotomy.

73. Which nursing interventions should be included for the client diagnosed with full-thickness and deep partial-thickness burns to 50% of their body? **Select all that apply.**
    1. Perform meticulous hand hygiene.
    2. Screen visitors for infections.
    3. Provide a low-cholesterol, low-protein diet.
    4. Change invasive lines once a week.
    5. Administer prophylactic antibiotics as prescribed.

74. Which nursing task should the RN delegate to a UAP for the client diagnosed with **full-thickness burns over their right leg?**
    1. Instruct the UAP to take the client's pulse oximeter reading.
    2. Tell the UAP to change the dressing on the right leg.
    3. Ask the UAP to apply mafenide acetate to the right leg.
    4. Request the UAP to complete the admission assessment.

75. The nurse is caring for a client diagnosed with deep partial-thickness and full-thickness burns to their chest area. Which assessment data **warrant** notifying the HCP?
    1. The client is reporting pain rated 9 on a 1 to 10 pain scale.
    2. The client's pulse oximeter reading is 90%.
    3. The client's vital signs are T 100.4°F (38°C), P 100 bpm, R 24 breaths/min, and BP 102/60 mm Hg.
    4. The client's urinary output is 150 mL (5.1 oz) in 4 hours.

76. The charge nurse is teaching community members about fire safety. A participant asks, "What should I do if I get hot grease burns on my hand?" Which statement is the nurse's **best** response?
    1. "Apply an ice pack directly to the hand."
    2. "Place the hand under cool tap water."
    3. "Put burn ointment on the hand."
    4. "Go immediately to the doctor's office."

77. The RN charge nurse is teaching a group of new UAPs about burn care. Which information regarding skin care should be emphasized?
   1. Keep the skin moist by leaving the client's skin damp after the bath.
   2. Ensure the client is premedicated before the whirlpool.
   3. Tell the UAPs to turn the client from side to side at least every 2 hours.
   4. Instruct the UAPs not to implement any interventions regarding skin care.

78. Which action by the UAP **warrants** intervention by the RN charge nurse?
   1. The UAP decreases the IV rate of the client when their total parenteral nutrition bag is almost empty.
   2. The UAP elevates the head of the bed for a client receiving continuous tube feeding.
   3. The UAP assists the client diagnosed with full-thickness burns on their upper extremities in eating a high-protein meal.
   4. The UAP mixes a thickener into a glass of water for a client having difficulty swallowing.

79. The charge nurse is caring for clients on the burn unit. After the shift report, which client should the charge nurse assess **first**?
   1. The client diagnosed with full-thickness and deep partial-thickness burns having pain rated 8 on a 1 to 10 pain scale
   2. The client diagnosed with full-thickness burns and a urinary output of 120 mL (4.1 oz) in the past 8 hours
   3. The client diagnosed with full-thickness burns on their chest having difficulty breathing
   4. The client diagnosed with full-thickness burns on their right leg with no palpable pedal pulse

INTEGUMENTARY CASE STUDY

(0515) The triage nurse in the ED receives a call from the Emergency Medical Services (EMS) with report on a client being brought in via ambulance. The paramedic states that the client is a 46-year-old male who re-entered his burning house to rescue his three children, ages 4, 5, and 7. Two children are being transferred to the local children's hospital for evaluation and treatment; the client was able to get the 4- and 5-year-old out of the house before collapsing; the 7-year-old was rescued by EMS but pronounced dead at the scene. According to the neighbor, the client's spouse is a night shift nurse at "your hospital." The client is currently unresponsive and has severe burns over much of his body. Two IV lines, 18-gauge, in the left antecubital and hand, have been started and are running 0.9% NaCl at 150 mL/hr.

Vital Signs	Client Values
Blood pressure	84/52 mm Hg
Heart rate	114 bpm
Respirations	16 breaths/min
Temperature	101.5°F (38.6°C)
SpO₂	89% on room air
Pain	Unresponsive

The nurse announces a "Trauma Alert" via the overhead paging system, and places a call to the hospital's burn unit per hospital protocol.

(0540) Client arrives via cart and is unresponsive to name called. No sternal rub was performed due to the extent of burns on the chest. Color is pale with black soot around mouth and nose. Initial assessment reveals third-degree burns anteriorly over the face, chest, right arm and hand, and bilateral thighs; posteriorly over the neck and back. ED bed weight: 192 pounds (87.3 kg). There is minimal facial edema. The nurse quickly uses the *Rule of Nines* to calculate the total body surface area (TBSA) of the burns to be 63%.

Vital Signs	Client Values
Blood pressure	82/50 mm Hg
Heart rate	120 bpm
Respirations	32 breaths/min
Temperature	101.5°F (38.6°C)
SpO_2	84% on room air
Pain	Unresponsive

1. **Recognize cues. What matters most?** Select the **priority** client data that should be reported to the HCP.
    1. Hypotension
    2. Tachycardia
    3. Tachypnea
    4. Temperature
    5. Pulse oximetry
    6. Level of consciousness
    7. Death of 7-year-old child
    8. Transfer of 4- and 5-year-old children to children's hospital
    9. Next of kin situation
    10. TBSA

(0555) The nurse asks the ancillary staff to page the nursing supervisor to follow up on finding the client's spouse. The physician writes orders.

PROVIDER ORDERS:

CBC, BMP, serum carbon monoxide (CO), and ABGs STAT
PICC to be placed STAT
IV lines: (1) D_5NS at 150 mL/hr, and (2) lactated Ringer's solution at 150 mL/hr
Respiratory therapist (RT) to intubate and manage mechanical ventilation to ensure $PaO_2 \geq 90\%$
At time of intubation, administer: etomidate 0.3 mg/kg IV, fentanyl 5 mg/kg IV, and succinylcholine 1.5 mg/kg IV; maintain sedation per ICU protocol upon transfer
Continuous telemetry with vital signs every 15 minutes
Contact next of kin

(0615) Complete blood count (CBC), basal metabolic panel (BMP), carbon monoxide (CO), and ABGs obtained. Peripherally inserted central venous catheter (PICC) was placed in left upper arm and portable chest x-ray confirmed placement. Respiratory therapist (RT) intubated the client, established baseline ventilator settings, and will remain in ED.

Vital Signs	Client Values
Blood pressure	81/50 mm Hg
Heart rate	104 bpm
Respirations	22 breaths/min on the ventilator
Temperature	101.5°F (38.6°C)
SpO_2	85% on 100% oxygen via ventilator
Pain	Unresponsive

(0630) Current vital signs are taken.

Vital Signs	Client Values
Blood pressure	83/51 mm Hg
Heart rate	105 bpm
Respirations	22 breaths/min on the ventilator
Temperature	100°F (37.8°C)
SpO_2	86% on 100% oxygen via ventilator
Pain	Unresponsive

(0640) Diagnostic and laboratory results are posted.

Laboratory Test	Client Values	Reference Values
Hemoglobin (Hgb)	18 g/dL	Male: 14–17.3 g/dL Female: 11.7–15.5 g/dL
Hematocrit (Hct)	57%	Male: 42%–52% Female: 36%–48%
White blood cell (WBC) count	13.8	4.5 to 11.1×10^3/microL
Platelets	410	140 to 400×10^3/microL
Creatinine	0.9 mg/dL	Male: 0.61 to 1.21 mg/dL Female: 0.51 to 1.11 mg/dL
Glucose	182 mg/dL	Fasting: Less than 100 mg/dL Random: Less than 200 mg/dL
Potassium	5.3 mEq/L	3.5 to 5 mEq/L or mmol/L
Sodium	150 mEq/L	135 to 145 mEq/L or mmol/L
Blood urea nitrogen (BUN)	25 mg/dL	8 to 21 mg/dL Adult over 90 years: 10 to 31 mg/dL
Carbon monoxide	160 ppm	0 ppm

Laboratory Tests: ABGs	Client Values	Reference Values
pH	7.29	7.35–7.45
Pao$_2$	68 mm Hg	80–100 mm Hg
Paco$_2$	51 mm Hg	35–45 mm Hg
HCO$_3$	17 mEq/L	21–28 mEq/L

(0645) Chest x-ray: Evidence of distal tip of left upper arm PICC line resting in superior vena cava. Current vital signs:

Vital Signs	Client Values
Blood pressure	81/50 mm Hg
Heart rate	100 bpm
Respirations	22 breaths/min on the ventilator
Temperature	101.5°F (38.6°C)
Spo$_2$	88% on 100% oxygen via ventilator
Pain	Unresponsive

2. **Analyze cues. What could it mean?** For each client finding, indicate whether it is consistent with the listed disease process(es). Each finding may support more than one condition.

Finding	Interstitial Fluid Shift	Respiratory Compromise
Hemoglobin and hematocrit		
Tachypnea		
Serum pH		
Hyperkalemia		
BUN level		
Paco$_2$		
Pao$_2$		
Carbon monoxide		

3. **Prioritize hypotheses. Where do I start?** What are the top priorities for the care of the client at this time? **Select two answers.**
   1. Cardiopulmonary monitoring
   2. Emotional distress
   3. Grief and loss
   4. Hemodynamic instability
   5. Intake and output monitoring
   6. Wound care to burn sites

(0700) The nursing supervisor and the client's spouse arrive in the ED.

4. **Generate solutions. What can I do?** For each intervention, specify whether the intervention is **indicated** or **not indicated** for the client's care.

Potential Nursing Intervention	Indicated	Not Indicated
Prepare intubation medications		
Apply sterile dressings loosely over burns		
Monitor sedation level		
Provide emotional support to client's spouse		
Ask the spouse if they had working fire alarms in the home		
Monitor telemetry		
Request an order for an indwelling urinary catheter		
Suggest the spouse go to the local children's hospital		
Obtain client's health history from spouse		
At the bedside, inform the spouse of death of 7-year-old		

The physician discussed the plan with the spouse and has ordered the client to be transferred from the ED to the hospital's Burn Center intensive care unit (ICU). The nurse obtains a bed assignment from the admissions office.

5. **Take action. What will I do?** Which actions are appropriate for the nurse to take? **Highlight one answer choice from each column.**

A	B
1. Decrease the client's sedation	1. Accompany RT to transfer the client to the Burn Center ICU
2. Call the children's hospital for an update	2. Assign a student nurse to accompany RT to transfer the client to the Burn Center ICU
3. Call report to the Burn Center ICU	3. Increase the client's sedation

(1800) The off-going Burn Center ICU nurse prepares a report for the next shift and conducts a reassessment of the client.

6. **Evaluate outcomes. Did it help?** For each assessment finding, indicate whether the client's condition has improved, declined, or no change.

Reassessment Findings	Improved	Declined	No Change
Blood pressure: 94/58 mm Hg			
Heart rate: 100 bpm			
Moaning when repositioned			
Potassium: 5.0 mEq/L			
Carbon monoxide: 160 ppm			
Facial edema: +3			

ANSWERS AND RATIONALES

The correct answer number and rationale are in **boldface purple type.** Rationales for why other answer options are incorrect are also given.

1. 1. If the client's INR is elevated, the antidote for the oral anticoagulant warfarin (Coumadin) is vitamin K (AquaMephyton), but this is not the nurse's first intervention.
   2. The client should use a soft-bristle toothbrush, but this is not the nurse's first intervention.
   3. The nurse can always check the client's vital signs, but it is not the first intervention when addressing the client's report of gums bleeding.
   4. **The nurse should first check the client's INR to determine whether the bleeding is secondary to an elevated INR level. An INR level above 3 or 3.5, in the case of a mechanical valve, can cause bleeding.**

CLINICAL JUDGMENT GUIDE: This is an alternate type of question included in the NCLEX-RN® test plan. The test taker must be able to read an MAR, be knowledgeable of medications, and decide on the nurse's most appropriate intervention.

2. 1. This client needs assistance being removed from the CPM machine, but it is not a priority over a client needing pain medication before a very painful procedure. Equipment is not a priority over the client's body.
   2. This is a psychosocial need and should be addressed, but it is not a priority over a physiological need.
   3. This temperature is elevated and the client should be seen, but the nurse should medicate the client going to the whirlpool first, then assess this client. Pain is a priority over an elevated temperature.
   4. **The client must be medicated with a narcotic medication before being taken to the whirlpool, which is a physiological need; therefore, the nurse should see this client first.**

CLINICAL JUDGMENT GUIDE: When deciding which client to assess first, the nurse should utilize Maslow's Hierarchy of Needs, in which physiological needs are the priority over psychosocial needs. The alleviation of pain, actual or potential, is a priority need.

3. 1. The client having pain when ambulating after an ORIF of the hip is expected; this client would not need to be assessed first.
   2. The client should be ambulating and moving the left leg while in bed and would not need to be in the CPM machine 10 days postoperatively.
   3. **Numbness and tingling of the legs are findings of possible neurovascular compromise. This client should be assessed first.**
   4. The client being transferred should be assessed but would be considered stable; therefore, this client would not be assessed before a client experiencing possible neurovascular compromise.

CLINICAL JUDGMENT GUIDE: The nurse must determine which clinical manifestation is unexpected for the disease process or surgical procedure. The nurse should assess the client first if the clinical manifestation is not expected. This question determines whether the nurse is knowledgeable of the clinical manifestations of various disease processes.

4. 1. **An absent pulse is not uncommon in a client diagnosed with arterial occlusive disease. No further action should be taken if the client can move the toes and denies tingling or numbness.**
   2. To identify the location of the pulse, the nurse should use a Doppler device to amplify the sound, but this is not the first intervention if the client can move the toes and denies numbness and tingling.
   3. Placing the client's leg in a dependent position will increase blood flow and may help the nurse palpate the pulse, but it is not the nurse's first intervention.
   4. Warming will dilate the arteries and may help the nurse to find the pedal pulse, but this is not the first intervention. (Cooling, in contrast, causes vasoconstriction and decreases the ability to palpate the pulse.)

CLINICAL JUDGMENT GUIDE: When the question asks which intervention should be implemented first, it means all the options are something a nurse could implement, but only one should be implemented first. The nurse should use the nursing process to determine the appropriate intervention: If the client is in distress, do not assess; if the client is not in distress, then the nurse should assess.

5. 1. The NSAID is routine and is not a priority medication.
   2. The client needs to receive the IV antibiotic, but this is not a priority over the client reporting an acute problem of itching and hives.
   3. The client should receive the antiviral agent, but not before a client exhibiting hives and itching, which is an acute problem.
   4. **The client diagnosed with urticaria (hives) and pruritus (itching) is having an allergic reaction and should receive the antihistamine first.**

   CLINICAL JUDGMENT GUIDE: The client exhibiting an acute reaction or problem should receive medical treatment first. Routine scheduled medications are not a priority over medications addressing acute client needs.

6. 1. Corticosteroid cream will not treat potential melanoma, which is what the client is explaining to the nurse.
   2. SPF 15 is recommended to help prevent skin cancer, but it will not help treat a melanoma.
   3. **The client should consult their HCP immediately if a mole or lesion shows any findings of melanoma—asymmetry, border irregularity, color change or variation, and diameter of 6 mm or more (ABCD).**
   4. Dark, woven clothing helps prevent skin cancer but it will not do anything for a mole change.

   CLINICAL JUDGMENT GUIDE: The test taker must read all the options carefully before choosing the option that says, "Notify the HCP." If any of the options will provide information the HCP needs to know to make a decision, the test taker should choose that option. If the HCP does not require any additional information to make a decision and the nurse suspects the condition is serious or life-threatening, the priority intervention is to notify the HCP.

7. 1. **The nurse should implement the first intervention, ensuring the client does not move the leg because doing so may cause further injury. The client should not attempt to move or stand on the injured extremity.**
   2. The client should elevate the leg to decrease edema, but this is not the first intervention. Remember to do no harm.
   3. The application of ice will help decrease edema and pain, but the first intervention is to do no harm.
   4. Assessment is usually the first intervention, but when at the scene of an accident, the nurse should ensure the accident victim does not cause further injury before assessing.

   CLINICAL JUDGMENT GUIDE: The nurse should use the nursing process when answering questions that ask which intervention to implement first. Assessment is the first step in the nursing process, but in an emergency, remember the nurse should ensure the client does not further injure themself.

8. 1. The nurse should obtain the needed equipment, but that is not the first intervention.
   2. The nurse should remove the old dressing with nonsterile gloves, but not before determining whether the client has been premedicated.
   3. The nurse should explain the procedure before performing the dressing change, but that is not the first intervention.
   4. **Dressing changes for a stage III pressure injury will be painful for the client. The nurse should ensure the client receives pain medication at least 30 minutes before the procedure. This shows client advocacy.**

   CLINICAL JUDGMENT GUIDE: There will be management questions on the NCLEX-RN® addressing client advocacy. A client advocate acts as a liaison between clients and HCPs to help improve or maintain a high quality of healthcare.

9. 1. **The Hgb and Hct are low, which requires the nurse to assess this client first. The nurse must take the client's vital signs, check the surgical dressing, and determine whether the client is symptomatic for hypovolemia.**
   2. The client diagnosed with rheumatoid arthritis should have a positive rheumatoid factor (RF). The positive RF factor confirms the diagnosis of this disease process.
   3. A client diagnosed with a stage IV pressure injury would frequently have an infection; therefore, the nurse would expect an elevated WBC count.
   4. Corticosteroids elevate the client's glucose level; therefore, the nurse would not assess this client first.

   CLINICAL JUDGMENT GUIDE: The nurse must know normal laboratory values and be able to determine whether the laboratory value is normal for the client's disease process or the medications the client is taking.

10. 1. The nurse should complete a report documenting the client's fall, but this is not the first intervention.
    2. The nurse should notify the clinical manager, but this is not the nurse's first intervention.
    3. **The nurse must determine whether the client has injuries before taking any other action. This is the first intervention the nurse must implement before moving the client.**
    4. The nurse should determine why the client was ambulating alone, but it is not the priority nursing intervention. Determining whether the client has any injuries is the most critical intervention.

CLINICAL JUDGMENT GUIDE: Assessment is the first step of the nursing process, and the test taker should use the nursing process or some other systematic process to assist in determining priorities.

11. 1. The triple-lumen lines should be flushed with heparin solution, and this task cannot be delegated to a UAP.
    2. This is teaching, and the nurse should not delegate teaching of the client.
    3. **The UAP can assist the client to the bathroom as part of the bowel training; the RN is responsible for the training, but the nurse can delegate this task.**
    4. Corticosteroid cream is a medication, and the RN cannot delegate medication to a UAP.

CLINICAL JUDGMENT GUIDE: The RN cannot delegate assessment, evaluation, teaching, administering medications, or an unstable client to a UAP.

12. 1. Because the UAP is informing the RN of pertinent information, the nurse should assess the client to determine which action to take.
    2. The client may be hemorrhaging; therefore, the nurse cannot delegate assessing the vital signs of an unstable client.
    3. The nurse should not remove the dressing. The nurse should reinforce the dressing and notify the HCP if the bleeding does not stop or if the client is showing signs of hypovolemia. Reinforcing the dressing would help decrease bleeding, but the nurse must assess first.
    4. **The client is potentially unstable; therefore, the RN should not delegate care to the UAP.**

CLINICAL JUDGMENT GUIDE: Any time the nurse receives information from another staff member about a client experiencing a possible complication, the nurse must assess the client. The nurse should not make decisions about a client's needs based on another staff member's information.

13. 1. **Tying a client to a chair is a form of restraint, and the client cannot be restrained without an HCP order; therefore, the nurse should immediately free the client. This is a legal issue.**
    2. The UAP is not hired to smoke with the client, and the RN should talk to the UAP, but this does not warrant an immediate response. The client being illegally restrained warrants immediate intervention.
    3. Bringing a beverage to the client would not warrant immediate intervention.
    4. The UAP can assist the client in ambulating.

CLINICAL JUDGMENT GUIDE: Delegation means the RN is responsible for the UAP's actions and performance. The nurse must correct the UAP's performance to ensure the client is cared for safely and legally in the hospital or the home.

14. 1. Tinea corporis is commonly known as ringworm and should have cool compresses applied, not warm compresses.
    2. **The LPN can apply medication to the client's athlete's foot; therefore, this is an appropriate assignment for the LPN.**
    3. Onychomycosis is a fungal infection of the toenails (crumbly, discolored, and thickened nails); the HCP, not the UAP, should remove the toenail.
    4. Isotretinoin (Accutane), used to treat acne, is contraindicated in pregnant women or women intending to become pregnant while on the drug.

CLINICAL JUDGMENT GUIDE: When the test taker is deciding which option is the most appropriate task to delegate or assign, the test taker should choose the task that allows each staff member to function within their full scope of practice. Do not assign a task to a staff member that requires a higher level of expertise than the staff member has.

15. 1. The UAP can assist a client in eating a regular meal; this would not warrant immediate action.
    2. The UAP's request for assistance is appropriate because it ensures client safety. This action would not warrant immediate intervention.
    3. The UAP is attempting to move a client weighing 400 lb (181.4 kg) to the bedside commode. The UAP should request assistance to ensure client safety and protect

the UAP's back. This situation is dangerous and requires intervention by the RN.
4. This action ensures client safety and does not require immediate intervention by the nurse.

CLINICAL JUDGMENT GUIDE: Delegation means the RN is responsible for the UAP's actions and performance. The nurse must correct the UAP's performance to ensure the client is cared for safely and legally in the hospital or the home.

16. 1. The client with a lower extremity amputation should be placed prone to prevent contractures.
    2. **The RN should praise the UAP for taking the initiative and placing the client in the prone position. The prone position will help prevent residual limb contractures, making it easier to apply a prosthetic device.**
    3. This action is appropriate and should not be reported to the charge nurse. The RN should first praise the UAP and then report this behavior to the charge nurse to reward the UAP for appropriate behavior.
    4. The client with a lower extremity amputation presents one of the few times a client should be placed on the stomach, the prone position.

CLINICAL JUDGMENT GUIDE: Delegation means the RN is responsible for the UAP's actions and performance. The nurse should praise the UAP's action when warranted or must correct the UAP's performance to ensure the client is cared for safely and legally in the hospital or the home.

17. 1. Stockings should be applied after the legs have been elevated for a period of time when the amount of blood in the leg vein is at its lowest. Applying the stockings when the client sits in a chair indicates that the UAP does not understand the correct procedure for applying the elastic compression stockings.
    2. The top of the stocking should not be too tight. The UAP should be able to insert two to three fingers under the proximal end of the stocking. Not allowing this much space indicates the UAP does not understand the correct procedure for applying compression stockings.
    3. **Stockings should be applied after the legs have been elevated for a period of time when the amount of blood in the leg vein is at its lowest. Having the client elevate the legs before placing the stockings on the legs indicates that the UAP** understands the procedure for applying the elastic compression stockings.
    4. The toe opening should be positioned on the bottom of the foot; therefore, this indicates the UAP does not understand the correct procedure for applying the elastic compression stockings.

CLINICAL JUDGMENT GUIDE: Delegation means the RN is responsible for evaluating the UAP's actions and performance. The nurse should praise the UAP's action when warranted or must correct the UAP's performance to ensure the client is cared for safely and legally in the hospital or the home.

18. 1. The client needs to be told the importance of therapy, but this is not the most critical client; therefore, this client does not need to be assigned to the most experienced nurse.
    2. Bone pain and fever are expected clinical manifestations of the client diagnosed with osteomyelitis, so this client is stable and does not need to be assigned to the most experienced nurse.
    3. **Deep, unrelenting pain is a sign of compartment syndrome, an acute, potentially life-threatening complication, in a client diagnosed with a fracture; therefore, this client should be assigned to the most experienced nurse.**
    4. The client diagnosed with low back pain and radiating pain should be assessed, but this is not a sign of an acute complication; therefore, this client does not need to be assigned to the most experienced nurse.

CLINICAL JUDGMENT GUIDE: The test taker must determine which client is the most unstable and would require the most experienced nurse, thus making this type of question an "except" question. Three clients are either stable or have non–life-threatening conditions.

19. 1. The LPN should not be sent to the ED because the LPN's expertise is needed to care for the clients in the busy rehabilitation unit.
    2. The RN has 8 years of experience in the rehabilitation unit, and the charge nurse does not want to send a nurse vital to the rehabilitation team.
    3. The UAP completing orientation should stay on the unit, and a UAP cannot do as much in the ED as a licensed nurse.
    4. **The RN with medical unit experience would be the most appropriate nurse to send to the ED because this nurse has experience that would be helpful in the**

ED. The nurse is also an RN and would be more useful in the ED than a UAP or an LPN.

CLINICAL JUDGMENT GUIDE: The charge nurse must be able to determine which staff member is most appropriate to float to another unit. The charge nurse does not want to leave their unit unsafe by sending the most experienced nurse, but wants to send the most helpful staff member for the other unit.

20. 1. The UAP cannot teach the client; therefore, this task cannot be delegated.
    2. The client is confused and should be assessed before being placed in an inclusion bed, used when a client wanders. The client should be assessed, and assessment cannot be delegated.
    3. The UAP cannot administer medications; therefore, this task cannot be delegated.
    4. **The UAP is a vital part of the healthcare team and should be encouraged to attend the multidisciplinary team meeting and provide input into the client's care.**

CLINICAL JUDGMENT GUIDE: The test taker must know the roles of all multidisciplinary healthcare team members and HIPAA rules and regulations. These topics will be tested on the NCLEX-RN® examination.

21. 1. The nurse should monitor the PCA pump, but remember that equipment is not a priority over the client's body.
    2. **Logrolling clients when turning is essential and a priority to maintain proper body alignment.**
    3. The client with spinal surgery is on bedrest until the first postoperative day; therefore, this is not a priority intervention.
    4. The nurse can place pillows under the client's thighs, but the priority postoperative intervention is to prevent postoperative complications; this means ensuring the client is logrolled when turning.

CLINICAL JUDGMENT GUIDE: When answering questions about a specific surgery or procedure, the nurse should identify an intervention that is specific to the surgery or procedure.

22. 1. **This client would benefit from a home healthcare nurse's evaluation of the client's home and the spouse's ability to care for the client.**
    2. The nurse should help the spouse care for the client in their home. Placing them in a nursing home may be a possibility if they cannot care for them, but the most appropriate response would be to try to help the spouse care for the client in their home.
    3. The HCP can talk to the spouse but cannot address concerns about taking care of the client when discharged home.
    4. The nurse could allow the spouse to vent feelings, but the first intervention is to address concerns and do something to alleviate those concerns.

CLINICAL JUDGMENT GUIDE: The test taker must know the roles of all multidisciplinary healthcare team members and HIPAA rules and regulations. These topics will be tested on the NCLEX-RN® examination.

23. 1. This is a formal step in filing a grievance, but the nurse's next action should be following the chain of command and making an informal complaint with the clinical manager.
    2. The nurse has already told the offending colleague this makes them uncomfortable; therefore, this action is inappropriate.
    3. If a direct request to the perpetrator does not stop the comments, then an informal complaint may be effective, especially if both parties realize a problem exists. The offended nurse should utilize the chain of command and notify the clinical manager.
    4. **The offended nurse should follow the chain of command and notify the clinical manager as the next action.**

CLINICAL JUDGMENT GUIDE: The nurse is responsible for knowing and complying with local, state, and federal standards of care, especially regarding sexual harassment.

24. 1. Assisting the client to become independent in self-care is the occupational therapist's role.
    2. The client must be in therapy at least 3 hours a day, but the 3-hour period includes all types of therapy, not just physical therapy. This statement is true but does not answer the client's question.
    3. A multidisciplinary team decides which therapy the client should receive, but this does not answer the client's question.
    4. **The physical therapist will assist in improving the circulation, strengthening muscles, and ambulating and transferring the client from a bed to a chair. This is the nurse's best response to explain why the client goes to physical therapy daily.**

CLINICAL JUDGMENT GUIDE: The test taker must know the roles of all multidisciplinary healthcare team members and HIPAA rules and regulations.

These topics will be tested on the NCLEX-RN® examination.

25.
1. The physical therapist addresses crutch walking, using a walker, gait training, or transferring techniques, and is the most appropriate team member to address the problem.
2. The social worker addresses the client's concerns outside the acute care arena, such as financial concerns or referrals.
3. The occupational therapist addresses the upper extremity activities of daily living, not walking difficulties.
4. The HCP can order the physical therapist to see the client to teach the client about crutch walking but would not be the one doing the instruction.

CLINICAL JUDGMENT GUIDE: The test taker must know the roles of all multidisciplinary healthcare team members and HIPAA rules and regulations. These topics will be tested on the NCLEX-RN® examination.

26.
1. The nurse can discuss this situation with the healthcare team, but the most helpful intervention is to explain the rights of people with disabilities according to the ADA.
2. The ADA was passed in 1990 and ensures that a client diagnosed with a disability has a right to be employed. Employers must make "reasonable accommodations," such as equipment or access ramps, to facilitate the employment of a person diagnosed with a disability.
3. The nurse should not interfere and contact the client's employer. The nurse should empower clients to care independently for themselves.
4. This client might be able to do this, but the most helpful intervention is to contact the EEOC. The employer is violating the 1990 Americans with Disabilities Act.

CLINICAL JUDGMENT GUIDE: The nurse is responsible for knowing and complying with local, state, and federal standards of care.

27.
1. The UAP can escort clients to different rehabilitation therapies. This action would not warrant immediate intervention.
2. The family members are an integral part of the healthcare team. This action would not warrant intervention by the charge nurse.
3. The primary nurse cannot ask another nurse to administer medication prepared by the primary nurse. The nurse preparing the injection must administer the medication. This action requires the charge nurse to intervene.
4. Ensuring someone watches the nurse's assigned clients is an appropriate action and would not require intervention by the charge nurse.

CLINICAL JUDGMENT GUIDE: There will be management questions on the NCLEX-RN®. Concepts of Management are included under the category Safe and Effective Care Environment and subcategory Management of Care.

28.
1. This response does not address the client's fears and concerns.
2. This statement will allow the client to vent feelings of helplessness and fear. It is the nurse's best response.
3. The client is not verbalizing that they will kill themself; therefore, this is not the nurse's best response.
4. This negates the client's feelings; therefore, this is not the nurse's best response.

CLINICAL JUDGMENT GUIDE: The NCLEX-RN® test plan includes Therapeutic Communication as a subcategory under Psychosocial Integrity. The nurse should allow clients and families to vent their feelings.

29.
1. Nonmaleficence is the duty to prevent or avoid doing harm. The nurse asking not to be assigned to the NICU because of a lack of experience in caring for critically ill infants is supporting the ethical principle of nonmaleficence.
2. The NICU is a specialized unit requiring the nurse to know about equipment and care for critically ill infants. Accepting the assignment may cause harm to one of the neonates.
3. This is challenging the charge nurse's assignment and does not support the ethical principle of nonmaleficence.
4. This blatantly violates the charge nurse's authority and does not support the ethical principle of nonmaleficence.

CLINICAL JUDGMENT GUIDE: The NCLEX-RN® test plan includes nursing care addressing ethical principles, including autonomy, beneficence, justice, and veracity, to name a few.

30.
1. This therapeutic response encourages the spouse to vent feelings, but the client's spouse needs specific information.

2. According to the National Council of State Boards of Nursing (NCSBN), case management is content included in the management of care. The case manager is responsible for collaborating with and coordinating the services provided by all healthcare team members, including the home healthcare nurse. The home healthcare nurse directs the client's care after discharge from the rehabilitation unit. This is the nurse's best response.
3. This does not address the spouse's concern, and sometimes the client is discharged when the family and client are not ready, in the client's opinion. This is a false reassurance and is not the nurse's best response.
4. In rehabilitation, the HCP is part of the team and is not the only team member to determine the discharge date. This is not the nurse's best response.

CLINICAL JUDGMENT GUIDE: The test taker must know the roles of all multidisciplinary healthcare team members and HIPAA rules and regulations. These topics are tested on the NCLEX-RN® examination.

31. 1. The nurse's comment does not address the client's question and concern. This is not an appropriate response.
    2. **The rehabilitation commission of each state will help evaluate and determine whether the client can receive training or education for another occupation after injury.**
    3. This client is not asking about disability. The client is concerned about employment. The nurse needs to refer the client to the appropriate agency.
    4. This does not address the client's concern about gainful employment. This therapeutic response will allow the client to vent feelings, but the client is asking for information.

CLINICAL JUDGMENT GUIDE: There will be management questions on the NCLEX-RN®. In many instances, there is no test-taking strategy. The nurse must know management issues and comply with local, state, and federal requirements.

32. 1. The client is confiding in the nurse about a doctor, and the nurse should address the client's concern, not tell the client to talk to the doctor. Many clients do not feel comfortable talking to a doctor.
    2. **The nurse should determine what is concerning the client. It could be a** misunderstanding or an actual situation in which the client's care is unsafe or inadequate.
    3. After the nurse determines whether the client's concern warrants a new doctor, the nurse should talk to the nursing supervisor and help the client get a second opinion. The nurse is the client's advocate.
    4. The choice of doctor is ultimately the client's, and the client has a right to another doctor.

CLINICAL JUDGMENT GUIDE: The nurse should always try to support the client's or the family's request if it does not violate any local, state, or federal rules and regulations. The client has a right to request a second opinion if the client does not like the HCP's care.

33. 1. An abductor pillow is used for a client with a total hip replacement to help prevent hip dislocation; the UAP can place the pillow between the client's legs. This task is appropriate to delegate.
    2. The client should be out of bed and ambulating by the third postoperative day to help prevent complications secondary to immobility, such as deep vein thrombosis (DVT) or pneumonia.
    3. Just because the client is elderly does not mean the client must be fed. Nothing in the stem of the question would indicate the client could not feed themselves. The RN should encourage independence as much as possible and delegate feeding the client to a UAP only when necessary.
    4. The RN cannot delegate assessment to the UAP; therefore, checking the surgical dressing is not appropriate delegation.

CLINICAL JUDGMENT GUIDE: An RN cannot delegate assessment, teaching, evaluation, medications, or an unstable client to a UAP. Tasks that cannot be delegated are nursing interventions requiring nursing judgment.

34. 1. Closing the door and cubicle curtain protects the client's privacy and would not warrant immediate intervention from the nurse.
    2. **The client with spinal surgery should be logrolled with at least two, if not three, staff members assisting with the turning from side to side. Logrolling the client ensures proper body alignment. Asking the client to turn would warrant intervention by the nurse.**
    3. Checking the temperature of the bath water prevents scalding the client with water that is

too hot or making the client uncomfortable with water that is too cold. This action would not warrant immediate intervention.
4. The UAP must perform the skill safely; putting the side rails upright ensures the client will not fall out of the bed.

CLINICAL JUDGMENT GUIDE: The RN must ensure the UAP can perform any delegated tasks. It is the nurse's responsibility to demonstrate or teach the UAP how to perform the task and then evaluate the task performed.

35. Correct answers are 3, 4, and 5.
    1. The right leg should not be elevated in the rehabilitation unit because it can cause contracture of the right leg, leading to the prosthetic leg not fitting properly. The leg should be elevated for the first 48 hours to decrease edema and then kept straight.
    2. The occupational therapist addresses the client's activities of daily living and upper extremity problems, not lower extremity problems.
    3. Pushing the residual limb against a pillow will help toughen the end of the limb, which is needed when wearing a prosthetic limb.
    4. The expected treatment for a client diagnosed with impetigo is warm saline followed by soap and water to remove crusts, followed by topical antibiotic cream.
    5. Impetigo is very contagious, so wearing gloves and practicing meticulous hygiene are essential when caring for this client.

CLINICAL JUDGMENT GUIDE: This is an alternate type of question included in the NCLEX-RN®. The nurse must be able to select all the options that answer the question correctly.

36. 1. The procedure for tornadoes is to have all clients, staff, and visitors stay in the hallway and close the doors to all the rooms to help prevent flying debris or glass from hurting anyone.
    2. This may be recommended for individuals in the home, but it is not the hospital protocol for tornadoes.
    3. The procedure for tornadoes is to have all clients, staff, and visitors stay in the hallway and close the doors to all the rooms to prevent flying debris or glass from hurting anyone.
    4. The client and visitors should be in the client's room with the door closed for a fire, but this is not the correct procedure for a tornado.

CLINICAL JUDGMENT GUIDE: The nurse must be knowledgeable of emergency preparedness. Employees receive this information during orientation and are responsible for correctly implementing procedures. The NCSBN NCLEX-RN® test plan includes questions on a Safe and Effective Care Environment.

37. 1. The finance office is responsible for discussing the cost and insurance issues with the client.
    2. The physiatrist is a medical HCP caring for clients in the rehabilitation area.
    3. The vocational counselor would assist the client with employment training if needed.
    4. The case manager is responsible for coordinating the total rehabilitative plan and collaborating with and coordinating the services provided by all healthcare team members, including the home healthcare nurse responsible for directing the client's care after discharge from the rehabilitation unit.

CLINICAL JUDGMENT GUIDE: The test taker must know the roles of all the multidisciplinary healthcare team members and HIPAA rules and regulations. These topics will be tested on the NCLEX-RN® examination.

38. 1. The rehabilitation nurse must recognize and address sexual issues to promote feelings of self-worth that are essential to total rehabilitation. The client's age should not matter, but this client is young; therefore, this is a priority.
    2. This is not a psychosocial intervention; the social worker or occupational therapist usually addresses the home situation.
    3. This is not necessarily a psychosocial intervention but should be addressed so the client can be independent. The social worker usually addresses transportation.
    4. The client may or may not need psychological counseling, but the priority psychosocial intervention of the rehabilitation nurse is to discuss the client's sexual needs.

CLINICAL JUDGMENT GUIDE: The NCLEX-RN® test plan includes Therapeutic Communication as a subcategory of Psychosocial Integrity. The nurse should allow clients and families to vent their feelings and address psychosocial concerns.

39. 1. The RN could apologize for the UAP's comments, but this is not the first intervention.

2. This is a violation of HIPAA, and the RN should tell the UAP about this, but it is not the first intervention.
3. The RN should not allow the conversation to continue. The UAP is violating confidentiality and is gossiping about another client.
4. **The RN should stop the conversation immediately and ask the UAP to go to the nurse's station, not to embarrass the UAP. Gossiping about clients violates their privacy and breaches protected health information under HIPAA.**

CLINICAL JUDGMENT GUIDE: There will be management questions on the NCLEX-RN®. In many instances, there is no test-taking strategy. The nurse must be knowledgeable of management issues. The Health Insurance Portability and Accountability Act (HIPAA) was passed into law in 1996 to standardize the exchange of information between HCPs and to ensure client record confidentiality.

40. 1. After two verbal warnings, the clinical manager should document the behavior and start formal proceedings to correct the staff nurse's behavior.
2. The human resources department would not need to be notified until the clinical manager has decided to terminate the staff nurse's employment.
3. **Every hospital has a procedure for termination if the employee is not performing as expected. After two verbal warnings, the clinical manager should document the employee's actions in writing and implement the hospital policy for possible termination.**
4. The clinical manager cannot allow the nurse to go home because this will affect the care of the clients during the shift and cause hardship for the other staff members.

CLINICAL JUDGMENT GUIDE: There will be management questions on the NCLEX-RN®. In many instances, there is no test-taking strategy. The nurse must be knowledgeable of management issues.

41. 1. The LPN's scope of practice allows the LPN to take telephone orders.
2. The LPN's scope of practice does not include an admission assessment.
3. The registered dietitian would be the most appropriate team member to teach about diets.
4. The UAP could obtain the intake and output; therefore, this is not an appropriate assignment for an LPN.

CLINICAL JUDGMENT GUIDE: The RN cannot assign assessment, teaching, evaluation, or an unstable client to an LPN. The LPN can transcribe HCP orders and call HCPs on the phone to obtain orders for a client.

42. 1. The client diagnosed with COPD would be expected to have low oxygen and high CO_2 levels in the arterial blood; therefore, this laboratory result would not warrant intervention from the charge nurse.
2. This WBC level is within normal limits; therefore, this client does not warrant immediate intervention from the charge nurse.
3. **Antibiotic therapy can result in a superinfection that destroys the normal bacterial flora of the intestines and produces diarrhea. Diarrhea, in turn, causes an increased excretion of potassium, resulting in hypokalemia. This K+ level is below normal, and the charge nurse should notify the HCP.**
4. This glucose level is slightly elevated, and TPN is high in glucose; therefore, this laboratory result does not require immediate intervention.

CLINICAL JUDGMENT GUIDE: The nurse must be knowledgeable of normal laboratory values and be able to determine whether the laboratory value is normal for the client's disease process or the medications the client is taking.

43. 1. The nurse is an employee of the hospital and cannot witness client documents.
2. **This is the correct action to take; the nurse is an employee of the hospital directly involved in providing care and cannot witness client documents.**
3. This is incorrect information; the document should be witnessed by individuals other than family members or employees of the hospital providing direct care.
4. The living will must be witnessed by two individuals when the client is signing it, but it does not have to be notarized.

CLINICAL JUDGMENT GUIDE: The NCLEX-RN® test plan includes nursing care ruled by legal requirements. The nurse must be knowledgeable of these issues.

44. 1. The nurse should ensure the client has appropriate shoes when ambulating, but the priority is the safety of the client, which means using a gait belt.
2. The nurse's priority is to ensure the safety of the client, and placing a safety gait belt

around the client's waist before ambulating the client helps to ensure safety. The gait belt provides a handle to hold onto the client securely during ambulation.
3. The nurse should explain the procedure to the client, but it is not a priority over ensuring safety for the client while walking in the hall.
4. The nurse should ensure a clear path to walk, but the priority intervention is to protect the client if they fall, which can be prevented by placing a gait belt around the client's waist.

CLINICAL JUDGMENT GUIDE: The NCLEX-RN® test plan includes adhering to safety standards when caring for clients.

45.
1. Being a client advocate means the nurse will support the client's wishes, but in some situations the nurse must adhere to the medical regimen. Saying the client does not have to attend therapy is detrimental to the client's recovery and is not being a client advocate.
2. Being a client advocate means the nurse will support the client's wishes, but the nurse must adhere to the medical regimen in some situations. Talking to the physical therapist will not help the client's recovery.
3. Finding ways for the client to perform the exercises with the physical therapist supports the medical regimen. This action supports client advocacy. Physical therapists cannot prescribe.
4. Discussing the client's concerns does not help the client's recovery; therefore, this statement does not support client advocacy.

CLINICAL JUDGMENT GUIDE: There will be management questions on the NCLEX-RN® addressing client advocacy. A client advocate acts as a liaison between clients and HCPs to help improve or maintain a high healthcare quality.

46.
1. As long as the client gives permission, the nurse can discuss the client's condition with anyone.
2. The nurse can answer questions over the phone with the client's permission. It may be difficult for the client's spouse to come to the rehabilitation unit.
3. The client and spouse are allowed and encouraged to attend the multidisciplinary team meeting, but the nurse should talk to the spouse on the phone.
4. The nurse can talk to anyone the client requests and it is not a violation of HIPAA as long as the client permits the nurse to share information.

CLINICAL JUDGMENT GUIDE: There will be management questions on the NCLEX-RN®. In many instances, there is no test-taking strategy. The nurse must be knowledgeable of management issues.

47. Correct answers are 1, 2, and 3.
1. An antibiotic ointment, such as Polysporin, should be applied thinly four times daily. Polysporin can be purchased without a prescription.
2. Children should be kept home from school until the lesions crust over.
3. Use separate towels for the client. The client's towels, pillowcases, and sheets should be changed after the first day of treatment. The clothing should be changed and laundered daily for the first 2 days.
4. Crusts should be removed before the ointment is applied. Soak a soft, clean cloth in one-half cup of white vinegar and a quart of lukewarm water. Press a cloth on the crusts for 10 to 15 minutes three or four times daily. Then, gently wipe off the crusts and apply a little antibiotic ointment.
5. The child does not have to wear sterile gloves.

CLINICAL JUDGMENT GUIDE: This is an alternate type of question included in the NCLEX-RN®. The nurse must be able to select all the options that answer the question correctly.

48.
1. The nurse's scope of practice includes teaching the client how to use equipment.
2. This is a violation of HIPAA. The client's right to confidentiality is compromised because anyone could read the client's record on the computer. The charge nurse should intervene.
3. The nurse can discuss a client situation with the HCP; therefore, this action does not require intervention.
4. The nurse should refer a client with a spiritual need to the chaplain. It is not necessary to know what the need is; only the chaplain needs to see the client.

CLINICAL JUDGMENT GUIDE: There will be management questions on the NCLEX-RN®. There is often no test-taking strategy; the nurse must be knowledgeable of management issues. HIPAA was passed into law in 1996 to standardize the exchange of information between HCPs and to ensure client record confidentiality.

49. 1. Vitiligo is a common skin disorder in which white spots appear on the skin, usually occurring on both sides of the body in the same location. The client would not need an immediate appointment.
    2. Allergic contact dermatitis occurs when skin comes in contact with an allergen to which the client is sensitive or allergic. Clinical manifestations include redness, swelling, blistering, itching, and weeping. This client has an acute dermatological condition and should be seen immediately.
    3. Angiomas are not dangerous or contagious and do not need to be treated unless they bleed or bother the client. This client does not need an immediate appointment.
    4. The client may have shingles, but this cannot be determined at this time. The rash of shingles begins as red patches that soon develop blisters, often on one side of the body. It is treated with acyclovir (Zovirax), but the nurse would not need to make an appointment immediately.

CLINICAL JUDGMENT GUIDE: The test taker must determine which clinical manifestation is unexpected for the disease process. If the clinical manifestation is unexpected, the nurse should assess the client first. This question determines whether the nurse is knowledgeable of clinical manifestations of various disease processes.

50. 1. An MRI is not the diagnostic test used to confirm the diagnosis of basal cell carcinoma.
    2. A washing is not used to confirm the diagnosis of basal cell carcinoma.
    3. The only way to determine whether skin growth is cancerous is to biopsy it.
    4. A biopsy will definitively diagnose the skin cancer.

CLINICAL JUDGMENT GUIDE: The nurse must know about normal diagnostic tests pre- and postprocedure. These interventions must be memorized, and to ensure client safety, the nurse must be able to determine whether the client can have the diagnostic procedure and postprocedure care.

51. Correct order is 5, 3, 1, 2, 4.
    5. The gait belt is applied to ensure the safety of the client and the person assisting the client to ambulate.
    3. The client should use the strong hand to control the assistive device.
    1. The client should move the cane forward to provide stable support for the weaker leg when it is moved.
    2. The client should move the weaker leg even with the supportive cane while maintaining the stronger leg in place.
    4. Finally, the stronger leg can move to a position even with the weak leg and cane.

CLINICAL JUDGMENT GUIDE: The NCLEX-RN® has alternate questions, including ranking interventions. The test taker must put the interventions in the correct order to get the answer correct.

52. 1. Adequate skin care is an appropriate intervention to help prevent pressure injuries, but it is not the priority intervention.
    2. The priority interventions to prevent skin impairment are frequent position changes, skin care, and nutritional support.
    3. Sufficient nutritional intake will help prevent pressure injuries, but it is not the priority intervention.
    4. Using any mechanical device does not eliminate the need for turning and repositioning the client to help prevent pressure injuries.

CLINICAL JUDGMENT GUIDE: Test questions asking the test taker to select the priority intervention mean all the options may be plausible. The test taker has to determine the most important.

53. 1. Assessing the client's breath sounds is an appropriate intervention, but if the client is distressed, the nurse should help the client's body.
    2. The client should be encouraged to cough and deep breathe, but it will not help oxygenate the client, which is the priority for the client diagnosed with a fat embolism.
    3. Oxygen must be administered to treat hypoxia, which occurs after a fat embolism; therefore, this is the nurse's first intervention.
    4. The HCP may or may not administer heparin therapy, but it would not be the first intervention the nurse would implement.

CLINICAL JUDGMENT GUIDE: The nurse should use the nursing process when answering questions asking which intervention the nurse should implement first. If the client is in distress, do not assess; the nurse needs to address the client's physiological needs. The nurse should use Maslow's Hierarchy of Needs, which states that oxygenation needs are the priority.

54. 1. The wounds need to be kept sterile to decrease the chance of infection, but the priority for electrical burn wounds is to monitor for cardiac problems.

2. All clients need to have vital signs assessed, but the priority for electrical burn wounds is to monitor for cardiac problems.
3. The client's oxygenation level should be monitored, but the priority for electrical burns is cardiac problems.
4. The electrical current in the body bounces off the bone and goes through the muscle. The heart is a muscle; therefore, the priority intervention is for the nurse to apply cardiac monitors to assess for lethal dysrhythmias that may occur.

CLINICAL JUDGMENT GUIDE: The test taker should determine what is different about the client's disease process or disorder. All clients need to have vital signs assessed and oxygenation levels monitored. What is different for clients diagnosed with electrical burns?

55. 1. The nurse should have another staff member to assist with the lift, but it is not a priority over the safety of the client in the equipment.
    2. This is a priority because client safety must be ensured. If the client is not placed correctly in the lift sleeve, the client could fall. A standard electrical outlet or a rechargeable battery powers electric client Hoyer lifts. The lifting is completely controlled by hand, eliminating any physical exertion by the caregiver.
    3. The nurse should lift the client slowly, but this is not a priority.
    4. The stretcher should be locked and ready for the transfer, but the client is the priority.

CLINICAL JUDGMENT GUIDE: If the test taker is trying to determine the correct answer between options 2 and 4, the test taker should select the client's body over any equipment. All these options are plausible for a nurse to implement, but the safety of the client is the priority.

56. 1. Grade 6 indicates the client is independent in feeding, bathing, and toileting.
    2. Grade 4 indicates the client has some functioning areas of ADLs.
    3. Grade 3 indicates the client will need more assistance with ADLs.
    4. Grade 0 indicates the client is dependent on all six functions: bathing, feeding, toileting, continence, dressing, and transferring. This client would require the RN to delegate ADLs to the UAP.

CLINICAL JUDGMENT GUIDE: This is a knowledge-based question pertinent to rehabilitation nursing.

The test taker must realize that a score of 6 or 0 would be the answer because on most scales, but not all, the higher the number, the more severe the condition.

57. 1. The arm should be elevated to decrease edema, not placed in the dependent position, lower than the heart.
    2. Moist heat, immobilization, elevation, and systemic antibiotics are the treatments for cellulitis, an inflammation of subcutaneous tissue.
    3. Anti-staphylococcal soap (Hibiclen, Lever 2000, Dial) is prescribed for staph infection.
    4. The affected area should be left open to air, not wrapped by elastic (ACE) bandages.

CLINICAL JUDGMENT GUIDE: The nurse must know the expected medical treatment for the client. This is a knowledge-based question.

58. Correct order is 2, 5, 3, 4, 1.
    2. The wheelchair should be ready for the client to transfer to, which is the first step.
    5. The brakes should be locked so the chair will not move during the transfer.
    3. The client should use the stronger side of the body for support when moving.
    4. The client shifts the weight forward to pivot into the chair.
    1. The client should not attempt to sit until the chair is felt on the back of the legs so the client knows where the chair is.

CLINICAL JUDGMENT GUIDE: The NCLEX-RN® has alternate questions, including ranking interventions in priority order. The test taker must put the interventions in the correct order to get the answer correct.

59. 1. The residual limb should be elevated after 48 hours to help prevent contractures. Because the client is in the rehabilitation unit, it is past 48 hours.
    2. The LPN could give the HS snacks to the clients, but the UAP could also do this; therefore, it is not appropriate for the LPN to do this task.
    3. The UAP cannot perform sterile procedures, so this cannot be delegated to a UAP.
    4. The RN cannot assign the assessment to the LPN.

CLINICAL JUDGMENT GUIDE: The RN cannot delegate assessment, teaching, evaluation, medications, or an unstable client to the UAP. The RN cannot assign assessment, teaching, evaluation, or an unstable client to the LPN.

60. 1. The RN cannot delegate assessment to the UAP.
    2. The UAP can clean the client's dentures, so this task should be delegated.
    3. The UAP should not perform passive ROM exercises because it could lead to harm if not done correctly. The RN should perform passive ROM.
    4. The client's right leg should be elevated to decrease edema, not in a dependent position, which is hanging off the bed.

    CLINICAL JUDGMENT GUIDE: The RN cannot delegate assessment, teaching, evaluation, medication, or an unstable client to a UAP. The nurse must be knowledgeable about interventions that cannot be delegated, and in some cases, the intervention should not be implemented at all—such as option 4.

61. 1. A sterile environment should be maintained, but the priority is fluid volume because the client is at risk for hypovolemia.
    2. The priority intervention in the first 24 hours for the client diagnosed with a third-degree burn is maintaining intravascular volume so the client will not die from hypovolemic shock.
    3. Preventing infection is essential, but maintaining fluid volume is the priority.
    4. The nurse should assess the client's pain, but for a client diagnosed with third-degree burns over both the legs, the priority is maintaining fluid volume.

    CLINICAL JUDGMENT GUIDE: The nurse must know the expected medical treatment for the client. This is a knowledge-based question.

62. 1. Orthostatic hypotension is a side effect of administering the beta blocker medication atenolol (Tenormin); therefore, this medication should be questioned.
    2. Ceftriaxone (Rocephin) is an antibiotic, and these clinical manifestations do not warrant questioning this medication.
    3. Bisacodyl (Dulcolax) is a laxative, and lightheadedness would not warrant questioning this medication.
    4. Lightheadedness is a side effect of beta blockers which should not be administered until further assessment and notification of the HCP.

    CLINICAL JUDGMENT GUIDE: The NCLEX-RN® has alternate types of questions such as this one. It is an application-style question, and the test taker needs to be able to read a medication administration record (MAR) and know the side effects of medications.

63. Correct answers are 1, 2, and 4.
    1. Acupuncture is traditional Chinese medicine that involves using sharp, thin needles inserted in the body at precise points and is believed to adjust and alter the body's energy flow into healthier patterns.
    2. Guided imagery is the use of relaxation and mental visualization to improve mood or physical well-being.
    3. A compression sequential device is a pneumatic device to prevent DVT from the legs and arms. This is medically approved and is not CAM.
    4. Music therapy is a technique of CAM that uses music prescribed in a skilled manner by trained therapists. Programs are designed to help clients overcome physical, emotional, intellectual, and social challenges.
    5. Muscle-strengthening exercise is not CAM. It is performed as physical therapy and is a medical treatment.

    CLINICAL JUDGMENT GUIDE: This is an alternate type of question in which the test taker must select all options to get the question correct. According to the NCLEX-RN® tests plan, CAM is tested.

64. 1. This is why a client is referred to a vocational counselor.
    2. This describes the physiatrist, a physician specializing in rehabilitative care.
    3. This is why a client is referred to an occupational therapist.
    4. This is why a client is referred to the recreational therapist.

    CLINICAL JUDGMENT GUIDE: The nurse must know the role of the client's multidisciplinary team in rehabilitation. The nurse must be able to refer the client to the appropriate team member to help with rehabilitation.

65. 1. This question may be asked, but it does not assess daily schedules and habits.
    2. Assessment of daily schedules and habits includes questions concerning hygiene practices, eating, elimination, sexual activity, sleep, work, exercise, and recreational activities.
    3. Asking about insurance does not help the nurse assess the client's daily schedules and habits.
    4. This question can be asked but it does not address daily schedules and habits.

CLINICAL JUDGMENT GUIDE: The nurse must be able to ask appropriate questions when completing assessments, especially in rehabilitation nursing.

66. 1. The vancomycin must have a peak and trough drawn every third or fourth dose, depending on the HCP's order.
    2. Pantoprazole (Protonix) does not have a required laboratory test on a routine basis.
    3. Silver sulfadiazine (Silvadene) does not require a routine laboratory test.
    4. Morphine does not have a required laboratory test on a routine basis.

CLINICAL JUDGMENT GUIDE: This is an alternate type of question included in the NCLEX-RN® test plan. The test taker must be able to read an MAR, be knowledgeable of medications, and decide on the nurse's most appropriate intervention.

67. Answer: 1 tablet.
    The routine diuretic medication furosemide (Lasix) comes in 40-mg tablets. On M/W/F the client should receive ½ tablet, on Su/T/Th/Sa the client should receive 1 whole tablet.

CLINICAL JUDGMENT GUIDE: The NCLEX-RN® test plan includes dosage calculations under Pharmacological and Parenteral Therapies. This category is included under Physiological Integrity, which promotes physical health and wellness by providing care and comfort, reducing client risk potential, and managing health alterations.

68. Correct answers are 1, 2, and 3.
    1. The home health aide can weigh a client and document the finding.
    2. A home health aide can offer the significant other time away from the home to do personal business.
    3. Taking and recording vital signs are within the home health aide's capabilities.
    4. Taking the client to personal business in the home health aide's vehicle crosses boundaries, particularly when the business involves finances.
    5. The home health aide cannot perform assessments and make nursing judgments based on the findings.

CLINICAL JUDGMENT GUIDE: This is an alternate type of question included in the NCLEX-RN®. The nurse must be able to select all the options that answer the question correctly.

69. 1. Emergency services must come to the mall immediately. This person is having an allergic reaction to something, and this is a potentially life-threatening emergency.
    2. The nurse should determine whether the person has an epinephrine autoinjector (EpiPen) available that will save their life. If not, the nurse will have to wait for the ambulance.
    3. The client diagnosed with allergies should wear a medical alert bracelet to let anyone know what they are allergic to. Still, the first intervention is to try to save the person's life by giving epinephrine to the client.
    4. The nurse should protect the client's head, but this is not the priority intervention.

CLINICAL JUDGMENT GUIDE: When the question asks which intervention should be implemented first, it means all the options are something a nurse could implement, but only one should be implemented first. The nurse should use the nursing process to determine the appropriate intervention: If the client is in distress, do not assess; if the client is not in distress, then the nurse should assess.

70. Correct order is 3, 1, 5, 2, 4.
    3. This client has a change in normal sputum production. Frequently, clients diagnosed with obstructive pulmonary diseases are placed on steroid therapy. Steroid therapy can mask an infection. The only clinical manifestation of an infection may be a change in the color of the sputum.
    1. This client has a deep wound that needs to be assessed.
    5. The nurse can perform this test with a portable machine. The HCP may need to adjust the client's medication based on the results.
    2. Filgrastim (Neupogen) is a medication that increases the client's WBC production.
    4. This is expected behavior for a client diagnosed with Alzheimer's disease.

CLINICAL JUDGMENT GUIDE: This is an alternate question requiring the nurse to assess clients in order of priority. The nurse must evaluate each client's situation and determine which are life-threatening, which conditions are expected for the client's situation, or which client has a psychosocial problem.

71. 1. Sunburn is an example of this depth of burn; a superficial partial-thickness burn affects the epidermis; the skin is reddened and blanches with pressure.
    2. Deep partial-thickness burns are scalds and flash burns that injure the epidermis,

upper dermis, and portions of the deeper dermis. This causes pain, blistered and mottled red skin, and edema.
3. Full-thickness burns are caused by flame, electric current, or chemicals and include the epidermis, entire dermis, and sometimes subcutaneous tissue, and may also involve connective tissue, muscle, and bone.
4. First-degree burn is another name for a superficial partial-thickness burn.

CLINICAL JUDGMENT GUIDE: This is a knowledge-based question requiring the test taker to know the appropriate classifications of burns.

72. 1. After the airway, the most urgent need is preventing irreversible shock by replacing fluids and electrolytes.
    2. This is important but not a priority over fluid volume balance. Curling's ulcer is an acute peptic ulcer of the duodenum resulting as a complication from severe burns when reduced plasma volume leads to sloughing of the gastric mucosa.
    3. Infection prevention is a priority, but not before maintaining fluid and electrolyte balance for the first 48 to 72 hours. The client will die if fluid and electrolyte balance is not maintained.
    4. An escharotomy is an incision that releases the scar tissue, which prevents the body from being able to expand, and enables chest excursion in circumferential chest burns. The client has not had time to develop eschar.

CLINICAL JUDGMENT GUIDE: When the question asks which intervention is a priority, it means all the options are something a nurse could implement, but only one should be implemented first. The nurse should use the nursing process to determine the appropriate intervention: If the client is in distress, do not assess; if the client is not in distress, then the nurse should assess.

73. Correct answers are 1, 2, and 5.
    1. **Hand washing is the number one intervention used to prevent infection, a priority for the client diagnosed with a burn.**
    2. **The client is at risk for infection, and visitors diagnosed with infections should not be allowed to visit the client.**
    3. The client must have a high-protein diet to help with tissue growth.
    4. Invasive lines and tubing should be changed daily.
    5. **Prophylactic antibiotics are administered to help prevent infection.**

CLINICAL JUDGMENT GUIDE: This is an alternate type of question included in the NCLEX-RN®. The nurse must be able to select all the options that answer the question correctly.

74. 1. **The UAP can put the pulse oximeter on the client's finger and record the number. The RN must evaluate the reading to determine whether it is within normal limits.**
    2. The dressing change is a sterile procedure; therefore, this cannot be delegated to the UAP.
    3. Mafenide acetate (Sulfamylon) is a medication, and the RN cannot delegate medication administration to a UAP.
    4. The RN cannot delegate assessment to the UAP.

CLINICAL JUDGMENT GUIDE: Delegation means the RN is responsible for the UAP's actions and performance. The nurse must correct the UAP's performance to ensure the client is cared for safely and legally in the hospital or the home.

75. 1. Severe pain would be expected in a client diagnosed with these types of burns; therefore, it would not warrant notifying the HCP.
    2. **A pulse oximeter reading greater than 93% is within normal limits. Therefore, a 90% reading indicates the client is in respiratory distress and requires the nurse to notify the HCP.**
    3. The client's vital signs show an elevated temperature, pulse, and respiration, along with low blood pressure. Still, these vital signs would not be unusual for a client diagnosed with severe burns.
    4. Fluid and electrolyte balance must be evaluated to ensure the output is at least 30 mL/hr. This output is within normal limits; therefore, the data do not warrant notifying an HCP.

CLINICAL JUDGMENT GUIDE: The test taker must read all the options carefully before choosing the option that says, "Notify the HCP." If any of the options will provide information the HCP needs to know to make a decision, the test taker should choose that option. If the HCP does not require any additional information to make a decision and the nurse suspects the condition is serious or life-threatening, the priority intervention is to notify the HCP.

76. 1. Ice should never be applied to a burn because this will worsen the tissue damage by causing vasoconstriction.

2. Cool water gives immediate and striking relief from pain and limits local tissue edema and damage.
3. Burn ointment should not be applied until the burning has stopped. The client should first put the hand in cool water.
4. The client should be told to go to the ED, not the doctor's office, for burn care.

CLINICAL JUDGMENT GUIDE: This is a knowledge-based question requiring the test taker to know the appropriate care for burns.

77. 1. The skin should be kept dry and patted completely dry after each bath.
2. The client should be premedicated, but it is not the responsibility of the UAPs to ensure this intervention is implemented.
3. Clients should be turned at least every 1 to 2 hours to prevent pressure areas on the skin. Prevention of pressure areas is a priority for a client diagnosed with a burn.
4. All employees in any healthcare facility are responsible for providing care within their scope of services. UAPs can turn clients to help prevent pressure injuries.

CLINICAL JUDGMENT GUIDE: This is a knowledge-based question requiring the test taker to know the appropriate care for burns.

78. 1. The UAP cannot give TPN; it is administered via a subclavian line and should be considered a medication. The RN cannot delegate assessment, teaching, evaluation, medications, or an unstable client to a UAP.
2. The UAP can care for a client receiving a continuous tube feeding and should elevate the HOB to prevent aspiration pneumonia.
3. The UAP can assist a client with a meal.
4. The UAP can add a beverage thickener (Thick-It) to water before giving it to a client; it will help prevent the client from choking.

CLINICAL JUDGMENT GUIDE: The RN must ensure the UAP can perform any delegated tasks. It is the nurse's responsibility to demonstrate or teach the UAP how to perform the task and then evaluate the task performed.

79. 1. The client diagnosed with full- and partial-thickness burns is expected to have pain, and it should be assessed, but not before a client having difficulty breathing.
2. The client does not have 30 mL urine output an hour (this should be 240 mL/8 hours), and the client should be assessed but not before a client diagnosed with airway problems.
3. When determining which client to see first, the charge nurse should use Maslow's Hierarchy of Needs and assess the client diagnosed with airway problems first.
4. No palpable pulse indicates neurovascular compromise, but it is not a priority over airway problems.

CLINICAL JUDGMENT GUIDE: When deciding which client to assess first, the nurse should utilize Maslow's Hierarchy of Needs, in which physiological needs are the priority over psychosocial needs.

CASE STUDY ANSWERS

1. Correct answers are 1, 2, 3, 4, 5, 6, 9, and 10. When caring for a severe burn victim, the nurse should prioritize using the ABCs (A = airway, B = breathing, C = circulation). The nurse should report the hypotension, tachycardia, tachypnea, temperature, pulse oximetry reading, level of consciousness, TBSA, and the next of kin (spouse) situation. The status of the client's children are psychosocial findings and not a priority at this time. While the next of kin situation would also be considered psychosocial, the spouse is a nurse who may be working within the hospital. Since the client is unresponsive, unless another person has been designated to make healthcare decisions (unknown), the spouse will make decisions regarding the client's care.

2. Correct answers are marked.

Finding	Interstitial Fluid Shift	Respiratory Compromise
Hemoglobin and hematocrit increased	X	
Tachypnea	X	X
Serum pH lower		X
Hyperkalemia	X	
BUN level increased	X	
$Paco_2$	X	X
Pao_2	X	X
Serum CO		X

The client with significant injuries from burns will have rapid fluid shifts due to increased capillary permeability. All fluid components of the blood begin to leak out of the vascular system, causing edema, hypotension, and hemoconcentration (higher hemoglobin and hematocrit, hyperkalemia, and elevated BUN levels). The lungs may become congested as the fluid moves out of the vascular system. In this case, the soot noted around the client's nose and mouth indicates underlying smoke inhalation, which is why tachypnea is present and $Paco_2$ and Pao_2 are impacted by both the fluid shift and the respiratory compromise. Finally, the serum CO indicates inhalation of toxic fumes, and the low pH further indicates severe respiratory distress.

3. Correct answers are 1 and 4.
Cardiopulmonary monitoring and attempting to achieve hemodynamic stability are the top two priorities for the nurse. Remember, ABCs and physical needs are priority over psychosocial needs in a severe burn injury. Intake/output monitoring is a circulatory answer choice, but it is much narrower and only a part of stabilizing the client. Avoiding infection during wound care is essential, but ABCs take priority. The nurse will anticipate the family's emotional distress, including grieving related to the house fire, the death of their 7-year-old child, and the condition of the other two children; however, the client's physical needs take priority.

4. Correct answers are marked.

Potential Nursing Intervention	Indicated	Not Indicated
Prepare intubation medications	X	
Apply sterile dressings loosely over burns	X	
Monitor sedation level	X	
Provide emotional support to client's spouse	X	
Ask the spouse if they had working fire alarms in the home		X
Monitor telemetry	X	
Request an order for an indwelling urinary catheter	X	
Suggest the spouse go to the local children's hospital		X
Obtain client's health history from spouse	X	
At the bedside, inform the spouse of death of 7-year-old		X

The nurse should consider all "indicated" answer choices as appropriate. Assessing whether the family had functioning smoke alarms in the home is unimportant and irrelevant to the current situation. While the spouse may choose to go to the children's hospital, the nurse should ask if there is someone else they can call to help decide who stays with the client and who attends the children. The nurse or another healthcare professional should relay what is known regarding the couple's three children, but this should not be done at the client's bedside.

5. Correct answers are 3 then 1.

A	B
1. Decrease the client's sedation	1. Accompany RT to transfer the client to the Burn Center ICU
2. Call the children's hospital for an update	2. Assign a student nurse to accompany RT to transfer the client to the Burn Center ICU
3. Call report to the Burn Center ICU	3. Increase the client's sedation

Before transferring the client to the Burn Center ICU, the nurse needs to call report to ensure that the bed is ready and the receiving nurse is prepared. At the time of transfer to the unit, the nurse should accompany the RT to ensure the client remains safe and the team can intervene if his condition declines. The priority must remain with the physical needs of the client as he remains unstable and in critical condition.

6. Correct answers are marked.

Reassessment Findings	Improved	Declined	No Change
Blood pressure: 94/58 mm Hg	X		
Heart rate: 100 bpm	X		
Moaning when repositioned	X		
Potassium: 5.0 mEq/L	X		
Carbon monoxide: 160 ppm			X
Facial edema: +3		X	

The client's vital signs, potassium level, and level of consciousness have improved; there has been no change in CO level; and facial edema has increased markedly. Don't think that "moaning" is a decline in condition; the client has been unresponsive until now. The client may or may not need his sedation adjusted depending on his tolerance of the ventilator.

Hematological and Immunological Management

10

You have brains in your head. You have feet in your shoes. You can steer yourself any direction you choose.

—Dr. Seuss

QUESTIONS

1. The client diagnosed with breast cancer is positive for the *BRCA* gene and is requesting advice from the nurse about treatment options. Which statement is the nurse's **best** response?
   1. "If it were me in this situation, I would consider having a bilateral mastectomy."
   2. "What treatment options has your healthcare provider (HCP) discussed with you?"
   3. "You should discuss your treatment options with your HCP."
   4. "Have you talked with your significant other about available treatment options?"

2. The staff nurse answers the telephone on a medical unit, and the caller tells the nurse they planted a bomb in the facility. Which actions should the nurse implement? **Select all that apply.**
   1. Do not touch any suspicious object.
   2. Call 911, the emergency response system.
   3. Try to get the caller to provide additional information.
   4. Immediately pull the red emergency wall lever.
   5. Write down exactly what the caller says.

3. The new graduate nurse (GN) working on a medical unit night shift is concerned that the charge nurse is drinking alcohol on duty. On more than one occasion, the new GN smelled alcohol when the charge nurse returned from a break. Which action should the new GN implement **first?**
   1. Confront the charge nurse with the suspicions.
   2. Talk with the night supervisor about the concerns.
   3. Ignore the situation unless the nurse cannot do their job.
   4. Ask to speak to the nurse educator about the problem.

4. The nurse is completing a head-to-toe assessment on a client diagnosed with breast cancer and notes a systolic murmur that was not mentioned during report. Which action should the nurse implement **first?**
   1. Notify the HCP about the new cardiac complication.
   2. Document the finding in the client's electronic health record (EHR) and tell the charge nurse.
   3. Check the EHR to determine whether this is the first time a murmur has been identified.
   4. Ask the client whether they have ever been told they have an abnormal heart sound.

5. The nurse is reviewing the laboratory report for the client diagnosed with lung cancer. Which action should the nurse implement?

Laboratory Report

Laboratory Test	Client Values	Reference Values
WBC count	7.8	4.5 to 11.1 10^3/microL
Neutrophils	62%	40% to 75%
Hemoglobin (Hgb)	14.3	Male: 14 to 17.3 g/dL
		Female: 11.7 to 15.5 g/dL
Hematocrit (Hct)	43.1%	Male: 42% to 52%
		Female: 36% to 48%

1. Place the client in reverse isolation.
2. Notify the HCP.
3. Make sure no flowers are in the room.
4. Continue to monitor the client.

6. The RN charge nurse observes two unlicensed assistive personnel (UAPs) arguing in the hallway. Which action should the nurse implement **first** in this situation?
    1. Tell the manager to check on the UAPs.
    2. Instruct the UAPs to stop arguing in the hallway.
    3. Have the UAPs go to a private room to talk.
    4. Mediate the dispute between the UAPs.

7. The GN is working with a UAP, a 12-year hospital employee. However, tasks delegated to the UAP by the GN are frequently not completed. Which action should the GN take **first**?
    1. Tell the RN charge nurse the UAP will not do tasks as delegated by the nurse.
    2. Write a counseling record with objective data and give it to the manager.
    3. Complete the delegated tasks and do nothing about the insubordination.
    4. Address the UAP to discuss why the tasks are not completed as requested.

8. The client is diagnosed with laryngeal cancer and is scheduled for a laryngectomy next week. Which intervention would be a **priority** for the clinic nurse?
    1. Assess the client's ability to swallow.
    2. Refer the client to a speech therapist.
    3. Order the client's preoperative laboratory work.
    4. Discuss the client's operative permit.

9. The RN charge nurse is making assignments for the surgical unit. Which client should be assigned to the new GN?
    1. The 84-year-old client with a chest tube that is draining bright red blood
    2. The 38-year-old client 1-day postoperative with a temperature of 101.2°F (38.4°C)
    3. The 42-year-old client having just returned to the unit after a breast biopsy
    4. The 55-year-old client reporting unrelenting abdominal pain

10. Which task is **most** appropriate for the RN surgical nurse to assign to the licensed practical nurse (LPN)?
    1. Tell the LPN to administer the aminoglycoside antibiotic to the client.
    2. Request the LPN to empty the client's indwelling urinary catheter.
    3. Instruct the LPN to assess the client just transferred from the PACU.
    4. Ask the LPN to determine whether the client understands the discharge teaching.

11. The RN primary nurse informs the RN charge nurse that one of the UAPs is falsifying vital signs. Which action should the shift manager implement **first?**
    1. Notify the unit manager of the potential situation of falsifying vital signs.
    2. Take the assigned client's vital signs and compare them with the UAP's results.
    3. Talk to the UAP about the primary nurse's allegation.
    4. Complete a counseling record and place it in the UAP's file.

12. The client tells the nurse, "I am not sure my surgeon is telling me the truth about my prognosis." The nurse knows the client is diagnosed with terminal cancer, but the HCP is not telling the client per the family's request. Which statement is the nurse's **best** response?
    1. "I think you should know you have terminal cancer."
    2. "You do have a right to a second opinion."
    3. "You are concerned your surgeon is not telling you the truth."
    4. "I think you should talk to your surgeon about your concerns."

13. The nurse hung the wrong IV antibiotic for the postoperative client. Which intervention should the nurse implement **first?**
    1. Assess the client for any adverse reactions.
    2. Complete the incident or adverse occurrence report.
    3. Administer the correct IV antibiotic medication.
    4. Notify the client's HCP.

14. The 24-year-old male client diagnosed with testicular cancer is scheduled for a unilateral orchiectomy. Which **priority** intervention should the clinic nurse implement?
    1. Teach the client to turn, cough, and deep breathe.
    2. Discuss the importance of sperm banking.
    3. Explain about the testicular prosthesis.
    4. Refer the client to the American Cancer Society (ACS).

15. The female client in the preoperative holding area tells the nurse about a reaction to a latex diaphragm. Which intervention should the nurse perform **first?**
    1. Notify the operating room personnel.
    2. Label the client's EHR with the allergy.
    3. Place a red allergy band on the client.
    4. Inform the client to tell all HCPs of the allergy.

16. The RN critical care nurse, an LPN, and the UAP are caring for clients in a critical care unit (CCU). Which task would be **most** appropriate for the RN to assign or delegate?
    1. Instruct the UAP to obtain the client's serum glucose level.
    2. Request the LPN to change the central line dressing.
    3. Ask the LPN to bathe the client and change the bed linens.
    4. Tell the UAP to obtain urine output for the 12-hour shift.

17. Which task should the RN critical care nurse delegate to the UAP?
    1. Check the pulse oximeter reading for the client on a ventilator.
    2. Take the client's sterile urine specimen to the laboratory.
    3. Obtain the vital signs for the client in an Addisonian crisis.
    4. Assist the HCP with performing a paracentesis at the bedside.

18. The CCU charge nurse is making client assignments. Which client should the charge nurse assign to the pregnant nurse?
    1. The client with intracavity radiation for cervical cancer with ARDS
    2. The HIV-positive client admitted for chest pain to rule out (R/O) myocardial infarction
    3. The immunosuppressed client diagnosed with cytomegalovirus (CMV)
    4. The client on I-131 iodine for hyperthyroidism in a motor vehicle accident

19. The intensive care unit (ICU) nurse is caring for a client and notes blood oozing out from under the transparent dressing covering the peripheral IV site, bleeding gums, and blood in the indwelling urinary catheter bag. Which intervention should the nurse implement **first**?
    1. Check the client's hemoglobin/hematocrit (H&H) level.
    2. Monitor the client's pulse oximeter reading.
    3. Apply pressure to the IV site.
    4. Notify the client's HCP.

20. A client diagnosed with AIDS dementia is angry and yells at everyone entering the room. None of the critical care staff want to be assigned to this client. Which intervention would be **most** appropriate for the nurse manager to resolve this situation?
    1. Explain that this attitude violates the client's rights.
    2. Request the HCP to transfer the client to the medical unit.
    3. Discuss some possible options with the nursing staff.
    4. Try to find a nurse unaffected by being assigned to the client.

21. Which situation would prompt the healthcare team to utilize the client's advance directive when making decisions for the client?
    1. The client diagnosed with a head injury exhibiting decerebrate posturing
    2. The client diagnosed with a C6 spinal cord injury and on a ventilator
    3. The client diagnosed with end-stage renal disease being placed on dialysis
    4. The client diagnosed with terminal cancer and intellectually disabled

22. Which staff nurse should the charge nurse in the ICU send to the medical unit?
    1. The nurse having worked in the ICU for 18 months
    2. The nurse orienting to the ICU
    3. The nurse having worked at the hospital for 2 months
    4. The nurse with 12 years of experience in this ICU

23. The confused client in the CCU is attempting to pull out the IV line and the indwelling urinary catheter. Which action should the RN nurse implement **first**?
    1. Ask a family member to stay with the client.
    2. Request the UAP to stay with the client.
    3. Place the client in a chest restraint.
    4. Notify the HCP to obtain a restraint order.

24. Which tasks should the RN long-term care nurse delegate to the UAP? **Select all that apply.**
    1. Instruct the UAP to perform the a.m. care for the clients.
    2. Tell the UAP to wash the hair of the clients.
    3. Ask the UAP to cut the toenails of the clients.
    4. Request the UAP to turn the clients every shift.
    5. Instruct the UAP to empty the clients' wastebaskets.

25. The RN long-term care nurse notes the UAP tied a sheet around the client in the chair so the client would not fall out. Which action should the nurse implement **first**?
    1. Praise the UAP for being concerned about the safety of the client.
    2. Remove the sheet from the client immediately.
    3. Explain to the UAP that the sheet is a form of restraint.
    4. Assess the client's need for restraints and notify the HCP for an order.

26. The RN charge nurse in the long-term care center is making assignments for LPNs and UAPs on the day shift. Which task is **most** appropriate to assign to the LPN?
    1. Instruct the LPN to place antiembolism hose on the client.
    2. Ask the LPN to escort the client outside to smoke a cigarette.
    3. Tell the LPN to administer the tube feeding to the client.
    4. Request the LPN to change the client's colostomy bag.

27. The RN staff nurse is caring for clients in a skilled nursing unit. Which task should the staff nurse delegate to the UAP? **Select all that apply.**
    1. Instruct the UAP to apply sequential compression devices to the client on strict bedrest.
    2. Ask the UAP to assist the radiology tech in performing a STAT portable chest x-ray.
    3. Request the UAP to prepare the client for a wound débridement at the bedside.
    4. Tell the UAP to obtain the intakes and outputs for all the clients on the unit.
    5. Have the UAP help the client move from the bed to their chair for meals.

28. The older adult client receiving chemotherapy reports that food does not taste how it used to. Which intervention should the medical unit nurse implement **first?**
    1. Ask the dietitian to consult with the client on food preferences.
    2. Medicate the client before meals with an antiemetic medication.
    3. Ask the HCP to suggest an over-the-counter nutritional supplement.
    4. Check the client's current weight with the client's usual weight.

29. The nurse is assigned to a quality improvement committee to decide on a quality improvement project for the unit. Which issue should the nurse discuss at the committee meetings?
    1. Systems that make it difficult for the nurses to do their job
    2. How unhappy the nurses are with their current pay scale
    3. Collective bargaining activity at a nearby hospital
    4. The number of medication errors committed by another nurse

30. The nurse is discussing an upcoming surgical procedure with a 76-year-old client diagnosed with cancer. Which action is an example of the ethical principle of fidelity?
    1. The nurse ensures the client understands the procedure before signing the permit.
    2. The nurse refuses to disclose the client's personal information to the chief nursing officer.
    3. The nurse tells the client their diagnosis when the family did not want them to know.
    4. The nurse tells the client they are uninformed about their diagnosis.

31. Which client laboratory data should the nurse report to the HCP **immediately?**
    1. The elevated amylase report on a client diagnosed with acute pancreatitis
    2. The elevated white blood cell (WBC) count on a client diagnosed with a septic leg wound
    3. The urinalysis report showing many bacteria in a client receiving chemotherapy
    4. The serum glucose level of 235 mg/dL on a client diagnosed with type 1 diabetes

32. The RN charge nurse in a long-term care facility is reviewing the male resident's laboratory data.

Laboratory Report

Laboratory Test	Client Values	Reference Values
WBC count	5.25	4.5 to 11.1 × 10^3/microL
Red blood cell (RBC) count	4.3	Male: 4.51 to 6.01 × 10^6 cells/microL
		Female: 4.01 to 5.51 × 10^6 cells/microL
Hemoglobin (Hgb)	13	Male: 14 to 17.3 g/dL
		Female: 11.7 to 15.5 g/dL
Hematocrit (Hct)	39	Male: 42% to 52%
		Female: 36% to 48%
Platelets	39	150 to 450 × 10^3/microL

Which instructions should the nurse give to the UAP caring for the client?
1. Place the client in reverse isolation immediately.
2. Administer oxygen during strenuous activities.
3. Do not shave the resident with a safety razor.
4. Check the resident's temperature every 4 hours.

33. The clinic RN manager is discussing osteoporosis with the clinic staff. Which activity is an example of a secondary nursing intervention regarding osteoporosis?
    1. Obtain a bone density evaluation test on a female client older than 50.
    2. Perform a spinal screening examination on all female clients.
    3. Encourage the client to walk 30 minutes daily on a hard surface.
    4. Discuss risk factors for developing osteoporosis.

34. A client had an allergic reaction to penicillin and was admitted to the hospital 2 weeks ago. The client is being seen at the clinic for a follow-up visit. Which **priority** intervention should the nurse implement?
    1. Recommend the client wear a medical alert bracelet.
    2. Encourage the client to tell the pharmacy about their allergy.
    3. Tell the client not to be around any person taking penicillin.
    4. Allow the client to vent feelings about the hospitalization.

35. Which action would be **most** appropriate for the clinic nurse suspecting another staff nurse of stealing narcotics from the clinic?
    1. Confront the staff nurse with the suspicion.
    2. Call the state board of nurse examiners.
    3. Notify the director of nurses immediately.
    4. Report the suspicion to the clinic's HCP.

36. The clinic nurse administered 200,000 units of intramuscular penicillin to a client. Which **priority** intervention should the nurse implement?
    1. Place a bandage over the intramuscular injection site.
    2. Tell the client to put a warm compress over the injection site.
    3. Document the medication injection in the client's EHR.
    4. Inform the client to stay in the waiting room for 30 minutes.

37. The home health aide calls the office and reports pain after feeling a pulling sensation in their back when transferring the client from the bed to the wheelchair. Which **priority** action should the RN tell the home health aide?
    1. Explain how to perform isometric exercises.
    2. Instruct the home health aide to go to the local emergency department (ED).
    3. Tell the home health aide to complete an occurrence report.
    4. Recommend the home health aide apply an ice pack to their back.

38. The client diagnosed with osteoarthritis is 6 weeks postoperative for open reduction and internal fixation of the right hip. The home health aide tells the RN the client will not get in the shower in the morning because they "hurt all over." Which action would be **most** appropriate by the nurse?
    1. Tell the home health aide to allow the client to stay in bed until the pain subsides.
    2. Instruct the home health aide to get the client up to a chair and bathe them.
    3. Explain to the home health aide that the client should get up and take a warm shower.
    4. Arrange an appointment for the client to visit their HCP.

39. The RN is discussing the care of a client with a home health aide. Which task can the nurse delegate to the home health aide?
    1. Instruct the home health aide to assist the client with a shower.
    2. Ask the home health aide to prepare the breakfast meal for the client.
    3. Request the home health aide to take the client to an HCP appointment.
    4. Tell the home health aide to show the client how to use a glucometer.

40. The RN home healthcare agency director is teaching a class to the home health aides concerning safety in home health nursing. Which statement by the home health aide indicates the director needs to **reteach** safety information?
    1. "It is all right to call the agency if I am afraid of going into the home."
    2. "I should wear my uniform and name tag when I enter the home."
    3. "I must take my cellular phone when visiting the client's home."
    4. "It is all right if I don't wear gloves when touching bodily fluids."

41. The home health RN director is making assignments. Which client should be assigned to the **most** experienced home health nurse?
    1. The client recovering from Guillain-Barré syndrome reporting being tired all the time
    2. The client with multiple stage 3 and 4 pressure injuries on the sacral area
    3. The client 2 weeks postoperative for laryngectomy secondary to laryngeal cancer
    4. The client being discharged from service within the next week

42. The home health nurse is visiting a client diagnosed with colon cancer after a sigmoid colostomy. The client is crying and tells the nurse they were told the cancer has spread and they expect to die very soon. Which intervention should the nurse implement?
    1. Discuss the possibility of being placed on hospice services.
    2. Contact the client's oncologist to discuss the client's prognosis.
    3. Ask the client whether they planned funeral services.
    4. Recommend the client get a second opinion concerning the prognosis.

43. The client tells the home health nurse, "My oncologist told me they can't do anything else for my cancer. I do not want my children to know, but I had to tell someone. You won't tell them, will you?" Which statement is the nurse's **best** response?
    1. "Because you told me about the prognosis, I must talk to your children."
    2. "I don't think it is a good idea not to tell your children; they should know."
    3. "I will not say anything to your children, but I will contact the home health doctor."
    4. "You are concerned I might talk to your children about your prognosis."

44. The hospice nurse is making rounds. Which client should the nurse assess **first**?
    1. The client diagnosed with end-stage heart failure and increasing difficulty breathing
    2. The client with family planning to surprise them with an early birthday party
    3. The client reporting being tired and irritable all the time
    4. The client diagnosed with chronic lung disease having not eaten for 3 days

45. A client diagnosed with cancer and receiving chemotherapy is brought to the ED after vomiting bright red blood. Which intervention should the nurse implement **first?**
    1. Check to see which antineoplastic medications the client has received.
    2. Start an IV of normal saline with an 18-gauge IV catheter.
    3. Investigate to see whether the client has a do not resuscitate (DNR) order documented.
    4. Call the oncologist to determine what laboratory work to order.

46. The nurse is called to the room of a client diagnosed with lung cancer by the client's spouse because the client is not breathing. The client has discussed having a DNR order written but has not decided on it. Which interventions should the nurse implement **first?**
    1. Ask the spouse whether they want the client to be resuscitated.
    2. Tell the spouse to leave the room and perform a slow code.
    3. Assess the client's breathing and call a code from their room.
    4. Notify the oncologist the client has arrested.

47. The dying client asks to see their child, but the child refuses to come to the hospital. Which action should the nurse implement **first?**
    1. Call the child and tell them they must come to see their parent before it is too late.
    2. Ask the social worker to call and see whether the child will come to the hospital.
    3. Check with the family to see whether they can discuss the issue with the child.
    4. Do nothing because intervening in a private matter would be boundary crossing.

48. The nurse is caring for clients on an oncology unit. Which client should the nurse assess **first?**
    1. The afebrile client diagnosed with leukemia and a WBC count of 100×10^3/microL
    2. The client after undergoing four rounds of chemotherapy and feeling nauseated
    3. The client diagnosed with lung cancer with absent breath sounds in the lower lobes
    4. The client diagnosed with R/O breast cancer and a negative biopsy this a.m.

49. The nurse caring for clients on an oncology unit is administering medications. Which medication should the nurse administer **first?**
    1. The antinausea medication to the client anticipating getting sick
    2. The pain medication to the client with pain rated at a 2 on a 1 to 10 scale
    3. The loop diuretic to the client with an output greater than their intake
    4. The nitroglycerin paste to the client diagnosed with angina pectoris

50. The client, informed they have 6 months to live, tells the nurse, "This can't be happening. I am too young to die." Which statement is the nurse's **best** response?
    1. "I can contact the chaplain to come talk to you."
    2. "I will leave you alone and return shortly."
    3. "Is there anyone I can call to be with you?"
    4. "If it is all right with you, I will sit here with you."

51. The nurse administered pain medication 30 minutes ago to a client diagnosed with terminal cancer. Thirty minutes after the medication, the client tells the nurse, "I don't think you gave me anything. My pain is even worse than before." Which interventions should the nurse implement? **Select all that apply.**
    1. Attempt to determine whether the client is experiencing spiritual distress.
    2. Ask the client to rate their pain on the numeric pain scale.
    3. Reposition the client to relieve pressure on the pain site.
    4. Call the HCP to request an increase in pain medication.
    5. Explain to the client that they should relax and let the medication take effect.

52. Which member of the healthcare team should be assigned to a dying client having frequent symptoms of distress?
    1. The UAP available to sit with the client
    2. The LPN having grown attached to the family
    3. The RN with experience as a hospice nurse
    4. The RN having graduated 2 months ago

53. During the morning assessment, the client diagnosed with cancer reports nausea most of the time.

Client's Name: Mr. B	**Admit Number:** 543216	**Allergies:** NKDA
Date: Today	**Height:** 67 in (170.2 cm)	**Weight:** 74.2 kg (163 lb)
Diagnosis: Cancer of the pancreas		

Medication	0701–1900	1901–0700
Morphine sulfate 2 mg IVP q 2 hours PRN		
Promethazine 12.5 mg IVP q 4 hours PRN		
Prochlorperazine 5 mg PO TID PRN		
Hydrocodone 5 mg PO q 4–6 hours PRN		
Signature/Initials	Day Nurse DN/RN	Night Nurse NN/RN

Based on the client's medication administration record (MAR), which intervention should the day nurse implement **first**?
1. Administer the prescribed promethazine PRN.
2. Administer the prescribed prochlorperazine AC.
3. Discuss changing the order for prochlorperazine to routine with the HCP.
4. Assess the client to see whether pain is the cause of the nausea.

54. The infection control nurse notices a rise in nosocomial infection rates in the surgical unit. Which action should the infection control nurse implement **first**?
1. Hold an in-service for the staff on the proper hand washing method.
2. Tell the unit manager to decide on a corrective measure.
3. Arrange to observe the staff at work for several shifts.
4. Form a hospital-wide quality improvement project.

55. The UAP is preparing to provide postmortem care to a client with a questionable diagnosis of anthrax. Which instruction is the **priority** for the RN staff nurse to provide to the UAP?
1. The UAP is not at risk for contracting an illness.
2. The UAP should wear a mask, gown, and gloves.
3. The UAP may skip performing postmortem care.
4. Ask whether the UAP is pregnant before entering the client's room.

56. The client on a medical unit died of a communicable disease. Which information should the RN staff nurse provide to the mortuary workers?
1. No information can be released to the mortuary service.
2. The nurse should tell the funeral home the client's diagnosis.
3. Ask the family for permission to talk with the mortician.
4. Refer the funeral home to the HCP for information.

57. The RN medical-surgical nurse and UAP are caring for a group of clients on a medical unit. Which action by the UAP **warrants immediate** intervention by the nurse?
1. The UAP dons unsterile gloves before emptying a urinary catheter bag.
2. The UAP places clean linen in all the clients' rooms for the day.
3. The UAP uses a different plastic bag for every client when getting ice.
4. The UAP massages the client's trochanter when turning the client.

58. The charge nurse is making assignments on a surgical unit. Which client should be assigned to the **least** experienced nurse?
1. The client after vaginal hysterectomy with an indwelling catheter
2. The client after open cholecystectomy with gray drainage in the tube
3. The client after a hip replacement reporting something popped while walking
4. The client after a Whipple procedure reporting being thirsty all the time

59. The unit manager on an oncology unit receives a negative report about a client's care from the assigned night shift nurse. Which action should the unit manager implement **first**?
    1. Ask the night charge nurse to ensure the nurse does the work.
    2. Request the nurse to come in and discuss the care provided.
    3. Discuss the situation with the client making the report.
    4. Document this occurrence in the nurse's employee file.

60. The client was admitted to the orthopedic unit for injuries received during an argument with their partner. The client tells the nurse, "I am afraid my partner will kill me if I leave. It was my fault anyway." Which statement is the nurse's **best** response?
    1. "What did you do to set them off that way?"
    2. "Do you have a plan for safety if you go back?"
    3. "Why do you think it was your fault?"
    4. "You should leave before it is too late."

61. The spouse of a client on the surgical unit comes to the desk and asks the nurse, "What does the biopsy report say?" Which intervention is the nurse's **best** action?
    1. Check the EHR to see whether the client has allowed the spouse to have information.
    2. Obtain the pathology report and tell the spouse the biopsy results.
    3. Call the HCP and arrange a time for the spouse to meet with the HCP.
    4. Inform the client and spouse of the biopsy results simultaneously.

62. The RN oncology nurse and LPN are caring for clients on an oncology unit. Which client should be assigned to the LPN?
    1. The client diagnosed with acute leukemia on a continuous infusion of antineoplastic medications.
    2. The client, newly diagnosed with lung cancer, being admitted for placement of an implanted port
    3. The client diagnosed with an ovarian tumor weighing 22 pounds being prepared for surgery in the morning
    4. The client diagnosed with pancreatic cancer reporting frequent, unrelenting abdominal pain

63. The nurse has received the morning shift report on an oncology unit. Which client should the nurse assess **first**?
    1. The client diagnosed with leukemia and a WBC count of 1.2×10^3/microL
    2. The client diagnosed with a brain tumor reporting a headache rated as a 2 on a pain scale of 1 to 10
    3. The upset and crying client diagnosed with breast cancer
    4. The client diagnosed with lung cancer and dyspneic on exertion

64. The RN staff nurse is caring for a client diagnosed with systemic lupus erythematosus (SLE). Which client-reported data have **priority**?
    1. The client reports trouble finding makeup to cover the rash across their nose.
    2. The client tells the UAP to close the drapes because sunlight harms them.
    3. The client notices a bright red color in the bedside commode.
    4. The client reports joint stiffness and requests pain medication.

65. The nurse is caring for a client newly diagnosed with protein-calorie malnutrition secondary to acquired immune deficiency syndrome (AIDS). Which nursing interventions should the nurse implement? **Select all that apply.**
    1. Place the client on daily weights.
    2. Have the client identify preferred foods.
    3. Refer to the dietitian.
    4. Monitor bedside glucose levels four times a day.
    5. Perform central line dressing changes every 72 hours.

66. The client diagnosed with congestive heart failure and iron deficiency anemia is prescribed a unit of packed red blood cells (PRBCs). **Rank in order of performance.**
    1. Administer furosemide between units.
    2. Check the client's hemoglobin and hematocrit.
    3. Assess the client's lung sounds and periphery.
    4. Have the client sign a permit to receive blood.
    5. Return the empty blood bags to the laboratory.

67. The nurse in a rheumatology clinic is teaching a 34-year-old female client diagnosed with rheumatoid arthritis (RA) about methotrexate. Which information has the **highest priority?**
    1. Teach the client to take measures to prevent a pregnancy.
    2. Inform the client to keep the follow-up appointments with the clinic.
    3. Have the client see a dietitian for any loss of appetite.
    4. Tell the client to keep a diary of symptoms to bring to appointments.

68. The 28-year-old female client in the outpatient clinic has been told their test for human immunodeficiency virus (HIV) is positive. Which interventions should the nurse implement? **Select all that apply.**
    1. Discuss having regular gynecological examinations.
    2. Assist the client in making funeral arrangements.
    3. Refer the client to a social worker.
    4. Encourage the client to take the highly active antiretroviral therapy (HAART).
    5. Teach the client to follow a healthy lifestyle.

69. The RN oncology nurse and LPN are caring for clients. Which client should be assigned to the LPN?
    1. The 47-year-old client newly diagnosed with chronic lymphocytic leukemia
    2. The young adult client 4 hours postprocedure for bone marrow biopsy
    3. The 30-year-old client receiving PRBCs with a hemoglobin of 6 g/dL
    4. The elderly client receiving antineoplastic medications

70. Which client should the charge nurse assign to the medical-surgical nurse being sent to work on the oncology unit for this shift?
    1. The middle-aged client diagnosed with non-Hodgkin's lymphoma having complications from daily radiation treatments
    2. The 36-year-old client diagnosed with Hodgkin's disease being prepared for a bone marrow transplant
    3. The malnourished client diagnosed with leukemia with petechiae covering both anterior and posterior body surfaces
    4. The young adult female client diagnosed with ovarian cancer 1-day postoperative total abdominal hysterectomy

71. The RN oncology nurse and the UAP are caring for a group of clients. Which information provided by the UAP **warrants immediate** intervention by the nurse?
    1. The elderly client diagnosed with bladder cancer having bright red blood in the urinal
    2. The obese client receiving chemotherapy reporting pain in their mouth
    3. The 50-year-old client with a biological response modifier and vital signs of T 99.2°F (37.3°C), P 68 bpm, R 24 breaths/min, and BP of 198/102 mm Hg
    4. The client receiving a steroid reporting having a rounded swollen face

72. The RN oncology nurse is caring for a middle-aged client 1-day postoperative sigmoid resection and notes bright red bleeding on the midline abdominal incision. Which intervention should the nurse implement **first**?
    1. Assess the client's vital signs.
    2. Reinforce the abdominal dressing.
    3. Notify the HCP.
    4. Place the client in the Trendelenburg position.

73. Which nursing task should the RN oncology nurse delegate to the UAP?
    1. Discontinue the elderly client's subclavian IV catheter.
    2. Empty the Jackson-Pratt (JP) drainage tube and record the amount.
    3. Determine whether the client's pain medication has been effective.
    4. Perform irrigation for the obese client 2 days postoperative abdominoperineal resection.

74. The 79-year-old client is 2 days postoperative ureterosigmoidostomy for cancer of the bladder. Which assessment data **warrant** the RN oncology nurse notifying the HCP?
    1. The client has excreted urine from the rectum.
    2. The client's abdominal incision is slightly reddened.
    3. The client has an apical pulse of 98 bpm and BP 114/80 mm Hg.
    4. The client has a low-grade fever and a hard, rigid abdomen.

75. The RN oncology nurse is caring for an elderly female client diagnosed with stage 4 ovarian cancer and showing signs of grieving. Which nursing intervention is the **priority** for this client?
    1. Request that the client be referred to hospice.
    2. Encourage the client to make plans for their funeral.
    3. Allow the client to verbalize feelings about having cancer.
    4. Discuss an advance directive and a power of attorney for healthcare.

76. The 57-year-old female client diagnosed with ovarian cancer has had five courses of chemotherapy. Which laboratory data **warrant immediate** intervention by the RN oncology nurse?
    1. Absolute neutrophil count (ANC) of 681 cells/microL
    2. Platelet count of 175,000/microL
    3. Red blood cell count of 5.0×10^6 cells/microL
    4. Hemoglobin of 11.2 g/dL and hematocrit 37%

77. The RN oncology nurse is performing a head-to-toe assessment on an elderly client diagnosed with prostate cancer. The nurse notes an irregular-shaped lesion with some scabbed-over areas surrounding the lesion. Which intervention should the nurse implement **first**?
    1. Take no action because this is a common lesion found on the skin.
    2. Assess the lesion by completing the ABCDs of skin cancer.
    3. Document the findings in the client's EHR.
    4. Instruct the client to make sure the HCP checks the lesion.

78. The 39-year-old client diagnosed with pancreatic cancer has an advance directive (AD) stipulating no cardiopulmonary resuscitation. Which intervention should the RN oncology nurse implement **first**?
    1. Notify the client's HCP about the AD.
    2. Determine whether the client has discussed the AD with their significant other.
    3. Scan a copy of the AD into the client's EHR.
    4. Give the original AD to the client.

HEMATOLOGICAL/IMMUNOLOGICAL CASE STUDY

(1015) The triage nurse in the ED assesses a 39-year-old female client brought in by her spouse. The client reports extreme fatigue, headache, and pain in the chest with a cough. She states, "I had a cold last week, but it's gotten worse." Alert and oriented to person, place, time, and situation, she appears anxious, stating, "We have to get out of here before the bus drops our children off after school." The spouse reassures the client that they will make arrangements for child care if needed. The client's skin is pale and clammy, but the face is flushed. Coarse cough is present, with green sputum; lung sounds are diminished in the bases with rales auscultated in lower and mid posterior lungs. The abdomen is soft, and the client denies any change in bowel or bladder patterns. No pedal edema, (+) pedal pulses, and hand grasps bilaterally equal. Vital signs are populated in the chart.

Vital Signs	Client Values
Blood pressure	108/62 mm Hg
Heart rate	102 bpm
Respirations	26 breaths/min
Temperature	102.6°F (39.2°C)
Spo$_2$	89% on room air
Pain	Chest 7/10 with cough; headache 5/10

1. **Recognize cues. What matters most?** The nurse prepares to call the ED physician. Which **priority** data should be reported to the HCP? **Select all that apply.**
   1. Reports of extreme fatigue
   2. Pain in the chest with cough
   3. Worry about child-care arrangements
   4. Pale clammy skin with flushed face
   5. Course cough with thick green sputum
   6. Adventitious lung sounds
   7. Blood pressure
   8. Respiratory rate
   9. Temperature
   10. Oxygen saturation

(1040) The ED physician visits the client, obtains a brief health history and assessment; notes the presence of a "butterfly rash" and places orders below in the EHR.

PROVIDER ORDERS:

CBC, BMP, ESR
Sputum culture and sensitivity
Nasal antigen test for COVID-10; **if positive,** obtain and send a serum polymerase chain reaction (PCR)
Chest x-ray STAT
IV 5% dextrose in normal saline (D$_5$NS) at 150 mL/hr
Oxygen 2–4 L via nasal cannula; maintain pulse oximetry ≥93%
Droplet precautions
Acetaminophen 1,000 mg every 6 hours as needed for fever >100.5°F (38°C)

Past History: Recent diagnosis of systemic lupus erythematosus (SLE), tubal ligation at age 35, and COVID-19 approximately 8 months ago. The client has not traveled outside the country in the past year. No known allergies, exercises 1–2 times per week, and denies use of alcohol or illicit drugs. Spouse states that the client had the third of three doses of IV belimumab at the infusion center last week. The client reports shortness of breath with stairs. Weight of 134.2 lb (61 kg).

(1100) Complete blood count (CBC), basal metabolic panel (BMP), erythrocyte sedimentation rate (ESR) are obtained and sent to the lab. The nasal antigen test for COVID-19 was negative. A portable chest x-ray was done, and the client was instructed on the need for a sputum culture and sensitivity.

(1140) Diagnostic and laboratory results are received.

Laboratory Test	Client Values	Reference Values
Hemoglobin (Hgb)	10.8	Male: 14–17.3 g/dL Female: 11.7–15.5 g/dL
Hematocrit (Hct)	34	Male: 42–52% Female: 36–48%
White blood cell (WBC) count	1.8	4.5 to 11.1 × 10^3/microL
Absolute neutrophil count	400	2,500–7,000 neutrophils/microL
Platelets	165	140 to 400 × 10^3/microL
Creatinine	0.9	Male: 0.61 to 1.21 mg/dL Female: 0.51 to 1.11 mg/dL
Glucose	182	Fasting: Less than 100 mg/dL Random: Less than 200 mg/dL
Potassium	3.7	3.5 to 5 mEq/L or mmol/L
Sodium	136	135 to 145 mEq/L or mmol/L
Blood urea nitrogen	20	8 to 21 mg/dL Adult over 90 years: 10 to 31 mg/dL
Erythrocyte sedimentation rate (ESR)	62	<20 mm/hr

Chest x-ray results: Bilateral opacities and patchy areas in bases. *Impression:* Bilateral pneumonia.

2. **Analyze cues. What could it mean?** For each client finding, indicate whether it is consistent with the listed disease process of SLE, pneumonia, or COVID-19. Each finding may support more than one condition.

Finding	SLE	Pneumonia	COVID-19
Extreme fatigue			
Coarse cough			
Fever			
Butterfly rash			
Leukopenia			
Elevated ESR			
Tachycardia			
Hypoxia			
Tachypnea			
Shortness of breath			

(1220) The physician reviews the test results with the client and spouse and plans to admit the client for acute pneumonia treatment and consultation with an immunologist. The client and spouse verbalize understanding and agree to the plan. The spouse leaves to arrange child care for the couple's four children: two daughters, ages 9 and 5, and 18-month-old twin sons. The physician writes orders:

PROVIDER ORDERS:

Admit. Diagnosis: Bilateral pneumonia and recent onset SLE
Consult hematologist/immunologist
Oxygen 2–4 L via nasal cannula PRN to maintain pulse oximetry of ≥94%
Continuous pulse oximetry
CBC with differential, BMP every a.m.
Notify physician with sputum culture and sensitivity results
Strict intake and output
IV D_5NS @ 125 mL/hr
Ciprofloxacin 200 mg IV STAT then every 12 hours
Hydrocortisone 100 mg IV STAT then every 6 hours
Acetaminophen 1,000 mg every 6 hours as needed for fever >100.5°F (38°C)
Diet: Regular, encourage PO fluids
Activity: As tolerated

3. **Prioritize hypotheses. Where do I start?** Complete the sentence by choosing from the drop-down list of options. Based on the client's condition at this time, the nurse recognizes that the client is at the highest risk for _____

Select ▼
1. Bleeding
2. Dehydration
3. Sepsis

and will require _____

Select ▼
1. Anticoagulants
2. Antibiotics
3. Antineoplastics

(1410) The client is transferred from ED to the medical-surgical unit. The nurse assesses the client, reviews the ED notes and transfer orders, and establishes the initial plan of care.

4. **Generate solutions. What can I do?** For each intervention, specify whether the intervention is **indicated** or **not indicated** for the client's care.

Potential Nursing Intervention	Indicated	Not Indicated
Elevate the head of the bed at least 45°.		
Ensure the client is on fluid restriction.		
Discourage the client's children from visiting.		
Place the client in a private room.		
Increase oxygen from 2 L to 3 L with pulse oximetry 89%.		
Ensure ciprofloxacin and hydrocortisone were given.		
Draw and send serum PCR.		

(Day 2, 0700) Laboratory results: CBC with differential and BMP posted to the medical record. Values unchanged except for glucose = 194 mg/dL, WBC count = 1.2×10^3/microL, and absolute neutrophil count = 180 neutrophils/microL. The admitting physician discusses the results with the client's hematologist/immunologist and agrees on a plan.

(1030) The client's hematologist/immunologist visited and spoke with the client regarding the need to start a 7-day course of treatment with filgrastim 5 mcg/kg daily subcutaneously once the client is home. They explained that if an additional biologic treatment is needed in the future, an alternative to belimumab will be considered. It was requested that the nurse provide teaching regarding this medication before anticipated discharge in 2 or 3 days.

5. **Take action. What will I do?** Which actions are appropriate for the filgrastim teaching of this client? **Drag and drop one correct action from the options listed in the left column into the right column.**

Possible Actions	Correct Actions
Provide written instructions.	
Provide hands-on demonstration.	
Provide written and hands-on demonstration.	
Explain that the route is PO.	
Explain that the route is IV.	
Explain that the route is subcutaneous.	
Instruct that the client may stop the filgrastim at any time.	
Instruct that the client should complete the 7-day course of treatment.	
Instruct that the client may take the filgrastim every other day if desired.	
With the client's permission, include the spouse in teaching sessions.	
With the client's permission, include the oldest child in the teaching sessions.	
Teach the client before or after visiting hours.	

(Day 4 of hospitalization; 0900) The client has stabilized and will be discharged late this afternoon, and the nurse has provided discharge instructions.

6. **Evaluate outcomes. Does the client understand the teaching?** For each client statement, indicate whether the teaching regarding the new medication, filgrastim, was effective or ineffective.

Client Statement	Teaching Effective	Teaching Ineffective
"Filgrastim will not help cure my SLE."		
"I will swallow the filgrastim with a full glass of water."		
"I should avoid crowds."		
"I will need to take the filgrastim every day for 7 days."		
"Since I am afraid of needles, my oldest daughter can give me the filgrastim."		

ANSWERS AND RATIONALES

The correct answer number and rationale are in **bold-face purple type.** Rationales for why other answer options are incorrect are also given.

1. 1. This is boundary crossing because the nurse does not have breast cancer. The nurse should assess what information the client is seeking and then explain the treatment or refer the client, as appropriate.
   2. **The nurse must assess what information the client needs. To do this, the nurse must know what treatment options have been suggested to the client. Assessment is the first step in the nursing process.**
   3. This may be needed after the nurse further assesses the situation, but this is not the first intervention.
   4. The client needs information about treatment options from a designated HCP; the significant other would not have such information or suggestions.

   CLINICAL JUDGMENT GUIDE: The test taker should answer the question with factual information. Assessment is the first step of the nursing process, and the nurse should assess the client's current understanding of treatment options.

2. Correct answers are 1, 3, and 5.
   1. The nurse should begin a systematic search of the unit after activating the bomb scare emergency plan, and if any suspicious objects are found, the nurse should not touch them and notify the bomb squad.
   2. The nurse should notify the house supervisor and administration because they are responsible for informing the police department.
   3. The nurse should stay calm and keep the caller on the telephone. The nurse should attempt to get as much information from the caller as possible. The nurse can notify someone nearby to initiate the bomb scare procedure.
   4. Hospital red emergency levers are to notify the fire department of a fire, not a bomb scare.
   5. The nurse should try to transcribe exactly what the caller says; this may help identify the caller and where a bomb might be placed.

   CLINICAL JUDGMENT GUIDE: The nurse must be knowledgeable of hospital emergency preparedness. Students and new employees receive this information in hospital orientations and are responsible for correctly implementing procedures. The NCLEX-RN® test plan includes questions on the Safe and Effective Care Environment.

3. 1. The new GN must work under this RN charge nurse; confronting the nurse would not resolve the issue because the nurse can ignore the new GN. Someone in authority over the charge nurse must address this situation with the nurse.
   2. **The night supervisor or the unit manager can require the charge nurse to submit to drug screening. In this case, the supervisor on duty should handle the situation.**
   3. The nurse practice act binds the new graduate to report potentially unsafe behavior regardless of the nurse's position.
   4. The nurse educator would not be in authority over the charge nurse.

   CLINICAL JUDGMENT GUIDE: When the nurse is deciding on a course of action involving other staff members, a rule of thumb is this: If the individual about which the nurse is concerned is superior in job title to the nurse, then the nurse should go through the chain of command to the next-level superior. If the individual is subordinate in job title to the nurse, then the nurse should confront the individual.

4. 1. This should be done if the murmur is new; however, the nurse should investigate the finding further before notifying the HCP.
   2. This should be done, but assessing the client's situation is the nurse's priority.
   3. **Although the client was not admitted for a cardiac problem, they may have had a murmur for a while, and the previous nurse did not pick it up or did not mention it in the report because it was a long-standing physiological finding in this client. The nurse should research the EHR for a current history and physical examination to determine whether the HCP is aware of the condition.**
   4. The nurse should not ask the client because this could scare or alarm the client needlessly.

   CLINICAL JUDGMENT GUIDE: Assessment is the first step of the nursing process. The next step is for the nurse to investigate the assessment findings in the EHR without alarming the client.

5. 1. The client's laboratory work does not indicate an increased risk for infection. The client

does not need to be placed in reverse isolation.
2. The laboratory work is within normal limits. The nurse does not need to notify the HCP.
3. The client is not at an increased risk for infection; therefore, the client may have flowers in the room.
4. This client's laboratory work is within normal limits. The nurse should continue to monitor the client.

CLINICAL JUDGMENT GUIDE: This is an alternate type of question included in the NCLEX-RN® test plan. The test taker must be able to read an EHR, be knowledgeable of laboratory data, and make decisions concerning the nurse's most appropriate action.

6. 1. The nurse should stop the behavior from occurring in a public place. The RN charge nurse can discuss the issue with the UAPs and determine whether the manager should be notified.
   2. The first action is to stop the argument from occurring publicly. The RN charge nurse should not discuss the UAPs' behavior in public.
   3. The second action is to have the UAPs go to a private area before resuming the conversation.
   4. The charge nurse may need to mediate the disagreement; this would be the third step.

CLINICAL JUDGMENT GUIDE: In any business, including a healthcare facility, arguments or discussions of confidential information should not occur among staff of any level where clients, visitors, or other staff can see or hear it.

7. 1. The GN should handle the situation directly with the UAP first before notifying the RN charge nurse.
   2. This may need to be completed, but not before directly discussing the behavior with the UAP.
   3. The GN must address the insubordination with the UAP, not just complete the tasks that are the responsibility of the UAP.
   4. The GN must first discuss the insubordination directly with the UAP. The nurse must give objective data as to when and where the UAP did not follow through with the completion of assigned tasks.

CLINICAL JUDGMENT GUIDE: When the nurse is deciding on a course of action involving other staff members, a rule of thumb is this: If the individual about which the nurse is concerned is superior in job title to the nurse, then the nurse should go through the chain of command to the next-level superior. If the individual is subordinate in job title to the nurse, then the nurse should confront the individual.

8. 1. The client's swallowing ability is not impaired before the surgical procedure.
   2. The client will not be able to speak after removing the larynx; therefore, referral to the speech therapist to discuss an alternate means of communication is a priority.
   3. The HCP, not the nurse, is responsible for ordering the preoperative laboratory work.
   4. The HCP, not the nurse, is responsible for discussing the operative permit.

CLINICAL JUDGMENT GUIDE: The test taker must know the setting that ultimately dictates the appropriate intervention. The adjectives will clue the test taker to the setting. In this question, the phrase "clinic nurse" clues the test taker to the setting. The test taker must also remember the nurse's scope of practice and realize that options 3 and 4 are outside the nurse's scope of practice.

9. 1. This client is unstable and requires a more experienced nurse.
   2. An elevated temperature indicates a potential complication of surgery; therefore, this client requires a more experienced nurse.
   3. Of the four clients, the one most stable is the client after a breast biopsy; therefore, this client would be the most appropriate to assign to a new graduate nurse.
   4. Unrelenting pain requires further assessment; therefore, the client should be assigned to a more experienced nurse.

CLINICAL JUDGMENT GUIDE: When the test taker is deciding which client should be assigned to a new graduate, the most stable client should be assigned to the least experienced nurse.

10. 1. The LPN can administer IV antibiotic medication according to the LPN scope of practice.
    2. The UAP, not the LPN, should be instructed to empty the indwelling urinary catheter.
    3. The LPN should not be assigned to assess a client.
    4. The LPN should not be assigned to evaluate the client's understanding of the discharge teaching.

CLINICAL JUDGMENT GUIDE: The RN cannot assign assessment, teaching, evaluation, or an unstable client to an LPN.

11. 1. This should not be implemented until the allegation is verified and the RN charge nurse has discussed the situation with the UAP.
    2. The RN charge nurse should have objective data about the allegation of falsifying vital signs before confronting the UAP; therefore, the charge nurse should take the client's vital signs and compare them with the UAP's results before taking any other action.
    3. The RN charge nurse should not confront the UAP until objective data are obtained to support the allegation.
    4. Written documentation should be the last action when resolving staff issues.

CLINICAL JUDGMENT GUIDE: Management and legal questions will be asked on the NCLEX-RN® examination. There is often no test-taking strategy; the nurse must be knowledgeable of management issues.

12. 1. If the nurse tells the client the truth, the client may ask, "What happens now? How long do I have to live?" In this situation, the nurse should not tell the client the truth.
    2. The client does have a right to a second opinion, but in this situation, the nurse should encourage the client to talk to the surgeon.
    3. This therapeutic response encourages the client to vent their feelings, but the client needs answers. This is not the best response by the nurse.
    4. Because the nurse knows the client is terminal, it would be best for the nurse to encourage the client to talk to the surgeon. The client needs the truth, and the surgeon is the person who tells the client.

CLINICAL JUDGMENT GUIDE: The nurse needs to guide clients to the correct person when they have questions about their healthcare.

13. 1. The nurse should first assess the client before taking any other action to determine whether the client is experiencing any untoward reaction.
    2. The nurse must complete an incident report, but not before taking care of the client.
    3. The nurse should administer the correct medication, but not before assessing the client.
    4. The client's HCP must be notified, but the nurse should be able to provide the HCP with pertinent client information, so this is not the first intervention.

CLINICAL JUDGMENT GUIDE: Whenever something happens to the client, the nurse should assess the client before taking any other action.

14. 1. The client must be taught postoperative care, but this is not the priority intervention of the clinic nurse.
    2. Sperm banking will allow the client's sperm to be kept until the time the client wants to conceive a child. This is a priority because it must be done between the clinic visit and admission to the hospital for the procedure. The unilateral orchiectomy will not result in sterility, but the subsequent treatments may cause sterility.
    3. The nurse can discuss the testicular prosthesis, but this is not a priority over sperm banking because the prosthesis may or may not be inserted at the time of surgery.
    4. A referral to the ACS is appropriate, but is not the most important information a 24-year-old male client needs at this time.

CLINICAL JUDGMENT GUIDE: All options are plausible in questions that ask the test taker to identify a priority intervention. The test taker must identify the most important intervention.

15. 1. Because the client is in the preoperative holding area, the immediate safety need is to inform the operating room personnel so that no latex gloves or equipment will contact the client. Person-to-person communication for a safety issue ensures that the information is not overlooked.
    2. The nurse should document the allergy in the EHR, but this is not the first intervention because the client is in the preoperative holding area.
    3. The nurse should place a red allergy band on the client, but this is not the first intervention.
    4. The nurse should always teach the client, but the first intervention is the client's safety, which is why the operating room team should be notified.

CLINICAL JUDGMENT GUIDE: When the test question asks the test taker to determine which intervention should be implemented first, it means that all the options could be possible. In this situation, informing the operating room personnel ensures the client's safety.

16. 1. The serum blood glucose level requires a venipuncture, which is not within the scope of the UAP's expertise. The laboratory

technician would be responsible for obtaining a venipuncture.
2. This is a sterile dressing change and requires assessing the insertion site for infection; therefore, this would not be the most appropriate task to assign to the LPN.
3. The RN should ask the UAP to bathe the client and change bed linens because this is a task the UAP can perform. The LPN could be assigned higher-level tasks.
4. The UAP can add up the urine output for the 12-hour shift; however, the RN is responsible for evaluating whether the urine output is expected for the client.

CLINICAL JUDGMENT GUIDE: When the test taker is deciding which option is the most appropriate task to delegate or assign, the test taker should choose the task that allows each member of the staff to function at their full scope of practice. Do not assign a task to a staff member that requires a higher level of expertise than the staff member has, and do not assign a task to a staff member when another staff member with a lower level of expertise can do it.

17. 1. The client on the ventilator is unstable; therefore, the RN should not delegate these tasks to the UAP.
2. The UAP can take specimens to the laboratory; it is not a medication.
3. The client in an Addisonian crisis is unstable; therefore, the RN should not delegate these tasks to the UAP.
4. The UAP cannot assist the HCP with an invasive procedure at the bedside.

CLINICAL JUDGMENT GUIDE: The RN cannot delegate assessment, teaching, evaluation, medication, or an unstable client to a UAP.

18. 1. The client with intracavity radiation could cause problems with the pregnant nurse's fetus, so she should not be assigned to this client.
2. The pregnant nurse can be assigned to an HIV-positive client. The nurse must adhere to Standard Precautions.
3. The cytomegalovirus could harm the nurse's fetus, so the pregnant nurse should not be assigned to this client.
4. The I-131 is radioactive iodine, and a pregnant nurse should not be near radiation.

CLINICAL JUDGMENT GUIDE: The NCLEX-RN® has questions asking the test taker to address making assignments on units. Pregnant nurses should not care for clients with conditions that can harm the fetus.

19. 1. The nurse will need to check the client's H&H, but not before notifying the HCP. The client is exhibiting signs of disseminated intravascular coagulation (DIC).
2. Monitoring the client's pulse oximeter reading would be an intervention the nurse could implement, but it is not the first intervention for a client exhibiting signs of DIC.
3. Applying pressure to the IV site will not help stop the bleeding because the client's coagulation factors have been exhausted. The client must receive heparin therapy.
4. The client is exhibiting findings of DIC, which requires IV therapy. This is a life-threatening complication that requires immediate medical intervention, so the nurse must notify the HCP first.

CLINICAL JUDGMENT GUIDE: When the question's stem provides all the data needed to determine whether the client is in life-threatening distress, the nurse must contact the client's HCP.

20. 1. The staff's feelings are not a violation of the client's rights. Refusing to care for the client violates the client's rights.
2. Transferring the client to the medical unit solves the problem for the CCU, but the healthcare team should address the client's behavior. This is not the most appropriate intervention for the nurse manager.
3. This would be the most appropriate intervention because it allows the staff to have input into resolving the problem. When staff have input into resolving the situation, there is ownership of the problem.
4. One nurse cannot be on duty 24 hours a day. The nurse manager should try to allow the staff to identify options to address the client's behavior.

CLINICAL JUDGMENT GUIDE: Management questions will be asked during the NCLEX-RN® examination. There is often no test-taking strategy; the nurse must be knowledgeable of management issues.

21. 1. The client must have lost decision-making capacity because of a condition that is not reversible or must be in a condition specified under state law, such as a terminal, persistent vegetative state; irreversible coma; or as specified in the advance directive. A client exhibiting decerebrate posturing is unconscious and unable to make decisions.
2. The client on a ventilator has not lost the ability to make healthcare decisions.

The nurse can communicate by asking clients to blink their eyes to yes or no questions.
3. The client receiving dialysis is alert and does not lose the ability to make decisions; therefore, the advance directive should not be consulted to make decisions for the client.
4. An intellectual disability does not mean the client cannot make decisions unless the client has a legal guardian with a durable power of attorney for healthcare. If the client has a legal guardian, then the client cannot complete an advance directive.

CLINICAL JUDGMENT GUIDE: There will be legal and management of care questions on the NCLEX-RN® examination. Advance directives are included under the category Safe and Effective Environment and the subcategory of Management of Care.

22. 1. This nurse should be sent to the medical unit because, with 18 months' experience, the nurse is familiar with the hospital routine and would be helpful to the medical unit but is not the most experienced ICU nurse on duty.
    2. The nurse still orienting to the unit should not be sent to the medical unit. The nurse should be kept in contact with the nurse preceptor during orientation.
    3. The nurse new to the hospital should not be sent to an unfamiliar unit.
    4. The nurse with 12 years of experience should be kept in the ICU because this level of expertise would be more helpful for client care than a nurse with 18 months of experience.

CLINICAL JUDGMENT GUIDE: The nurse needs to know management issues for the NCLEX-RN® examination. The nurse with experience in certain areas of nursing would be most appropriate to float to the areas with related types of clients. Still, the ICU must maintain appropriate staff levels and experience.

23. 1. The family may or may not be able to control the client's behavior, but the nurse should not ask a family member first. The CCU usually has mandated visiting hours.
    2. The nurse should first ensure the client's safety by having someone stay at the bedside with the client, then call the HCP, and finally apply mitt restraints.
    3. This form of restraint is against the law unless the nurse has an HCP order. This is the least restrictive form of restraint but would not be helpful if the client is pulling at tubes.
    4. The nurse must notify the HCP before putting the client in restraints; restraints must be used only in an emergency, for a limited time, and for the protection of the client.

CLINICAL JUDGMENT GUIDE: The nurse should address the client's safety needs first and know legal compliance with local, state, and federal requirements, such as The Joint Commission Standards on Restraints and Seclusion.

24. Correct answers are 1 and 2.
    1. The UAP can perform a.m. care; therefore, this can be delegated to the UAP.
    2. Washing the hair of clients can be delegated to the UAP.
    3. The UAP should not cut clients' toenails; this should be referred to a podiatrist.
    4. The clients should be turned every 2 hours, not every shift.
    5. The housekeeping department should empty the wastebaskets, not the UAP.

CLINICAL JUDGMENT GUIDE: The RN cannot delegate assessment, teaching, evaluation, medications, or an unstable client to the UAP.

25. 1. The RN can praise the UAP for safety concerns, but first, the sheet must be removed because it is a form of restraint and is illegal.
    2. The nurse must remove the sheet because it is a restraint. An HCP order must be obtained before restraining a client.
    3. The RN should discuss the restraint policy with the UAP, but not before removing the restraint.
    4. The nurse should determine whether the client needs restraints for safety and then call and obtain the order, but not before removing the sheet. If needed, a chest restraint could be used to secure the client to the chair.

CLINICAL JUDGMENT GUIDE: The RN must ensure the UAP provides legal and ethical nursing care to the clients in the long-term care facility.

26. 1. The UAP could place antiembolism hose on the client.
    2. The UAP should not escort the client outside to smoke a cigarette; the UAP will be off the unit, and this encourages poor health habits.
    3. The LPN, not the UAP, should administer a tube feeding.
    4. The UAP can change a colostomy bag on a client after an extended period, which is implied because the client is in a long-term care center.

CLINICAL JUDGMENT GUIDE: The RN charge nurse should not assign a task to the LPN that a UAP could implement.

27. Correct answers are 1, 2, 4, and 5.
    1. The UAP can apply sequential compression devices to the client on strict bedrest.
    2. The UAP can assist with a portable STAT chest x-ray if she is not pregnant.
    3. The client must be premedicated for wound débridement; therefore, this task cannot be delegated to the UAP.
    4. The UAP can obtain intake and output for clients.
    5. The UAP can assist the client in transferring from the bed to the chair.

CLINICAL JUDGMENT GUIDE: The RN cannot delegate assessment, teaching, evaluation, medications, and an unstable client to the UAP. The nurse cannot delegate premedicating the client.

28.
    1. Asking the dietitian to consult with the client is a good intervention, but the nurse should assess the impact of the change in taste on the client.
    2. The client did not report nausea. Antiemetic medication prevents nausea associated with food odors and attempting to eat.
    3. The nurse can recommend an over-the-counter supplement to increase nutrition, but the nurse should first assess the impact of the problem. Over-the-counter supplements are expensive, and the nurse should suggest the client try malts, milkshakes, and fortified soups. Then, if the client does not like or gets tired of the taste, a family member can consume the food, and it is not wasted.
    4. Checking the client's weight change over time is the first step in assessing the client's nutritional status and the impact of the taste changes on the client.

CLINICAL JUDGMENT GUIDE: The test taker should employ a systematic approach to problem-solving. The nursing process is a systematic approach, and assessment is the first step of the nursing process.

29.
    1. A quality improvement project looks at how tasks are performed and attempts to see whether the system can be improved. A medication delivery system that takes a long time for the nurse to receive a STAT or "now" medication is an example of a system that needs improvement and should be addressed by a quality improvement committee.
    2. Financial staff reimbursement is a management issue, not a quality improvement issue.
    3. Collective bargaining is an administrative issue, not a quality improvement issue.
    4. The number of medication errors a nurse commits is a management-to-nurse issue and does not involve a systems issue unless several nurses have committed the same error because the system is not functioning appropriately.

CLINICAL JUDGMENT GUIDE: The NCLEX-RN® examination test plan includes management of care principles such as performance or quality improvement. The nurse should be knowledgeable of research and quality improvement initiatives.

30.
    1. This is an example of autonomy. The client needs all pertinent information before making an informed choice.
    2. This is an example of fidelity. Fidelity is the duty to be faithful to commitments, which involves keeping information confidential and maintaining privacy and trust.
    3. This is an example of veracity, the duty to tell the truth.
    4. This is an example of nonmaleficence, the duty to do no harm. This avoids telling a client facing surgery that he has cancer.

CLINICAL JUDGMENT GUIDE: The NCLEX-RN® test plan includes nursing care that addresses ethical principles, including autonomy, fidelity, veracity, and nonmaleficence, to name a few.

31.
    1. An elevated amylase level would be expected in a client diagnosed with acute pancreatitis. The nurse would not need to call the HCP immediately.
    2. An elevated WBC count would be expected in a client diagnosed with a septic (infected) leg wound. The nurse would not need to call the HCP immediately.
    3. The urinalysis report showing many bacteria is indicative of an infection. Clients receiving chemotherapy are at high risk of developing an infection. The nurse should notify the HCP immediately.
    4. This blood glucose level is above normal range but would not be particularly abnormal for a client diagnosed with type 1 diabetes. The nurse would not need to call the HCP immediately.

CLINICAL JUDGMENT GUIDE: The nurse must be knowledgeable of normal laboratory values and be able to determine whether the laboratory value is normal for the client's disease process or the medications the client is taking. The nurse must be able to determine which laboratory values require immediate notification of the HCP.

32. 1. The resident's WBC count is within normal limits and indicates an ability to resist infection. The nurse should not place this resident in reverse isolation.
    2. The resident's H&H is slightly lower than normal but not low enough to cause dyspnea during activity. The resident does not need oxygen.
    3. **The resident's platelet count is very low and could cause the resident to bleed. The nurse should initiate bleeding precautions that include not using sharp blades to shave the resident and using soft-bristle toothbrushes.**
    4. The client is not at risk for developing an infection. The client does not need their temperature checked every 4 hours.

CLINICAL JUDGMENT GUIDE: This is an alternate type of question included in the NCLEX-RN® test plan. The test taker must be able to read the EHR, be knowledgeable of laboratory data, and make decisions concerning the nurse's most appropriate action.

33. 1. **A secondary nursing intervention includes screening for early detection. The bone density evaluation will determine the density of the bone and is diagnostic for osteoporosis.**
    2. Spinal screening examinations are performed on adolescents to detect scoliosis. This is a secondary nursing intervention, but not to detect osteoporosis.
    3. Teaching the client is a primary nursing intervention. This is an appropriate intervention to help prevent osteoporosis but not a secondary intervention.
    4. Discussing risk factors is an appropriate intervention but not a secondary nursing intervention.

CLINICAL JUDGMENT GUIDE: The test taker should know primary, secondary, and tertiary interventions. Primary nursing interventions focus on the prevention of a disease or injury. Secondary nursing interventions aim to detect and treat a disease or injury early. Tertiary nursing interventions are centered on the management of chronic health problems.

34. 1. **This is the nurse's priority intervention because any emergency personnel coming into contact with the client should be aware of the client's allergy. Allergic reactions to penicillin, an antibiotic, can kill the client.**
    2. The client's pharmacy can be made aware of the allergy, but this is helpful only when the client is having prescriptions filled.
    3. Unless the client has an allergy to penicillin dust, which is rare, coming into contact with another person taking penicillin will not cause the client to have an allergic reaction.
    4. Therapeutic communication allows the client to vent feelings, which is an appropriate intervention, but it is not a priority over teaching the client how to prevent a potentially life-threatening reaction.

CLINICAL JUDGMENT GUIDE: All the options are plausible in questions that ask the test taker to identify a priority intervention. The test taker should identify the most important intervention.

35. 1. The clinic nurse should not confront the staff nurse without objective data that support the allegation.
    2. The state board of nurse examiners cannot do anything to the nurse until the nurse has been convicted of the crime. Many states have programs to help addicted nurses, and some states may revoke the nurse's license to practice nursing.
    3. **The clinic nurse should report the suspicions so that appropriate actions can be taken, such as a urine drug screen for the nurse, watching the nurse for the behavior, and possibly notifying the police department.**
    4. The nurse should follow the chain of command, which does not include the HCP.

CLINICAL JUDGMENT GUIDE: Management and legal questions will be asked on the NCLEX-RN® examination. There is often no test-taking strategy; the nurse must be knowledgeable of management issues.

36. 1. The nurse can or cannot place a bandage over the injection site. This is not a priority intervention.
    2. Warm compresses will help increase the absorption of the medication, but this is not the priority nursing intervention.
    3. The medication injection must be documented in the client's EHR in a clinic, just as it must be in an acute care area. Still, documentation is not a priority over a possible life-threatening allergic reaction.
    4. **The client is at risk of having an allergic reaction to the penicillin, which is a life-threatening complication. Therefore,**

the client must stay in the waiting room for at least 30 minutes so the nurse can determine whether an allergic reaction is occurring.

CLINICAL JUDGMENT GUIDE: The nurse must be knowledgeable of interventions when administering medications to clients and be able to make appropriate decisions to best evaluate the client's response to medications given.

37. 1. Isometric exercises such as weight lifting increase muscle mass. The RN should not instruct the home health aide to do these exercises.
    2. The home health aide may go to the ED, but the RN should address the aide's back pain. The person with back pain often does not need to be seen in the ED.
    3. An occurrence report explaining the situation is important documentation and should be completed. It provides the staff member with the required documentation to begin a workers' compensation case for payment of medical bills. However, the RN on the phone should help decrease the home health aide's pain, not worry about paperwork.
    4. The home health aide is in pain, and applying ice to the back will help decrease pain and inflammation. The RN should be concerned about a coworker's pain. Remember: Ice for acute pain and heat for chronic pain.

CLINICAL JUDGMENT GUIDE: The test taker should apply the nursing process when selecting the priority action. The home health aide is experiencing pain; therefore, the RN should offer an action to relieve the distress.

38. 1. Allowing the client to stay in bed is inappropriate because a client diagnosed with osteoarthritis should be encouraged to move, which will decrease the pain.
    2. A bath at the bedside does not require as much movement from the client as getting up and walking to the shower. This is not an appropriate action for a client diagnosed with osteoarthritis.
    3. Movement and warm or hot water will help decrease the pain; the worst thing the client can do is not to move. The home health aide should encourage the client to get up and take a warm shower or bath.
    4. Osteoarthritis is a chronic condition, and the HCP could not do anything to keep the client from "hurting all over."

CLINICAL JUDGMENT GUIDE: This question requires the test taker to know basic disease processes and interventions to assist the client in postoperative recovery.

39. 1. The home health aide's responsibility is to care for the client's needs, including assisting with a.m. care.
    2. The home health aide is not responsible for cooking the client's meals.
    3. The home health aide is not responsible for taking the client to appointments. This also presents an insurance problem because the client is in the home health aide's car.
    4. Even in the home, the home health nurse should not delegate teaching.

CLINICAL JUDGMENT GUIDE: The RN cannot delegate assessment, evaluation, teaching, medications, or care of an unstable client to a UAP, including a home health aide.

40. 1. If the home health aide is fearful, the home health aide should not go into the home and should notify the agency. The employee's safety is important. This statement does not require reteaching.
    2. The home health aide should be clearly identified when entering the client's neighborhood and home for safety purposes. This statement does not require reteaching.
    3. The home health aide should be able to contact the RN or agency about any potential or actual concerns. This is for the safety of the client as well as the employee. This statement does not require reteaching.
    4. Standard Precautions apply in the home as in the hospital. If the home health aide has the potential to touch the client's bodily fluids, then the aide should wear gloves and wash hands. The statement indicates the home health aide needs reteaching.

CLINICAL JUDGMENT GUIDE: According to the NCLEX-RN® test plan, staff education and serving as a resource person to other staff is a component of the management of care.

41. 1. The client diagnosed with Guillain-Barré syndrome would have been on bedrest for days to weeks and would be in a debilitated state; therefore, reports of being tired all the time would be expected. This client would not require the most experienced nurse.
    2. The client diagnosed with pressure injuries requires meticulous nursing care and a nurse experienced with wounds.

The most experienced nurse should be assigned this client.
3. The client with a laryngectomy has received teaching before and after the procedure and would not require extensive teaching or nursing care; therefore, this client would not require the most experienced nurse.
4. Discharge teaching starts on admission into the home healthcare agency; therefore, most of the teaching would have been completed, and this client would not need the most experienced nurse.

CLINICAL JUDGMENT GUIDE: The test taker must determine which client is the most unstable and would require the most experienced nurse.

42. 1. Hospice is a service for clients with fewer than 6 months to live. If the client has been told they will die "very soon," then this is probably fewer than 6 months. If the client does not die within the 6 months, they will not automatically be discharged from hospice. Each client is assessed individually for the need to remain in hospice care. If the client does not want any heroic measures and wants to die at home, then hospice will provide these services. This intervention would be appropriate for the nurse.
2. The nurse is not responsible for discussing the client's prognosis. The oncologist would have to write a letter stating the client had fewer than 6 months to live to be placed on hospice services. The client should discuss this with the oncologist, not the nurse.
3. Because the client is crying and upset, it would be more appropriate for the nurse to discuss a plan for living and hospice services than to discuss what is going to happen after they die. This should be done at some point, but this is not an appropriate time.
4. The client does have a right to a second opinion, but the nurse should not tell the client this unless the client is questioning the diagnosis.

CLINICAL JUDGMENT GUIDE: The test taker should be familiar with hospice and hospice services.

43. 1. The client is an adult, and the nurse must respect the client's confidentiality. The nurse does not have to tell the children.
2. This is giving advice and is not the nurse's role.
3. The nurse not telling the children respects the client's wishes and confidentiality, but the HCPs should be told of new client circumstances, as the information applies to the client's care.
4. This is a therapeutic response, but the client did not indicate an understanding that the nurse would talk about the client's status to the children. The client just wanted to tell someone.

CLINICAL JUDGMENT GUIDE: When the test taker is deciding on a therapeutic response, then the test taker must determine whether a response that directly addresses the problem or whether a therapeutic conversation is indicated.

44. 1. This client may need oxygen or an intervention to keep the client comfortable. This client should be seen first.
2. This client does not have priority over difficulty breathing.
3. This client does not have priority over difficulty breathing.
4. This client does not have priority over difficulty breathing.

CLINICAL JUDGMENT GUIDE: The test taker should apply some systematic approach when answering priority questions. Maslow's Hierarchy of Needs should be used when determining which client to assess first. The test taker should start at the bottom of the pyramid, where physiological needs are a priority.

45. 1. The medications are not important at this time. The client is bleeding.
2. The client is at risk for shock. The nurse should take steps to prevent vascular collapse. Starting the IV is the priority.
3. This is not important in the emergency department.
4. Prevention of circulatory collapse is the priority. The nurse could anticipate an order for a complete blood count (CBC) and a type and crossmatch.

CLINICAL JUDGMENT GUIDE: The test taker must be aware of the setting, which dictates the appropriate intervention. The adjectives will cue the test taker to the setting, in this case, the ED. The test taker must also remember the nurse's scope of practice. Starting an IV line with normal saline is within a nurse's scope of practice.

46. 1. It is too late to ask this question. This decision must be made before an arrest situation.
2. The nurse should not hesitate to call a code; a full code must be performed, not a slow one.
3. These are the first steps of a code.

4. This should be done by someone at the desk, not by the nurse responding to the emergency.

CLINICAL JUDGMENT GUIDE: The nurse must react immediately in an emergency and should not hesitate. The nurse should immediately begin cardiopulmonary resuscitation (CPR) and follow the hospital's protocol.

47. 1. The child has a right to refuse to come to the hospital regardless of what the nurse thinks they should do. The nurse is unaware of the family dynamics that led to this dilemma.
    2. This only places another healthcare professional in the picture and would not be the best option.
    3. **Other family members are more likely to understand the family dynamics and would be the best ones to intervene.**
    4. The nurse should attempt to assist in reconciliation between the client and their child if possible.

CLINICAL JUDGMENT GUIDE: The nurse should always try to support the client if it does not violate any local, state, or federal rules and regulations. Presenting the client's request to the family does not violate any regulations.

48. 1. This is an expected laboratory value for a client diagnosed with leukemia. The client's bone marrow overproduces immature white blood cells and clogs the bloodstream.
    2. **This client is reporting nausea, which is an uncomfortable experience. The nurse should attempt to intervene and treat the nausea. This client should be seen first.**
    3. Absent breath sounds are expected in a client diagnosed with lung cancer.
    4. A negative biopsy is a good result. This client does not need to be seen first.

CLINICAL JUDGMENT GUIDE: When deciding which client to assess first, the test taker should determine whether the clinical manifestations the client is exhibiting are normal or expected for the client's situation. After eliminating the expected options, the test taker should determine which situation is unexpected or causing the client distress.

49. 1. **Anticipatory nausea is a very real problem for clients diagnosed with cancer and undergoing treatment. If this problem is not rectified quickly and progresses to vomiting, the client may not get relief. This medication should be administered first.**
    2. This is considered mild pain and can be treated after the anticipatory nausea.
    3. This is expected and indicates the medication is working. This medication does not have priority.
    4. This routine medication can be administered after the nausea and pain medications. Sublingual nitroglycerin is administered for acute chest pain, or angina.

CLINICAL JUDGMENT GUIDE: The test taker should know which medications are a priority and should be administered first by the nurse.

50. 1. The nurse should address the client's spiritual faith, but this is not the nurse's best response at this time.
    2. The nurse should not leave the client alone after receiving this news.
    3. The nurse should ensure someone is with the client, but it is not the nurse's best response.
    4. **The nurse's best response is to stay with the client and allow the client to vent feelings of denial, fear, and hopelessness.**

CLINICAL JUDGMENT GUIDE: The nurse needs to address the client's psychosocial needs, and allowing the client to vent feelings is an appropriate intervention. A nurse with good listening skills is a very special nurse.

51. Correct answers are 1, 3, and 4.
    1. **Spiritual distress can significantly affect the perception of pain. If the client is not receiving relief from pain medication, the nurse should explore other variables that could affect pain perception.**
    2. Clients experiencing chronic pain may or may not be able to rate their pain on a scale. The client has provided all the information about the pain that is currently needed. The pain is greater than it was before the medication.
    3. **This alternative to medication may provide minimal relief while other interventions are being attempted.**
    4. **The nurse should notify the HCP that the current pain regimen is ineffective.**
    5. This is a condescending statement and would tend to agitate the client more than help.

CLINICAL JUDGMENT GUIDE: This is an alternate type of question included in the NCLEX-RN®. The nurse must be able to select all the options that answer the question correctly.

52. 1. The RN charge nurse should not assign a UAP to care for a client in spiritual distress. This is outside the UAP's functions.

2. The charge nurse should not delegate or assign care based on a personal relationship of the nurse with the family. The nurse most qualified to care for the client's needs should be assigned to the client.
3. A hospice nurse has experience managing clinical manifestations associated with the dying process. This is the best nurse to care for this client.
4. A new graduate would not have the experience or knowledge to manage the clinical manifestations as effectively as an experienced hospice nurse.

CLINICAL JUDGMENT GUIDE: When the test taker is deciding which option is the most appropriate task to delegate or assign, the test taker should choose the task that allows each member of the staff to function within their full scope of abilities.

53. 1. The nurse could administer the antiemetic, promethazine (Phenergan), as a one-time medication administration or whenever the client asks for it, but this is not a proactive intervention.
    2. Administering the PRN antiemetic, prochlorperazine (Compazine), prophylactically before meals is a proactive stance and assists the client in maintaining nutrition goals. This is the best action. If the client responds well to the regimen, the nurse should discuss changing the order to become a routine medication.
    3. If the client responds well to the PRN prochlorperazine (Compazine), the nurse should discuss changing the order to become a routine medication instead of just PRN.
    4. The client did not report pain. Nausea can be caused by pain, but any number of other reasons can also cause it. The nurse should be concerned with controlling the symptom.

CLINICAL JUDGMENT GUIDE: This is an alternate type of question included in the NCLEX-RN® test plan. The test taker must be able to read a medication administration record (MAR), be knowledgeable of medications, and make decisions about the nurse's most appropriate intervention.

54. 1. The infection control nurse should evaluate the problem thoroughly before deciding on an action.
    2. The infection control nurse should assess the staff member's delivery of care and use standard nursing practice before deciding on a course of action with the unit manager.
    3. This action will allow the infection control nurse to observe compliance with standard nursing practices such as hand washing. Once the nurse has attempted to determine a cause, then a corrective action can be implemented.
    4. The entire hospital has not shown an increased infection rate; only one unit has shown an increase.

CLINICAL JUDGMENT GUIDE: The test taker should use a systematic process to determine priority interventions. Assessment is the first step in the nursing process. The infection control nurse should assess the surgical unit to determine possible causes of the increased nosocomial infection rates.

55. 1. The UAP may be at risk of contracting the illness.
    2. The UAP should wear appropriate personal protective equipment when providing care.
    3. The UAP should not be told to skip performing assigned tasks.
    4. The fetus is not affected by anthrax, so a pregnant nurse could care for the client, taking the same precautions as a nurse who is not pregnant.

CLINICAL JUDGMENT GUIDE: The nurse must always prioritize standard precautions when caring for all clients, especially when blood and body fluids are present.

56. 1. The mortuary service is considered part of the healthcare team in this case. The personnel in the funeral home should be made aware of the client's diagnosis.
    2. The mortuary service is considered part of the healthcare team. In this case, the personnel in the funeral home should be made aware of the client's diagnosis.
    3. The nurse does not need to ask the family for permission to protect the funeral home workers.
    4. The nurse, not the HCP, releases the body to the funeral home.

CLINICAL JUDGMENT GUIDE: The test taker must know the members and roles of each multidisciplinary healthcare team member and the Health Insurance Portability and Accountability Act (HIPAA) rules and regulations. The client is being placed under the care of the mortuary service, and they should be aware of the client's diagnosis.

57. 1. This procedure is correct for contacting blood and body fluids. The nurse does not need to intervene.

2. This may be wasteful if the linens are not used because the client is discharged, but it does not warrant immediate intervention by the RN until the unit has a problem with linen over usage. This action saves the UAP time.
3. This is the correct procedure for getting ice. The nurse does not need to intervene.
4. Massaging pressure points increases tissue damage and skin breakdown risk. The RN should intervene and stop this action by the UAP.

CLINICAL JUDGMENT GUIDE: When the question asks, "Which warrants immediate intervention?" it is an "except" question. Three comments indicate the UAP is performing appropriate interventions, and one indicates the intervention is not correct and should be stopped. The RN must ensure the UAP performs tasks correctly and intervene if the UAP is unsafe.

58. 1. **This client has had a common surgical procedure and is not experiencing a complication. The least experienced nurse could care for this client.**
2. Green bile in a T-tube is expected, but a gray tint to the drainage indicates an infection. An experienced nurse should be assigned to this client.
3. A popping feeling when ambulating indicates the hip joint may have dislocated. An experienced nurse should be assigned to this client.
4. A Whipple procedure involves removing most of the pancreas. The findings indicate the client is not metabolizing glucose (symptom of diabetes mellitus). An experienced nurse should be assigned to this client.

CLINICAL JUDGMENT GUIDE: The test taker must determine which client is the most stable to be assigned to the least experienced nurse.

59. 1. The unit manager should talk to the client first, not ask the night charge nurse to watch the nurse. This step may be needed if a doubt about the nurse's performance arises.
2. This is the second step if the manager determines the report is valid.
3. **The first step is to discuss the report with the client. This step lets the client know that the client is being heard, and the manager can ask any questions to clarify the report.**
4. The occurrence may need to be documented and placed in the employee's file, but this is not the unit manager's first intervention.

CLINICAL JUDGMENT GUIDE: The nurse needs to know management issues for the NCLEX-RN® examination. The first step is for the unit manager to seek further information from the client making the negative report.

60. 1. This is blaming the client. No one has the right to abuse the client.
2. **The nurse must assess the client's risk from intimate partner violence (IPV) and provide the client with a referral to a women's center if applicable. This is the nurse's best response.**
3. The client does not owe the nurse an explanation of their feelings. This is not a good response to the client.
4. The nurse is advising. The decision whether to leave the abuser or not must be the client's decision.

CLINICAL JUDGMENT GUIDE: The nurse should assist the client to remain free from harm. The nurse should be knowledgeable about appropriate referrals and implement the referral to the most suitable person or agency.

61. 1. **Even though the client's spouse is making the request, the nurse should still check to ensure that the client has listed the spouse as being allowed to receive information. The HIPAA regulations do not allow releasing information to anyone not explicitly designated by the client.**
2. The nurse cannot do this unless the client has designated that their spouse can receive information.
3. The HCP, as well as the nurse, must abide by HIPAA.
4. The HCP is responsible for divulging biopsy results. If the spouse is present when the HCP enters the room and the client allows the spouse to stay, then consent for receiving information is implied.

CLINICAL JUDGMENT GUIDE: The nurse should know the HIPAA and follow the guidelines related to exchanging personal healthcare information to ensure client medical record confidentiality.

62. 1. The infusion of antineoplastic medications is limited to chemotherapy- and biotherapy-competent RNs. A qualified RN should be assigned to this client.
2. This client should be assigned to an RN able to answer the client's questions about cancer and cancer treatments.

3. This client is preoperative, and the LPN can prepare a client for surgery.
4. An experienced RN should be assigned to this client because the client is unstable, with unrelenting pain.

CLINICAL JUDGMENT GUIDE: The test taker must determine which client is the most stable to assign to the LPN. The expected care of the client should be included in the LPN's scope of practice.

63. 1. A low WBC count is expected in a client diagnosed with leukemia. This client does not need to be assessed first.
    2. A client diagnosed with a brain tumor would be expected to have a mild headache. This client does not need to be assessed first.
    3. The client is upset and crying. When all the information in the options is expected and not life-threatening, then psychological issues have priority. This client should be seen first.
    4. Dyspnea on exertion is expected in a client diagnosed with lung cancer. This client does not need to be assessed first.

CLINICAL JUDGMENT GUIDE: The nurse should use some tool as a reference to guide the decision-making process. In this situation, Maslow's Hierarchy of Needs is applied. Physiological needs are prioritized over psychosocial needs, but the other clients in the stem question are not experiencing clinical manifestations unrelated to their diagnosis, so the nurse can address the client with a psychosocial need first.

64. 1. A butterfly rash is one of the clinical manifestations of SLE; this statement does not alert the nurse to a new finding.
    2. Photosensitivity is a clinical manifestation of SLE and does not alert the nurse to a new problem.
    3. Bright red coloration in the bedside commode indicates blood, alerting the nurse to possible renal involvement. The HCP must be notified to order diagnostic tests and steps taken to limit kidney damage.
    4. Joint stiffness is related to the SLE and is a clinical manifestation. The nurse will medicate the client for pain, but the priority is to limit damage to the kidneys.

CLINICAL JUDGMENT GUIDE: When deciding on the priority, the test taker must decide between clinical signs and symptoms normally found in clients with the diagnosis that are not life-threatening and those that can be life-threatening or life-altering.

65. Correct answers are 1, 2, and 3.
    1. The client's daily weights will provide information on fluid balance and nutrition deficits.
    2. The client's preferred foods can be used to help increase the client's appetite and should be provided whenever possible on the meal trays.
    3. The dietitian can be the nurse's best ally when caring for a client diagnosed with nutritional problems.
    4. Glucose levels are monitored when a client is on total parenteral nutrition (TPN), not for a client newly diagnosed with a nutritional problem.
    5. This would be appropriate for a client on TPN.

CLINICAL JUDGMENT GUIDE: The test taker must note words hinting at a problem's extent, such as "newly," in the question's stem. This eliminates options 4 and 5. Words matter. "Left" or "right," "only," and "all" are words that can eliminate or define the option.

66. Correct order is 2, 4, 3, 1, 5.
    2. The nurse should check the client's hemoglobin and hematocrit first of the steps listed. Most healthcare facilities have a procedure to administer PRBCs only when the H&H are lower than 8 g/dL and 24%, respectively. Blood is a scarce commodity, and unless the client is scheduled for surgery, there are other means of providing care for the client without the administration of blood products.
    4. The client must consent to receiving blood and blood products. If the client refuses to allow the blood to be administered, the procedure stops there.
    3. The nurse must determine the client's physical status before picking up the blood in case the nurse assesses a client situation requiring the nurse to contact the HCP.
    1. If furosemide (Lasix), a loop diuretic, is ordered, it usually will be administered between the units of blood to prevent fluid volume overload.
    5. The blood bags can be returned to the laboratory after the blood has infused.

CLINICAL JUDGMENT GUIDE: Rank order questions can be answered by test takers by "placing" themselves at the client's bedside and asking, "What would I do first?"

67. 1. The disease-modifying antirheumatic drug methotrexate can cause fetal abnormalities or loss of the fetus. The client should be placed on birth control for the duration of administration of this medication and 2 years after.
    2. This is a standard instruction for many disease processes, but it is not a priority over the prevention of pregnancy.
    3. This medication can produce nausea, and nutritional intake is important, but not over preventing a pregnancy and possible complications.
    4. Keeping a diary of symptoms and questions is a good idea, but the priority is to prevent an unplanned pregnancy.

CLINICAL JUDGMENT GUIDE: If the question's stem gives an age, then it is usually an important indication of what the question is asking. In this question an age and a gender, female, are both given. Any time the client is a female of childbearing age, the test taker must consider there may be another potential client, the fetus.

68. Correct answers are 1, 4, and 5.
    1. HIV-positive females are at risk for multiple gynecological problems.
    2. This is not in the nurse's scope of practice, and clients newly diagnosed are living 20 years or longer with the virus.
    3. Nothing in the stem indicated a need for this referral.
    4. HAART regimens are responsible for the improved prognosis of HIV-positive clients.
    5. A healthy lifestyle will improve the client's ability to maintain her health.

CLINICAL JUDGMENT GUIDE: When answering "select all" questions, each option is answered as a true or false question. One option cannot rule out another.

69. 1. The newly diagnosed client must be taught about the disease and treatment options. The RN cannot delegate teaching to an LPN.
    2. This is postprocedure care for a stable client; therefore, the RN could assign the LPN to care for this client. The RN cannot assign assessment, teaching, evaluation, or an unstable client to the LPN.
    3. This client has a hemoglobin of 6 g/dL, which is extremely low; this client is unstable and should not be assigned to the LPN.
    4. The LPN cannot administer antineoplastic (chemotherapy) medications to the client. The chemotherapy nurse must be an RN with additional education in chemotherapy medication.

CLINICAL JUDGMENT GUIDE: The test taker must determine which client is the most stable to assign to the LPN. The expected care of the client should be included in the LPN's scope of practice.

70. 1. This client is receiving treatments that can have life-threatening side effects; the nurse is not experienced with this type of client.
    2. Bone marrow transplants are very specific to oncology clients; therefore, this client would not be appropriate to assign to a float nurse.
    3. This is expected in a client diagnosed with leukemia, but it indicates a severely low platelet count; a nurse with more experience should care for this client.
    4. A medical-surgical nurse should be able to care for a client 1-day postoperative abdominal surgery; therefore, this client can be assigned to a floating nurse.

CLINICAL JUDGMENT GUIDE: The nurse needs to know management issues for the NCLEX-RN® examination. The nurse with experience in certain areas of nursing would be most appropriate to float to the areas with related types of clients.

71. 1. This is expected from this client and does not warrant immediate attention.
    2. This is stomatitis and is expected with a client receiving chemotherapy.
    3. Biological response modifiers that stimulate the bone marrow can increase the client's blood pressure to dangerous levels. This BP is very high and warrants immediate attention.
    4. This client is experiencing steroid toxicity, which is called "moon" face, and is expected; therefore, this client does not warrant immediate intervention.

CLINICAL JUDGMENT GUIDE: The test taker should apply some systematic approach when answering priority questions. Maslow's Hierarchy of Needs should be used when determining which client to assess first. The test taker should start at the bottom of the pyramid, where physiological needs are a priority.

72. 1. The RN should assess the client's vital signs to determine whether the client is hemorrhaging. Hypotension and tachycardia indicate hemorrhaging, potentially a life-threatening emergency.
    2. The nurse may need to reinforce the dressing if the dressing becomes too saturated, but

this would be after a thorough assessment is completed.
3. The nurse should assess the situation before notifying the HCP.
4. The client may be put in the Trendelenburg position.

CLINICAL JUDGMENT GUIDE: The test taker should employ a systematic approach to problem-solving. The nursing process is a systematic approach, and assessment is the first step of the nursing process.

73. 1. The UAP cannot discontinue a subclavian line; this is a higher-level nursing intervention.
    2. The UAP can empty the JP drainage tube and reapply negative pressure. The RN cannot delegate assessment, teaching, evaluation, medications, or an unstable client.
    3. The nurse must do evaluation of the effectiveness of a PRN medication.
    4. The UAP should not do the initial colostomy irrigation, but the client would not have fecal output 2 days postoperative surgery.

CLINICAL JUDGMENT GUIDE: The RN cannot delegate assessment, teaching, evaluation, medications, or an unstable client to the UAP.

74. 1. A ureterosigmoidostomy is a surgical procedure wherein the ureters, which carry urine from the kidneys, are diverted into the sigmoid colon. It is done as a treatment for bladder cancer, in which the urinary bladder had to be removed. This is expected; therefore, it does not warrant notifying the HCP.
    2. This may indicate the client has an incisional infection, but the HCP can be notified of this on rounds because this is not life-threatening.
    3. The apical pulse and blood pressure are within normal range; therefore, this does not warrant notifying the HCP.
    4. This client is exhibiting clinical manifestations of peritonitis, which is a life-threatening complication secondary to abdominal surgery; therefore, the nurse should notify the HCP.

CLINICAL JUDGMENT GUIDE: The test taker must be able to identify life-threatening complications and notify the HCP immediately.

75. 1. Referral to hospice is an appropriate intervention for this client, but it does not apply to the client's grieving.
    2. At this time, the client should consider funeral arrangements, but the priority intervention is to assist the client to deal with the loss of their life. That is accomplished by therapeutic communication.
    3. Therapeutic communication is the priority intervention for a client diagnosed with stage 4 cancer and grieving. Allowing the client to work through the steps of grieving is accomplished by encouraging the client to express feelings.
    4. An advance directive and a durable power of attorney for healthcare are appropriate interventions for a client diagnosed with stage 4 cancer, but this does not address the grieving.

CLINICAL JUDGMENT GUIDE: The nurse needs to address the client's psychosocial needs, and allowing the client to vent feelings is an appropriate intervention. A nurse with good listening skills is a very special nurse.

76. 1. An absolute neutrophil count of 681/microL indicates the client does not have sufficient mature white blood cells or granulocytes to act as a defense against infections. This client needs to be placed in reverse isolation and receive pegfilgrastim (Neulasta), a biological response modifier.
    2. A platelet count of 175,000/microL is within normal range. Thrombocytopenia is lower than 100,000/microL; therefore, the RN does not need to intervene.
    3. A red blood cell count of 5,000,000 is within normal limits (3.61 to 5.11×10^6 cells/microL).
    4. H&H are a little low but not life-threatening; therefore, this does not warrant intervention.

CLINICAL JUDGMENT GUIDE: The nurse must be knowledgeable of normal laboratory values and be able to determine whether the laboratory value is normal for the client's disease process or the medications the client is taking. The nurse must be able to determine which laboratory values require immediate notification of the HCP.

77. 1. The nurse should complete an assessment of the lesion. This is not a common lesion found on clients.
    2. This is part of assessing the lesion and should be completed. The ABCDs of skin cancer detection include the following: (1) Asymmetry—Is the lesion balanced on both sides with an even surface? (2) Borders—Are the borders rounded and smooth or notched and indistinct? (3) Color—Is the color a uniform light brown or is it variegated and darker or reddish purple? (4) Diameter—A

diameter exceeding 4–6 mm is considered suspicious.
3. The nurse should document the findings in the EHR, but it is not the RN's first nursing intervention.
4. Instructing the client also to notify the HCP to assess the lesion should be done, but does not have priority.

CLINICAL JUDGMENT GUIDE: The test taker should apply some systematic approach when answering priority questions. Maslow's Hierarchy of Needs should be used when determining which client to assess first. The test taker should start at the bottom of the pyramid, where physiological needs are a priority.

78. 1. The HCP should be aware of the AD so a do not resuscitate (DNR) order can be written. Only the HCP can write this order. The RN should notify the HCP to get the DNR order written immediately. The order must be written before an arrest occurs, or CPR will be initiated.
2. The AD should be discussed between the client and the significant others, but the AD is still valid even if the significant others do not agree and the HCP can write the DNR order based on the client's wishes.
3. A copy is placed in the client's EHR to notify all healthcare team members of the client's decisions, but this is not the priority intervention.
4. Giving the client a copy of the AD is good, but it is not the priority intervention.

CLINICAL JUDGMENT GUIDE: Management and legal questions will be asked on the NCLEX-RN® examination. There is often no test-taking strategy; the nurse must be knowledgeable of management issues.

CASE STUDY ANSWERS

1. Correct answers are 1, 2, 4, 5, 6, 8, 9, and 10. The abnormal clinical findings and subjective data should be reported to the HCP. The report does not need the worry about child-care arrangements and the normal blood pressure.

2. Correct answers are marked.

Finding	SLE	Pneumonia	COVID-19
Extreme fatigue	X	X	X
Coarse cough		X	X
Fever		X	X
Butterfly rash	X		
Leukopenia	X		
Elevated ESR	X		
Tachycardia		X	X
Hypoxia		X	X
Tachypnea		X	X
Shortness of breath		X	X

Except for extreme fatigue, findings are clustered into autoimmune related or infectious related. The butterfly rash is specific to SLE and is supported by immunosuppression findings (leukopenia), and the ESR indicates the associated chronic inflammation. The remaining findings are indicative of a respiratory infection.

3. Correct answers are 3 and 2.
Based on the client's condition, the nurse recognizes that the client is at the highest risk for

3. Sepsis

and will require

2. Antibiotics

The client is being admitted for bilateral pneumonia. She is immunocompromised due to her recent SLE treatment with belimumab, so her ability to fight the infection is limited. Her care should focus on monitoring her condition and observing for early recognition of sepsis. Initially, the client's respiratory status may seem like the highest priority; however, the other options listed were bleeding and dehydration. Ensure the condition selected in the first part coincides with the treatment.

4. Correct answers are marked.

Potential Nursing Intervention	Indicated	Not Indicated
Elevate the head of the bed at least 45°.	X	
Ensure the client is on a fluid restrictions.		X
Discourage visitors.	X	
Place the client in a private room.	X	
Increase oxygen from 2 L to 3 L with pulse oximetry 89%.	X	
Ensure the first dose of ciprofloxacin and hydrocortisone given.	X	
Draw and send serum PCR.		X

Elevating the head of the bed and increasing oxygen will ease the breathing process. The nurse should discourage visitors, especially young children and the elderly, from visiting because of the client's pneumonia and compromised immune status. While the ciprofloxacin and hydrocortisone were ordered STAT in the ED, they should be selected to confirm order completion.

The client should be encouraged to drink as much liquid as possible to aid in thinning respiratory secretions. The PCR order was written to only indicate whether the nasal antigen COVID test was positive.

5. Correct answers are marked.

Possible Actions	Correct Actions
Provide written instructions. Provide hands-on demonstration.	Provide written and hands-on demonstration.
Explain that the route is PO. Explain that the route is IV.	Explain that the route is subcutaneous.
Instruct that the client may stop the filgrastim at any time. Instruct that the client may take the filgrastim every other day if desired.	Instruct that the client should complete the 7-day course of treatment.
With the client's permission, include the oldest child in the teaching sessions. Teach the client before or after visiting hours.	With the client's permission, include the spouse in teaching sessions.

Providing both written and hands-on education will help the client retain information. Filgrastim is only administered subcutaneously and is ordered for 7 days. Including the family in teaching is helpful if the client gives permission, and in this case, the spouse rather than the daughter, would be appropriate.

6. Correct answers are marked.

Client Statement	Teaching Effective	Teaching Not Effective
"Filgrastim will not help cure my SLE."	X	
"I will swallow the filgrastim with a full glass of water."		X
"I should avoid crowds."	X	
"I will need to take the filgrastim every day for 7 days."	X	
"Since I am afraid of needles, my oldest daughter can give me the filgrastim."		X

Filgrastim is a biosynthetic colony-stimulating factor used to generate neutrophils in clients with extremely low immune status; it is not used to cure SLE. Until the client's immunity has improved, she should avoid large crowds. Filgrastim is ordered to be administered for 7 consecutive days.

Filgrastim is administered subcutaneously, not orally, and the client's oldest daughter is 9 and should not be taught to give injections.

Women's Health Management

The journey of a thousand miles begins with one step.
—Lao Tzu

QUESTIONS

1. Which client should the postpartum nurse assess **first** after receiving the a.m. shift report?
   1. The client reporting perineal pain when urinating
   2. The client saturating multiple peri-pads during the night
   3. The client refusing to have their newborn in the room
   4. The client crying because the baby will not nurse

2. Which newborn infant would **warrant immediate** intervention by the nursery nurse?
   1. The 1-hour-old newborn with abundant lanugo
   2. The 6-hour-old newborn with respirations of 52 breaths/min
   3. The 12-hour-old newborn turning red and crying
   4. The 24-hour-old newborn who has not passed meconium

3. The client in labor is showing late decelerations on the fetal monitor. Which intervention should the nurse implement **first**?
   1. Notify the healthcare provider (HCP) immediately.
   2. Instruct the client to take slow, deep breaths.
   3. Place the client in the left lateral position.
   4. Prepare for an immediate delivery of the fetus.

4. The nurse walks into the client's room to check on the mother and her newborn. The client states another nurse just took her baby back to the nursery. Which intervention should the nurse implement **first**?
   1. Initiate an emergency Code Pink, indicating an infant abduction.
   2. Ask the mother to describe the nurse who took the baby.
   3. Determine whether the infant was returned to the nursery.
   4. Ask the mother whether the nurse asked for the code word.

5. The women's health clinic nurse is returning telephone calls. Which client should the nurse contact **first**?
   1. The 16-year-old client reporting severe lower abdominal cramping
   2. The 27-year-old primigravida client reporting blurred vision
   3. The 48-year-old perimenopausal client expelling dark-red blood clots
   4. The 68-year-old client thinking her uterus is falling out of her vagina

6. The charge nurse has received laboratory results for clients on the postpartum unit. Which client would **warrant** intervention by the nurse?
   1. The client with white blood cell count 18,000/mm^3
   2. The client with serum creatinine level 0.8 mg/dL
   3. The client with platelet count of 410,000/mm^3
   4. The client with serum glucose level of 280 mg/dL

7. The nurse on the postpartum unit is administering a.m. medications. Which medication should the nurse administer **first**?
   1. The sliding scale insulin to the client diagnosed with type 1 diabetes
   2. The stool softener to the client reporting severe constipation
   3. The non-narcotic analgesic to the client reporting a headache, rated as a 3 on a pain scale of 1 to 10
   4. The rectal suppository for the client reporting hemorrhoidal pain

8. The labor and delivery nurse is performing a vaginal examination and assesses a prolapsed cord. Which intervention should the nurse implement **first**?
   1. Place the client in the Trendelenburg position.
   2. Ask the father to leave the delivery room.
   3. Request the client not to push during contractions.
   4. Prepare the client for an emergency cesarean section (C-section).

9. Which newborn infant would the nursery nurse assess **first**?
   1. The 3-hour-old newborn weighing 6 lb 2 oz (2.8 kg)
   2. The 4-hour-old newborn delivered at 42 weeks' gestation
   3. The 6-hour-old newborn measuring 22 in (55.9 cm) long
   4. The 8-hour-old newborn delivered at 40 weeks' gestation

10. Which antepartum client should the charge nurse assign to the **most** experienced nurse?
    1. The 34-week gestation client receiving terbutaline and on strict bedrest
    2. The 36-week gestation client in active labor with a fetal biophysical profile of 10
    3. The 38-week gestation client dilated to 10 cm and 100% effaced
    4. The 42-week gestation client after pushing for 4 hours and showing yellow amniotic fluid

11. A registered nurse (RN) has been floated from the medical unit to the postpartum unit. Which client should be assigned to this nurse?
    1. The 4-hour postpartum client whose fundus is not midline
    2. The 8-hour postpartum client saturating three peri-pads in 1 hour
    3. The 14-hour postpartum client after experiencing eclampsia during delivery
    4. The 23-hour postpartum client being discharged home this morning

12. Which **priority** intervention should the nurse implement for the 38-weeks' gestation client receiving epidural anesthesia?
    1. Place the client in the fetal position.
    2. Assess the client's respiratory rate.
    3. Prehydrate the client with IV fluid.
    4. Ensure the client has been NPO for 4 hours.

13. The 28-year-old female client is being scheduled for an emergency appendectomy. Which **priority** question should the emergency department nurse ask the client?
    1. "Are you currently breastfeeding?"
    2. "Have you ever had general anesthesia?"
    3. "Do you have any medication allergies?"
    4. "Is there any chance you are pregnant?"

14. Which client should the labor and delivery RN charge nurse assign to the **most** experienced nurse?
    1. The client with a fetal heart rate of 130 bpm
    2. The client with nonreassuring fetal heart rate patterns
    3. The client scheduled for a cesarean section
    4. The client having a vaginal birth and has been pushing for 1 hour

15. The UAP informs the RN postpartum nurse she has helped the 1-day postpartum client change her peri-pad three times in the last 4 hours. Which action should the nurse implement?
    1. Ask the UAP why the nurse was not notified earlier.
    2. Go to the room and check the client immediately.
    3. Instruct the UAP to massage the client's uterus.
    4. Document the finding in the client's electronic health record (EHR).

16. The UAP is assisting the RN nursery nurse in the newborn nursery. Which action by the UAP would **warrant** intervention?
    1. The UAP swaddles the infant securely in a blanket.
    2. The UAP uses gloves when changing the infant.
    3. The UAP is bathing the newborn with a bar of soap.
    4. The UAP wipes down the crib with a disinfectant.

17. The charge nurse is making assignments in the labor and delivery department. Which client should be assigned to the **most** experienced nurse?
    1. The 26-week gestational client having Braxton Hicks contractions
    2. The 32-week gestational client having triplets and on bedrest
    3. The 38-week gestational client with contractions 3 minutes apart
    4. The 39-week gestational client with late decelerations on the fetal monitor

18. Which tasks should the RN postpartum nurse delegate to the UAP? **Select all that apply.**
    1. Instruct the UAP to prepare a sitz bath for the client.
    2. Ask the UAP to call the laboratory for a STAT complete blood count (CBC).
    3. Tell the UAP to show the mother how to breastfeed.
    4. Direct the UAP to check the client's fundus.
    5. Have the UAP take the breakfast tray to the client.

19. A nurse from the medical-surgical unit is assigned to the postpartum unit. Which client should the charge nurse assign to the medical-surgical nurse?
    1. The client diagnosed with mastitis and trying to breastfeed
    2. The client postsurgical vaginal hysterectomy and oophorectomy
    3. The client having difficulty bonding with her infant
    4. The unmarried client giving her child up for adoption

20. The UAP responds to a code in the newborn nursery. Which task should the RN house supervisor delegate to the UAP?
    1. Tell the UAP to sit in the waiting room with the family.
    2. Give medication to the nurse from the crash cart.
    3. Assist the nurse anesthetist with intubation.
    4. Instruct the UAP to obtain supplies needed during the code.

21. Which action by the RN nursery nurse would **warrant immediate** intervention by the charge nurse?
    1. The nurse allows an experienced volunteer to rock an infant.
    2. The nurse puts a gloved finger into the newborn's mouth.
    3. The nurse performs the Ortolani maneuver on the newborn.
    4. The nurse requests the licensed practical nurse (LPN) to bathe the newborn infant.

22. The RN and UAP are caring for clients on a postpartum unit. Which task would be **most** appropriate for the RN to assign to the UAP?
    1. Perform an in-and-out catheterization.
    2. Complete the client's discharge instructions.
    3. Escort the client to the car and check for a car seat.
    4. Spray anesthetic foam on the client's episiotomy.

23. The RN charge nurse is making assignments on the postpartum unit. Which client should be assigned to the LPN?
    1. The client delivering her sixth baby now returning to her room
    2. The client postsurgical C-section yesterday running a low-grade fever
    3. The client postvaginal delivery this morning with foul-smelling lochia
    4. The client 1-day postvaginal delivery and ambulating in the hall

24. The RN nursery nurse and UAP are caring for babies in the newborn nursery. Which action by the UAP would **warrant immediate** intervention?
    1. The UAP does not check the mother's identification (ID) band with the infant's ID band.
    2. The UAP brings the mother a full package of newborn diapers.
    3. The UAP applies baby lotion to the newborn while the mother is watching.
    4. The UAP tells the father to support the newborn's head.

25. Which tasks should the RN postpartum nurse delegate to the UAP? **Select all that apply.**
    1. Tell the UAP to assess the vital signs of the 4 hours postvaginal delivery client.
    2. Request the UAP to pass out the breakfast trays to the clients.
    3. Instruct the UAP to administer Rho(D) immune globulin to the Rh-negative client.
    4. Ask the UAP to remove the client's indwelling urinary catheter.
    5. Direct the UAP to assist the client to breastfeed her infant.

26. Which behavior by the UAP **warrants immediate** intervention by the RN postpartum nurse?
    1. The UAP helped the client with an episiotomy apply an ice pack to the perineal area.
    2. The UAP pushes the PCA button for the 8-hour postoperative C-section client.
    3. The UAP uses nonsterile gloves to remove the client's peri-pad.
    4. The UAP encourages the client to eat all the food on the breakfast tray.

27. The RN charge nurse is making assignments on a postpartum unit that has two RNs, two LPNs, and two UAPs. Which task or assignment is **most** appropriate?
    1. Instruct the UAP to evaluate how the mother and infant are bonding.
    2. Tell the RN to change the sharps container in the medication room.
    3. Ask the LPN to administer ibuprofen to the client experiencing afterbirth pains.
    4. Request the LPN to care for the 6-hours postpartum client after eclampsia.

28. The RN postpartum nurse instructed the UAP to provide a sitz bath to the postpartum client diagnosed with hemorrhoids. Which **priority** intervention should the nurse implement?
    1. Document the sitz bath in the client's nurse's notes.
    2. Follow up to ensure the UAP gave the sitz bath.
    3. Assess the client's hemorrhoids every 4 hours.
    4. Discuss the importance of not getting constipated.

29. Which newborn should the RN charge nurse in the nursery assign to the LPN?
    1. The 4-hour neonate born at 42 weeks
    2. The jittery and irritable 8-hour newborn
    3. The 18-hour newborn with a mother addicted to heroin
    4. The 22-hour neonate born vaginally after 2 hours of pushing

30. The client being seen in the obstetric (OB) clinic tells the nurse, "I don't think it is right that the judge is making me get a contraceptive implant just because they don't think I am a good mother." Which ethical principle does the requirement **violate**?
    1. Autonomy
    2. Justice
    3. Fidelity
    4. Beneficence

31. The client in labor is diagnosed with gestational hypertension and has preeclampsia. Which interventions should the nurse implement? **Select all that apply.**
    1. Monitor the IV magnesium sulfate.
    2. Check the client's telemetry monitor.
    3. Assess the client's deep tendon reflexes.
    4. Administer furosemide IV push (IVP).
    5. Notify the nursery when delivery is imminent or has occurred.

32. The father of a newborn infant tells the nurse excitedly, "Someone just took our baby and they removed the infant security bracelet." Which action should the nurse implement **first?**
    1. Tell the father to remain calm and return to the newborn's mother.
    2. Assign staff members to block all exits from the unit.
    3. Page a Code Pink, indicating an infant abduction.
    4. Question the father about what exactly happened in the room.

33. The client after delivering twins 3 days ago calls the women's health clinic and tells the nurse, "I am having hip pain that makes it difficult to walk." Which statement is the nurse's **best** response?
    1. "I will make you an appointment to see the HCP today."
    2. "This often occurs a few days after delivery and will disappear with time."
    3. "Make sure you perform the Kegel exercises 10 to 20 times daily."
    4. "The pain may decrease if you empty your bladder every 2 hours."

34. The 36-week gestational client has just delivered a stillborn infant. To whom should the nurse refer the client at this time?
    1. The sudden infant death syndrome (SIDS) support group
    2. The maternal-child case manager
    3. The hospital chaplain
    4. Child Protective Services

35. The client is 20 weeks pregnant and comes to the women's health clinic. The nurse notices bruises on her abdomen and back. Which response is **most** appropriate for the nurse?
    1. "Please tell me the name of your abuser."
    2. "This could cause you to lose your baby."
    3. "How did you get these bruises?"
    4. "Do you feel safe in your home?"

36. The client's partner comes to the postpartum unit and demands the girlfriend's room number. The nurse can smell alcohol on the person's breath, and they are acting erratically. Which action should the nurse implement?
    1. Explain to the client her partner is causing problems.
    2. Give the client's room number to the significant other.
    3. Contact hospital security to come to the unit.
    4. Tell the partner they cannot be here while intoxicated.

37. The nurse is caring for a Jehovah's Witness postpartum client needing a Rho(D) immune globulin injection. Which question should the nurse ask the client?
    1. "Rho(D) immune globulin is a blood product. Do you want the injection?"
    2. "Do you know what blood type your spouse has?"
    3. "Did you know that you have Rh-negative blood?"
    4. "Do you know whether your insurance will pay for the shot?"

38. The nurse is administering medications to clients on a postpartum floor. Which medication should the nurse **question** administering?
    1. The rubella vaccine to the postpartum client with a negative titer
    2. The yearly flu vaccine to a client reporting an allergy to eggs
    3. The PPD to a client with recent tuberculosis exposure concerns
    4. The hepatitis B vaccine to a breastfeeding client

39. Which client would the newborn nursery nurse assess **first** after receiving shift report?
    1. The newborn diagnosed with chignon
    2. The neonate diagnosed with caput succedaneum
    3. The newborn diagnosed with a cephalohematoma
    4. The neonate with a port-wine stain

40. Which statement indicates to the postpartum nurse the discharge teaching for the first-time mother is **effective?**
    1. "I should contact my baby's doctor if she refuses two or more feedings."
    2. "My baby will have green liquid stools for at least 1 month after I take her home."
    3. "I must administer vitamin K elixir daily with formula to my daughter."
    4. "If my daughter has thick, dark-colored stool I will call her doctor."

41. Which primigravida client should the RN clinic nurse report to the certified nurse midwife?
    1. The 12-week gestation client reporting nausea and vomiting
    2. The 24-week gestation client reporting ankle edema
    3. The 32-week gestation client reporting facial edema
    4. The 38-week gestation client reporting urinary frequency

42. The nurse is caring for a postpartum client in the "taking in" phase. Which intervention is **most** appropriate for the nurse to implement?
    1. Ask the client to demonstrate how to change the infant's diaper.
    2. Determine whether the client's blood is Rh-negative or Rh-positive.
    3. Allow the client to express feelings about the birth of her infant.
    4. Discuss the advantages of breastfeeding over bottle feeding.

43. Which data should the nurse assess on the 2-hour postpartum client who delivered vaginally? **Select all that apply.**
    1. Palpate the client's breasts.
    2. Check the client's vaginal discharge.
    3. Assess the client's pedal pulses.
    4. Inspect the client's surgical incision.
    5. Check the client's pupillary response.

44. Which interventions should the postpartum nurse teach the client who is breastfeeding her infant to avoid developing mastitis? **Select all that apply.**
    1. Clean nipples and breasts with soap before each breastfeeding.
    2. Ensure the infant latches on correctly to the breast when feeding.
    3. Apply a nipple shield between breastfeeding attempts.
    4. Perform hand washing before breastfeeding the infant.
    5. Wear a breast binder when not breastfeeding.

45. The nurse volunteering in a free clinic has cared for a female client for several weeks. The client states, "My partner and I have been trying to have a baby for 6 years. What can we do?" Which statement is the nurse's **best** response?
    1. "You should discuss your concerns with the doctor when they come in."
    2. "Infertility treatments are very expensive, and you would have to pay for it."
    3. "You are concerned because you have been unable to get pregnant."
    4. "Have you tried the rhythm method to try and conceive a child?"

46. Which client should the labor and delivery nurse assess **first** after receiving the shift report? **Rank in order of priority.**
    1. The client "needing to push," is 10 cm dilated, and 100% effaced
    2. The client exhibiting early decelerations on the fetal monitor
    3. The client hesitating about whether or not to have an epidural
    4. The upset client because her obstetrician is on vacation
    5. The client in the latent phase of labor and ambulating in the hallway

47. The nurse is caring for clients in a women's health clinic. Which client **warrants** intervention by the nurse?
    1. The pregnant client with hemoglobin and hematocrit levels of 11 g/dL and 33%.
    2. The pregnant client with a fasting blood glucose level of 100 mg/dL
    3. The pregnant client with 3+ protein in her urine
    4. The pregnant client with white blood cell count of 11.5×10^3/microL

48. The client is 1 day postpartum, and the nurse notes the fundus is displaced laterally to the right. Which nursing intervention should be implemented **first?**
    1. Prepare to perform an in-and-out catheterization.
    2. Assess the bladder using the bladder scanner.
    3. Massage the client's fundus for 2 minutes.
    4. Assist the client to the bathroom to urinate.

49. The 27-year-old female client is being scheduled for a chest x-ray. Which question should the nurse ask the client?
    1. "Have you ever had a chest x-ray before?"
    2. "Is there any chance you may be pregnant?"
    3. "When was the date of your last period?"
    4. "Do you have any allergies to shellfish?"

50. The clinical manager is reviewing hospital occurrence reports and notes that the nurse on the postpartum unit has documented three medication errors in the last 2 months. Which action should the clinical manager implement **first?**
    1. Initiate the formal counseling procedure for multiple medication errors.
    2. Continue to monitor the nurse for any further medication errors.
    3. Discuss the errors with the nurse to determine whether there is a medication system problem.
    4. Arrange for the nurse to attend a medication administration review course.

51. The nursery nurse is assessing newborns. Which newborn warrants **immediate** intervention by the nurse?
    1. The newborn remaining in the fetal position when lying supine
    2. The newborn with toes flaring out when the lateral heel is stroked
    3. The newborn turning their head toward the cheek being stroked
    4. The newborn extending their arms when hearing a loud noise

52. The client on the postpartum unit tells the nurse, "My partner thinks he is the father of my baby, but he is not. What should I tell him?" Which response supports the ethical principle of nonmaleficence?
    1. "You should tell the truth before he becomes attached to the infant."
    2. "How do you think your partner will feel knowing he is not the father?"
    3. "I know my partner would want to know whether my child was theirs or not."
    4. "Do you know what the real father is planning on doing about the baby?"

53. The hospital's chief nursing officer instructed the RN clinical manager of the postpartum unit to research a change in the care delivery system. Which statement **best** describes modular nursing?
    1. Nurses are designated the primary responsible persons for client care.
    2. The RN and UAP are assigned a group of postpartum clients.
    3. Nursing staff members are divided into groups responsible for client care.
    4. Nurses are assigned specific tasks rather than specific clients.

54. Which action by the postpartum clinical manager would be **most effective** in producing a smooth transition to the new medication delivery system?
    1. Counsel any nurses unable to adapt to the change.
    2. Ask the staff to vote on accepting the new system.
    3. Have an open-door policy to discuss the change.
    4. Send written documentation of the change by hospital e-mail.

55. During an interview, the pregnant client at the women's health clinic hesitantly tells the nurse, "I think I should let someone know that I can't stop eating dirt. I crave it all the time." Which action should the nurse implement **first**?
    1. Explain that the behavior is normal.
    2. Ask whether the client is taking the prenatal vitamins.
    3. Check the client's hemoglobin and hematocrit.
    4. Determine whether there is a history of pica in the family.

56. The client is 16 weeks pregnant and tells the office nurse, "My partner's insurance has changed, and they say I can't use you anymore." Which statement is the nurse's **best** response?
    1. "If we continue to see you, it will cost you much more money."
    2. "Because you are already pregnant your insurance company must pay."
    3. "You are concerned you don't want to change doctors now?"
    4. "Can your partner get a supplemental policy to cover this pregnancy?"

57. The 16-year-old mother of a 1-day-old infant wants her son circumcised. Which intervention should the nurse implement?
    1. Request the client's mother to sign the permit.
    2. Determine whether the insurance will pay for the procedure.
    3. Refer the client to the social worker to apply for Medicaid.
    4. Have the 16-year-old client sign for informed consent.

58. Which client should the RN newborn nurse refer to the hospital ethics committee?
    1. The anencephalic newborn with parents wanting everything done
    2. The newborn with a 16-year-old mother wanting to place the infant up for adoption
    3. The newborn with a known cocaine user mother who is positive for HIV
    4. The newborn needing a unit of blood with parents refusing consent

59. The client has delivered a 37-week gestation infant with the cord wrapped around its neck. The infant died in utero. Which interventions should the nurse implement? **Select all that apply.**
    1. Allow the mother to hold and cuddle the infant.
    2. Have the mother transferred to the medical unit.
    3. Encourage the father to talk about his child with the nurse.
    4. Recommend to the parents that the child be cremated.
    5. Discourage the client from giving the infant a name.

60. Which action would be **most** important for the RN clinical manager to take regarding a primary nurse receiving numerous compliments from clients and their families for excellent care they provide?
    1. Ask the nurse what they do that makes their care so special.
    2. Document the comments on the nurse's performance evaluation.
    3. Acknowledge the comments with a celebration on the station.
    4. Take no action because excellent care is expected by all nurses.

61. The client asks the nurse in the women's health clinic, "I am so miserable during my premenstrual syndrome I can't even go to work. What can I do?" Which teaching interventions should the nurse implement? **Select all that apply.**
    1. Increase the amount of colas and coffee daily.
    2. Avoid simple sugars such as cakes and candy.
    3. Drink at least two glasses of red wine nightly.
    4. Decrease the intake of foods high in salt.
    5. Adhere to a regular schedule for sleep.

62. The nurse is completing the admission assessment for a 12-week pregnant client visiting the women's health clinic. The client tells the nurse, "Being a vegan, I will not drink milk or eat meat." Which intervention should the nurse implement?
    1. Recommend the client eat grains, legumes, and nuts daily.
    2. Suggest that the client eat at least two eggs every day.
    3. Discuss not adhering to the vegan diet during pregnancy.
    4. Explain that a vegan diet does not require iron supplements.

63. The RN charge nurse of the postpartum unit is making assignments. Which clients should be assigned to the medical-surgical nurse assigned to the unit for the day? **Select all that apply.**
    1. The client reporting pain after delivering 4 hours ago
    2. The client being discharged and needing discharge teaching about breastfeeding
    3. The client being treated for HELLP syndrome
    4. The client on a fetal monitor at 30 weeks' gestation
    5. The client on a Pitocin drip and gravida 8

64. The labor and delivery nurse is assisting the anesthetist preparing to insert an epidural catheter in a client nearing delivery. Which picture indicates the correct position for the client?
    1. Position one

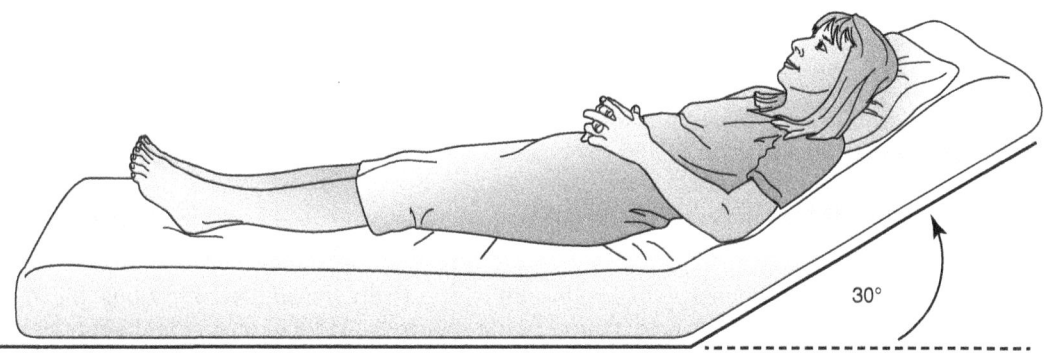

    2. Position two

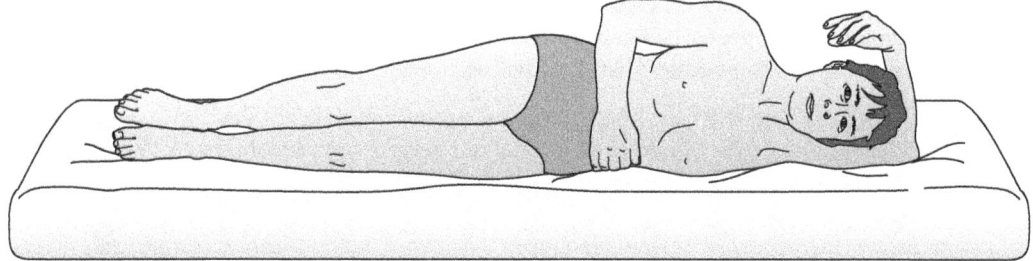

    3. Position three

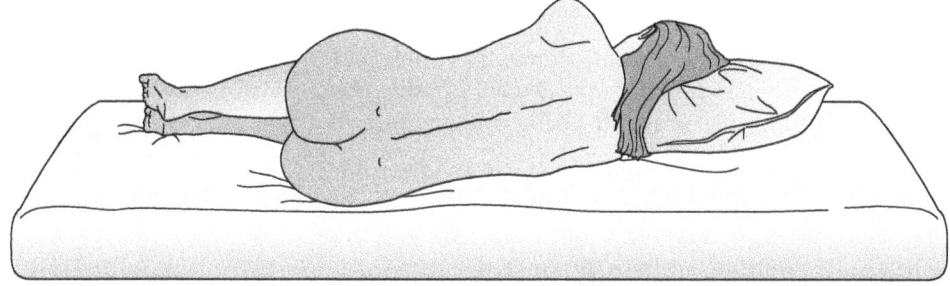

4. Position four

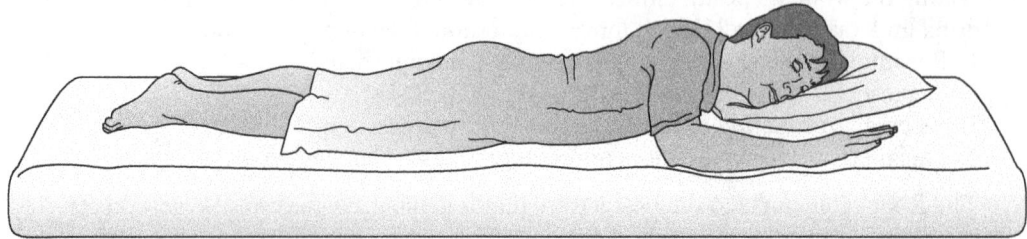

65. The 34-week pregnant client in the labor and delivery unit is on magnesium sulfate IV drip for eclampsia. The labor and delivery nurse assesses the client's reflexes as absent with repeated stimulation.

Deep Tendon Reflex Scale
0 = absent despite reinforcement
1 = present only with reinforcement
2 = normal
3 = increased but normal
4 = markedly hyperactive, with clonus

Which nursing intervention should the nurse implement **first?**
1. Notify the obstetrician.
2. Document the finding as absent.
3. Have another nurse assess the reflexes.
4. Turn off the magnesium drip.

66. The public health nurse works at the clinic for sexually transmitted infections (STIs). The female client has been diagnosed with gonorrhea. Which nursing interventions should the nurse implement? **Rank in order of performance.**
1. Notify the client's sexual partners of potential exposure to an STI.
2. Complete the report to the Centers for Disease Control and Prevention.
3. Teach the client safe sex procedures and precautions.
4. Administer the prescribed antibiotic to the client.
5. Ask the client to provide a list of sexual partners.

67. The emergency department nurse observed a motor vehicle accident on the way home from work. The driver of one of the vehicles is several months pregnant. Which nursing intervention should the nurse implement **first?**
1. Determine the length of gestation.
2. Assess the driver for signs of trauma.
3. Check to see whether the client was wearing a seat belt.
4. Monitor for fetal heart tones.

68. Which postpartum client should the charge nurse assign to the new graduate nurse?
1. The client reporting pain and with hemorrhoids
2. The client, during the night, saturated multiple peri-pads
3. The client refusing to have the newborn in the room
4. The client crying because the baby will not nurse

69. Which newborn infant would **warrant immediate** intervention by the nursery nurse?
1. The 1-hour-old newborn with tiny, white, hard spots on the nose
2. The 6-hour-old newborn with a respiratory rate of 24
3. The 12-hour-old newborn turning red and crying
4. The 18-hour-old newborn with a viscous, sticky tar, odorless stool

70. The laboring client is showing late decelerations on the fetal monitor. After placing the client in the left lateral position, which intervention should the labor and delivery nurse implement **first**?
    1. Notify the client's obstetrician immediately.
    2. Encourage the client to pant when contractions occur.
    3. Administer oxytocin intravenously.
    4. Prepare for an immediate delivery of the fetus.

71. The charge nurse is monitoring laboratory results for clients on the postpartum unit. Which client would **warrant** intervention by the postpartum nurse?
    1. The client after a vaginal delivery with a white blood cell count of 15×10^3/microL
    2. The client after a C-section with a serum potassium level of 4.8 mEq/L
    3. The client diagnosed with preeclampsia and a platelet count of 90×10^3/microL
    4. The client diagnosed with gestational diabetes and a serum glucose level of 140 mg/dL

72. The charge nurse is making assignments in the labor and delivery department. Which client should be assigned to the **most** experienced nurse?
    1. The 26-week gestational client having Braxton Hicks contractions
    2. The 32-week gestational client having twins and on bedrest
    3. The 38-week gestational client 100% effaced and 10 cm dilated
    4. The 39-week gestational client with early decelerations on the fetal monitor

73. Which task should the RN postpartum nurse delegate to the UAP?
    1. Instruct the UAP to take the client having a fundus not midline to the bathroom.
    2. Ask the UAP to take the vital signs for the client diagnosed with HELLP syndrome.
    3. Tell the UAP to assist the new mother with breastfeeding her infant daughter.
    4. Request the UAP to administer Rho(D) immune globulin to the Rh-negative mother.

74. A float nurse from the medical-surgical unit is assigned to the postpartum unit. Which client should the charge nurse assign to the float nurse?
    1. The client with a fetal demise at 34 weeks' gestation
    2. The client with a boggy fundus that massaging has not helped
    3. The client with six saturated peri-pads in the last shift
    4. The unmarried client giving her child up for adoption

75. The postpartum nurse is administering medications to clients on a postpartum floor. Which medication should the nurse **question** administering?
    1. The yearly flu vaccine to the client reporting an allergy to tomatoes
    2. The hepatitis B vaccine to a breastfeeding client
    3. The Rho(D) immune globulin to the Rh-negative mother whose infant is Rh-positive
    4. The rubella vaccine to the postpartum client with a positive titer

76. Which client should the newborn nursery nurse assess **first** after receiving the shift report?
    1. The Asian newborn with purple splotches on the lower back
    2. The Caucasian newborn with a purple area on the right side of the face
    3. The Hispanic newborn with a red rash, "flea bites," on the chest
    4. The Black newborn with edema between suture lines

77. The nursery nurse is assessing newborns. Which newborn would require **further** assessment by the nurse?
    1. The newborn remaining in the fetal position when lying supine
    2. The newborn whose toes flare out when the lateral heel is stroked
    3. The newborn acting as if they are walking when their feet are placed on a hard surface
    4. The newborn grasping the finger placed in their hand

MATERNAL-CHILD CASE STUDY

(1000) The postpartum nurse assumes care of a 37-year-old gravida 6 para 6 (G6P6) who vaginally delivered 1 hour ago, following an 8-hour labor. The client had a 4,600-g (10.1-lb) baby girl at 40 weeks' gestation.

Vital Signs	Client Values
Blood Pressure	126/78 mm Hg
Pulse	78 bpm
Respirations	20 breaths/min
Temperature	98.6°F (37°C)
SpO₂	99% (room air)

The client is alert, oriented, and cooperative. Heart rate regular, no gallops, rubs, or murmurs. Pulses 2+, capillary refill less than 3 seconds in all extremities. PERRLA. Lungs clear bilaterally. Abdomen rounded. Fundus midline, at the umbilicus, soft, and tender with pain reported as 4/10. Perineum intact, no edema. Skin warm, dry, no abrasions noted. Deep tendon reflexes (DTRs) 2+, no clonus present.

Prenatal Record:

Prenatal history: No history of tobacco, alcohol, or drug use. No known drug allergies (NKDA). No current medications. Regular prenatal care received beginning at 8 weeks' gestation. Last visit 1 week ago: BP 128/60 mm Hg, pulse 76 bpm, respirations 18 breaths/min, afebrile. Height: 65 inches (165 cm). Weight: 120 kg (265 lb); body mass index (BMI) 44.1.

Labs: Blood type O; Rh positive; rapid plasma reagin (RPR) nonreactive.

Ultrasound: At 19 weeks' gestation showed no evidence of fetal growth restriction, no fetal anomalies, the amniotic fluid volume within normal limits, and the placenta anterior and distal to the internal os.

1. **Recognize cues. What matters most?** The postpartum nurse prepares to call the obstetrician. Which **priority** client data would require follow-up by the HCP? **Select all that apply.**
    1. BP 126/78 mm Hg
    2. Fundus midline, soft, tender
    3. Heart rate 78 bpm
    4. 40 weeks' gestation
    5. G6P6
    6. 4,600-g baby
    7. O₂ saturation 99%, room air
    8. Pain 4/10
    9. RPR nonreactive
    10. BMI 44.1

2. **Analyze cues. What could it mean?** What **at-risk** issues should the nurse be concerned about the client developing? **Select three answers.**
   1. Puerperal infection
   2. Congenital syphilis
   3. Postpartum hemorrhage
   4. Thromboembolic disease
   5. Cystitis
   6. Rh isoimmunization

(1030) The postpartum nurse assesses the client, who reports an increase in pain 5/10 and a backache. The fundus is soft, 2 cm above the umbilicus and left of midline. Lochia is bright red, two perineal pads soaked. The client is drowsy and requesting the newborn to be taken to the nursery so she can sleep.

Vital Signs	Client Values
Blood Pressure	110/60 mm Hg
Pulse	99 bpm
Respirations	20 breaths/min
Temperature	100°F (37.8°C)
Spo$_2$	97% (room air)

3. **Prioritize hypotheses. Where do I start?** Complete the sentence by choosing from the drop-down list of options. Based on the client's condition at the time, the nurse recognizes that the client is at the **highest** risk for _____

   Select ▼
   1. DVT
   2. Endometritis
   3. Hemorrhage

and will require _____.

   Select ▼
   1. IV cephalosporins
   2. Crystalloid fluids
   3. Unfractionated heparin

4. **Generate solutions. What can I do?** For each intervention, specify whether the intervention is **indicated** or **not indicated** for the client's care.

Potential Nursing Intervention	Indicated	Not Indicated
Massage uterine fundus until firm.		
Obtain vital signs hourly.		
Insert catheter to empty bladder.		
Assess blood glucose before meals and at bedtime.		
Place in Trendelenburg position.		
Perform vaginal examinations hourly.		
Maintain large-bore IV access.		
Provide sips of clear liquids.		
Obtain continuous pulse oximetry readings.		

(1045) The nurse receives additional orders. The physician orders are populated in the chart.

PROVIDER ORDERS:

Oxytocin 40 units in 1,000 mL NS infuse at 50 mU/min
Methylergonovine maleate 0.2 mg IM STAT
Indwelling urinary catheter to continuous drainage
Labs: CBC, CMP, fibrinogen, PT, aPTT
Type and crossmatch for 4 units PRBCs
Hydrocodone 2.5 mg/acetaminophen 325 mg 1–2 tablets PO q 4–6 hours PRN; acetaminophen not to exceed 4 g/day

5. **Take action. What will I do?** Which provider orders should the nurse perform **right away**? **Select all that apply.**
   1. Initiate oxytocin infusion.
   2. Administer methylergonovine maleate.
   3. Insert an indwelling urinary catheter.
   4. Draw laboratory tests.
   5. Notify blood bank of type and cross.
   6. Administer hydrocodone tablets.

(1400) The obstetrician arrives, performs a bimanual massage, and removes a placental fragment. Following a new order for misoprostol, 800 mcg sublingual is administered to the client.

(1430) The client's fundus is 1 cm below umbilicus, midline, and firm to palpation. Rubra lochia is noted with a moderate amount on the perineal pad placed 30 minutes ago. The client is oriented to person, place, and time. Heart rate regular, no gallops, rubs, or murmurs. Pulses 2+, capillary refill less than 3 seconds in all extremities. PERRLA. Lungs clear bilaterally. Hypoactive bowel sounds ×4. The client rates pain as 2/10. Skin warm, dry, no abrasions noted. DTRs 2+.

Vital Signs	Client Values
Blood pressure	118/65 mm Hg
Heart rate	90 bpm
Respirations	20 breaths/min
Temperature	99.6°F (37.6°C)
Spo_2	97% (room air)

6. **Evaluate outcomes. Did it help?** For each assessment finding, indicate whether the client's condition has **improved**, **declined**, or **no change**.

Finding	Improved	Declined	No Change
Blood pressure			
Heart rate			
Spo_2			
Temperature			
Firm fundus			
Moderate rubra lochia			
DTRs			
Lungs clear bilaterally			

ANSWERS AND RATIONALES

The correct answer number and rationale are in **bold-face purple type.** Rationales for why other answer options are incorrect are provided.

1. 1. This pain may be related to an episiotomy or perineal tear, but this client is not a priority over a client who may be hemorrhaging.
   2. **Saturating multiple peri-pads indicates heavy bleeding, which may indicate hemorrhaging. The nurse should assess this client first.**
   3. The nurse needs to assess this client for possible maternal and infant bonding problems, but this is a psychosocial issue that should be addressed after a physiological issue, such as possible hemorrhaging.
   4. This client will require some time to be taught, but this is not a priority over a hemorrhaging client.

   CLINICAL JUDGMENT GUIDE: The test taker should apply a systematic approach when answering a priority question. Maslow's Hierarchy of Needs should be used when determining which client to assess first. The test taker should start at the bottom of the pyramid, and physiological needs are the priority.

2. 1. The newborn diagnosed with lanugo is normal and would not warrant immediate intervention by the nurse.
   2. The normal respiratory rate for a newborn is 30 to 60 breaths/min; therefore, this would not warrant immediate intervention.
   3. The newborn turning red when crying is not in distress; therefore, this would not warrant immediate intervention.
   4. **The newborn who has not passed meconium 24 hours after birth must be evaluated for intestinal obstruction or a congenital abnormality. This finding could be caused by an imperforate anus, Hirschsprung's disease, cystic fibrosis, or several other possibilities. This newborn warrants immediate intervention.**

   CLINICAL JUDGMENT GUIDE: When deciding which client to assess first, the test taker should determine whether the client's signs and symptoms are normal or expected for the client's situation. After eliminating the expected options, the test taker should determine which situation is more life-threatening.

3. 1. The nurse should first intervene to increase blood supply to the fetus; therefore, notifying the HCP is not the nurse's first intervention.
   2. Slow, deep breaths may help decrease the mother's anxiety, but the nurse's first intervention is to increase the blood supply to the fetus.
   3. **The left lateral position will improve the fetus's placental blood flow and oxygen supply. This should be the nurse's first intervention.**
   4. The nurse should prepare for an emergency C-section, but this is not the nurse's first intervention.

   CLINICAL JUDGMENT GUIDE: When the test taker is deciding when to notify an HCP, the test taker should look at the other three options and determine whether one of the options should be implemented before notifying the HCP. Another option may, for example, provide information the HCP will need to make a decision.

4. 1. Once the nurse determines the infant is not in the nursery, a Code Pink should be initiated. A Code Pink notifies all hospital personnel of a possible infant abduction.
   2. This will be done if the infant was not returned to the nursery, but this is not the first intervention.
   3. **The nurse should first determine whether another staff member returned the infant to the nursery. Most hospitals have infant security bracelets to prevent abduction from the hospital. The alarm has not sounded and the nurse should not call a false alarm.**
   4. There are many safety precautions to prevent infant abductions, and most facilities have a code word that is changed daily. The mother must ask anyone who wants to take the infant out of the mother's room for the code word. This is not the nurse's first intervention.

   CLINICAL JUDGMENT GUIDE: The test taker should apply the nursing process when the question asks, "Which intervention should the nurse implement first?" All answers are plausible; the test taker must identify the most critical intervention.

5. 1. The client reporting severe lower abdominal cramping should be called to determine whether she is currently menstruating, but this is not a priority over a pregnant client with symptoms of preeclampsia.
   2. **Blurred vision is a symptom of preeclampsia, and this is the client's first pregnancy. This client should be contacted first and**

343

told to come into the clinic for further evaluation.
3. The expulsion of dark-red blood clots indicates the client is going through menopause. This is not a life-threatening situation because dark red blood does not indicate frank bleeding.
4. This is uncomfortable for the client and indicates the need for a hysterectomy or instructions in the insertion and use of a pessary device to hold the uterus in place, but it is not life-threatening.

CLINICAL JUDGMENT GUIDE: When deciding which client to assess first, the test taker should determine whether the signs and symptoms the client exhibits are expected for the client's situation. After eliminating the expected options, the test taker should determine which situation is more life-threatening.

6. 1. The white blood cell count usually rises during labor and postpartum—up to $25 \times 10^3/microL$; therefore, this does not warrant intervention.
   2. The serum creatinine level is within normal limits; therefore, this client does not warrant immediate intervention.
   3. Platelets show a marked increase 3 to 5 days after birth, but the client who is 1 to 2 days postpartum would have a slightly increased platelet count. Normal platelet count is 150 to $450 \times 10^3/microL$, so this client's count is within normal limits.
   4. **This glucose level is elevated, and the nurse should investigate further to determine why the glucose level is abnormal. The normal fasting glucose level is lower than 100 mg/dL and random levels are lower than 200 mg/dL.**

CLINICAL JUDGMENT GUIDE: The test taker must be knowledgeable of laboratory data and be able to make appropriate decisions based on the information.

7. 1. **The client diagnosed with type 1 diabetes must receive insulin before eating; therefore, this must be administered first.**
   2. The stool softener will take several days to soften the stool; therefore, this medication does not need to be administered first.
   3. The client reporting a headache is not a priority over a type 1 diabetic client who needs sliding scale coverage. This client should receive medication after the insulin-dependent diabetic receives insulin.
   4. The rectal suppository is administered to shrink the hemorrhoids and has a local anesthetic effect, but it would not be a priority over the sliding scale insulin.

CLINICAL JUDGMENT GUIDE: The test taker should know which medications are a priority, such as life-sustaining medications, insulin, and mucolytics (Carafate). These medications should be administered first by the nurse.

8. 1. **A prolapsed cord is an emergency because the prolapsed cord could compromise the fetus's blood supply. Placing the client in the Trendelenburg position will cause the fetus to shift in the uterus and take the pressure off the umbilical cord. The safety of the fetus is the priority.**
   2. In emergencies, the nurse may request visitors to leave the delivery room, depending on how visitors act during the crisis, but this is not the first intervention.
   3. This is an appropriate intervention, but the nurse's priority is getting pressure off the umbilical cord.
   4. The fetus is in distress and the nurse must prepare for an emergency C-section, but it is not the nurse's first intervention.

CLINICAL JUDGMENT GUIDE: The test taker should apply the nursing process when the question asks the nurse, "Which intervention should be implemented first?" If the client is in distress, the nurse should do something. In this question, the fetus is in distress and the nurse should manipulate the mother's position to increase blood flow through the umbilical cord.

9. 1. The newborn who weighs 6 lb and 2 oz (2.8 kg) is within normal weight for a newborn; therefore, the nurse would not need to assess this baby first.
   2. **The newborn delivered at 42 weeks is postmature and is at risk for hypoglycemia and hypothermia because the placenta begins to deteriorate after 40 weeks and subcutaneous fat is utilized to support the infant's life. The nurse should assess this baby first just because of the 42-week gestation.**
   3. The newborn who is 22 inches (55.9 cm) long is longer than most infants, but this infant would not need to be assessed first.
   4. The newborn delivered at 40 weeks' gestation is within normal gestation time; therefore, the nurse would not need to assess this baby first.

CLINICAL JUDGMENT GUIDE: When deciding which client to assess first, the test taker should determine whether the client's signs and symptoms are normal for the client's situation. After eliminating the expected options, the test taker should determine which situation is more life-threatening.

10. 1. This client is preterm but is stable according to the data in the option. Terbutaline (Brethine) is a uterine relaxant and the client should be on strict bedrest.
    2. A biophysical profile is used to determine whether the fetus is ready to make the trip down the vaginal canal. Up to two points each are given for fetal breathing movements, gross body movements, fetal tone (flexion), amniotic fluid volume, and reactive (or not) nonstress test, with a score of 10 being the best.
    3. This client is ready to deliver the fetus; therefore, the most experienced nurse would not need to be assigned to this client.
    4. This client is postmature, and the fetus is at risk for meconium aspiration; therefore, this client should be assigned to the most experienced nurse.

CLINICAL JUDGMENT GUIDE: The test taker must determine the least stable client and assign this client to the most experienced nurse.

11. 1. This client needs to urinate because the number one reason for a displaced fundus is a full bladder. Because a medical nurse may not know how to palpate a fundus, this client should be assigned to a more experienced nurse.
    2. This client may be hemorrhaging and should be assigned to a more experienced nurse.
    3. This client is still at risk for a seizure, but a medical nurse should be able to care for a client who has a seizure. This client should be assigned to the medical nurse.
    4. This nurse must evaluate the mother's ability to care for the new infant or complete discharge teaching; therefore, a more experienced nurse should be assigned to this client.

CLINICAL JUDGMENT GUIDE: The test taker must determine which client is most stable or may be at risk for a complication a medical nurse could care for safely.

12. 1. The client should be in the fetal position, but the possibility of anesthesia ascending the spinal cord is the priority.
    2. If the anesthesia ascends the spinal cord, the client will quit breathing; therefore, this is the priority intervention.
    3. The client should be prehydrated, but it is not a priority over the airway.
    4. Clients are made NPO to prevent aspiration pneumonia secondary to vomiting if the client is undergoing general anesthesia, not epidural anesthesia.

CLINICAL JUDGMENT GUIDE: The test taker should apply Maslow's Hierarchy of Needs. Airway is the priority. Remember that priority intervention means all the options are something the RN can implement, but there is only one correct option.

13. 1. Nothing in the question's stem suggests the client has an infant. It is a question the nurse could ask the female client, but it is not a priority.
    2. This is a question the nurse could ask the client, but because the question states the client is a 28-year-old female, age and gender are pertinent to which option the test taker should select.
    3. This is a question all clients should be asked, but the adjectives describing the client as "a 28-year-old" and "female" should identify the fourth option as the most priority question.
    4. Because the client will have to have anesthesia for the surgery and is within childbearing age, the nurse should determine whether the client is pregnant.

CLINICAL JUDGMENT GUIDE: The test taker must acknowledge adjectives in questions when determining the correct answer. When the stem gives the client a gender and an age, it is pertinent to the correct answer.

14. 1. Normal fetal heart rate is 110 to 160 bpm, so this client is stable.
    2. Nonreassuring fetal heart rate patterns indicate the fetus is in danger, which requires a more experienced nurse.
    3. A scheduled C-section is a stable client, so a less experienced nurse could care for this client.
    4. Pushing for 1 hour before a vaginal birth is normal; therefore, a less experienced nurse could care for this client.

CLINICAL JUDGMENT GUIDE: The most experienced nurse should be assigned to the most critical client. Nonreassuring fetal heart patterns indicate the infant is in distress.

15. 1. The RN should first assess the client to determine whether the UAP was negligent in reporting before talking to the UAP.
    2. This client may or may not be experiencing excessive bleeding, but the nurse's first intervention is to assess the client.
    3. Excessive bleeding could indicate the uterus is boggy, which would require the RN to massage the uterus. This assessment and intervention cannot be delegated to a UAP.
    4. The nurse should not document any information before verifying the client's situation.

    CLINICAL JUDGMENT GUIDE: Any time the nurse receives information from another staff member about a client who may be experiencing a complication, the nurse must assess the client. The nurse should not make decisions about the client's needs based on another staff member's information.

16. 1. The infant should be securely swaddled in a blanket to maintain body heat.
    2. The UAP should wear nonsterile gloves when exposed to blood or body fluids.
    3. When bathing a newborn, soap is not necessary. Soap can dry the skin; therefore, this action warrants intervention by the nurse.
    4. The UAP should wipe the crib with disinfectant to decrease the potential for contamination.

    CLINICAL JUDGMENT GUIDE: When the question asks, "Which warrants immediate intervention?" it is an "except" question. Three actions are appropriate for the UAP, and one is incorrect.

17. 1. Braxton Hicks contractions are irregular contractions of the uterus throughout the pregnancy and are not true labor. This client would not need to be assigned to the most experienced nurse.
    2. The client having triplets on bedrest is not in imminent danger; therefore, this client would not need the most experienced nurse.
    3. This client is progressing normally and would not require the most experienced nurse.
    4. Late decelerations on the fetal monitor indicate fetal distress; this is a life-threatening situation, and an emergency C-section may be necessary. The charge nurse should assign the most experienced nurse to this client.

    CLINICAL JUDGMENT GUIDE: The test taker must determine which client is the most unstable and assign this client to the most experienced nurse.

18. Correct answers are 1 and 5.
    1. The UAP can provide hygiene care to the client. A sitz bath requires the UAP to check the temperature of the water and does not require nursing judgment.
    2. The UAP's primary responsibility is direct client care. The unit secretary, not the UAP, should call the laboratory.
    3. The RN cannot delegate teaching to the UAP.
    4. The RN cannot delegate assessment; therefore, the UAP cannot check the client's fundus.
    5. The UAP can take the meal tray to the client.

    CLINICAL JUDGMENT GUIDE: This is an alternate type of question included in the NCLEX-RN®. The RN must be able to select all the options that answer the question correctly. There are no partially correct answers. Remember, the nurse cannot delegate assessment, evaluation, teaching, administration of medications, or care of an unstable client to a UAP.

19. 1. A client diagnosed with mastitis who is trying to breastfeed requires a nurse experienced in the postpartum unit who can teach the client about breastfeeding and assess for complications.
    2. This routine surgical procedure would not require the nurse to have any specialized postpartum experience. For this client, it would be most appropriate to assign the float nurse with experience in the medical-surgical unit.
    3. A client who is having difficulty bonding would require a nurse with experience in the postpartum unit to care for the client and document pertinent information if bonding does not occur.
    4. There are many legal issues surrounding adoption as well as caring for the mother who is giving up her child; this client should be assigned a nurse more experienced in postpartum care.

    CLINICAL JUDGMENT GUIDE: The test taker must determine which client requires the least specialized knowledge and assign the float nurse to that client. Legal issues, teaching, and psychosocial concepts require the more experienced nurse.

20. 1. An experienced nurse, a chaplain, or social worker should be assigned to sit with the family during this crisis.
    2. Even though the UAP is not administering the medication, the UAP should not

be handling the RN medication in a crisis situation.
3. The UAP cannot assist with intubation; this must be assigned to a registered nurse or respiratory therapist.
4. **The UAP can stand by and be ready to obtain any supplies needed for the code. This would be a most appropriate task to delegate in an emergency.**

CLINICAL JUDGMENT GUIDE: The RN cannot delegate assessment, teaching, evaluation, medications, or an unstable client to a UAP. Tasks that cannot be delegated are nursing interventions that require nursing judgment.

21. 1. Volunteers are often asked to rock irritable infants so that the nurse can have more time to perform higher-level nursing care. This action would not warrant immediate intervention by the charge nurse.
    2. The nurse is using palpation to determine whether the newborn has a cleft palate. This assessment is within the scope of practice for the newborn nursery nurse.
    3. **The Ortolani maneuver is performed to assess developmental hip dysplasia. Only a pediatrician or a nurse practitioner should perform this maneuver because it can cause further damage if done incorrectly.**
    4. The LPN can bathe a newborn infant; therefore, this would not warrant immediate intervention by the RN charge nurse.

CLINICAL JUDGMENT GUIDE: When the question asks, "Which warrants immediate intervention?" it is an "except" question. Three of the actions are appropriate, whereas one action is not.

22. 1. This client cannot urinate, which may or may not be a complication of the delivery and anesthesia. Catheterization is a sterile procedure, and many facilities do not allow the UAP to perform sterile procedures. The RN should not delegate this task.
    2. This is teaching, and the RN cannot delegate teaching to the UAP.
    3. **The infant must be transported in a car safety seat. The UAP can determine whether there is a car seat and take the appropriate action if there is not one.**
    4. Anesthetic foam is a topical medication, and the RN cannot delegate medication administration to the UAP.

CLINICAL JUDGMENT GUIDE: The RN cannot delegate assessment, evaluation, teaching, medications, or an unstable client to a UAP.

23. 1. The more pregnancies the client has had, the more likely it will be that the uterus will not contract to prevent bleeding. The RN should be assigned to this client.
    2. A client diagnosed with a fever and a surgical incision may be experiencing a complication and should be assigned to an RN.
    3. Foul-smelling lochia indicates the client has an infection; therefore, this client should not be assigned to the LPN.
    4. **The ambulating client is stable and has no complications; therefore, this client should be assigned to the LPN.**

CLINICAL JUDGMENT GUIDE: The test taker must determine which client is the most stable, which makes this an "except" question. Three clients are either unstable or have potentially life-threatening conditions.

24. 1. **The Joint Commission and safety standards mandate that all hospital personnel check the parent's ID band with the infant's ID band before releasing the infant to the mother's or father's care.**
    2. The UAP can bring diapers to the mother; therefore, this would not warrant immediate intervention.
    3. The UAP can put lotion on the infant while the mother watches because this is not teaching.
    4. This may be teaching, but the UAP ensures the newborn is safe; therefore, this action would not warrant immediate intervention.

CLINICAL JUDGMENT GUIDE: When the question asks, "Which warrants immediate intervention?" it is an "except" question. Three of the actions are appropriate, whereas one action is not.

25. Correct answers are 1, 2, and 4.
    1. The UAP can take vital signs on a stable client.
    2. The UAP can pass out breakfast trays.
    3. Rho(D) immune globulin (RhoGAM) is a medication that cannot be delegated to the UAP.
    4. The UAP can remove an indwelling urinary catheter. It is not a medication.
    5. The UAP should not assist with breastfeeding. The RN must perform teaching and evaluate breastfeeding.

CLINICAL JUDGMENT GUIDE: The RN cannot delegate assessment, teaching, evaluation, medication, or an unstable client to a UAP.

26. 1. Ice packs are applied to acute injuries, so this intervention is appropriate for the UAP.
    2. Only the client pushes the PCA (patient-controlled analgesia) pump; therefore, this action requires immediate intervention by the nurse.
    3. Using nonsterile gloves is appropriate when handling blood and body fluids, so this intervention is appropriate for the UAP.
    4. The UAP can encourage a client to eat the food on the breakfast tray; therefore, this behavior does not warrant immediate intervention.

CLINICAL JUDGMENT GUIDE: The phrase "warrants immediate intervention" means one of the options is inappropriate for the UAP to perform or the UAP is performing the task inappropriately.

27. 1. The UAP cannot assess, teach, evaluate, administer medications, or care for an unstable client.
    2. A housekeeper, a UAP, or an LPN can change the sharps container, which is not an appropriate task to assign to the RN.
    3. The LPN can administer medications, and ibuprofen has an antiprostaglandin effect that is appropriate for a client experiencing afterbirth pains.
    4. The RN charge nurse should not assign an LPN to an unstable client. This client may have another seizure and should be monitored closely for at least 24 to 48 hours postdelivery.

CLINICAL JUDGMENT GUIDE: The RN must know what can be delegated and assigned to the UAP and LPN. There will be numerous questions on the NCLEX-RN® concerning delegation and assignment. Remember that the nurse may not delegate the following to the UAP: assessment, teaching, evaluation, administering medications, or caring for an unstable client.

28. 1. The RN should document the sitz bath, but it is not a priority over ensuring the UAP gave the sitz bath.
    2. The most critical intervention for the nurse when delegating a task is to follow up to ensure it is done.
    3. The RN should assess the client, but the priority intervention is to ensure the UAP completes the assigned task.
    4. The nurse should ensure the client does not get constipated, but the test taker must read the question's stem to determine how to answer it correctly.

CLINICAL JUDGMENT GUIDE: When the question asks which option is the priority intervention, it means one or more of the options are something a nurse can implement. The test taker must determine what the question is asking to select the right answer. There is always something in the question stem that will help the test taker choose the correct option.

29. 1. This newborn is postmature and may have complications, so she should be assigned to an RN.
    2. The newborn is experiencing hypoglycemia and should be assigned to an RN.
    3. The newborn is at risk for going through heroin withdrawal and should be assigned to an RN.
    4. The newborn born vaginally after 2 hours of labor is stable and should be assigned to the LPN.

CLINICAL JUDGMENT GUIDE: The test taker must decide which newborn is the most stable and which is the most critical. Once the test taker makes this decision, the most stable newborn should be assigned to the LPN.

30. 1. This requirement violates the client's autonomy, which is a client's right to self-determination without outside control. This approach has been used as a condition of probation, to allow women accused of child abuse or neglect to get out of a jail term.
    2. Justice is the duty to treat all clients fairly, regardless of age, socioeconomic status, and other variables.
    3. Fidelity is the duty to be faithful to commitments.
    4. Beneficence is the duty to do good actively for the clients.

CLINICAL JUDGMENT GUIDE: The nurse must be aware of ethical principles that guide nursing and healthcare practices. The judge is acting under legal guidelines that can supersede the client's rights.

31. Correct answers are 1, 3, and 5.
    1. Magnesium sulfate, a uterine relaxant, is the drug of choice to help prevent seizures. The medication relaxes smooth muscles and reduces vasoconstriction, thus promoting circulation to the mother's vital organs and increasing placental circulation to the fetus.
    2. The mother is not placed on telemetry, but continuous electronic fetal monitoring is required to identify fetal heart rate patterns that suggest fetal compromise.

3. The deep tendon reflexes are monitored to evaluate for magnesium sulfate toxicity.
4. After delivery, the mother will excrete large volumes of fluid, a sign of recovery from preeclampsia. However, the loop diuretic furosemide (Lasix) would not be given before delivery because it may lead to hypovolemia.
5. The nursery should be notified of the delivery to prepare for the neonate. Because the client is in labor, the baby will be born within a reasonable time frame.

CLINICAL JUDGMENT GUIDE: This is an alternate format type of question included in the NCLEX-RN® examination. The nurse must be able to select all the options that answer the question correctly. There are no partially correct answers.

32. 1. The nurse should encourage the father to remain calm for his wife in this crisis, but this is not the first intervention.
    2. Assigning staff members is part of the Code Pink protocol but is not the nurse's first intervention.
    3. **The nurse's first intervention is to call a Code Pink. Then, the nurse should institute all other nursing interventions. The infant's safety is the priority.**
    4. The nurse should question the father for exact details, but the nurse should first call the Code Pink to find the person who took the infant.

CLINICAL JUDGMENT GUIDE: The nurse is responsible for knowing and complying with hospital protocols and the local, state, and federal standards of care.

33. 1. This pain is normal and does not require seeing the HCP today.
    2. **During the first few days after delivery, hormone levels and the ligaments and cartilage of the pelvis return to their prepregnancy position. These changes cause hip and joint pain that interferes with ambulation. The mother should understand that the pain is temporary and does not indicate a problem.**
    3. Kegel exercises tone up the client's peritoneal muscles after pregnancy. These exercises would not help hip and joint pain.
    4. Emptying the bladder will not help the client's joint and hip pain.

CLINICAL JUDGMENT GUIDE: The test taker should know the physiological process of pregnancy and postpartum care and provide factual information to the client.

34. 1. SIDS occurs among infants who are living, not fetuses in utero.
    2. The case manager coordinates care between disciplines for clients diagnosed with chronic illnesses. This client has lost a baby and would not need a referral to a case manager.
    3. **According to the NCLEX-RN® test plan, management of care includes appropriate use of referrals. The chaplain is responsible for intervening in a case where there is spiritual distress. The loss of a child is devastating.**
    4. Child Protective Services (CPS) are notified only if the child is being abused. This baby died in utero; therefore, CPS would not be notified, except in states where the mother is a drug abuser or has chronic alcoholism.

CLINICAL JUDGMENT GUIDE: The nurse must be knowledgeable about referrals and implement the referral to the most appropriate person or agency.

35. 1. This statement makes the assumption the client is being abused—which is probably true—but the nurse should not put words in the client's mouth. Because this is a legal issue, the nurse cannot suggest in any manner to the client that verbal or physical abuse is occurring. If the client is being abused and decides to file charges, then the accused can use the defense that, indeed, this is not abuse and that the client decided to consider the actions as abuse only after the nurse suggested it.
    2. This statement is true but judgmental and would not encourage a therapeutic relationship with the client.
    3. Research indicates that abusive situations escalate during pregnancy, particularly with the woman being hit in the abdominal area; therefore, this question is not necessary. These bruises suggest that abuse is occurring.
    4. **The nurse's best intervention is to assess the safety of the client and infant and provide information to the client about a safe haven.**

CLINICAL JUDGMENT GUIDE: The nurse is responsible for knowing and complying with local, state, and federal standards of care.

36. 1. The nurse should not upset the client by telling her that her partner is creating problems.
    2. The nurse should not allow a person displaying this behavior to remain on the unit.

3. The nurse should first contact hospital security to intervene and escort the partner off the unit.
4. Confronting a drunken individual could escalate the situation. The nurse should contact security to take care of this situation.

CLINICAL JUDGMENT GUIDE: There will be legal and management questions on the NCLEX-RN®. In many instances, there is no test-taking strategy; the nurse should protect the safety of the client.

37. 1. Jehovah's Witnesses do not believe in accepting blood products, but it is the individual's choice. The nurse is a client advocate and should make sure the client is aware that without the injection, her next pregnancy could result in erythroblastosis fetalis. However, with the injection, her religious belief may be compromised because Rho(D) immune globulin (RhoGAM) is a blood product.
    2. The baby's father must be Rh-positive; otherwise, the baby would not be Rh-positive, and the mother would not require the Rho(D) immune globulin (RhoGAM) injection. The baby's blood type determines whether the mother needs the RhoGAM injection.
    3. This question is not pertinent when administering RhoGAM to the client. Rho(D) immune globulin (RhoGAM) is prescribed only for Rh-negative mothers who have Rh-positive babies or within 72 hours of a miscarriage.
    4. The client's insurance status is not pertinent information for the nurse caring for the client.

CLINICAL JUDGMENT GUIDE: Any time there is a cultural or religious factor in the question, the test taker should know that this will affect the correct answer.

38. 1. The nurse would not question administering this medication because a negative titer means the client is not immune to rubella (German measles). This vaccine prevents rubella infection and possible severe congenital disabilities in a fetus in a subsequent pregnancy.
    2. The flu vaccine is made using egg-based technology; therefore, the nurse should question the administration of this vaccine to a client who is allergic to eggs.
    3. A positive PPD (purified protein derivative) test determines whether the client was exposed to tuberculosis.
    4. The nurse would not question administering the hepatitis B vaccine to a breastfeeding mother because 1-day-old infants receive the vaccine.

CLINICAL JUDGMENT GUIDE: The nurse must be aware of the indications for specific medications, appropriate interventions when administering medications, and adverse side effects that can occur from medications. This is a knowledge-based question.

39. 1. A chignon is newborn scalp edema created by vacuum extraction and will resolve within a few days of delivery. This infant would not need to be assessed first.
    2. Caput succedaneum appears over the vertex of the newborn's head because of pressure against the mother's cervix during labor. The edematous area crosses suture lines, is soft, and varies in size. It resolves quickly and disappears within 12 hours to several days after birth. This newborn would not need to be seen first.
    3. A cephalohematoma results when there is bleeding between the periosteum and the skull from pressure during birth. The firm swelling is absent at birth but develops within 24 to 48 hours. Any time a client is bleeding, it warrants intervention by the nurse.
    4. A port-wine stain, nevus flammeus, is a permanent, flat, reddish purple mark that varies in size and location and does not blanch with pressure. This would not require immediate intervention from the nurse.

CLINICAL JUDGMENT GUIDE: When deciding which client to assess first, the test taker should determine which conditions or signs and symptoms the client is exhibiting are expected for the client's situation. After eliminating the expected option, the test taker should determine which situation is more life-threatening.

40. 1. Refusal of two or more feedings indicates the infant has a problem that requires the mother to notify the HCP. This indicates the mother understands the discharge teaching.
    2. Green liquid stool indicates a problem and requires the mother to notify the HCP.
    3. Vitamin K is administered intramuscularly to the infant in the newborn nursery to prevent the infant from bleeding. The gastrointestinal tract is sterile when the infant is born and requires bacteria to synthesize vitamin K from the food eaten by the infant.

4. The infant will have meconium stool for a few days after birth, so the mother should not notify the HCP.

CLINICAL JUDGMENT GUIDE: When the question asks, "Which statement indicates the teaching is effective?" the test taker must select the option with the correct information.

41. 1. Nausea and vomiting are typical for a 12-week gestation client.
    2. Ankle edema is expected in a 24-week gestation client.
    3. **Facial edema is a sign of gestational hypertension requiring the clinic nurse to contact the certified nurse midwife.**
    4. The increasing size of the uterus compresses the bladder, leading to increased frequency of urination, so this is an expected finding.

CLINICAL JUDGMENT GUIDE: The test taker should ask, "Is it normal for this client?" For example, "Is it normal for the 12-week gestation client to have nausea and vomiting?" If this is normal, the nurse would not need to notify anyone of this finding.

42. 1. The "taking in" phase is the first phase the mother goes through after the delivery. The mother is not ready to learn or be taught anything in this phase.
    2. This nursing intervention is not part of the "taking in" phase.
    3. **During the "taking in" phase, the client is self-absorbed and needs to be cared for, so allowing the client to talk about her own experience is the most appropriate intervention.**
    4. The client in the "taking in" phase is not ready to learn or be taught anything.

CLINICAL JUDGMENT GUIDE: The test taker must know the "taking in" phase and apply the knowledge appropriately. Remembering information is not the same as being able to apply the information.

43. Correct answers are 1 and 2.
    1. **The breasts should be palpated to assess for fullness or engorgement.**
    2. **The nurse should check for the amount, color, and consistency of vaginal discharge.**
    3. The nurse should assess for deep vein thrombosis (DVT), but this does not include assessing pedal pulses.
    4. The client, following a vaginal delivery, will not have a surgical incision.
    5. The nurse does not need to check the pupillary response for a postpartum client; this would be appropriate for a client diagnosed with a neurological disorder.

CLINICAL JUDGMENT GUIDE: This is an alternate type of question included in the NCLEX-RN®. The nurse must be able to select all the options that answer the question correctly. There are no partially correct answers. The key to the assessment data is a "postpartum" client.

44. Correct answers are 2 and 4.
    1. Soap will dry out the nipples, which can cause cracking and openings in the skin for possible bacterial entry.
    2. **Mastitis results from bacterial invasion of the breast tissue from cracks or fissures in the nipples, overdistention of the breasts, or milk stasis. These issues can be avoided by frequent breastfeeding with the proper technique.**
    3. Nipple shields are used for inverted nipples, not mastitis prevention.
    4. **Hands can carry bacteria such as *Staphylococcus aureus* and *Escherichia coli* that can cause mastitis; therefore, hand washing should be performed to reduce the risks.**
    5. A breast binder is utilized for lactation suppression, not to reduce the risk of mastitis.

CLINICAL JUDGMENT GUIDE: This is an alternate type of question included in the NCLEX-RN®. The nurse must be able to select all the options that answer the question correctly. There are no partially correct answers.

45. 1. The HCP in a free clinic could not refer this client to an infertility clinic because of cost. The nurse can discuss this with the client.
    2. **If the couple cannot conceive in 6 years, then a referral to an infertility clinic would be appropriate. Still, the tests and treatment for infertility are costly. The client is being seen in a free clinic, which indicates a lack of funds. The nurse has a relationship with this client over the period of "several weeks." The nurse should answer the client's question.**
    3. This therapeutic response does not answer the client's question, "What can we do?"
    4. If the client has not conceived in 6 years, this is not a probable solution to the client's concern.

CLINICAL JUDGMENT GUIDE: The test taker should know the physiological process of pregnancy and infertility and provide factual information to the client.

46. The correct order is 1, 2, 3, 5, 4.
    1. The client who is 10 cm dilated, 100% effaced, and "needing to push" is ready to deliver the fetus; therefore, the nurse should assess this client first.
    2. Early decelerations are not associated with fetal compromise but indicate head compression. The nurse should assess this client second to determine whether delivery is imminent.
    3. This client does not have an immediate need, although epidurals are offered to clients in active labor; therefore, the nurse should assess this client third.
    5. The latent phase of labor is early labor when cervical dilation is 3 cm or less. This client is stable and ambulating but should be assessed fourth.
    4. Although this information is causing distress to the mother, there is nothing the nurse can do about this situation. The on-call obstetrician or certified nurse midwife will have to deliver the fetus. This client should be assessed fifth.

CLINICAL JUDGMENT GUIDE: This is an alternate type of question included in the NCLEX-RN®. The nurse must be able to determine the order to assess clients.

47. 1. The pregnant client has an increased circulating blood volume, which slightly decreases the hemoglobin and hematocrit; therefore, this client would not warrant intervention.
     2. The normal fasting blood glucose level is lower than 100 mg/dL; therefore, this client does not warrant intervention by the nurse.
     3. Protein in the urine indicates the client is at risk for gestational hypertension; therefore, this client warrants intervention and further assessment by the nurse.
     4. The white blood cell count increases during pregnancy; the normal range is 5 to 12×10^3/microL and rises during labor. This client does not warrant intervention.

CLINICAL JUDGMENT GUIDE: The nurse must be knowledgeable of normal laboratory values. These values must be memorized and the nurse must be able to determine whether the laboratory value is normal for the client's disease process or medications the client is taking.

48. 1. If the client is unable to urinate, then the nurse will have to perform an in-and-out catheterization to empty the bladder. However, the nurse should implement the least invasive intervention.
     2. The nurse could use a bladder scanner to determine whether the bladder is full, but the first intervention is to ask the client to urinate.
     3. Massaging the fundus will not put the fundus in a midline position until the bladder is empty.
     4. A full bladder is the most common reason for a displaced fundus. The nurse should always do the least invasive procedure, asking the client to attempt to void. Emptying the bladder should allow the fundus to return to the midline position.

CLINICAL JUDGMENT GUIDE: The nurse must know the expected medical treatment for a client. This is a knowledge-based question.

49. 1. The nurse does not need to know when the client had her last chest x-ray when scheduling this chest x-ray.
     2. The nurse should ask whether the client may be pregnant because if there is a chance of pregnancy, the client should not have an x-ray. Any time a female client is of childbearing age and has any x-ray, this question should be asked.
     3. The date of the client's last period would not affect the client's having a chest x-ray.
     4. This question would be asked if the client was receiving some type of contrast or dye.

CLINICAL JUDGMENT GUIDE: The test taker must know about diagnostic tests and client screening before the procedure. This is a knowledge-based question.

50. 1. The clinical manager should first talk to the nurse to determine what is causing the medication error.
     2. Three medication errors in a short period require the clinical manager to investigate the cause.
     3. This should be the clinical manager's first intervention to assess whether the system is responsible for the medication errors or whether it is a nursing error problem. For example, a system error problem would be when the medication is unavailable at the prescribed time.
     4. This may be needed but is not the clinical manager's first intervention. If the clinical manager determines the nurse is at fault, this is a possible action.

CLINICAL JUDGMENT GUIDE: The nurse needs to know management issues for the NCLEX-RN® and appropriate interventions.

51. 1. When the infant is placed supine, the infant should extend the arm and leg on the side to which the head is turned and then flex the extremities on the other. This is known as the tonic-neck reflex or fencing reflex, which is normal for the newborn. The newborn remaining in a fetal position when supine warrants further intervention to assess for neurological problems.
    2. The Babinski reflex is elicited by stroking the lateral sole of the foot from the heel forward. Normal reflexes are the toes flare outward and the big toe dorsiflexes. This is a normal response for an infant but is abnormal in an adult, indicating neurological deficit in the adult. Therefore, this does not warrant immediate intervention.
    3. This is the rooting reflex, which is normal for a newborn. This would not warrant immediate intervention.
    4. The Moro reflex or the startle reflex is a sharp extension and abduction of the arm with thumbs and forefingers in a C-position followed by flexion and adduction to embrace position. This response occurs with loud noise or when the newborn is startled. This would not warrant immediate intervention.

CLINICAL JUDGMENT GUIDE: When the question asks which client warrants "immediate intervention" it is an "except" question. Three of the clients exhibit normal responses, whereas one does not.

52. 1. This is the ethical principle of veracity, which is truth-telling.
    2. Nonmaleficence is the duty to do no harm. Many ethicists think that the principle of nonmaleficence has priority over other ethical principles except for autonomy. Nonmaleficence allows the nurse to answer a question or make a decision that does not create further complications for the client.
    3. This is paternalism, which gives advice and tells the client what is best for her.
    4. This assessment question could guide the nurse in helping the client make a decision, but it does not demonstrate the ethical principle of nonmaleficence.

CLINICAL JUDGMENT GUIDE: The NCLEX-RN® test plan describes nursing care that addresses ethical principles, including autonomy, beneficence, justice, veracity, and others.

53. 1. This statement describes primary care, a type of nursing care delivery.
    2. Modular nursing is frequently called care pairs, in which nurses are paired with lesser-trained caregivers to provide nursing care to a group of clients.
    3. This statement describes team nursing, which is a type of nursing care delivery.
    4. This statement describes functional nursing, in which there is a charge nurse, a medication nurse, and a treatment nurse.

CLINICAL JUDGMENT GUIDE: Management and research questions will be on the NCLEX-RN®. In many instances, there is no test-taking strategy for these questions.

54. 1. Threatening and attempting to manipulate the staff will create distrust and anger, which will not facilitate a smooth transition for the medication delivery system.
    2. This action is unfair because the new system is being implemented whether the staff members vote for it or not. Some situations, resulting from financial or other constraints, require the clinical manager to implement a change without the staff's input.
    3. To be an effective change agent, the manager must develop trust, establish common goals, and facilitate effective communication.
    4. Sending the documentation by hospital e-mail is pertinent to ensure all staff members receive the information. Still, it is ineffective in producing a smooth transition and reducing resistance to change.

CLINICAL JUDGMENT GUIDE: Management and research questions will be on the NCLEX-RN®. In many instances, there is no test-taking strategy for these questions.

55. 1. This behavior may be normal for some individuals and may not be detrimental to the infant or mother, but the nurse must investigate the situation first before making this statement.
    2. Clay and dirt in the gut may decrease the absorption of nutrients such as iron. Therefore, asking this question is appropriate, but the first intervention should be to determine whether complications are related to pica.
    3. Pica, ingesting substances not normally considered food, may decrease food intake

and, therefore, essential nutrients. Iron deficiency was once thought to cause pica but is now considered a result. Before further action is taken, the nurse must first assess whether the behavior is detrimental to the mother or infant.
  4. Pica may be related to cultural beliefs about materials that will ensure a healthy mother and infant. This should not be the nurse's first intervention. The safety of the mother and fetus is the priority. If the H&H are within normal limits, the nurse should support the cultural belief.

CLINICAL JUDGMENT GUIDE: The test taker should apply the nursing process when the question asks, "Which action should the nurse implement first?" If the client is in distress, do something. In this case, the test taker should select an option that directly assesses the client's condition.

56. 1. **Insurance companies contract with specific providers to provide care to the client at a reduced rate. Using this doctor, who is not a preferred provider of care, will result in a more significant out-of-pocket expense for the client.**
  2. This is not a true statement, and the nurse should not give the client false information, especially about money.
  3. This therapeutic response is to encourage the client to vent feelings. This client needs factual information.
  4. Some insurance companies will not cover a preexisting condition for 1 year after the policy is initiated; therefore, this pregnancy may not be covered.

CLINICAL JUDGMENT GUIDE: The nurse should be aware of insurance guidelines to provide factual information to the client.

57. 1. The 16-year-old client must sign for her child's care. The grandmother has no authority to sign informed consent for the procedure.
  2. The procedure cost should not be a factor for the nurse when discussing a medical procedure with the client.
  3. The client is not requesting assistance to pay the medical bills; therefore, this intervention is inappropriate.
  4. **A 16-year-old mother has the right to make decisions for her child; therefore, the mother must sign the informed consent for the procedure.**

CLINICAL JUDGMENT GUIDE: The test taker should know legal rights and responsibilities and understand best practices for obtaining informed consent.

58. 1. **Anencephaly is a congenital abnormality that entails an absence of all or a major part of the brain. The infant has no chance of life outside a healthcare institution. The healthcare team refers situations to the ethics committee to help resolve dilemmas when caring for clients.**
  2. This is not an ethical dilemma because the 16-year-old client has a right to place her infant up for adoption. This situation would not need to be referred to an ethics committee.
  3. If the nurse wants to take the child away from the mother, then this must be reported to Child Protective Services. Therefore, this is not an ethical dilemma. The nurse has a law that directs the decision. This situation would not need to be referred to an ethics committee.
  4. This is a legal issue, not an ethical issue. The healthcare team can request the hospital attorney to take these parents to court and request a court order to administer blood. The parents do not have the right to refuse life-sustaining treatment for their child.

CLINICAL JUDGMENT GUIDE: The NCLEX-RN® test plan identifies that the nurse must know ethical practices, recognize ethical dilemmas, and take appropriate actions.

59. Correct answers are 1, 2, and 3.
  1. The mother should be encouraged to hold and cuddle the infant to help with grieving.
  2. The mother should not be required to stay on a unit where she can hear crying infants and happy families. The nurse should transfer the client to another unit.
  3. The nurse should remember the father has lost the baby, too. Acknowledging and encouraging the father to talk about the loss will help with the grieving process.
  4. The nurse's beliefs about funerals should not be imposed on the client. This is a boundary-crossing violation.
  5. Grief support groups recommend giving the infant a name because it acknowledges the infant's existence.

CLINICAL JUDGMENT GUIDE: This is an alternate format type of question included in the NCLEX-RN® examination. The nurse must be able to select all the options that answer the question correctly. There are no partially correct answers.

60. 1. The clinical manager could ask the primary nurse why she provides such excellent care, but it is not the most important action. Excellence in care should be documented in writing in the nurse's personnel file to support merit raises, transfers, and promotions.
    2. The clinical manager should recognize the comments of clients and families during the performance evaluation. Excellence in care should be documented in writing in the nurse's personnel file to support merit raises, transfers, and promotions. Many healthcare facilities have employee recognition programs.
    3. This is a possible action, but this could single out the nurse and cause dissension among the other staff. Parties on the unit should celebrate the unit's accomplishments, not a single individual.
    4. Excellent care is expected of all primary nurses, but when multiple clients and families recognize the nurse's care, there should be documentation in the nurse's personnel file.

CLINICAL JUDGMENT GUIDE: Management and research questions will be on the NCLEX-RN®. In many instances, there is no test-taking strategy for these questions.

61. Correct answers are 2, 4, and 5.
    1. The client should decrease the amount of caffeine, which includes coffee, tea, cola, and chocolate because caffeine increases irritability, insomnia, anxiety, and nervousness.
    2. Avoiding simple sugars will prevent rebound hypoglycemia and exacerbation of the signs and symptoms of premenstrual syndrome (PMS).
    3. Alcohol is a central nervous system depressant and aggravates the depression associated with PMS. This is not an appropriate intervention.
    4. Decreasing salt intake will decrease fluid retention, thereby decreasing edema.
    5. Insomnia is a symptom of PMS, and a regular sleep schedule will help decrease the severity of PMS.

CLINICAL JUDGMENT GUIDE: This is an alternate format type of question included in the NCLEX-RN® examination. The nurse must be able to select all the options that answer the question correctly. There are no partially correct answers.

62. 1. Vegans avoid animal proteins, which are complete proteins that contain all the essential amino acids the body cannot synthesize from other sources. Vegetable proteins lack one or more essential amino acids, so the vegan must combine different plant proteins, grains, legumes, and nuts to allow for the intake of all essential amino acids. Vegans avoid all animal products and have difficulty meeting adequate nutritional protein needs.
    2. Vegans avoid animal products. If she does not drink milk, she will not eat eggs.
    3. The nurse should assist the client in adhering to cultural, spiritual, or personal beliefs. The nurse should not try to convince the client to change her beliefs unless it is a danger to the fetus or the mother.
    4. A vegan diet requires extra iron supplements; iron in the vegetarian diet is poorly absorbed because of the lack of heme iron from meat.

CLINICAL JUDGMENT GUIDE: The nurse must attempt to support a client's cultural beliefs. This is a knowledge-based question, and the nurse must know the client's cultural beliefs.

63. Correct answers are 1 and 4.
    1. This client has delivered her infant and has pain. The medical-surgical nurse can care for this client.
    2. This client requires teaching, a knowledge base the medical-surgical nurse should not be assumed to have encountered on a medical-surgical unit.
    3. HELLP syndrome stands for H—hemolysis (the breakdown of red blood cells), EL—elevated liver enzymes, LP—low platelet count. HELLP syndrome is a group of symptoms that occur in pregnant women who have preeclampsia or eclampsia. Symptoms include fatigue or feeling unwell, fluid retention and excess weight gain, headache, nausea and vomiting that continues to get worse, pain in the upper right part of the abdomen, blurry vision, nosebleeds or other bleeding that won't stop easily (rare), and seizures or convulsions (rare). A medical-surgical nurse does not have the expertise required to care for this client.
    4. This is a preterm client who is on a monitor. The medical-surgical nurse can care for this client. If something occurs on the monitor or the client goes into labor, the nurse can get help.

5. Pitocin is a medication that stimulates uterine contraction; it is used to induce labor or administered postpartum to help a boggy uterus contract. It must be administered by a nurse familiar with the medication and its potential adverse effects.

CLINICAL JUDGMENT GUIDE: The test taker must decide on each option individually. Would the medical-surgical nurse have the knowledge and skill to care for the client or should the client be cared for by a nurse familiar with the specialized area of antepartum and postpartum care?

64.
  1. This is a semi-Fowler's position, useful for increasing ease of breathing, and so on, but it does not provide access to the epidural space.
  2. This is the Sims position used for administering an enema.
  3. This position allows for a space to be created between the vertebrae and allows the anesthetist to insert the catheter into the epidural space.
  4. The laboring client could not lie on her stomach.

CLINICAL JUDGMENT GUIDE: The test taker should assess which position would allow access to the anatomical area needed to insert the catheter. Remember that the epidural space is part of the central nervous system.

65.
  1. The nurse should notify the HCP after ensuring that no more magnesium is administered to the client.
  2. Documenting the data is essential but does not come before safety of the client or notifying the HCP.
  3. It is not necessary for the nurse to have the findings verified before protecting the client.
  4. The adverse effects of parenterally administered magnesium sulfate, an anticonvulsant, usually are the result of magnesium intoxication. These include flushing, sweating, hypotension, depressed reflexes, flaccid paralysis, hypothermia, circulatory collapse, and cardiac and central nervous system depression proceeding to respiratory paralysis. This client is demonstrating magnesium toxicity. The nurse should immediately discontinue the magnesium and administer the antidote, calcium gluconate.

CLINICAL JUDGMENT GUIDE: The test taker should carefully read all graphs, charts, or legends when choosing an option. Absent reflexes should indicate a need for an action on the part of the nurse. Documentation, although important, is not directly taking care of the client and should only be chosen first when the data supplied are normal.

66. Correct order is 4, 5, 3, 1, 2.
  4. The client came to the clinic for treatment, which should be the first intervention.
  5. All sexual partners of the client should be notified of possible exposure to an STI. This is the responsibility of the public health nurse.
  3. The nurse's only opportunity to teach the client about safe sex practices may be this clinic visit.
  1. The nurse should attempt to notify the sexual partners of the client to prevent the spreading of the disease to other unsuspecting individuals.
  2. The report is filed monthly or quarterly.

CLINICAL JUDGMENT GUIDE: The test taker must logically deduce the steps for the nurse to implement. Care of the client is first. Next, the nurse must consider other clients who may be affected and get the names and contact information of the sexual partners; this must be done to contact the individuals. Reports and documentation are last.

67.
  1. At the scene of an accident, it is not important how far along the driver is.
  2. The driver must be assessed for signs of trauma before anything else can be done. If the client dies, then the fetus will die, too.
  3. Whether or not the driver was wearing a seat belt is a legal matter, and possible assessment data for the labor and delivery nurse to determine potential trauma to the fetus, but not at the scene of the accident.
  4. This might be done if the nurse has a stethoscope, but the mother's status is first because the fetus's life depends on her.

CLINICAL JUDGMENT GUIDE: The nurse has two clients in this scenario, the mother and the fetus, but one life depends on the status of the other. All the options in this question have words that can be used to indicate assessment, so the test taker must choose the first assessment to make.

68.
  1. This pain must be assessed and medication administered. A new graduate would be able to care for this client safely.
  2. Saturating multiple peri-pads indicates heavy bleeding, which may indicate hemorrhaging. A more experienced nurse should be assigned to this client.

3. The nurse needs to assess this client for possible maternal and infant bonding problems and would require a nurse who has experience with psychosocial problems. This client should be assigned to a more experienced nurse.
4. This client requires a nurse who is knowledgeable and experienced in breastfeeding; therefore, a more experienced nurse should be assigned to this client.

CLINICAL JUDGMENT GUIDE: The test taker must determine which client is most stable and assign this client to the new graduate nurse with the least experience.

69. 1. These are called milia and look similar to pimples; they will fade within a few days and do not warrant immediate intervention.
    2. **The normal respiratory rate for a newborn is 30 to 60; therefore, this information warrants immediate intervention.**
    3. The newborn who is turning red when crying is not in distress; therefore, this would not warrant immediate intervention.
    4. The newborn should pass meconium within 24 hours of birth. It is viscous, sticky (similar to tar), and odorless. This would not warrant intervention by the nursery nurse.

CLINICAL JUDGMENT GUIDE: The test taker must know normal vital signs for clients of all ages.

70. 1. **The fetus is in distress; after increasing blood supply by placing the client in the left lateral position, the labor and delivery nurse needs to contact the obstetrician for immediate C-section.**
    2. Panting during contractions will help prevent the client from pushing, but it is not the first intervention. This client needs immediate evaluation by an obstetrician.
    3. Oxytocin (Pitocin) is a uterine stimulant; this fetus is in distress and does not need uterine contractions. This is an inappropriate intervention.
    4. The nurse needs to prepare for immediate delivery of the fetus but not before contacting the obstetrician. The nurse cannot perform a C-section.

CLINICAL JUDGMENT GUIDE: When the test taker is deciding when to notify an HCP, the test taker should look at the other three options and determine whether one of the options should be implemented before notifying the HCP. In this question, the nursing interventions to address the late decelerations have been implemented. The HCP must be notified now.

71. 1. The white blood cell count rises normally during labor and postpartum—up to 25×10^3/microL; therefore, this does not warrant intervention.
    2. The serum potassium level is within normal limits, 3.5 to 5.3 mEq/L, so this client does not warrant immediate intervention by the charge nurse.
    3. **HELLP syndrome is a group of symptoms that occur in pregnant women who have hemolysis (H), elevated liver enzymes (EL), and low platelet count (LP), which occurs in women who are severely preeclamptic and eclamptic. Normal platelet count is 150 to 450 $\times$ 10^3/microL, so this client's platelet count requires immediate intervention.**
    4. This glucose level is elevated, but because the client had gestational diabetes this blood glucose level does not require immediate intervention.

CLINICAL JUDGMENT GUIDE: The test taker must be knowledgeable of laboratory data and be able to make appropriate decisions based on the information.

72. 1. Braxton Hicks contractions are irregular contractions of the uterus throughout the pregnancy and are not true labor. This client would not need to be assigned to the most experienced nurse.
    2. The client having twins on bedrest is not in imminent danger; therefore, this client would not be assigned to the most experienced nurse.
    3. **This client is ready to deliver; therefore, the most experienced nurse should be assigned to this client because the other three clients are not experiencing any life-threatening complications.**
    4. Early decelerations on the fetal monitor do not indicate fetal distress; therefore, this client does not need to be assigned to the most experienced nurse.

CLINICAL JUDGMENT GUIDE: The test taker must determine which client is most at risk for complications and assign this client to the most experienced nurse.

73. 1. The UAP can assist the client to the bathroom to urinate. The UAP cannot assess the client's fundus. The most common reason for a non-midline fundus is a full bladder.
    2. The client diagnosed with HELLP syndrome is unstable; therefore, the RN should not delegate these vital signs to the UAP.

3. The RN cannot delegate teaching to the UAP.
4. The RN cannot delegate medication administration to the UAP.

CLINICAL JUDGMENT GUIDE: The RN must know what can be delegated and assigned to the UAP. There will be numerous questions on the NCLEX-RN® concerning delegation and assignment. Remember that the nurse may not delegate the following to the UAP: assessment, teaching, evaluation, administering medications, or caring for an unstable client.

74. 1. The float nurse should be able to address the psychosocial concerns of the mother and family. The client has no physiological problems, so the float nurse could care for this client. Often, following a fetal demise, the mother is transferred to a medical-surgical unit so she does not have to hear babies crying.
    2. A boggy uterus indicates a potentially life-threatening situation and requires an experienced postpartum nurse to care for this client.
    3. This client is potentially hemorrhaging and requires a more experienced nurse to care for her.
    4. There are many legal issues surrounding adoption as well as caring for the mother who is giving up her child; this client should be assigned a nurse more experienced in postpartum care.

CLINICAL JUDGMENT GUIDE: The test taker must determine which client is most at risk for complications or has the highest need and assign this client to the most experienced nurse.

75. 1. The flu vaccine is made using duck eggs; therefore, the nurse should question the administration of this vaccine to a client who is allergic to eggs, not tomatoes.
    2. The nurse would not question administering the hepatitis B vaccine to a breastfeeding mother because 1-day-old infants receive the vaccine.
    3. Rho(D) immune globulin (RhoGAM) should be administered to the client because the baby is Rh-positive. This will help prevent erythroblastosis fetalis in the woman's next pregnancy.
    4. The nurse would question administering this medication because a positive titer means the client is immune to rubella (German measles).

CLINICAL JUDGMENT GUIDE: The test taker must be knowledgeable of laboratory data and be able to make appropriate decisions based on the information, including which laboratory information impacts vaccinations.

76. 1. Mongolian spots are blue or purple splotches on the baby's lower back and buttocks. The spots are caused by a concentration of pigmented cells that usually disappear in the first 4 years of life. This newborn does not need to be assessed first.
    2. A port-wine stain is a flat pink, red, or purple birthmark. They are caused by a concentration of dilated tiny blood vessels called capillaries. The most effective way of treating port-wine stains is with a special laser procedure when the baby is older. This newborn does not need to be assessed first.
    3. Erythema toxicum is a red rash on newborns often described as "flea bites." The rash is common on the chest and back but may be found all over. It does not require any treatment and disappears by itself in a few days; therefore, the nurse does not need to assess this newborn first.
    4. A cephalohematoma results when there is bleeding between the periosteum and the skull from pressure during birth. The firm swelling, edema, is not present at birth but develops within the first 24 to 48 hours. Any time a client is bleeding, it warrants intervention by the nurse.

CLINICAL JUDGMENT GUIDE: When deciding which client to assess first, the test taker should determine whether the client's signs and symptoms are expected for the client's situation. After eliminating the expected options, the test taker should determine which situation is more life-threatening.

77. 1. When the infant is placed supine, the infant should extend the arm and leg on the side to which the head is turned and then flex the extremities on the other. This is known as the tonic-neck reflex or fencing reflex, which is normal for the newborn. The newborn remaining in a fetal position when supine warrants further intervention to assess for neurological problems.
    2. The Babinski reflex is elicited by stroking the lateral sole of the foot from the heel forward. Normal reflexes are toes flared outward and the big toe dorsiflexes. This is a normal response for an infant but is abnormal in an adult, indicating neurological deficit in

the adult. Therefore, this does not warrant immediate intervention.
3. The stepping reflex is intact when the nurse places the baby on a flat surface. The baby will "walk" by placing one foot in front of the other. This is expected and does not warrant intervention by the nurse.
4. The grasp reflex is elicited by placing a finger on the infant's open palm. The hand will close around the finger. Newborn infants have strong grasps and can almost be lifted from the examination table with both hands. This would not warrant intervention.

CLINICAL JUDGMENT GUIDE: The test taker should know about relex assessment and corresponding neurological disorders for clients of all ages.

CASE STUDY ANSWERS

1. Correct answers are 2, 5, 6, and 10.
   The fundus should be firm and nontender; this finding should be reported. The client is a grand multipara, represented by a client having five or more births at 20 weeks' gestation or more. This information places the client at higher risk for complications and should be reported to the HCP. A newborn weighing more than 4,500 g is referred to as having macrosomia. The client delivered a 4,600-g baby and is at risk for complications. This information should be reported. The client has a BMI of 44.1, is obese, and places the client at risk for complications. This information should be reported. Normal data does not need to be reported.

   CLINICAL JUDGMENT GUIDE: The test taker should examine each answer option individually. Alternative question formats, such as this extended multiple responses or select all that apply questions, can have one to all correct answers.

2. Correct answers are 1, 3, and 4.
   1. Puerperal infection is an infection of the reproductive tract in the postpartum period. The client is at risk for a puerperal infection owing to obesity and uterine tenderness.
   2. The client's RPR is nonreactive, indicating no syphilis infection. Congenital syphilis would be seen in the infant, not the mother.
   3. Postpartum hemorrhage has traditionally been defined as blood loss greater than 500 mL after childbirth. The client is at risk for postpartum hemorrhage because of grand multiparity and obesity. Several assessment findings, i.e., soft fundus and moderate lochia, could indicate postpartum hemorrhage.
   4. This client is at risk for thromboembolic disease owing to obesity, multiparity, and advanced maternal age (over 35 years).
   5. Cystitis is a lower urinary tract infection. The client shows no symptoms of this disease.
   6. The client is Rh positive, so not at risk for Rh isoimmunization (also called Rh alloimmunization).

3. Correct answers are 3 and 2.
   Based on the client's condition, the nurse recognizes that the client is at the highest risk for

   | 3. Hemorrhage |

   and will require

   | 2. Crystalloid fluids |

4. Correct answers are marked.

Potential Nursing Intervention	Indicated	Not Indicated
Massage uterine fundus until firm.	X	
Obtain vital signs hourly.		X
Insert catheter to empty bladder.	X	
Assess blood glucose before meals and at bedtime.		X
Place in Trendelenburg position.		X
Perform vaginal examinations hourly.		X
Maintain large-bore IV access.	X	
Provide sips of clear liquids.		X
Obtain continuous pulse oximetry readings.	X	

The client's fundus should be massaged, bladder emptied, IV maintained, and continuous pulse oximetry readings should be evaluated. Hourly vital signs are not frequent enough. There is no indication that the blood glucose needs to be assessed. The client should be placed in a reclining position with legs elevated to a 20- to 30-degree angle to increase venous return without compromising breathing or cardiac function. Vaginal examinations are not indicated postpartum. The client should be kept NPO in case of potential surgical intervention.

5. Correct answers are 1, 2, 3, 4, and 5.
   1. The oxytocin infusion is the first-line treatment of postpartum hemorrhage and is a priority intervention.
   2. The methylergonovine maleate administration can reverse postpartum hemorrhage caused by uterine atony. This intervention is a priority.
   3. The indwelling urinary catheter will keep the bladder empty and is a priority intervention because a full bladder can inhibit the uterus from contracting.
   4. Laboratory tests help guide client care decisions and are a priority intervention.
   5. Notifying the blood bank of a type and cross is essential to have blood available for a potential transfusion.
   6. Hydrocodone tablets for pain are essential for client comfort but are not a priority intervention.

6. Correct answers are marked.

Finding	Improved	Declined	No Change
Blood pressure	X		
Heart rate	X		
SpO_2			X
Temperature	X		
Firm fundus	X		
Moderate rubra lochia	X		
DTRs			X
Lungs clear bilaterally			X

The client's blood pressure, heart rate, and temperature have decreased since treatment. The fundus is now firm and moderate rubra lochia is noted, which are expected findings and indicate improvement in the client's condition. SpO_2, DTRs, and lung sounds remain unchanged.

Pediatric Health Management

People are like stained-glass windows. They sparkle and shine when the sun is out but when the darkness sets in, their true beauty is revealed only if there is light from within.

—Elisabeth Kübler-Ross

QUESTIONS

1. The nurse is working in the emergency department (ED) of a children's medical center. Which client should the nurse assess **first**?
    1. The 1-month-old infant crying and with colic
    2. The 2-year-old toddler bitten by another child at the day-care center
    3. The 6-year-old school-age child hit by a car while riding a bicycle
    4. The 14-year-old adolescent suspected by the parent of being sexually active

2. The 8-year-old client diagnosed with a vaso-occlusive sickle cell crisis is reporting a severe headache. Which intervention should the nurse implement **first**?
    1. Administer 6 L of oxygen via nasal cannula.
    2. Assess the client's neurological status.
    3. Administer a narcotic analgesic by IV push (IVP).
    4. Increase the client's IV rate.

3. The 6-year-old client recovering from abdominal surgery is attempting to make a pinwheel spin by blowing on it with the nurse's assistance. The child starts crying because the pinwheel won't spin. Which action should the nurse implement **first**?
    1. Praise the child for the attempt to make the pinwheel spin.
    2. Notify the respiratory therapist to implement incentive spirometry.
    3. Encourage the child to turn from side to side and cough.
    4. Demonstrate how to make the pinwheel spin by blowing on it.

4. The nurse is caring for clients on the pediatric medical unit. Which client should the nurse assess **first**?
    1. The child diagnosed with type 1 diabetes with a blood glucose level of 180 mg/dL
    2. The child diagnosed with pneumonia, coughing, and a temperature of 100°F (37.8°C)
    3. The child diagnosed with gastroenteritis with a potassium (K^+) level of 3.9 mEq/L
    4. The child diagnosed with cystic fibrosis with a pulse oximeter reading of 90%

5. The nurse has received the a.m. shift report for clients on a pediatric unit. Which medication should the nurse administer **first**?
   1. The third dose of antibiotic to the child diagnosed with methicillin-resistant *Staphylococcus aureus* (MRSA)
   2. The IVP methylprednisolone to the child diagnosed with asthma
   3. The sliding scale insulin to the child diagnosed with type 1 diabetes mellitus
   4. The methylphenidate to a child diagnosed with attention deficit-hyperactivity disorder (ADHD)

6. The nurse enters the client's room and realizes the 9-month-old infant is not breathing. Which interventions should the nurse implement? **Rank in order of priority.**
   1. Perform cardiac compressions at a rate of 30:2.
   2. Check the infant's brachial pulse.
   3. Administer two puffs to the infant.
   4. Determine unresponsiveness.
   5. Open the infant's airway.

7. The 3-year-old client has been admitted to the pediatric unit. Which task should the registered nurse (RN) instruct the unlicensed assistive personnel (UAP) to perform **first**?
   1. Orient the parents and child to the room.
   2. Obtain an admission kit for the child.
   3. Post the child's height and weight at the head of the bed.
   4. Provide the child with a meal tray.

8. The clinic nurse is preparing to administer an intramuscular (IM) injection to the 2-year-old toddler. Which intervention should the nurse implement **first**?
   1. Immobilize the child's leg.
   2. Explain the procedure to the child.
   3. Cleanse the area with an alcohol swab.
   4. Administer the medication in the thigh.

9. Which data would **warrant immediate** intervention from the pediatric nurse?
   1. Proteinuria for the child diagnosed with nephrotic syndrome
   2. Petechiae for the child diagnosed with leukemia
   3. Drooling for a child diagnosed with acute epiglottitis
   4. Elevated temperature in a child diagnosed with otitis media

10. Which client should the pediatric nurse assess **first** after receiving the a.m. shift report?
    1. The 6-month-old child diagnosed with bacterial meningitis and crying and irritable
    2. The 9-month-old child diagnosed with tetralogy of Fallot with edema of the face
    3. The 11-month-old child diagnosed with Reye syndrome now vomiting and lethargic
    4. The 13-month-old child diagnosed with diarrhea, with sunken eyeballs and decreased urine output

11. The pediatric clinic nurse is triaging telephone calls. Which client's parent should the nurse call **first**?
    1. The 4-month-old child had immunizations yesterday and the parent is reporting a high-pitched cry with 103°F (39.4°C) fever.
    2. The 8-month-old's parent is reporting the child has a fever and is pulling on the right ear.
    3. The 2-year-old child was diagnosed with patent ductus arteriosus and the parent reports running out of digoxin.
    4. The 3-year-old's parent is reporting their child may have chickenpox.

12. The parent of a 12-year-old child with a left below-the-knee cast calls the pediatric clinic nurse and tells the nurse, "My child is saying their foot is cold and feels like it is asleep." Which action should the nurse implement **first?**
    1. Prepare to bifurcate the left below-the-knee cast.
    2. Tell the parent to bring the child to the office.
    3. Instruct the parent to elevate the left leg on two pillows.
    4. Notify the child's orthopedist of the situation.

13. Which child client requires the nurse to notify the healthcare provider (HCP)?
    1. The 1-year-old child diagnosed with iron deficiency anemia with dark-colored stool
    2. The 3-year-old child diagnosed with phenylketonuria (PKU) and not allowed to eat meat or milk products
    3. The 5-year-old child diagnosed with rheumatic heart fever having difficulty breathing
    4. The 7-year-old child diagnosed with acute glomerulonephritis with dark tea-colored urine

14. The pediatric nurse on the surgical unit has just received the a.m. shift report. Which client should the nurse assess **first?**
    1. The 3-week-old child 1-day postoperative repair of a myelomeningocele with bulging fontanels
    2. The 3-month-old child 2 days postoperative for a temporary colostomy secondary to Hirschsprung's disease with a moist, pink stoma
    3. The 9-month-old child with a cleft palate repair spitting up formula and refusing to eat
    4. The 4-year-old child 1-day postoperative for repair of hypospadias with clear amber urine draining from an indwelling catheter

15. The charge nurse has assigned a staff nurse to care for an 8-year-old client diagnosed with cerebral palsy. Which nursing action by the staff nurse would **warrant immediate** intervention by the charge nurse?
    1. The staff nurse performs gentle range-of-motion (ROM) exercises to extremities.
    2. The staff nurse puts the client's bed in the lowest position possible.
    3. The staff nurse takes the client in a wheelchair to the activity room.
    4. The staff nurse places the child in the semi-Fowler's position to eat lunch.

16. The RN and the UAP are caring for clients on the pediatric unit. Which action by the nurse indicates **appropriate** delegation?
    1. The nurse requests the UAP to check the circulation of the child with a cast.
    2. The nurse asks the UAP to feed an infant postoperative cleft palate repair.
    3. The nurse has the UAP demonstrate a catheterization for a child diagnosed with a neurogenic bladder.
    4. The nurse checks to make sure the UAP's delegated tasks have been completed.

17. The RN on a pediatric unit has received the a.m. shift report and tells the UAP to keep the 2-year-old child NPO (nothing by mouth) for a procedure. At 0830, the nurse observes the mother feeding the child. Which action should the nurse implement **first?**
    1. Determine whether the UAP did not understand the instructions.
    2. Tell the HCP the UAP did not follow the nurse's direction.
    3. Ask the mother why she was feeding her child if the child was NPO.
    4. Notify the dietary department to hold the child's meal trays.

18. The charge nurse on the six-bed pediatric burn unit is making shift assignments and has one RN, one scrub technician, one UAP, and a unit secretary. Which client care assignment indicates the **best** use of the hospital personnel?
    1. The RN performs daily whirlpool dressing changes.
    2. The unit secretary prints the discharge instructions for a client.
    3. The scrub technician medicates the client before dressing changes.
    4. The UAP evaluates the current laboratory results for the client.

19. The RN and the UAP are caring for clients on a pediatric surgical unit. Which tasks would be **most** appropriate to delegate to the UAP? **Select all that apply.**
    1. Pass dietary trays to the clients.
    2. Obtain routine vital signs on the clients.
    3. Complete the preoperative checklist.
    4. Change linens on the clients' beds.
    5. Document the clients' intake and output.

20. Which client should the charge nurse on the pediatric unit assign to the **most** experienced nurse?
    1. The 4-year-old child diagnosed with hemophilia receiving factor VIII
    2. The 8-year-old child diagnosed with headaches and scheduled for a CT scan
    3. The 6-year-old child recovering from a sickle cell crisis
    4. The 11-year-old child newly diagnosed with rheumatoid arthritis

21. The RN charge nurse is making shift assignments on a pediatric oncology unit. Which delegation or assignment would be **most** appropriate?
    1. Delegate the UAP to obtain routine blood work from the central line.
    2. Instruct the licensed practical nurse (LPN) to contact the leukemia support group.
    3. Assign the chemotherapy-certified RN to administer chemotherapeutic medication.
    4. Have the dietitian check the meal trays for the amount eaten.

22. The RN observes the UAP bringing a cartoon video to a 6-year-old child on bedrest to watch on the television. Which action should the nurse take?
    1. Tell the UAP that the child should not be watching videos.
    2. Explain that this is the responsibility of the child life therapist.
    3. Praise the UAP for providing the child with an appropriate activity.
    4. Notify the charge nurse that the UAP gave the child videos to watch.

23. Which newborn should the RN in the neonatal intensive care unit (NICU) assign to a new graduate nurse after just completing the NICU internship?
    1. The 1-day-old infant diagnosed with a myelomeningocele
    2. The 2-week-old infant born 6 weeks premature
    3. The 3-hour-old infant being evaluated for esophageal atresia
    4. The 1-week-old infant diagnosed with tetralogy of Fallot

24. The newly hired RN is working on a pediatric unit and needs the UAP to obtain a urine specimen on an 11-month-old infant. Which statement made to the UAP indicates the nurse **understands** the delegation process?
    1. "Be sure to weigh the diaper when obtaining the urine specimen."
    2. "Do you know how to apply the urine collection bag?"
    3. "Use a small indwelling catheter when obtaining the urine specimen."
    4. "I need for you to get a urine specimen on the infant."

25. Which task is **most** appropriate for the RN pediatric nurse to delegate to the UAP?
    1. Ask the UAP to orient the parents and child to the room.
    2. Tell the UAP to prepare the child for an endoscopy.
    3. Request the UAP to log roll the client recovering from spinal surgery.
    4. Instruct the UAP to assess the child's developmental level.

26. Which behavior by the UAP **warrants** intervention by the RN?
    1. The UAP weighs the child's diaper on a scale and records the urine output on the intake and output (I&O) sheet.
    2. The UAP sits with the child while the parent goes down to the cafeteria to get something to eat.
    3. The UAP bathes the child diagnosed with congenital dislocated hip with the Pavlik harness on the child.
    4. The UAP applies wrist restraints on the 7-month-old 1-day postoperative cleft palate repair.

27. The RN is caring for pediatric clients. Which tasks are **most** appropriate to assign to a UAP or an LPN? **Select all that apply.**
    1. Instruct the LPN to teach the parent of a child newly diagnosed with type 1 diabetes.
    2. Tell the UAP to apply an ice collar to the child 1-day postoperative tonsillectomy.
    3. Ask the UAP to place ointment on a child's diaper rash around the anal area.
    4. Request the LPN to double-check the medication dose for the child receiving an antibiotic.
    5. Tell the LPN to enter the HCP's orders into the EHR for the child diagnosed with cystic fibrosis.

28. The nurse is discharging a 4-month-old child with a temporary colostomy. Which intervention should the RN implement?
    1. Request the UAP to complete the discharge written documentation.
    2. Tell the LPN to show the parent how to irrigate the colostomy.
    3. Ask the UAP to remove the child's IV catheter.
    4. Request the UAP to escort the parent and child to their car.

29. The UAP tells the RN the child diagnosed with Down syndrome and 2 days postoperative appendectomy is having pain. Which intervention should the nurse implement **first?**
    1. Tell the UAP to check the child's vital signs.
    2. Assess the child's abdominal dressing and pain level.
    3. Notify the HCP immediately.
    4. Check the MAR for the last time pain medication was administered.

30. The 8-year-old child in the pediatric unit is refusing to ambulate postoperatively. Which intervention would be **most** appropriate?
    1. Give the child the option to ambulate now or after lunch.
    2. Ask the parents to insist the child ambulate in the hall.
    3. Refer the child to the child developmental therapist.
    4. Tell the child they can play a video game after ambulating.

31. The clinic nurse overhears a parent in the waiting room tell the 6-year-old child, "If you don't sit down and be quiet, I am going to get the nurse to give you a shot." Which action should the nurse implement?
    1. Do not take any action because the parent is attempting to discipline their child.
    2. Tell the child the nurse would not give them a shot because the parent said to.
    3. Report this verbally abusive behavior to Child Protective Services.
    4. Tell the parent this behavior will cause the child to be afraid of nurses.

32. The parents of a newborn diagnosed with Down syndrome are holding their infant and crying. They ask, "Is it true that children with this condition are hard to take care of at home?" Which referral would be **most** appropriate for the parents?
    1. The National Down Syndrome Society Web site
    2. The hospital chaplain
    3. A Down syndrome support group
    4. A geneticist

33. The charge nurse on the pediatric unit hears the Code Pink (infant abduction) overhead announcement, newborn nursery. Which action should the charge nurse implement?
    1. Send a staff member to the newborn nursery.
    2. Explain the situation to the clients and visitors.
    3. Continue with the charge nurse's responsibilities.
    4. Station a staff member at all the unit exits.

34. The parent of a 4-year-old child diagnosed with Duchenne's muscular dystrophy is overwhelmed and asks the nurse, "I have been told a case manager will come and talk to me. What will they do for me?" Which statement indicates the nurse **understands** the role of the case manager?
    1. "You will have a case manager so that the hospital can save money."
    2. "They will make sure your child gets the right medication for muscular dystrophy."
    3. "They will help you find the resources you need to care for your child."
    4. "The case manager helps your child to have a normal life expectancy."

35. The nurse is assigned to the pediatric unit performance improvement committee. The unit is concerned with IV infection rates. Which action should the nurse implement **first** when investigating the problem?
    1. Contact central supply for samples of IV start kits.
    2. Obtain research to determine the best duration for IV dwell time.
    3. Identify how many IV infections have occurred in the last year.
    4. Audit the EHR to determine whether hospital policy is being followed.

36. The clinic nurse is discussing a tubal ligation with a 17-year-old adolescent diagnosed with Down syndrome. The adolescent does not want the surgery, but her parents (also in the room) are telling her she must have it. Which statement by the nurse would be an example of the ethical principle of justice?
    1. "I think this requires further discussion before scheduling this procedure."
    2. "You will not be able to have children after you have this procedure."
    3. "You should have this procedure because you could not care for a child."
    4. "You can refuse this procedure and your parents can't make you have it."

37. The school nurse has referred an 8-year-old student for further evaluation of vision. The single parent has told the school nurse they do not have money for the evaluation or glasses. Which action by the nurse would be an example of client advocacy?
    1. Tell the parent their child cannot read the board.
    2. Refer the parent to a local service organization.
    3. Ask the parent whether the family is on Medicaid.
    4. Loan the parent money for the examination.

38. The ED nurse is scheduling the 16-year-old client for an emergency appendectomy. Which intervention should the nurse implement when obtaining permission for the surgery?
    1. Withhold the narcotic pain medication until the client signs the permit.
    2. Have the client's parent or legal guardian sign the operative permit.
    3. Explain the procedure to the client and the parents in simple terms.
    4. Get a visitor from the ED waiting area to witness the parent's signature.

39. The unit manager has been notified by central supply that many client items are missing from stock and have not been charged to the client. Which action should the nurse manager implement regarding the lost charges?
    1. Send out a memo telling the staff to follow the charge procedures.
    2. Form a performance improvement committee to study the problem.
    3. Determine whether the items in question are being restocked daily.
    4. Schedule a staff meeting to discuss how to prevent further lost charges.

40. Which child's behavior **warrants** notifying the child developmental specialist?
    1. The 1-year-old child crying whenever the parent leaves the room
    2. The 2-year-old child talking in two- or three-word sentences
    3. The 3-year-old child who is bowel and bladder toilet traiied
    4. The 4-year-old child throwing frequent temper tantrums

41. Which child should the RN pediatric nurse assign to the new graduate nurse after completion of orientation to the pediatric unit?
    1. The 5-year-old child diagnosed with sickle cell crisis having uncontrolled pain using the patient-controlled analgesia (PCA) pump
    2. The 6-year-old child in Russell's traction for a fractured femur with insertion pin sites that are inflamed and infected
    3. The 12-year-old child newly diagnosed with type 1 diabetes needing medication teaching
    4. The 16-year-old client diagnosed with scoliosis being admitted for insertion of a spinal rod in the morning

42. Which action by the ED nurse **warrants** intervention by the charge nurse?
    1. The nurse is elevating the right arm of a child appearing to have a fractured wrist.
    2. The nurse is notifying Child Protective Services for a child suspected of being sexually abused.
    3. The nurse is assessing the tonsils on a 4-year-old drooling child with a sore throat.
    4. The nurse is obtaining a midstream urine specimen for the child reporting burning upon urination.

43. The day shift nurse is preparing to administer 0730 medications to the 12-year-old child diagnosed with type 1 diabetes. The child's 0730 blood glucose level is 252 mg/dL.

Client's Name: A.B. Allergies: NKA	Account Number: 134567 Date: Today	
Medication	0701–1900	1901–0700

Sliding scale regular insulin ac and hs
  Less than 150 no insulin
  151–200 4 units
  201–250 6 units
  251–300 8 units
  301 notify HCP		

10 units regular insulin 20 units isophane insulin	0730	
Signature/Initials	Day Nurse RN/DN	Night Nurse RN/NN

    Which insulin coverage should the nurse administer?
    1. Regular insulin 6 units
    2. Regular insulin 18 units and isophane insulin 20 units
    3. Regular insulin 10 units and isophane insulin 20 units
    4. Regular insulin 8 units

44. Which interventions should the nurse implement to help establish a nurse and parent relationship? **Select all that apply.**
    1. Include the parents when developing the plan of care for their child.
    2. Encourage the parents to hold their child as much as possible.
    3. Allow the parents to verbalize their feelings of fear and anxiety.
    4. Tell the parents to never leave while the child is hospitalized.
    5. Request the parents to bring toys from home the child will enjoy.

45. The nurse is caring for clients on the pediatric unit. Which child would **warrant** a referral to the early childhood development specialist?
    1. The 9-month-old child saying only "mama" or "dada"
    2. The 11-month-old child walking while hanging onto furniture
    3. The 8-month-old child sitting by leaning forward on both hands
    4. The 4-month-old infant turning from the abdomen to the back

46. The 10-year-old child diagnosed with leukemia is scheduled for a bone marrow aspiration. Which intervention is **most** important when obtaining informed consent for the procedure?
   1. Obtain assent from the child.
   2. Have the parent sign the permit.
   3. Refer any questions to the HCP.
   4. Witness the signature on the permit.

47. The 13-year-old client has just delivered a 4-pound baby boy. The stepfather of the client becomes verbally abusive to the nurse when asked to leave the room. The client is withdrawn and silent. Which **legal** action should the nurse implement?
   1. Call hospital security to come to the room.
   2. Contact Child Protective Services.
   3. Refer the child to the social worker.
   4. Ask the client whether she feels safe at home.

48. The fire alarm on the pediatric unit has just started sounding. Which action should the charge nurse implement **first**?
   1. Call the hospital operator to find out the location of the fire.
   2. Ensure that all visitors and clients are in their room with the door closed.
   3. Prepare to evacuate the clients and visitors down the stairs.
   4. Make a list of which clients are not currently on the unit.

49. A nurse overhears two other nurses talking about a client in the hospital dining room. Which action should the nurse implement **first**?
   1. Notify the HIPAA officer about the breach of confidentiality.
   2. Immediately report the two nurses to their clinical manager.
   3. Document and submit the situation in writing to the chief nursing officer (CNO).
   4. Tell the two nurses they are violating the client's confidentiality.

50. The nurse is caring for newborns in the nursery. Which newborn **warrants immediate** intervention by the nurse?
   1. The 8-hour-old newborn having yet to pass meconium
   2. The 15-hour-old newborn now slightly jaundiced
   3. The 4-hour-old newborn showing jittery and irritable behavior
   4. The 10-hour-old newborn crying nonstop

51. At 1300, the nurse is assessing a 12-year-old child reporting abdominal pain and rating it as a 5 on a scale of 1 to 10.

Client's Name: R.J. **Allergies:** NKDA	**Account Number:** 1023456 **Height:** 60 in (152.4 cm)	**Date:** Today **Weight:** 98 lb (44.5 kg)
Medication	1901–0700	0701–1900
Aluminum hydroxide; magnesium hydroxide 30 mL q 1 hour PRN		
Acetaminophen 650 mg PO q 6 hours PRN		
Hydrocodone 5 mg PO PRN pain q 4–6 hours	0600 NN	
Morphine 2 mg IVP PRN pain q 4 hours		
Signature/Initials	Night Nurse RN/NN	Day Nurse RN/DN

   Which intervention should the nurse implement?
   1. Administer 30 mL of aluminum hydroxide; magnesium hydroxide PO (oral).
   2. Administer 650 mg of acetaminophen PO.
   3. Administer 5 mg of hydrocodone PO.
   4. Administer 2 mg of morphine IVP.

Chapter 12 Pediatric Health Management

52. The nurse having never worked on the maternity ward has been pulled from the surgical unit to work in the newborn nursery. Which assignment would be **most** appropriate for the nurse to accept?
    1. Perform an assessment on the newborn.
    2. Assist the pediatrician with a circumcision.
    3. Gavage feed an 8-hour-old newborn.
    4. Transport newborns to their mothers' rooms.

53. The RN is instructing the UAP on gross motor skill activity that is appropriate for a developmentally delayed 9-month-old infant. Which activity should the RN delegate to the UAP?
    1. Help the child to sit without support.
    2. Teach the child to catch the beach ball.
    3. Reward the child with food for sitting up.
    4. Teach the child to blow a kiss.

54. Which incident should the primary nurse report to the clinical manager concerning a violation of information technology guidelines?
    1. The nurse keeps the computer screen turned away from public view.
    2. The nurse researches medications using the online formulary.
    3. The nurse shares their computer access code with another nurse.
    4. The nurse logs off the computer when leaving the terminal.

55. The nurse is caring for clients in a pediatric ED. Which client should the nurse assess **first**?
    1. The bleeding child diagnosed with a dog bite on the left hand
    2. The child with a laceration on the right side of the forehead
    3. The child diagnosed with a fractured tibia unable to move the foot
    4. The child having ingested a bottle of prenatal vitamins

56. The nurse is caring for a client in a children's medical center. Which behavior indicates the nurse **understands** the pediatric client's rights?
    1. The nurse administers an injection without talking to the child.
    2. The nurse covers the 5-year-old child's genitalia during a code.
    3. The nurse discusses the child's condition with the grandparents.
    4. The nurse leaves an uncapped needle at the client's bedside.

57. The nurse is administering IV fluids to a 3-year-old client. Which action by the nurse would **warrant** intervention by the charge nurse?
    1. The nurse places the IV on an infusion pump.
    2. The nurse does not use a volume-controlled device.
    3. The nurse does not check the child's IV site every 15 minutes.
    4. The nurse labels the IV tubing with date and time.

58. The nurse is caring for clients on a psychiatric pediatric unit. Which action by the nurse is **reportable** to the state board of nursing?
    1. The nurse leaves for lunch and does not return to complete the shift.
    2. The nurse fails to check the ID band when administering medications.
    3. The nurse has had three documented medication errors in the last 3 months.
    4. The nurse has admitted to having an affair with another staff member.

59. The nurse is working in a free healthcare clinic. Which client situation **warrants** further investigation?
    1. The child diagnosed with rheumatoid arthritis and wearing a copper bracelet
    2. The parent of a child diagnosed with sunburn using aloe vera plant juice on the burn
    3. The grandparent reporting rubbing mentholated ointment on the child's chest for a cold
    4. The parent telling the nurse that the child receives a variety of herbs every day

60. The UAP informs the RN primary nurse that the 4-year-old child is alone in the room because the parent went to the cafeteria to get something to eat. Which action should the nurse implement **first**?
    1. Arrange for the parent to have a tray sent to the room.
    2. Go to the cafeteria and ask the parent to return to the room.
    3. Tell the UAP to stay with the child until the parent returns.
    4. Notify social services that the parent left the child alone.

61. The nurse is evaluating an 18-month-old child in the pediatric clinic. Which data would indicate to the nurse that the child is meeting tasks according to Erikson's Stages of Psychosocial Development? **Select all that apply.**
    1. The child stamps their foot and says "no" frequently.
    2. The child does not interact with the parent.
    3. The child cries when the parent leaves the room.
    4. The child responds when called by name.
    5. The child smiles when successful at toilet training.

62. Which statement by the RN charge nurse indicates they have an autocratic leadership style?
    1. "You must complete all the a.m. care before you take your morning break."
    2. "I don't care how the work is done as long as it is completed on time."
    3. "I want to talk to you about your ideas on a new staffing mix."
    4. "I think we should have a potluck lunch tomorrow because it is Saturday."

63. The nurse is evaluating the care of a 5-year-old client diagnosed with a cyanotic congenital heart defect. Which outcome would support that discharge teaching has been **effective**?
    1. The parent makes the child get up when squatting.
    2. The child is playing in the dayroom without oxygen.
    3. The parent buys the child a baseball and a bat.
    4. The nurse finds unopened packs of salt on the meal tray.

64. The nurse is administering morning medications on a pediatric unit.

    Client Name: T.R.   **Account Number:** 5948726   **Date:** Today
    Allergies: Milk and dairy products
    Height: 21 in (53.3 cm)   **Weight:** 15 lb (6.8 kg)
    Date of Birth: 2 weeks ago

Medication	1901–0700	0701–1900
Digoxin 0.125 mg/5 mL q day PO		0900
250 mL 0.33% dextrose IV @ 10 mL/hr	0215 NN via buretrol setup and IV pump	
Signature/Initials	Night Nurse RN/NN	Day Nurse RN/DN

    Which action should the nurse take **first** when preparing to administer medication to the client?
    1. Check the client's apical pulse rate.
    2. Ask the parent for the baby's date of birth.
    3. Look to see whether a digoxin level has been drawn.
    4. Call the HCP to discuss the digoxin.

65. The nurse working in a pediatrician's office is preparing to administer the initial *Haemophilus influenzae* type b (Hib) vaccination to a 2-month-old infant. Which is the preferred site for the injection?

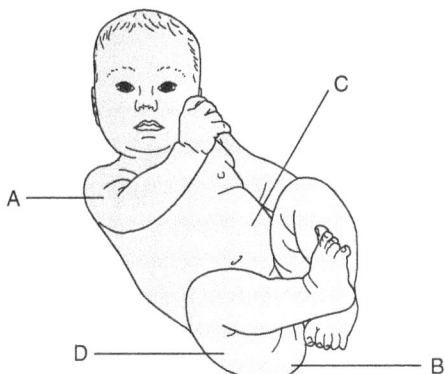

   1. A
   2. B
   3. C
   4. D

66. The nurse is preparing to administer an IV piggyback to an 8-year-old child. The child has an IV line running at 45 mL/hr. The medication comes prepared in 50 mL of normal saline (NS). At which rate should the nurse set the IV pump? _____

67. The unconscious 4-year-old child is brought to the ED by paramedics; the child has bruises covering the torso in varying stages of healing. The nurse notes small burn marks on the child's genitalia. Which actions should the nurse implement? **Select all that apply.**
   1. Notify Child Protective Services.
   2. Ask the parent how the child was injured.
   3. Perform a thorough examination for more injuries.
   4. Tell the parents that the police have been called.
   5. Prepare the child for skull x-rays and a CT scan.

68. The 24-month-old toddler is admitted to the pediatric unit diagnosed with vomiting and diarrhea. Which interventions should the nurse implement? **Rank in order of performance.**
   1. Teach the parent about weighing diapers to determine output status.
   2. Show the parent the call light and explain safety regimens.
   3. Assess the toddler's tissue turgor.
   4. Place the appropriate size diapers in the room.
   5. Take the toddler's vital signs.

69. Which child should the charge nurse assess **first**?
   1. The 1-month-old infant crying, inconsolable, with inspiratory retractions
   2. The 4-year-old toddler diagnosed with cystic fibrosis (CF) and pulse oximeter reading of 93%
   3. The 6-year-old child diagnosed with gastroenteritis and potassium level of 3.6 mEq/L
   4. The 14-year-old diagnosed with type 2 diabetes and blood glucose level of 210 mg/dL

70. Which task should the RN charge nurse delegate to the UAP?
   1. Take the vital signs of an African American child having a sickle cell crisis.
   2. Place oxygen via nasal cannula on a teenager diagnosed with cystic fibrosis.
   3. Obtain the weight of the restless child diagnosed with nephrotic syndrome.
   4. Escort the 9-year-old child diagnosed with traumatic brain injury to the ICU.

71. The charge nurse is observing the RN administer an IM injection to a 2-year-old toddler. Which action by the nurse **warrants** intervention by the charge nurse?
    1. The pediatric nurse immobilizes the child's leg.
    2. The nurse explains the procedure to the child.
    3. The pediatric nurse places the syringe in the sharps container.
    4. The nurse recaps the needle after administering the medication.

72. Which tasks should the RN delegate to the UAP? **Select all that apply.**
    1. Document the intake and output on the 15-year-old child diagnosed with congestive heart failure.
    2. Feed the 9-year-old child experiencing an acute exacerbation of inflammatory bowel disease (IBD).
    3. Elevate the child's leg having just had a cast applied for a fractured right ankle.
    4. Take the incapacitated child's catheterized urine specimen to the laboratory.
    5. Assess the vital signs of a 7-year-old child reporting ear pain.

73. Which client should the charge nurse assign to the **most** experienced pediatric ED nurse?
    1. The 1-year-old child tugging at their right ear with a temperature of 100.4°F
    2. The 6-year-old child wheezing and reporting chest tightness
    3. The 8-year-old child reporting burning when urinating
    4. The 11-year-old child diagnosed with bilateral crackles and a productive cough

74. The 13-year-old child is admitted to the ED with nucal rigidity, a positive Kernig's sign, a positive Brudzinki's sign, and an elevated temperature. Which intervention should the charge nurse implement **first**?
    1. Administer acetaminophen (Tylenol) PO with water.
    2. Place the teenage child in droplet isolation.
    3. Prepare the teenager for a lumbar puncture.
    4. Notify the hospital infection control nurse about this client.

75. The RN answers the phone and a distraught parent says, "My child just drank a bottle of cleaning solution." Which intervention should the nurse implement **first**?
    1. Instruct the parent to bring their child to the ED immediately.
    2. Ask the parent how old the child is and how much the child weighs.
    3. Inquire whether the parent has syrup of ipecac that could be given to the child.
    4. Ask the charge nurse to call poison control immediately.

76. The 9-year-old child has a pencil penetrating the right eye and is brought to the ED by the parents. Which intervention should the charge nurse implement **first**?
    1. Remove the harmful object with a lightly moistened gauze pad.
    2. Ask the parents about the child's medical history and any known allergies.
    3. Stabilize the pencil penetrating the right eye in place and patch the left eye.
    4. Assess the 9-year-old child's vital signs and pulse oximeter reading.

77. The RN is caring for a 7-year-old child admitted to the hospital for a hit on the head with a baseball. One hour ago, the child had a 15 on the Glasgow Coma Scale and now has a 12. Which intervention should the pediatric nurse implement **first**?
    1. Notify the hospital neurologist immediately.
    2. Document the findings in the EHR.
    3. Complete a Glasgow Coma Scale in 2 hours.
    4. Place the child in the high Fowler's position.

78. Which client should the charge nurse assign to the **least** experienced nurse in the pediatric ED?
    1. The drooling child with a sore throat reported by the parents
    2. The 4-year-old child with a distended abdomen and absent bowel sounds
    3. The 13-year-old child with an edematous and contused right ankle
    4. The child with blood in their urine reported by the parents

PEDIATRIC CASE STUDY

(1100) A 6-month-old male infant arrives at the ED with his parents. The parents report that the infant has had a runny nose, fever, and cough for several days. The parents state the cough has worsened, he is not eating much, and he seems to be struggling to breathe so they brought him to the ED.

(1115) Upon assessment the triage nurse finds a slightly lethargic and dyspneic infant. Skin is pink, warm, and dry. Anterior fontanel is soft and flat. Mucous membranes are moist. Nasal drainage is thin and clear. Nasal flaring is noted bilaterally. Chest retractions noted. Inspiratory and expiratory wheezing noted bilaterally throughout lung fields. Frequent dry cough is noted. Heart sounds are normal. Abdomen is soft and flat with bowel sounds present ×4.

Vital Signs	Client Values
Heart rate	180 bpm
Respirations	55 breaths/min
Temperature	101.5°F (38.6°C)
Spo$_2$	96% (room air)

The nurse takes a complete medical history and reviews the client's medications and places them in the EHR.

Medical history: The client was born prematurely at 36 weeks' gestation. He has chronic lung disease due to bronchopulmonary dysplasia (BPD) from his early birth. Mom reports the child is breastfed and feeds approximately every 3–4 hours for about 30 minutes.

All routine immunizations are up to date.

Weight: 15.1 lb (6.86 kg). Length: 24.2 inches (61.5 cm).

Allergies: No known allergies (NKA).

Medication List	
Medication	Time Taken
Acetaminophen 80 mg PO every 4 hours PRN	Last dose today at 1000

1. **Recognize cues. What matters most?** The nurse prepares to call the ED physician. Which **priority** client data should be reported to the HCP? **Select all that apply.**
    1. Heart rate of 180 bpm
    2. Fontanel assessment
    3. Respiratory assessment
    4. History of bronchopulmonary dysplasia
    5. Dyspnea
    6. Temperature of 101.5°F (38.6°C)
    7. Spo$_2$ 96% on room air
    8. Immunization status
    9. Bowel sounds
    10. Respirations: 55 breaths/min

2. **Analyze cues. What could it mean?** What at-risk issues should the nurse be concerned for the client developing? **Select three answers.**
    1. Impaired gas exchange
    2. Malnutrition
    3. Decreased skin integrity
    4. Fatigue
    5. Seizures

(1145) The physician visits the client and writes orders. The orders are populated in the chart.

PROVIDER ORDERS:

CBC, BMP, and a nasal swab for a rapid RSV antigen test STAT
Chest x-ray
Oxygen 1–2 L/min per nasal cannula to keep Spo$_2$ above 93%
Saline IV lock
Acetaminophen 80 mg PO every 4 hours PRN for fever greater than 101°F (38.3°C)
Suction

(1830) Diagnostic and laboratory results are posted.

Laboratory Test	Client Values	Reference Values	
Hemoglobin (Hgb)	13.4 g/dL	0–1 month	13.4–19.9 g/dL
		1–2 months	10.7–17.1 g/dL
		2–3 months	9.–14.1g/dL
		3–6 months	9.5–14.1 g/dL
		6–12 months	11.3–14.1g/dL
Hematocrit (Hct)	40%	0–1 month	42–65%
		1–2 months	33–55%
		2–3 months	28–41%
		3–6 months	29–41%
		6–12 months	31–41%
White blood cell count	18000 mm^3	0–1 month	9,000–30,000/mm^3
		1–3 months	5,000–19,500/mm^3
		3–12 months	6,000–17,500/mm^3
		1–2 years	6,000–17,000/mm^3
		2–4 years	5,500–15,500/mm^3
Platelets	300 × 10^3/microL	250 to 450 × 10^3/microL	
Creatinine	0.25 mg/dL	2–12 months	0.2 to 0.4 mg/dL
Glucose	99 mg/dL	Fasting: Less than 100 mg/dL	
		Random: Less than 200 mg/dL	
Potassium	3.8 mEq/L	3.5 to 5.3 mEq/L or mmol/L	
Sodium	144 mEq/L	135 to 145 mEq/L or mmol/L	
Blood urea nitrogen	10 mg/dL	8 to 21 mg/dL	
		Adult over 90 years: 10 to 31 mg/dL	
Rapid RSV antigen test	Positive	Negative	

3. **Prioritize hypotheses. Where do I start?** Complete the sentence by choosing from the drop-down list of options. Based on the client's condition at the time, the nurse recognizes that the client is at the **highest** risk for _____

> Select ▼
> 1. Malnutrition
> 2. Atelectasis
> 3. Anemia

and will require_____

> Select ▼
> 1. IV fluids
> 2. Oxygen
> 3. Transfusion

(1300) Chest x-ray study notes hyperinflation, patchy atelectasis, and peribronchial thickening in bilateral lung bases.

4. **Generate solutions. What can I do?** For each intervention, specify whether the intervention is **indicated** or **not indicated** for the client's care.

Potential Nursing Intervention	Indicated	Not Indicated
Implement droplet precautions.		
Provide a quiet and calm environment.		
Lay client flat.		
Start oxygen at 2 L via nasal cannula.		
Encourage short and frequent breastfeeding sessions.		
Encourage visitors.		
Provide deep suction before each feeding.		

5. **Take action. What will I do?** The client is admitted to the pediatric unit for observation. Which admission orders should the nurse consider a **priority** action? **Select all that apply.**
   1. Repeat complete blood count (CBC) and basic metabolic panel (BMP) in a.m.
   2. Obtain vital signs every 4 hours.
   3. Continue breastfeeding as tolerated.
   4. Educate family on disease prevention strategies.
   5. Record routine intake and output.
   6. Have suction available at bedside.

(0800) Client is awake in mom's arms. Skin is warm, dry, and pale. Fontanel is soft and flat. Mucous membranes are pink and moist. In lungs fine wheezes heard bilaterally throughout all lung fields. No chest retractions noted. Abdomen is soft with bowel sounds present ×4. Oxygen given at 1 L per nasal cannula. Mom states that the client's cough seems a little better and that he could breastfeed for 10 minutes twice during the night. Mom states she is still worried that he is not back to his normal happy self.

Vital Signs	Client Values
Heart rate	150 bpm
Respirations	40 breaths/min
Temperature	100°F (37.8°C)
SpO_2	94% (1 L)

6. **Evaluate outcomes. Did it help?** For each assessment finding, indicate whether the client's condition has **improved**, **declined**, or **no change**.

Finding	Improved	Declined	No Change
Temperature			
Heart rate			
Respirations			
Respiratory assessment			
SpO_2			

Two days later, the client is being ready for discharge. The client is awake, smiling in his crib, and playing with a toy with Dad. Skin is pink, warm, and dry. Lung sounds are clear. No dyspnea or retractions. Abdomen is soft with bowel sounds present ×4. Dad states client has been breastfeeding well for mom, he is only coughing occasionally, and his nose is running much less. The parents are excited to take their son home.

Vital Signs	Client Values
Heart rate	100 bpm
Respirations	30 breaths/min
Temperature	97.8 °F (36.6°C)
SpO_2	99% on room air

ANSWERS AND RATIONALES

The correct answer number and rationale are in **boldface purple type.** Rationales for why other answer options are incorrect are also given.

1. 1. The main sign of colic is intense crying; therefore, this is expected and would not warrant the nurse's assessing the child first.
   2. A human bite is dangerous but not life-threatening.
   3. **The child hit by a car should be assessed first because they may have life-threatening injuries that must be assessed and treated promptly.**
   4. This client is not a priority over a client diagnosed with a physiological problem.

   CLINICAL JUDGMENT GUIDE: When deciding which client to assess first, the test taker should determine whether the client's signs and symptoms are normal or expected for the client's situation. After eliminating the expected option, the test taker should determine which situation is more life-threatening.

2. 1. Administering oxygen may help decrease the sickling of the cells, but this should not be the first intervention to address the client's headache.
   2. **Because the client is reporting a headache, the nurse should first rule out cerebrovascular accident (CVA) by assessing the client's neurological status and then determine whether it is a headache that can be treated with medication.**
   3. Before administering any pain medication to a client, the nurse must first assess the client to determine whether the pain is expected with the disease process or a complication requiring further nursing intervention.
   4. Only after CVA has been ruled out should the nurse medicate the client. Adequate hydration will help decrease the sickling of the cells, but this is not the first intervention to address the client's pain.

   CLINICAL JUDGMENT GUIDE: Assessment is the first step of the nursing process, and the test taker should use the nursing process or some other systematic process to assist in determining priorities.

3. 1. **The nurse should always praise the child for attempts at cooperation even if the child did not accomplish what the nurse asked.**
   2. The nurse can take this action after praising the child for the attempt.
   3. This action is appropriate and should be implemented, but not before the nurse praises the child for the attempt.
   4. The nurse can demonstrate the correct technique for the child, but not before praising the child for the attempt.

   CLINICAL JUDGMENT GUIDE: All options are plausible in questions that ask the test taker to identify an intervention to implement first. The test taker must identify the most important intervention.

4. 1. A 180 mg/dL glucose level for a child diagnosed with type 1 diabetes is not life-threatening, and the nurse would not assess this child first.
   2. The nurse would expect the child diagnosed with pneumonia to have these signs and symptoms; therefore, the nurse would not assess this child first.
   3. This is a normal potassium level; therefore, the nurse would not assess this child first.
   4. **A pulse oximeter reading of lower than 93% is significant and indicates hypoxia, which is life-threatening; therefore, this child should be assessed first.**

   CLINICAL JUDGMENT GUIDE: When deciding which client to assess first, the test taker should determine whether the signs and symptoms the client is exhibiting are normal or expected for the client's situation. After eliminating the expected options, the test taker should determine which situation is more life-threatening.

5. 1. The third dose of an aminoglycoside antibiotic would not be a priority over sliding scale insulin because insulin must be administered before the breakfast meal.
   2. Routine medications have a 1-hour leeway before and after the scheduled time; therefore, the steroid methylprednisolone (Solu-Medrol) does not have to be administered first.
   3. **Sliding scale insulin is ordered ac, which is before meals; therefore, this medication must be administered first after receiving the a.m. shift report.**
   4. Routine medications have a 1-hour leeway before and after the scheduled time; therefore, the stimulant methylphenidate (Ritalin) does not have to be administered first.

   CLINICAL JUDGMENT GUIDE: The test taker should know which medications are a priority, such as insulin, mucolytics, etc. These medications should be administered first by the nurse.

6. Correct order is 4, 5, 3, 2, 1.
   4. The nurse must first determine the infant's responsiveness by flicking the baby's feet.
   5. The nurse should then open the child's airway using the head-tilt chin-lift technique, with care taken not to hyperextend the neck. Then the nurse should look, listen, and feel for respirations.
   3. The nurse then administers quick puffs of air while covering the child's mouth and nose, preferably with a rescue mask.
   2. The nurse should determine whether the infant has a pulse by checking the brachial artery.
   1. If the infant has no pulse, the nurse should begin chest compressions using two fingers at a rate of 30:2.

   CLINICAL JUDGMENT GUIDE: This is an alternate type of question included in the NCLEX-RN® test plan. The nurse must be able to perform skills in the correct order.

7. 1. The first intervention after the child is admitted to the unit is to orient the parents and child to the room, the call system, and the hospital rules, such as not leaving the child alone.
   2. This task is within the scope of the UAP, but it is not a priority over orienting the child and parents to the room.
   3. The height and weight should be posted in case the client codes, but this can be done after the child and parents are oriented to the room.
   4. The child should receive a meal tray, but not before orientation to the room.

   CLINICAL JUDGMENT GUIDE: All options are plausible in questions that ask the test taker to identify an intervention to implement first. The test taker must identify the most important intervention.

8. 1. The nurse should immobilize the child's leg, but it is not the first intervention.
   2. The nurse must explain any procedure in words the child can understand. It does not matter how old the child is.
   3. This is an appropriate intervention, but it is not the first intervention.
   4. This is an appropriate intervention, but it is not the first intervention.

   CLINICAL JUDGMENT GUIDE: All options are plausible in questions that ask the test taker to identify an intervention to implement first. The test taker must identify the most important intervention.

9. 1. The child diagnosed with nephrotic syndrome would be expected to have proteinuria.
   2. The child diagnosed with leukemia would be expected to have petechiae.
   3. Drooling indicates the child is having trouble swallowing, and the epiglottis is at risk of completely occluding the airway. This warrants immediate intervention. The nurse should notify the HCP and obtain an emergency tracheostomy tray for the bedside.
   4. A child diagnosed with an ear infection would be expected to have an elevated temperature.

   CLINICAL JUDGMENT GUIDE: When deciding which client to assess first, the test taker should determine whether the signs and symptoms the client is exhibiting are normal or expected for the client's situation. After eliminating the expected options, the test taker should determine which situation is more life-threatening.

10. 1. Irritability and crying are expected signs and symptoms for a child diagnosed with bacterial meningitis; therefore, this child does not need to be assessed first.
    2. The child diagnosed with tetralogy of Fallot would be expected to have signs of congestive heart failure, so this child would not be assessed first.
    3. The child diagnosed with Reye syndrome would present with lethargy and vomiting, so this child would not be assessed first.
    4. Sunken eyeballs and decreased urine output are signs of dehydration, which is a life-threatening complication of diarrhea; therefore, this child should be assessed first.

    CLINICAL JUDGMENT GUIDE: The test taker must determine whether the signs and symptoms are normal for the disease process; if the signs and symptoms are normal, then the nurse should not assess the child first. If two or more are not expected, then the nurse must determine which is more life-threatening, needs further assessment, or needs notification of the HCP.

11. 1. A high fever and high-pitched crying may indicate a reaction to the immunizations; therefore, this parent must be called first to bring the child to the clinic.
    2. This child probably has an ear infection, which needs to be seen but is not a priority over a reaction to immunizations.
    3. The nurse needs to call in a prescription for the digoxin, but not before calling the parent about their child reacting to an immunization.
    4. The child may need to be seen but primarily kept in isolation, so this parent does not need to be called first.

CLINICAL JUDGMENT GUIDE: The test taker must determine whether the signs and symptoms are normal for the disease process; if the signs and symptoms are not normal, then the nurse should call this parent first.

12. 1. These are signs and symptoms of neurovascular compromise, and the cast may need to be cut (bifurcated), but this is not the first intervention.
    2. The child should be brought to the office, but the parent should first attempt to decrease edema by elevating the extremity.
    3. **The nurse should first take care of the client's body by having the parent elevate the left leg.**
    4. The orthopedist should be notified, but it is not the first intervention.

CLINICAL JUDGMENT GUIDE: When the question asks the nurse which intervention should be implemented first, it means all the interventions are possible. The nurse should first implement an action that will help the client's situation.

13. 1. The child diagnosed with iron deficiency anemia would be taking an iron elixir, which causes the stool to be black.
    2. The child diagnosed with PKU should not eat any meats, milk, dairy, and eggs because the child lacks the enzyme that breaks down phenylalanine.
    3. **A complication of rheumatic heart disease is valvular disorders, which may be manifested by respiratory problems; therefore, the nurse should notify the child's HCP.**
    4. The child diagnosed with acute glomerulonephritis would be expected to have dark urine.

CLINICAL JUDGMENT GUIDE: The nurse should notify the HCP of any signs and symptoms that are not expected with the disease process or are signs of a complication.

14. 1. **Bulging fontanels is a sign of increased intracranial pressure, a complication of neurological surgery; therefore, this child should be assessed first.**
    2. A moist, pink stoma is normal; therefore, this child does not need to be assessed first.
    3. This child needs to be assessed but is not a priority over a child with a surgical, possibly life-threatening complication.
    4. The child will have an indwelling urinary catheter, and clear amber urine is normal, so this child does not need to be assessed first.

CLINICAL JUDGMENT GUIDE: The test taker must determine whether the signs and symptoms are expected for the surgical procedure. This child should be assessed first if the signs and symptoms are not expected. If two clients have signs and symptoms that are not expected, then the child diagnosed with a life-threatening complication should be assessed first.

15. 1. It is appropriate for the nurse to perform ROM exercises to help prevent contractures, specifically scissoring of the legs. This action would not require intervention.
    2. Safety issues should always be addressed, and keeping the bed in the lowest position may prevent injury to the child.
    3. Taking the child to the activity room is being a client advocate and would not warrant intervention.
    4. **The child should be positioned upright to prevent aspiration during meals; therefore, this action would require the charge nurse to intervene.**

CLINICAL JUDGMENT GUIDE: When the question asks, "Which nursing action warrants immediate intervention?" it is an "except" question. Three of the actions are appropriate, whereas one is not.

16. 1. The UAP cannot assess a client; therefore, this is an inappropriate delegation.
    2. The child with a cleft palate repair is at risk for choking or damaging the incision site; therefore, this task should not be delegated to a UAP.
    3. Demonstrating is teaching, and the UAP cannot teach a client.
    4. **The last step of delegating to a UAP is for the RN to evaluate and determine whether the delegated tasks have been completed and performed correctly. This action indicates the nurse has delegated appropriately.**

CLINICAL JUDGMENT GUIDE: When delegating to a UAP, the RN must follow the four rights of clinical delegation: the right task to the right person, using the right communication, and providing the right feedback. The right feedback includes determining whether the delegated tasks were performed correctly.

17. 1. **Communication to the UAP must be clear, concise, correct, and complete. The RN must determine why there was a lack of communication, which resulted in the child receiving food; therefore, this action should be implemented first.**
    2. The RN retains ultimate accountability for any delegated tasks and cannot blame the UAP for the child being fed by the mother. The HCP needs to be notified to cancel the procedure.
    3. The RN should talk to the mother about why the child was being fed, but the nurse

must first determine whether the UAP told the mother not to feed the child and that the child was to be given nothing by mouth.
4. This action is too late to take care of the situation.

CLINICAL JUDGMENT GUIDE: There will be communication and management questions on the NCLEX-RN®. The nurse should first assess the situation and determine whether there was a misunderstanding of the communication between the RN and the UAP.

18. 1. The scrub technician is assigned to perform daily whirlpool dressing changes, a lengthy procedure. Therefore, assigning the one RN to this task would be inappropriate because they cannot be unavailable for an extended period.
    2. One of the responsibilities of the unit secretary is to perform clerical duties to support the nurses. The unit secretary can print the discharge instructions for the RN, but the RN is totally responsible for the correctness and accuracy of the information.
    3. The scrub technician cannot administer medications.
    4. The UAP is not responsible for evaluating laboratory data for the clients. The UAP should be on the unit taking care of the clients.

CLINICAL JUDGMENT GUIDE: The test taker must know the roles and scope of practice for each healthcare team member. The nurse should not delegate tasks that are not appropriate for the level of licensure.

19. Correct answers are 1, 2, 4, and 5.
    1. The UAP can pass the dietary trays to the clients because it does not require judgment.
    2. One of the responsibilities of the UAP is taking routine vital signs on clients.
    3. The RN must complete the preoperative checklist because it requires nursing judgment to determine whether the client is ready for surgery.
    4. One of the responsibilities of the UAP is changing bed linens.
    5. The UAP can document the client's intake and output, but the UAP cannot evaluate the numbers.

CLINICAL JUDGMENT GUIDE: This is an alternative type of question included in the NCLEX-RN® examination. The nurse must be able to select all the options that answer the question correctly.

20. 1. The administration of blood products does not require the most experienced nurse.
    2. Preparing a child for a routine procedure does not require the most experienced nurse.
    3. The child recovering from a sickle cell crisis would not require the most experienced nurse.
    4. The child newly diagnosed with a chronic disease, which will have acute exacerbations, requires extensive teaching; therefore, the most experienced nurse should be assigned to this child and family.

CLINICAL JUDGMENT GUIDE: The test taker must determine which client is the most unstable and would require the most experienced nurse, thus making this type of question an "except" question. Three clients are either stable or have non-life-threatening conditions.

21. 1. Only the RN can withdraw blood from a central line.
    2. The social worker or case manager is responsible for referring clients to support groups. This task is not an expected responsibility of a floor nurse or LPN.
    3. Only chemotherapy-certified RNs can administer antineoplastic chemotherapeutic medications. According to the Oncology Nursing Society, this is a national minimal standard of care.
    4. The dietitian is responsible for ensuring that the proper food is provided along with evaluating the child's nutritional intake, not checking the amount of food eaten—this is the responsibility of the nursing staff.

CLINICAL JUDGMENT GUIDE: The test taker must know the role and scope of practice for each healthcare team member. The nurse should not delegate tasks that are not appropriate for the level of licensure or required experience.

22. 1. A 6-year-old child on bedrest needs an appropriate activity to help with distraction; a cartoon video would be an age-appropriate activity.
    2. The child life therapist is responsible for recreational and developmental activity for the hospitalized child, but any staff member should address the child's psychosocial needs.
    3. Part of the delegation process is to evaluate the UAP's performance of duties, and the RN should praise any initiative on the part of the UAP in being a client advocate.
    4. Videos are one of the few age-appropriate activities to occupy a 6-year-old on bedrest; therefore, there is no reason to notify the charge nurse.

CLINICAL JUDGMENT GUIDE: This is an "except" question. The test taker should ask which task is appropriate to delegate to the UAP. The RN is responsible for evaluating the UAP's actions.

23. 1. The newborn diagnosed with the myelomeningocele has a portion of the spinal cord and membranes protruding through the back and is at risk for hydrocephalus and meningitis; this client should be assigned to a more experienced nurse.
    2. **After completing the NICU internship, the new graduate nurse should be able to care for a premature infant because care is primarily supportive.**
    3. Esophageal atresia, a congenital anomaly in which the esophagus does not completely develop, is a clinical and surgical emergency. It puts the newborn at risk for aspiration because the upper esophagus ends in a blind pouch, with the lower part of the esophagus connected to the trachea. This newborn should be assigned to a more experienced nurse.
    4. Tetralogy of Fallot is a cyanotic congenital anomaly. It includes a combination of four defects of the heart, all of which result in unoxygenated blood being pumped into the systemic circulation. This newborn must be assigned to an experienced nurse.

CLINICAL JUDGMENT GUIDE: The test taker must determine which client is the most stable, which makes this an "except" question. Three clients are either unstable or have potentially life-threatening conditions.

24. 1. Weighing the diaper is the procedure for determining the infant's urinary output and is not part of obtaining a urine specimen.
    2. **The National Council of State Boards of Nursing (NCSBN) defined *delegation* as transferring the authority to perform a nursing task to a competent individual in a selected situation. The RN retains the accountability for the delegation. The nurse must determine whether the UAP has the ability and knowledge to perform a task. This question clarifies whether the UAP can obtain a urine specimen.**
    3. Obtaining a urine specimen with an indwelling catheter on an 11-month-old infant would require more expertise than a UAP would have on the pediatric unit. Furthermore, it does not determine whether the UAP understands how to do the procedure.
    4. This statement does not determine whether the UAP understands how to obtain a urine specimen from an 11-month-old infant.

CLINICAL JUDGMENT GUIDE: The nurse cannot delegate any task the UAP admits to being unable to perform. Delegation means the nurse is responsible for the UAP's actions; therefore, the nurse should confirm the UAP is knowledgeable of the appropriate procedure.

25. 1. The UAP can orient the parents and child to the room and demonstrate how to use the call light, how the bed works, or how the television works.
    2. The UAP cannot prepare a child for endoscopy; this requires assessment and evaluation to determine whether the child is ready for the procedure.
    3. There must be at least two people to log roll a child, and the UAP cannot do this procedure alone.
    4. The RN cannot delegate assessment to the UAP.

CLINICAL JUDGMENT GUIDE: The RN cannot delegate assessment, teaching, evaluation, medications, or an unstable client to a UAP.

26. 1. The UAP can weigh the diapers and obtain urine output. The RN must evaluate the output.
    2. A child under 12 cannot be left alone in the room, and the UAP could stay with the child while the parent gets something to eat.
    3. The Pavlik harness should not be removed, so bathing the child in the harness is appropriate and does not warrant intervention.
    4. **The 7-month-old should have elbow restraints, not wrist restraints. Elbow restraints prevent the child from putting fingers into the mouth, but allow the child to move the arms.**

CLINICAL JUDGMENT GUIDE: The RN supervises and evaluates the care the UAP provides to clients. The nurse must intervene and correct the UAP's behavior.

27. Correct answers are 2, 3, 4, and 5.
    1. The RN cannot assign teaching to the LPN.
    2. The UAP can apply an ice collar because the client is stable.
    3. The UAP can apply ointment to a diaper rash—it is a medication but the UAP can apply it.
    4. The LPN can double-check a dose of medication. The RN can assign medication administration to an LPN.
    5. The LPN can enter the HCP's orders into the EHR.

CLINICAL JUDGMENT GUIDE: This is an alternative type of question included in the NCLEX-RN®

examination. The nurse must be able to select all the options that answer the question correctly. The RN cannot delegate assessment, teaching, evaluation, medications, or an unstable client to a UAP. The RN cannot assign assessment, teaching, evaluation, or an unstable client to an LPN.

28.
1. The RN cannot delegate teaching to the UAP.
2. The LPN could teach a client how to irrigate a colostomy, but a 4-month-old is incontinent of stool; therefore, irrigating the colostomy is not done.
3. The LPN or RN should remove the IV catheter of a 4-month-old child, not the UAP.
4. **The UAP can escort the child and parents to the car.**

CLINICAL JUDGMENT GUIDE: The RN cannot delegate assessment, teaching, evaluation, medications, or an unstable client to a UAP. The RN cannot assign assessment, teaching, evaluation, or an unstable client to an LPN. Many questions on the NCLEX-RN® evaluate the test taker's knowledge of the disease process or surgical procedure, delegation, and assignments.

29.
1. **The UAP can take vital signs, but the RN should assess the child to determine whether this is routine postoperative pain (expected) or whether a complication is occurring.**
2. **A rule of thumb—if anyone else gives the RN information about a client, the nurse should assess the client before taking further action.**
3. The nurse may need to notify the HCP, but not before assessing the child.
4. The nurse may need to administer pain medication, but not before assessing the child.

CLINICAL JUDGMENT GUIDE: When the question asks, "Which intervention should the nurse implement first?" it means all or at least more than one option is plausible. Remember: If another person, a machine, or a laboratory datum provides information about the client, the RN should assess the client first.

30.
1. **The nurse should offer the child choices that ensure cooperation with the therapeutic regimen, such as asking when the child will ambulate, not whether the child will ambulate.**
2. The nurse could ask the parents for help to ensure the client ambulates, but this may cause a rift in the relationship between the nurse, parent, and child. This intervention is not the most appropriate intervention.
3. The child development therapist could assist with activities encouraging the client to ambulate, but the nurse should take control of the situation and ensure the client ambulates. This intervention is not the most appropriate intervention.
4. This is bribery, and the nurse should not use this technique to ensure cooperation with the therapeutic regimen.

CLINICAL JUDGMENT GUIDE: The test taker should know communication techniques appropriate to a child's developmental stages.

31.
1. The nurse must take action, or the child will fear the nurse.
2. The nurse should discuss the inappropriate comment with the parent, not the child.
3. If every nurse reported this type of comment to Child Protective Services, it would only unnecessarily increase the workload in an already overloaded system. Furthermore, reporting perceived potential abuse to Child Protective Services is a very serious accusation.
4. **The nurse should explain to the parent that threatening the child with a shot will cause the child to be frightened of healthcare professionals. This type of comment is inappropriate and should not be used to discipline a child.**

CLINICAL JUDGMENT GUIDE: The test taker should be familiar with communication techniques and tactfully discuss this statement with the parent.

32.
1. There is a Web site to obtain information about Down syndrome, but this type of referral would not be the most appropriate for parents needing to deal with the emotional aspects of having a child with special needs.
2. The hospital chaplain is an essential part of the multidisciplinary healthcare team but would not have specialized knowledge regarding caring for a special needs child.
3. **The most appropriate referral would be to a support group where other parents of children with special needs can share their feelings and provide advice on caring for their child in the home.**
4. Although Down syndrome results from a trisomy chromosome 21, it is primarily associated with a maternal age of more than 35 years. Furthermore, a geneticist would not have specialized knowledge regarding caring for a child with special needs.

CLINICAL JUDGMENT GUIDE: According to the NCLEX-RN® test plan, referrals are included in the management of care. The test taker must know the roles of each member of the multidisciplinary healthcare team and be prepared to make referrals for clients. These topics will be tested on the NCLEX-RN® examination.

33. 1. The newborn nursery does not need more people in the area. Personnel are needed to monitor all exits.
    2. The purpose of using code names to alert hospital personnel of emergencies is to avoid panic among the clients and visitors; therefore, the nurse should not explain the situation to the clients and visitors.
    3. Any time there is an overhead emergency announcement, the charge nurse is responsible for following the hospital emergency plan.
    4. **Code Pink means an infant has been abducted from the newborn nursery. The priority intervention is to prevent the abductor from taking the child from the hospital, which can be accomplished by placing a staff member at all the unit exits.**

CLINICAL JUDGMENT GUIDE: The nurse must be knowledgeable of hospital emergency preparedness. Students and new employees receive this information in hospital orientations and are responsible for correctly implementing procedures. The NCLEX-RN® test plan includes questions on the safe and effective care environment.

34. 1. Even though case management is a strategy to ensure coordination of care while reducing costs, the nurse should not share this with the parent.
    2. The case manager is not responsible for ensuring that the client receives the correct medication; it is the responsibility of the HCP.
    3. **The case manager will coordinate the care of a client diagnosed with a chronic illness with other members of the multidisciplinary healthcare team. This assignment attempts to prevent duplication of services and provides the parent with a specific individual to coordinate services to meet the child's needs.**
    4. The life expectancy of a child diagnosed with Duchenne's muscular dystrophy is approximately 25 years. The case manager is not responsible for helping the child have a normal life expectancy.

CLINICAL JUDGMENT GUIDE: According to the NCLEX-RN® test plan, questions on case management are included. The test taker must know the roles of all members of the multidisciplinary healthcare team. These will be tested on the NCLEX-RN® examination.

35. 1. Although this would not be the first step in investigating a problem, this action may be initiated if it is determined to cause an increase in infection rates.
    2. The nurse should utilize evidence-based practice research when proposing changes because it is part of the performance improvement process, but it is not the first intervention when investigating the problem.
    3. **The first intervention is to determine the extent of the problem and the problem owner.**
    4. This action may need to be implemented once it is determined whether there is a problem with IV infection rates. However, this would be the second step in the process.

CLINICAL JUDGMENT GUIDE: The NCLEX-RN® test plan includes performance improvement (quality improvement) in the management of care content. Performance improvement (quality improvement) activities are tested under the Management of Care section of the NCLEX-RN® test plan.

36. 1. The ethical principle of justice is to treat all clients fairly, regardless of age, socioeconomic status, or any other variable, including clients with special needs. This statement supports the adolescent's right to her opinion even though she has Down syndrome.
    2. If the adolescent needs clarification of the procedure, this would be an appropriate response, and an example of the ethical principle of veracity, or truth-telling.
    3. This statement exemplifies the ethical principle of paternalism, in which the nurse knows what is best for the client.
    4. **This is an example of autonomy, in which the client has the right to self-determination. The Nuremburg Code of Ethics supports explicitly the rights of individuals with special needs against being forced to participate in procedures they do not want.**

CLINICAL JUDGMENT GUIDE: The NCLEX-RN® test plan includes nursing care that addresses ethical principles, including autonomy, beneficence, justice, and veracity, to name a few.

37. 1. Although this may be the case, this is not client advocacy, and doing so may make the parent feel guilty about not being able to afford glasses for her child.
    2. **This is an example of client advocacy because many local service organizations, such as the Lions Club or the Rotary Club, will subsidize the cost of the vision test and glasses.**

3. Medicaid does not pay for glasses; it is not the school nurse's business whether the family is on Medicaid.
4. The nurse should not loan the parent money because this crosses professional boundaries.

CLINICAL JUDGMENT GUIDE: Advocating for a client's rights and needs is the responsibility of the RN and is tested under the Management of Care section of the NCLEX-RN® test plan. A client advocate acts as a liaison between clients and HCPs to help improve or maintain a high quality of healthcare.

38. 1. The 16-year-old client is not old enough to sign the permit; therefore, pain medication would not be withheld.
2. Legally, a child under 18 must have a parent or legal guardian sign for informed consent. The nurse should determine whether the child knows the situation and assents to the procedure.
3. The surgeon is responsible for explaining the procedure; the nurse is responsible for witnessing the signature on the operative permit.
4. The nurse is responsible for witnessing the signature. Having a visitor sign the operative permit is a violation of HIPAA.

CLINICAL JUDGMENT GUIDE: The test taker should know legal guidelines and informed consent. This information is included in the NCLEX-RN® test plan.

39. 1. A written memo does not allow the staff to have input into how to correct the problem. This memo might lead to blaming and arguments among the staff.
2. The performance improvement committee is designed to improve client care, not to address management issues.
3. This action implies that the unit manager does not believe the central supply lost charges. If the unit manager has this concern, it should be addressed directly with the central supply supervisor.
4. Because the staff is responsible for following the hospital procedure for charging for items used in client care, the unit manager should discuss this with the staff to determine what should be done to correct the problem.

CLINICAL JUDGMENT GUIDE: Management questions will be asked during the NCLEX-RN® examination. There is often no test-taking strategy; the nurse must be knowledgeable of management issues.

40. 1. A 1-year-old child crying when the parent leaves the room is developmentally on target.
2. The 2-year-old speaking in two- or three-word sentences is developmentally on target.
3. The 3-year-old should be toilet trained by this age.
4. **The toddler (age 1–3) is expected to throw temper tantrums, but a 4-year-old child should not be doing this; therefore, the child is not developmentally on target and the child developmental specialist should be notified.**

CLINICAL JUDGMENT GUIDE: The pediatric nurse must know the normal developmental tasks for each age. The Joint Commission mandates that all children in a pediatric unit have a developmental assessment and intervention if the child is not on task.

41. 1. The child diagnosed with uncontrolled pain would require a more experienced nurse.
2. Infected skeletal pin sites can lead to osteomyelitis, requiring a more experienced nurse.
3. This child and parents require extensive teaching and should be assigned to a more experienced nurse.
4. The new graduate nurse should be able to complete preoperative teaching and prepare the young client for surgery. This client is stable.

CLINICAL JUDGMENT GUIDE: An inexperienced nurse should be assigned the most stable client.

42. 1. Elevating the arm to help decrease edema is appropriate and does not warrant intervention.
2. The nurse is legally obligated to notify Child Protective Services of any suspected child abuse.
3. A drooling child may have epiglottitis, and opening the mouth may lead to respiratory distress. This action warrants intervention by the charge nurse.
4. The nurse must confirm a urinary tract infection by obtaining a urine specimen.

CLINICAL JUDGMENT GUIDE: The test taker must be able to apply assessment data and interventions to determine whether the action is appropriate. This question is an NCLEX-RN® style application question.

43. 1. The nurse must administer the scheduled insulin dose and the sliding scale coverage; therefore, this is the incorrect dose.
2. The nurse must administer the scheduled dose with an additional 8 units, so the total dose is 18 units of regular insulin and insulin isophane (NPH) 20 units. The nurse should not administer two injections to the child.

3. This is the scheduled dose, not including the sliding scale coverage.
4. This covers the sliding scale coverage but not the scheduled dose.

CLINICAL JUDGMENT GUIDE: This is an alternate type of question included in the NCLEX-RN® test plan. The test taker must be able to read a medication administration record (MAR), be knowledgeable of medications, and decide the most appropriate intervention.

44. Correct answers are 1 and 3.
    1. **Including the parents in developing the plan of care will help establish a positive relationship.**
    2. Holding their child will help with the child and parent relationship, but not with the nurse and parent relationship.
    3. **Allowing the parents to vent their feelings will help form a positive nurse and parent relationship.**
    4. The nurse must not make the parents feel guilty if they have to work while the child is hospitalized. A relative can stay with the child if the parents have to work.
    5. This will help the child and parent relationship, not the nurse and parent relationship.

CLINICAL JUDGMENT GUIDE: "Select all that apply" questions require the test taker to select all options that answer the question correctly.

45. 1. The 9-month-old infant's language and cognitive skills include imitating sounds, saying single syllables, and beginning to put syllables together. Using "mama" and "dada" indicates this child is developmentally on target.
    2. The 10- to 12-month-old infant can walk with one hand held by another or with one hand holding onto the furniture but will usually crawl to get places more rapidly. This behavior indicates the child is developmentally on target.
    3. **The 8-month-old infant should be able to sit steadily unsupported; therefore, this child is developmentally delayed and warrants a referral to the early childhood development specialist. Leaning forward on both hands to sit is normal for a 6-month-old.**
    4. The 4-month-old infant should be able to turn from the abdomen to the back; therefore, this child is developmentally on target.

CLINICAL JUDGMENT GUIDE: The pediatric nurse must know the normal developmental tasks for each age. The Joint Commission mandates that all children in a pediatric unit have a developmental assessment and intervention if the child is not on task.

46. 1. **The most important intervention for this child is to ensure the child has some control and input into the decision-making. Obtaining assent from children 7 years of age and older is customary. Assent means the child has been fully informed about the procedure and concurs with those giving the informed consent.**
    2. The parents must sign the permit because the child is under age 18, but the most important intervention is ensuring the child is included and aware of decisions about the child's body.
    3. The nurse may be able to clarify some of the child's or parent's questions and does not need to refer all questions to the HCP.
    4. Witnessing the signature on the permit is required before the child has surgery, but it is not the most important intervention.

CLINICAL JUDGMENT GUIDE: The NCLEX-RN® test plan indicates that the test taker should know the legal guidelines for informed consent.

47. 1. The nurse should call hospital security when a client or visitor is being abusive, but this is not a legal action.
    2. **Legally, the nurse is required to report any suspected child abuse. A 13-year-old child having a baby, withdrawn, and silent, along with a potential abuser trying to control access to the child, should make the nurse suspect child abuse.**
    3. Referring the client to a social worker is not a legal action.
    4. Asking the client whether she feels safe at home is an appropriate assessment question, but it is not a legal action.

CLINICAL JUDGMENT GUIDE: The NCLEX-RN® test plan indicates that the test taker should know legal guidelines and requirements.

48. 1. First, the charge nurse must ensure that clients and visitors are safe. Someone will notify the charge nurse about the location of the fire.
    2. **The safety of the clients and visitors is the priority; therefore, ensuring that they are in a room with the door closed is the first intervention.**
    3. The charge nurse may need to prepare for evacuation, but it is not the first intervention.
    4. Although making a list of clients not currently on the unit is an appropriate intervention, the charge nurse must first ensure the safety of the clients and visitors on the pediatric unit.

CLINICAL JUDGMENT GUIDE: The nurse must be knowledgeable of hospital emergency preparedness.

Students and new employees receive this information in hospital orientation and are responsible for correctly implementing procedures. The NCLEX-RN® test plan includes questions on the safe and effective care environment.

49.
1. The HIPAA officer can be notified of the breach of confidentiality, but the nurse must first confront the two nurses and correct the behavior.
2. The nurses can be reported to their clinical manager, but the nurse must first confront the two nurses and correct the behavior.
3. The situation can be documented in writing and turned into the HIPAA officer (not the CNO), but the nurse must first confront the two nurses and correct the behavior.
4. This is a violation of HIPAA; therefore, the nurse must first confront the two nurses and correct the behavior.

CLINICAL JUDGMENT GUIDE: There will be management questions on the NCLEX-RN®. There is often no test-taking strategy; the nurse must be knowledgeable of management issues. The Health Insurance Portability and Accountability Act (HIPAA) was passed in 1996 to standardize the exchange of information between HCPs and to ensure client record confidentiality.

50.
1. The nurse would not be concerned about not passing meconium until at least 24 hours after delivery.
2. The nurse would not be concerned about a slightly jaundiced newborn until after 24 hours postpartum; at this point, the HCP would investigate to determine whether the jaundice is pathological.
3. A jittery and irritable newborn must first be assessed for possible hypoglycemia. The nurse could feed the newborn glucose water or provide more frequent, regular feedings.
4. Although the nurse should determine why the newborn will not stop crying, the newborn showing signs of hypoglycemia warrants immediate intervention.

CLINICAL JUDGMENT GUIDE: When the question asks, "Which warrants immediate intervention?" it is an "except" question.

51.
1. Aluminum hydroxide; magnesium hydroxide (Maalox), an antacid, is administered to neutralize gastric acidity and help with heartburn, not abdominal pain.
2. A nonnarcotic analgesic, acetaminophen (Tylenol), treats mild pain, 2 to 4 on a pain scale.
3. The narcotic analgesic, hydrocodone (Vicodin), is used for moderate-to-severe pain; 5 is considered moderate pain. The child received a dose at 0600, which relieved the pain for 7 hours; therefore, this would be the most appropriate medication.
4. An IVP narcotic analgesic should be administered for severe pain, that is, pain greater than 7 on a pain scale of 1 to 10.

CLINICAL JUDGMENT GUIDE: This is an alternate type of question included in the NCLEX-RN® test plan. The test taker must be able to read a medication administration record (MAR), be knowledgeable of medications, and decide the nurse's most appropriate intervention.

52.
1. The nurse should not accept any assignment for which they are unqualified. A newborn assessment requires specialized knowledge and skills to detect potential complications.
2. The nurse unfamiliar with the procedure or the unit should not be assigned to assist a pediatrician in performing a procedure.
3. This is a dangerous procedure because the nurse must insert a tube into the newborn's stomach. A nurse unfamiliar with this procedure should refuse the assignment.
4. Any nurse can take an infant to the mother's room and check the bands to ensure the right infant is with the right mother. This task is appropriate for a nurse who has never worked in a nursery.

CLINICAL JUDGMENT GUIDE: The nurse should not accept any assignments that require knowledge, skills, or abilities beyond the nurse's expertise.

53.
1. The 9-month-old infant should be able to sit without support. Therefore, the RN should instruct the UAP to perform the developmental task of helping the child sit without support.
2. Teaching a child to catch a beach ball would be appropriate for a 15- to 18-month-old child, so the RN should not instruct the UAP to perform this task.
3. The UAP should not use food as a reward or comfort measure because it may lead to childhood obesity.
4. Teaching a child how to blow a kiss is a language or cognitive activity and will not help the child's gross motor development.

CLINICAL JUDGMENT GUIDE: An RN cannot delegate assessment, teaching, evaluation, medications, or an unstable client to a UAP. Interventions requiring clinical judgment cannot be delegated.

54. 1. Ensuring no one can view the screen is an appropriate information technology guideline.
    2. Researching medication online ensures safe and effective nursing care and shows that the nurse keeps abreast of new medications.
    3. According to the NCLEX-RN® test plan, the nurse must know about information technology. Giving another nurse their access code is a very serious violation of information technology guidelines and should be reported.
    4. Logging off the computer is an appropriate information technology guideline.

CLINICAL JUDGMENT GUIDE: The test taker must know information technology security and confidentiality. These topics will be tested on the NCLEX-RN® examination.

55. 1. A dog bite is an emergency but not life-threatening; therefore, the nurse will not assess this child first.
    2. The nurse must assess a child diagnosed with a head laceration, but not before a child at risk of a medication poisoning death.
    3. The child diagnosed with a fractured tibia would not be expected to move the foot.
    4. A child ingesting a bottle of prenatal vitamins is a potentially life-threatening medication poisoning. The nurse must first determine how many vitamins were taken, how long ago they were taken, and whether or not the vitamins contained iron. The child's neurological status must also be assessed.

CLINICAL JUDGMENT GUIDE: When deciding which client to assess first, the test taker should determine whether the signs and symptoms the client is exhibiting are normal or expected for the client's situation. After eliminating the expected option, the test taker should determine which situation is more life-threatening.

56. 1. The pediatric client has the right to an explanation of procedures being done to their body.
    2. The pediatric client has a right to be treated with dignity and respect. Just because the child is being coded does not mean the nurse should allow the child's body to be exposed to everyone in the room.
    3. The pediatric client has a right to confidentiality, and the parents or legal guardians are the only individuals with a right to the child's health information. Talking to the grandparents is a violation of HIPAA unless the parents have approved.
    4. The nurse is responsible and accountable to protect the health, safety, and rights of the pediatric client. Leaving an uncapped needle at the bedside could cause serious harm to the child.

CLINICAL JUDGMENT GUIDE: There will be management questions on the NCLEX-RN® addressing client advocacy. A client advocate acts as a liaison between clients and HCPs to help improve or maintain a high quality of care.

57. 1. Placing the IV line on an infusion pump helps ensure the client does not receive an overload of IV fluid. Most facilities require an IV pump and volume-controlled chamber when administering fluids in a pediatric clinic.
    2. A volume-controlled device (Buretrol) is an infusion device used with children when administering IV fluids. The chamber is filled with 1 hour's amount of fluid so that the child will not inadvertently receive an overload of fluid. Fluid volume overload is a potentially life-threatening situation in children.
    3. The nurse should assess the site frequently to ensure that the IV line does not infiltrate; however, every 15 minutes is unnecessary; therefore, this does not warrant intervention.
    4. The IV tubing should not be used longer than 72 hours; therefore, labeling the tubing with the date and time would not warrant intervention.

CLINICAL JUDGMENT GUIDE: When the question asks, "Which warrants immediate intervention?" it is an "except" question. Three of the statements indicate an appropriate intervention, whereas one does not.

58. 1. Abandonment is a reportable offense to the state board of nursing in every state. Reportable offenses could result in stipulations made to the nurse's license.
    2. This action is a failure to follow the five rights of medication administration, but it is not a reportable offense.
    3. Multiple medication errors are a management issue, not a reportable offense.
    4. Having an affair with a fellow employee is not a reportable offense.

CLINICAL JUDGMENT GUIDE: The NCLEX-RN® test plan includes nursing care ruled by legal requirements and scope of practice. The nurse must be knowledgeable of these issues. The nurse's actions should be documented then reported as necessary.

59.
1. A copper bracelet may or may not help the child diagnosed with rheumatoid arthritis, but it does not warrant further investigation because it will not hurt the child.
2. Aloe vera is used in many topical burn preparations; therefore, this practice would not warrant further investigation.
3. Mentholated topical ointment (Vick's VapoRub) may or may not help the child's cold, but it does not warrant further investigation because it will not hurt the child.
4. The Food and Drug Administration does not regulate herbal products, and there is very little (if any) research on herbal use with children. The nurse should investigate the herbs the child receives before taking action.

CLINICAL JUDGMENT GUIDE: The test taker should be knowledgeable about complementary and alternative medicine (CAM).

60.
1. This is an appropriate nursing intervention so the parent will not have to leave their child, but it is not the first intervention. The child's safety is the priority.
2. The RN could go to the cafeteria and tell the parent to return to the room, but the UAP should stay with the child during this time.
3. The child's safety is the priority; therefore, the RN should have the UAP stay with the child until the parent returns.
4. Social services would not need to be notified at this time. If the parent continually leaves the child alone, this would be appropriate.

CLINICAL JUDGMENT GUIDE: The test taker should apply the nursing process when the question asks the nurse, "Which intervention should be implemented first?" In this case, the safety of the client is the priority intervention.

61. Correct answers are 1, 3, 4, and 5.
1. An 18-month-old child should be throwing temper tantrums. This behavior indicates the child is developing a sense of autonomy.
2. An 18-month-old child should cling to the parent and interact continuously with the primary caregiver. A child not interacting with the parent is not meeting the task of developing a sense of autonomy.
3. The child has met the task of trust when they cry if the parent leaves the room.
4. When a child responds to their name, it indicates a sense of identity; therefore, the task is met.
5. When a child is smiling and happy with successful toilet training, it indicates the development of autonomy and independence.

CLINICAL JUDGMENT GUIDE: The pediatric nurse must know the normal developmental tasks for each age. The Joint Commission mandates that all children in a pediatric unit have a developmental assessment and intervention if the child is not on task.

62.
1. An autocratic manager uses an authoritarian approach to direct the activities of others. This individual makes most of the decisions alone without input from other staff members.
2. A laissez-faire manager maintains a permissive climate with little direction or control.
3. A democratic manager is people-oriented and emphasizes efficient group functioning. The environment is open, and communication flows both ways.
4. A democratic manager is people-oriented and emphasizes efficient group functioning.

CLINICAL JUDGMENT GUIDE: There will be management questions on the NCLEX-RN®. There is often no test-taking strategy; the nurse must be knowledgeable of management issues.

63.
1. Squatting relieves the hypoxic episodes, and the child should be able to remain in the squatting position.
2. The child diagnosed with a cyanotic congenital heart defect should have oxygen when being active.
3. This indicates the parent does not understand that the child will not be able to participate in active sports because of the stress on the heart.
4. This behavior indicates the parent understands the importance of salt restriction because of potential congestive heart failure.

CLINICAL JUDGMENT GUIDE: When the question asks, "Which outcome would support that teaching has been effective?" it is an "except" question. Three comments indicate that the client or family does not understand the teaching, and one indicates that the client or family does understand the teaching.

64.
1. This action is appropriate once the neonate's dose has been adjusted.
2. This action is appropriate once the neonate's dose has been adjusted.
3. At 2 weeks old, there probably will not be a level yet.

4. Digoxin can be administered to neonates, but this is an adult dose: The neonate maintenance dose is 4–8 mcg/kg; 0.125 mg equals 125 mcg. The dose for a 6.8-kg infant would be 27–54 mcg daily.

CLINICAL JUDGMENT GUIDE: This is an alternate type of question included in the NCLEX-RN® test plan. The test taker must be able to read a medication administration record (MAR), be knowledgeable of medications, and decide the nurse's most appropriate intervention.

65. 1. The infant's arm does not have enough tissue for an injection.
    2. The infant has a poorly developed dorsogluteal muscle, and the sciatic nerve is in this area of the body. Injecting a needle into the nerve could cause permanent damage.
    3. Vaccines are not administered into the abdomen.
    4. The anterior lateral thigh muscle (vastus lateralis) is the preferred site for an infant to receive an injection. It is the infant's largest muscle and is far away from nerves.

CLINICAL JUDGMENT GUIDE: The nurse must be aware of the appropriate location to administer medications based on the type of medication and the age or body size of the client.

66. Answer: 45 mL/hr.
    The IV pump is set at an hourly rate. Pediatric clients receive medications at the rate per hour prescribed by the HCP. Increasing the rate is not within scope of nursing judgment for this client. The medication should be administered at the rate determined by the HCP to be a safe volume.

CLINICAL JUDGMENT GUIDE: This is an alternate type of question included in the NCLEX-RN® examination. The nurse must know how to solve math questions.

67. Correct answers are 1, 3, and 5.
    1. This child has injuries consistent with child abuse. The nurse should notify Child Protective Services and the police.
    2. This could result in being unable to prosecute the perpetrator if the nurse is untrained in forensic medicine.
    3. The nurse should determine the full extent of the child's injuries.
    4. The nurse should not notify the parents of the potential involvement. The police are fully capable of doing this for themselves. The nurse could instigate an inflammatory situation with this action.
    5. The child needs x-ray studies to determine the extent of internal injuries.

CLINICAL JUDGMENT GUIDE: This is an alternative type of question included in the NCLEX-RN® examination. The nurse must be able to select all the options that answer the question correctly.

68. Correct order is 5, 3, 2, 4, 1.
    5. Taking the vital signs is part of the assessment and a beginning point for the nurse.
    3. Because the child has been losing fluids, the nurse should assess tissue turgor to determine whether the parents' fluid replacement has been adequate.
    2. The nurse should ensure that the parents do not leave the child alone in the room and that the parents are aware of any safety measures used to protect the toddler from abduction and how to call the nurse in case of need.
    4. The parents will need to change diapers so the child will not develop skin irritation problems.
    1. When the nurse provides diapers, it is an ideal opportunity to teach the parents about weighing them before and after the child soils them.

CLINICAL JUDGMENT GUIDE: This is an alternate type of question included in the NCLEX-RN® test plan. The nurse must be able to perform skills in the correct order.

69. 1. The child having respiratory difficulty and inspiratory retractions, should be assessed first. Remember Maslow's Hierarchy of Needs.
    2. A pulse oximeter reading of 93% is within normal limits (93%–100%). It is on the low side because CF causes chronic hypoxia, and a low arterial oxygen level is expected.
    3. This is a normal potassium level; therefore, the nurse would not assess this child first.
    4. A 210 mg/dL glucose level for a child diagnosed with type 2 diabetes is not life-threatening, and the nurse would not assess this child first.

CLINICAL JUDGMENT GUIDE: When deciding which client to assess first, the test taker should determine whether the client's signs and symptoms are normal or expected for the client's situation. After eliminating the expected option, the test taker should determine which situation is more life-threatening.

70. 1. The child in a sickle cell crisis is not stable; therefore, the RN charge nurse should not delegate this task to a UAP.
    2. Oxygen is considered a medication, and the RN cannot delegate medication administration to a UAP.

3. The child diagnosed with nephrotic syndrome experiences weight gain secondary to edema, which is expected with this disease process. This child is stable, and the UAP can obtain weights; therefore, the RN charge nurse can delegate this task to the UAP.
4. The child diagnosed with a traumatic brain injury is not stable; therefore, the UAP should not transfer this client to the ICU.

CLINICAL JUDGMENT GUIDE: When delegating to a UAP, the RN must follow the four rights of clinical delegation: the right task to the right person, using the right communication, and providing the right feedback.

71. 1. Immobilizing the child's leg is appropriate for the RN; therefore, this would not warrant intervention by the charge nurse.
    2. The RN should explain the procedure to the 2-year-old using age-appropriate terms; therefore, this would not warrant intervention by the charge nurse.
    3. The needle and syringe should be disposed of in the sharps container; therefore, this action does not warrant intervention.
    4. The RN should not recap the needle after administering the medication, so this warrants intervention by the charge nurse. The syringe and needle should be disposed of in the sharps container.

CLINICAL JUDGMENT GUIDE: When the question asks, "Which nursing action warrants immediate intervention?" it is an "except" question. Three of the actions are appropriate, whereas one is not.

72. 1. The UAP can document intake and output, and the child has a chronic illness; therefore, the child is stable. This task could be delegated safely.
    2. The child diagnosed with an acute exacerbation of IBD must be NPO; therefore, this task should not be delegated to the UAP.
    3. The UAP can elevate this child's leg and it is appropriate to elevate the leg to help decrease edema. This task could be delegated safely.
    4. The UAP can take laboratory specimens to the laboratory.
    5. The UAP can take the vital signs of a child reporting ear pain.

CLINICAL JUDGMENT GUIDE: When delegating to a UAP, the RN must follow the four rights of clinical delegation: the right task to the right person, using the right communication, and providing the right feedback. The right feedback includes determining whether the delegated tasks were performed correctly.

73. 1. The charge nurse should suspect this child has otitis media and would not have to assign the most experienced nurse to this child. A less experienced ED nurse could care for this client.
    2. The charge nurse should suspect this child is experiencing an acute exacerbation of reactive airway disease and assign the most experienced nurse to this child. This child is in a potentially life-threatening situation.
    3. The charge nurse should suspect this child has a urinary tract infection, which is not a life-threatening situation. The charge nurse should think about possible sexual abuse, but the most experienced nurse would not need to care for this child.
    4. The charge nurse should suspect the child has pneumonia, which is not life-threatening; therefore, the most experienced nurse does not need to be assigned to this child.

CLINICAL JUDGMENT GUIDE: The test taker must determine which client is the most unstable and would require the most experienced nurse, thus making this type of question an "except" question. Three clients are either stable or have non-life-threatening conditions.

74. 1. The child's temperature should be reduced by receiving an antipyretic medication such as acetaminophen (Tylenol), but it is not the first intervention the charge nurse should implement.
    2. The charge nurse should suspect bacterial meningitis and place the young teenage child in isolation until definitive diagnosis is made. The nurse must protect the child but also all the other clients, visitors, and staff in the ED. This intervention must be implemented first.
    3. The child will need to receive a lumbar puncture for definitive diagnosis of bacterial meningitis, but it is not the first intervention. Protecting others from this very contagious disease by placing the child in isolation is the priority.
    4. Notifying the infection control nurse is an important intervention, but not a priority over protecting other individuals in the ED.

CLINICAL JUDGMENT GUIDE: The test taker should apply the nursing process when the question asks the nurse, "Which intervention should be implemented first?"

75. 1. The parent should call 911 to give immediate medical treatment to the child.
    2. This is an appropriate question to ask to determine appropriate treatment, but the nurse should first have direct contact with Poison Control to determine the medical treatment for the child.
    3. Syrup of ipecac is no longer recommended because vomiting may cause more damage to the child, or lead to aspiration pneumonia.
    4. Contacting Poison Control is the first intervention. Poison Control will be able to provide the nurse with the correct instructions for the parent to help dilute this poison and remove it from their child's body.

CLINICAL JUDGMENT GUIDE: The test taker should apply the nursing process when the question asks the nurse, "Which intervention should be implemented first?" In this case, the safety of the client is the priority intervention and Poison Control can provide immediate instructions.

76. 1. The object should not be removed until surgery. Removing the object can cause more damage and possible hemorrhaging.
    2. The child's medical history and allergies should be determined, but it is not the charge nurse's first intervention.
    3. The charge nurse should stabilize the pencil in place so that further damage will not occur. The left eye should be patched to prevent eye movement. If the uninjured eye moves, the injured eye will also move involuntarily, possibly causing more damage.
    4. The child's vital signs and pulse oximeter reading should be assessed, but not before stabilizing the injury.

CLINICAL JUDGMENT GUIDE: The test taker should apply the nursing process when the question asks the nurse, "Which intervention should be implemented first?" In this case, ensuring the safety of the client by preventing further injury is the priority intervention.

77. 1. The best response on the Glasgow Coma Scale is 15, so a score of 12 indicates neurological deterioration and requires notifying the neurologist first. The nurse cannot implement any independent nursing interventions to help the child.
    2. The nurse should document the findings in the EHR, but first should notify the neurologist because this indicates a deteriorating condition.
    3. The nurse should continue to assess the client's Glasgow Coma Scale, but not before notifying the neurologist.
    4. Placing the child in the high Fowler's position will not help increased intracranial pressure; therefore, the nurse should not implement this intervention.

CLINICAL JUDGMENT GUIDE: The test taker should apply the nursing process when the question asks the nurse, "Which intervention should be implemented first?" In this case, the nurse should recognize the signs of a complication and notify the HCP.

78. 1. The charge nurse should suspect acute epiglottis, a potential medical emergency that should not be assigned to an inexperienced nurse.
    2. The charge nurse should suspect this child will be having emergency abdominal surgery and should not assign the child to an inexperienced nurse.
    3. This child is stable and will need an x-ray; therefore, an inexperienced nurse could care for this client.
    4. The charge nurse should realize this child may be hospitalized and should assign this child to a more experienced nurse.

CLINICAL JUDGMENT GUIDE: An inexperienced nurse should be assigned the most stable client.

CASE STUDY ANSWERS

1. Correct answers are 1, 3, 4, 5, 6, and 10. A heart rate of 180 bpm, respiratory rate of 55 breaths/min, and temperature of 101.5°F (38.6°C) are higher than expected. The client has dyspnea, chest retractions, inspiratory and expiratory wheezing throughout the lung fields, and a frequent dry cough. Abnormal results should be reported. The client's history of bronchopulmonary dysplasia is pertinent to the client's clinical findings and should be reported.

CLINICAL JUDGMENT GUIDE: The test taker should examine each answer option individually. Alternative question formats, such as this extended multiple response or "select all that apply" questions, can have one to all correct answers.

2. Correct answers are 1, 2, and 4.
    1. The client is experiencing chest retractions and wheezing throughout the lung fields. These findings place the client at risk for impaired gas exchange.
    2. The client is lethargic, dyspneic, and has chest retractions, which may lead to fatigue and ultimate malnutrition due to an inability to have the energy to breastfeed.
    3. No assessment information indicates this client is at risk for decreased skin integrity.
    4. The client is lethargic, dyspneic, and has chest retractions, which may lead to fatigue due to all energy sources being used to breathe.
    5. No assessment information indicates this client is at risk for seizures

3. Correct answers are 2 and 2.
    Based on the client's condition, the nurse recognizes that the client is at the highest risk for

    | 2. Atelectasis |

    and will require

    | 2. Oxygen |

4. Correct answers are marked.

Potential Nursing Intervention	Indicated	Not Indicated
Implement droplet precautions.	X	
Provide a quiet and calm environment.	X	
Lay client flat.		X
Start oxygen at 2 L via nasal cannula.	X	
Encourage short and frequent breastfeeding sessions.	X	
Encourage visitors.		X
Provide deep suction before feeding.		X

The nurse should not lay the client flat. Putting the client in a semi-Fowler's position will help facilitate respirations. The client has been diagnosed with respiratory syncytial virus (RSV), which is very contagious. Visitors should be limited. The client has a runny nose. No assessment data align with the need to deep suction. Nasal suction would be appropriate before feedings.

5. Correct answers are 2, 3, 5, and 6
    1. Scheduling routine blood work is not a priority for this client.
    2. Vital signs every 4 hours are a priority to allow the nurse to observe subtle changes in the client's condition.
    3. Breastfeeding as tolerated is a priority to ensure the client does not become dehydrated or malnourished.
    4. Education is important before discharge but is not a priority.
    5. Recording intake and output on a child is always a priority.
    6. Ensuring suction equipment is at the bedside is a priority for this client.

6. Correct answers are marked.

Finding	Improved	Declined	No Change
Temperature	X		
Heart rate	X		
Respirations	X		
Respiratory assessment	X		
SpO_2		X	

The client's SaO_2 is lower than on admission, and he is now on 1 L of oxygen by nasal cannula. This finding indicates that the client's condition has declined. The remaining findings indicate an improvement in the client's condition.

Mental Health Management

Learn from yesterday, live for today, hope for tomorrow.
—Albert Einstein

QUESTIONS

1. The nurse in the outpatient psychiatric unit is returning phone calls. Which client should the psychiatric nurse call **first?**
   1. The client diagnosed with histrionic personality disorder needing to talk to the nurse about something very important
   2. The client diagnosed with schizophrenia hearing voices telling them to hurt their mother
   3. The client diagnosed with major depression talking about killing themself, according to the spouse
   4. The client diagnosed with bipolar disorder, is manic, and has not slept for 2 days

2. The registered nurse (RN) is caring for children in a psychiatric unit. Which client requires **immediate** intervention by the psychiatric nurse?
   1. The 10-year-old child diagnosed with oppositional defiant disorder refusing to follow directions of the mental health worker (MHW)
   2. The 5-year-old child diagnosed with pervasive developmental disorder refusing to talk to the nurse and will not make eye contact
   3. The 7-year-old child diagnosed with conduct disorder throwing furniture against the wall in the day room
   4. The 8-year-old intellectually disabled child sitting on the playground eating dirt and sand

3. The client diagnosed with major depression is returning to the psychiatric unit from a weekend pass with their family. Which intervention should the nurse implement **first?**
   1. Ask the spouse for their opinion of how the visit went.
   2. Determine whether the client took their medication.
   3. Ask the client for their opinion of how the visit went.
   4. Check the client for sharps or dangerous objects.

4. The client on the psychiatric unit is yelling at other clients, throwing furniture, and threatening the staff members. The charge nurse determines the client is at imminent risk for harming the staff and clients. The charge nurse instructs the staff to place the client in seclusion. Which intervention should the RN charge nurse implement **first?**
   1. Document the client's behavior in the nurse's notes.
   2. Instruct the MHWs to clean up the day room area.
   3. Obtain a restraint or seclusion order from the HCP.
   4. Ensure that none of the other clients were injured.

5. A client comes to the emergency department (ED) and tells the triage nurse two people raped them. The client is crying and disheveled and has bruises on the face. Which action should the triage nurse implement **first**?
   1. Ask the client whether they want the police department notified.
   2. Notify a Sexual Assault Nurse Examiner (SANE) to see the client.
   3. Request an ED nurse to take the client to a room and assess for injuries.
   4. Assist the client in completing the ED admission form.

6. The nurse is working in an outpatient mental health clinic and returning phone calls. Which client should the psychiatric nurse call **first**?
   1. The client diagnosed with agoraphobia calling to cancel the clinic appointment
   2. The client diagnosed with a somatoform disorder with numbness in both legs
   3. The client diagnosed with hypochondriasis and afraid they may have breast cancer
   4. The client diagnosed with posttraumatic stress disorder (PTSD) threatening their spouse

7. The psychiatric nurse is working in an outpatient mental health clinic. Which client should the nurse intervene with **first**?
   1. The 2 months postpartum client sitting alone looking dejected
   2. The client whose spouse just died, and they want to go to heaven to be with them
   3. The client brought to the clinic because the parent thinks the client is anorexic
   4. The client rocking compulsively back and forth in a chair by the window

8. The ED nurse is assessing a client with a laceration on the forehead and a black eye. The nurse asks the person with the client to please leave the room. The person refuses to leave the room. Which action should the nurse take **first**?
   1. Tell the person the client must go to the x-ray department.
   2. Notify hospital security and have the person removed from the room.
   3. Explain that the person must leave the room while the nurse checks the client.
   4. Give the client a brochure about a shelter from intimate partner violence.

9. The charge nurse received laboratory data for clients in the psychiatric unit. Which client data **warrant** notifying the psychiatric HCP?
   1. The client on lithium with a serum lithium level 1 mEq/L
   2. The client on clozapine with a white blood cell (WBC) count of 13,000/microL
   3. The client on alprazolam with potassium level 3.7 mEq/L
   4. The client on quetiapine with a glucose level of 128 mg/dL

10. The client diagnosed with a panic attack disorder in the busy day room of a psychiatric unit becomes anxious, trembles, starts to hyperventilate, and is diaphoretic. Which intervention should the RN psychiatric nurse implement **first**?
    1. Administer alprazolam.
    2. Discuss what caused the client to have a panic attack.
    3. Escort the client from the day room to a quiet area.
    4. Instruct the UAP to take the client's vital signs.

11. The client diagnosed with a somatization disorder is reporting vomiting, diarrhea, and a fever. Which intervention should the nurse implement **first**?
    1. Assess the client's anxiety level on a scale of 1 to 10.
    2. Check the client's vital signs.
    3. Discuss problem-solving techniques.
    4. Notify the client's HCP.

12. Which nursing intervention is a **priority** for the client diagnosed with anorexia admitted to an inpatient psychiatric unit?
    1. Obtain the client's weight.
    2. Assess the client's laboratory values.
    3. Discuss family issues and health concerns.
    4. Teach the client about selective serotonin reuptake inhibitors.

13. Which client should the psychiatric clinic nurse assess **first**?
    1. The client diagnosed with long-term alcoholism and wanting to stop drinking
    2. The client diagnosed with cocaine abuse and reporting chest discomfort
    3. The client diagnosed with obsessive-compulsive disorder, constantly washing their hands
    4. The client believing they were given the "date rape drug" last night and raped

14. The client diagnosed with schizophrenia is being seen by the psychiatric clinic nurse for the initial visit. Which intervention should the nurse implement **first**?
    1. Develop a trusting nurse and client relationship.
    2. Determine the client's knowledge of medication.
    3. Assess the client's support systems.
    4. Allow the client to vent their feelings.

15. The client diagnosed with hypochondriasis is angry and yells at the psychiatric clinic nurse, "No one believes I am sick! Not my family, not my doctor, and not you!" Which statement is the nurse's **best** response?
    1. "Have you discussed your feelings with your family?"
    2. "I am sure your doctor believes you are sick."
    3. "I can see you are upset. Sit down and let's talk."
    4. "We cannot find any physiological reason for your illness."

16. The clinical manager assigned the psychiatric nurse a client diagnosed with major depression and attempted suicide. The client is being discharged tomorrow. Which discharge instruction by the psychiatric nurse would **warrant** intervention by the clinical manager?
    1. The nurse provides the client with phone numbers to call if needing assistance.
    2. The nurse makes the client a follow-up appointment in the psychiatric clinic.
    3. The nurse gives the client a prescription for a 1-month supply of antidepressants.
    4. The nurse tells the client not to take any over-the-counter (OTC) medications.

17. The RN charge nurse is caring for clients in an acute care psychiatric unit. Which client would be **most** appropriate for the charge nurse to assign to the licensed practical nurse (LPN)?
    1. The confused and disoriented client diagnosed with dementia
    2. The client diagnosed with schizophrenia experiencing tardive dyskinesia
    3. The client diagnosed with bipolar disorder and a lithium level of 2 mEq/L
    4. The client diagnosed with chronic alcoholism experiencing delirium tremens

18. Which task would be **inappropriate** for the RN psychiatric charge nurse to delegate to the MHW?
    1. Instruct the MHW to escort the client to the multidisciplinary team meeting.
    2. Ask the MHW to stay in the day room and watch the clients.
    3. Tell the MHW to take care of the client on a one-to-one suicide watch.
    4. Request the MHW to draw blood for a serum carbamazepine level.

19. The client in the psychiatric unit asks the MHW to mail a letter to their family for them. Which action would **warrant** intervention by the RN psychiatric nurse?
    1. The MHW tells the client to place the letter in the mailbox.
    2. The MHW informs the client they cannot send mail to their family.
    3. The MHW takes the letter and places it in the unit mailbox.
    4. The MHW reports the client mailed a letter at the team meeting.

20. The client admitted to the medical unit after a motor vehicle accident reveals using heroin. The UAP tells the RN the client is agitated, anxious, and has slurred speech. Which intervention should the nurse implement **first**?
    1. Assess the client for heroin withdrawal.
    2. Ask the UAP to take the client's vital signs.
    3. Notify the client's HCP.
    4. Administer chlordiazepoxide.

21. Which task would be **most** appropriate for the RN psychiatric nurse to delegate to the MHW?
    1. Request the MHW to take the client diagnosed with lithium toxicity to the ED.
    2. Have the MHW sit with a client diagnosed with bulimia for 1 hour after their meal.
    3. Encourage the MHW to teach the client how to express their anger positively.
    4. Ask the MHW to sit with the client while the client talks to their mother on the phone.

22. The RN psychiatric charge nurse is making shift assignments for the admission unit. The staff includes one RN, two LPNs, four MHWs, and a unit secretary. Which task would be **most** appropriate to assign to the LPNs?
    1. Update the clients' individualized care plans.
    2. Stay in the lobby area and watch the clients.
    3. Administer routine medications to the clients.
    4. Enter a laboratory order into the EHR for a client.

23. The MHW has tried to calm the angry client on the psychiatric unit, who is attempting to fight with another client. The RN observes the MHW "taking down" the client to the floor. Which intervention should the nurse implement?
    1. Assist the MHW with the "take down" of the client.
    2. Call hospital security to come and assist the MHW.
    3. Document the client's "take down" in the nurse's notes.
    4. Remove the other clients from the day room area.

24. The MHW reports to the RN psychiatric nurse that two clients were kissing each other while watching a movie in the lobby area. Which action should the nurse implement?
    1. Ask the MHW to tell the clients not to kiss each other again.
    2. Discuss the inappropriate behavior at the weekly team meeting.
    3. Transfer one of the clients to another psychiatric unit.
    4. Talk to the clients about kissing in the lobby area.

25. The nurse is caring for clients in the psychiatric unit. Which task would be **most** appropriate for the RN to delegate to the MHW?
    1. Instruct the MHW to walk with the agitated and anxious client.
    2. Ask the MHW to clean up the floor where the client has urinated.
    3. Tell the MHW to phone the HCP to obtain a PRN medication order.
    4. Request the MHW to explain seizure precautions to another staff member.

26. Which behavior by the MHW is an example of assault requiring **immediate** intervention by the RN psychiatric nurse?
    1. The MHW injures a client while forcibly putting them in the "quiet" room.
    2. The MHW refuses to let the client enter the day room without socks.
    3. The MHW escorts the client to the anger management class in another building.
    4. The MHW threatens to physically remove the client from bed since they have refused.

27. The RN charge nurse has assigned the LPN to administer medications for clients in an inpatient psychiatric unit. Which client should the LPN **require** that they take their prescribed medications?
    1. The client diagnosed with bipolar disorder declared incompetent in a court of law
    2. The client diagnosed with major depression and voluntarily admitted to the unit
    3. The client diagnosed with paranoid schizophrenia involuntarily admitted to the unit
    4. The client diagnosed with borderline personality disorder pending legal charges in court

28. Which client should the psychiatric charge nurse assign to the surgical unit nurse assigned to the psychiatric unit for the shift?
    1. The hallucinating and delusional client diagnosed with schizophrenia
    2. The client diagnosed with bipolar disorder being manic aggressive toward staff and clients
    3. The client diagnosed with chronic depression, talking to no one
    4. The angry client diagnosed with antisocial personality disorder

29. The psychiatric nurse assigned the MHW to stay with a client one-to-one because of the high risk for suicide. Which behavior by the MHW **warrants** intervention by the RN?
    1. The MHW stays with the client while in the bathroom.
    2. The MHW provides the client with plastic utensils for breakfast.
    3. The MHW stays outside the room during the client's group therapy.
    4. The MHW watches the client walking outside from the porch area.

30. Which MHW statement **warrants** intervention by the RN psychiatric nurse?
    1. "I assisted the client with dressing and hygiene this morning."
    2. "I am attending the team meeting for the next hour."
    3. "I gave the client diagnosed with heartburn some Maalox."
    4. "I am going to play cards with some clients in the day room."

31. The nurse in the substance abuse unit is administering medications. For which client would the nurse **question** administering their medication?
    1. The client admitted for alcohol detoxification receiving lorazepam with an apical pulse of 110 bpm
    2. The client admitted for heroin addiction receiving methadone with a respiratory rate of 22 breaths/min
    3. The client admitted for opioid withdrawal receiving clonidine with a blood pressure of 88/60 mm Hg
    4. The client diagnosed with Wernicke-Korsakoff syndrome receiving IV thiamine and with an oral temperature of 96.8°F (36°C)

32. The psychiatric nurse overhears an MHW telling a client diagnosed with schizophrenia, "You cannot use the phone while you are here on the unit." Which action should the RN psychiatric nurse take?
    1. Praise the MHW for providing correct information to the client.
    2. Tell the MHW this is not correct information in front of the client.
    3. Explain to the MHW that the client does not lose any rights.
    4. Discuss this situation at the weekly multidisciplinary team meeting.

33. The client diagnosed with bipolar disorder is admitted to the psychiatric unit in an acute manic state. The nurse must complete the admission assessment, but the client is restless, energetic, and agitated. Which intervention should the nurse implement?
    1. In a firm voice, ask the client to sit down.
    2. Administer lithium.
    3. Ask questions while walking and pacing with the client.
    4. Do not complete the admission assessment at this time.

34. The client in the psychiatric setting tells the nurse, "There were so many people at the team meeting; I am not sure what the psychiatric social worker is supposed to do for me." Which statement is the psychiatric nurse's **best** response?
    1. "The social worker evaluates the effectiveness of the client's medication."
    2. "This person provides activities that promote constructive use of leisure time."
    3. "The social worker will assist you in keeping your job or help you find a new one."
    4. "This person works with your family and community and makes referrals if needed."

35. The client diagnosed with paranoid schizophrenia is yelling, talking to themselves, and blocking the view of the television. The other clients in the day room are becoming angry. Which action should the RN take **first**?
    1. Obtain a restraint order from the HCP.
    2. Escort the other clients from the day room.
    3. Administer an intramuscular antipsychotic medication.
    4. Approach the client calmly with an MHW.

36. A child was admitted to the pediatric unit and diagnosed with a fractured jaw, bruises, and multiple cigarette burns to the arms. The mother reported their spouse hurt the child. An adult comes to the nurse's station saying, "I am the child's parent; can you tell me how they are doing?" Which statement is the nurse's **best** response?
    1. "Your child has a fractured jaw and some bruises but is doing fine."
    2. "I am sorry I cannot give you any information about your child."
    3. "You should talk to your spouse about your child's condition."
    4. "The social worker can discuss your child's condition with you."

37. The psychiatric nurse is caring for clients on a closed unit. Which client would warrant **immediate** intervention by the nurse?
    1. The client refusing to attend the anger management class
    2. The client requesting to go outside to smoke a cigarette
    3. The nauseated client who has vomited twice
    4. The client experiencing menses with abdominal cramping

38. The clinical manager wants to reward the staff on the psychiatric unit for having no tardies or absences for 1 month. Which action would be **most** appropriate for the clinical manager?
    1. Provide pizza, drinks, and dessert for all the shifts.
    2. Post a thank-you note on the board in the employee lounge.
    3. Individually acknowledge this accomplishment with the staff.
    4. Place official documentation in each staff's employee file.

39. The nurse is working in an outpatient psychiatric clinic. The client tells the nurse, "I am going to kill my spouse if they file for divorce. I know I can't live without them." Which action should the nurse implement?
    1. Take no action because this is confidential information.
    2. Document the statement in the client's nurse's notes.
    3. Inform the client's psychiatric HCP of the comment.
    4. Encourage the client to talk to their spouse about the divorce.

40. Which interventions should the inpatient RN psychiatric nurse implement for the client experiencing sleepwalking? **Select all that apply.**
    1. Encourage the client to exercise before going to bed.
    2. Place the client on elopement precautions.
    3. Instruct the client to drink decaffeinated beverages.
    4. Place an alarm on the bed that is activated when the client gets up.
    5. Tell the MHW to be on a one-to-one watch during the night.

41. The nurse is discussing the grieving process with the client. Which of the following stages make up Kübler-Ross's stages of grief? **Rank in the correct order.**
    1. Acceptance
    2. Bargaining
    3. Denial
    4. Anger
    5. Depression

42. The nurse is in the middle or working phase of the nurse and client relationship. Which statement is a task in the middle or working phase?
    1. Identify the client's strengths and weaknesses.
    2. Help the client identify problem-solving techniques.
    3. Evaluate the client's experience while in the group.
    4. Establish the rules for how meetings will be conducted.

43. Which situation requires **priority** intervention in an inpatient psychiatric unit?
    1. A client is threatening to throw the television at another client.
    2. A client wants to use the phone to call their spouse.
    3. A client sitting in a chair is delusional and hallucinating.
    4. A client has refused to eat anything for 2 days.

44. The client diagnosed with long-term alcoholism asks the nurse, "How does Alcoholics Anonymous help me quit drinking?" Which statements are the nurse's **best** responses? **Select all that apply.**
    1. "AA has sponsors to contact if you want to take a drink."
    2. "AA discusses medications used to help prevent drinking alcohol."
    3. "AA is a support group of alcoholics that successfully quit drinking."
    4. "AA helps you realize the power you have over your addiction to alcohol."
    5. "AA has professional guest speakers to address addictive personalities."

45. The client diagnosed with bipolar disorder is prescribed lithium and admitted to the psychiatric unit in an acute manic state. Which intervention should the nurse implement **first?**
    1. Have the laboratory draw a STAT serum lithium level.
    2. Evaluate what behavior prompted the psychiatric admission.
    3. Assess and treat the client's physiological needs.
    4. Administer a STAT dose of lithium to the client.

46. The psychiatric unit staff is upset about the new charge nurse sitting in their office all day. One of the staff members informs the clinical manager about the situation. Which statement by the clinical manager indicates a laissez-faire leadership style?
    1. "I will schedule a meeting to discuss the concerns of the charge nurse."
    2. "I hired the new charge nurse, and they are doing what I told them to do."
    3. "You and the staff should handle this situation independently."
    4. "I will talk to the charge nurse about your concerns and get back to you."

47. The MHW reports that one of the RNs threatened to force-feed the client diagnosed with schizophrenia if the client did not eat the meal on their lunch tray. Which action should the RN charge nurse take **first?**
    1. Tell the MHW that this intervention is part of the client's care plan.
    2. Request the nurse to come to the office and discuss the MHW's allegation.
    3. Ask the client what happened with the nurse during lunch.
    4. Ask the MHW to document the situation to submit to the head nurse.

48. The client diagnosed with paranoid schizophrenia is imminently aggressive and dangerous to themselves, the other clients, and the psychiatric staff members. The client is placed in a seclusion room. Which interventions should the RN psychiatric nurse implement? **Select all that apply.**
    1. Assess the client every 2 hours for side effects of medication.
    2. Teach the client what behavior will prompt the release from seclusion.
    3. Do not notify the client's family of the initiation of seclusion.
    4. Explain that the client will be in the seclusion room for 24 hours.
    5. Instruct the MHW to check the client every 10 to 15 minutes.

49. The psychiatric nurse overhears an MHW arguing with a client diagnosed with paranoid schizophrenia. Which action should the RN implement?
    1. Ask the MHW to go to the nurse's station.
    2. Tell the MHW to quit arguing with the client.
    3. Notify the clinical manager of the psychiatric unit.
    4. Report this behavior to the client abuse committee.

50. Which client should the RN psychiatric nurse working in a mental health clinic refer to the psychiatric social worker?
    1. The client wanting help getting on with their life as a rape victim
    2. The client scheduled for their first electroconvulsive therapy (ECT) treatment
    3. The client reporting having difficulty going to work every day
    4. The client unable to afford the prescribed antipsychotic medications

51. The psychiatric nurse took 15 minutes extra for their lunch break twice last week. Which action should the clinical manager implement?
    1. Take no action and continue to watch the nurse's behavior.
    2. Document the behavior in writing and place it in the nurse's file.
    3. Tell the nurse to check in and out with the manager during lunch.
    4. Talk to the nurse informally about taking 45 minutes for lunch.

52. The client diagnosed with Alzheimer's disease is in a special unit for cognitive disorders. Which assessment data would warrant **immediate** intervention by the psychiatric nurse?
    1. The client does not know their name, the date, or the place.
    2. The client is unable to dress themself without assistance.
    3. The client is difficult to arouse from sleep.
    4. The client needs assistance when eating a meal.

53. The mother of a client recently diagnosed with schizophrenia says to the nurse, "I was afraid of my child. Will they be all right?" Which response by the psychiatric nurse supports the ethical principle of veracity?
    1. "I can see your fear; you are concerned your child will not be all right."
    2. "If your child takes medication, the symptoms can be controlled."
    3. "Why were you afraid of your child? Did you think they would hurt you?"
    4. "Schizophrenia is a mental illness, and your child will not be all right."

54. The nurse is caring for clients in an outpatient psychiatric clinic. Which client would the nurse discuss with the HCP?
    1. The client diagnosed with bipolar disorder receiving carbamazepine
    2. The client diagnosed with schizophrenia reporting taking aluminum hydroxide and magnesium hydroxide daily for heartburn
    3. The client diagnosed with major depression receiving isoniazid
    4. The client diagnosed with anorexia nervosa receiving amitriptyline

55. The client in the psychiatric unit tells the nurse, "Someone just put a bomb under the couch in the lobby." Which action should the nurse implement **first?**
    1. Look under the couch for a bomb.
    2. Implement the bomb scare protocol.
    3. Have the staff evacuate the unit.
    4. Tell the client there is no bomb.

56. The new nurse on the psychiatric unit tells the RN charge nurse, "I don't like how the shift report is given." Which statement is the charge nurse's **best** response?
    1. "Because you're new, I think you should try it before commenting."
    2. "We have been doing the shift report this way for over 5 years."
    3. "Have you discussed your concerns about the shift report with the other nurses?"
    4. "I would be happy to listen to any ideas you have on how to give the shift report."

57. The client on the psychiatric unit tells the nurse, "I am so bored. I hate just sitting on the unit doing nothing." Which intervention should the nurse implement?
    1. Explain that the client can go to the activity area with time.
    2. Allow the client to vent feelings of boredom about the unit.
    3. Notify the psychiatric recreational therapist about the client's concerns.
    4. Tell the client that there is nothing that can be done about being bored.

58. The head nurse of a psychiatric unit in the county ED is assigning clients to the staff nurses. Which client should be assigned to the **most** experienced nurse?
    1. The crying client, upset because of being raped
    2. The agitated client diagnosed with bipolar disorder
    3. The dazed client found wandering the streets
    4. The hallucinating client diagnosed with schizophrenia

59. The client diagnosed with anorexia is refusing to eat and is lower than 20% of ideal body weight for their height and structure. The client has not eaten anything since admission 2 days ago. Which action should the nurse implement?
    1. Notify the psychiatrist to request a court order to feed the client.
    2. Take no action because the client can refuse treatment.
    3. Discharge the client because they are not complying with the treatment.
    4. Physically restrain the client and insert a nasogastric tube for feeding.

60. The client on a psychiatric involuntary admission is threatening to run away from the unit. Which intervention should the nurse implement **first?**
    1. Notify the police department of the client's threats.
    2. Place the unit on high alert for unauthorized departure.
    3. Talk to the client about their threat of running away.
    4. Have the client sign out against medical advice (AMA).

61. The nurse answers the client's phone in the lobby area, and the person asks, "May I speak to Mr. Jones?" Which action should the nurse implement?
    1. Ask the caller their name and interest in Mr. Jones.
    2. Tell the caller Mr. Jones cannot have phone calls.
    3. Request the caller to give the access code for information.
    4. Find Mr. Jones and tell him he has a phone call.

62. The client, seeing the psychiatric nurse in the mental health clinic, tells the nurse, "If I tell you something very important, will you promise not to tell anyone?" Which statement is the nurse's **best** response?
    1. "I promise I will not tell anyone if you don't want me to."
    2. "If it affects your care, I must contact someone for help."
    3. "If you don't want me to tell anyone, please don't tell me."
    4. "Why do you not want me to tell anyone if it is so important?"

63. Which situation would warrant **immediate** intervention by the RN charge nurse on the psychiatric unit after receiving the a.m. shift report?
    1. The client diagnosed with paranoid schizophrenia is delusional.
    2. The p.m. shift LPN called to say they cannot work today.
    3. The MHW reports losing their unit key card and identification badge.
    4. The unit secretary requests a supply order approval before processing it.

64. The client enters the mental health clinic with a gun and threatens to kill the nurse for telling their spouse to leave them. Which action should the nurse implement **first?**
    1. Instruct a staff member to call the local police department.
    2. Evacuate the clients and staff to a safe and secure place.
    3. Encourage the client to talk about their feelings of anger.
    4. Calmly and firmly ask the client to put the gun on the floor.

65. The charge nurse of the psychiatric unit is making assignments. Which clients should be assigned to the medical-surgical nurse working in the psychiatric unit for the day? **Select all that apply.**
    1. The client diagnosed with depression, having attempted suicide four times and refusing to go to therapy
    2. The client diagnosed with bipolar disease and diabetes requiring blood glucose monitoring
    3. The client diagnosed with dissociative identity disorder (DID) reporting false imprisonment
    4. The client diagnosed with schizophrenia blocking the screen of the television, refusing to allow others to watch television
    5. The client diagnosed with major depression having started antidepressant medication 2 days ago and wanting to remain in bed

66. The outpatient clinic psychiatric nurse is preparing to assist the HCP perform electroconvulsive therapy. **Rank in order of performance.**
    1. Attach the electrodes to the client.
    2. Check the client's name and date of birth against the EHR or orders.
    3. Start an IV line and run at a keep open rate.
    4. Verify that the client has not eaten or had liquids since midnight.
    5. Ask the HCP to begin the procedure.

67. The psychiatric nurse is reviewing client laboratory values. Which data require **immediate** intervention by the nurse?
    1. The client diagnosed with bipolar disease

    Client: A. N. **Allergies:** None
    Diagnosis: Bipolar Disease **Medical Records Number:** 123456

Laboratory Report		
Laboratory Test	Client Value	Reference Value
Lithium level	1.2	0.5 to 1.2 mEq/L

    2. The client diagnosed with mania

    Client: D.C. **Allergies:** Dilantin
    Diagnosis: Mania **Medical Records Number:** 109875

Laboratory Report		
Laboratory Test	Client Value	Reference Value
Valproic acid level	98	50 to 125 mcg/L

    3. The client diagnosed with schizophrenia

    Client: J.M. **Allergies:** NKDA
    Diagnosis: Schizophrenia **Medical Records Number:** 245689

Laboratory Report		
Laboratory Test	Client Value	Reference Value
White blood cell count	2.68	4.5 to 11.1 $\times$ 10^3/microL

    4. The client diagnosed with acute psychosis

    Client: S.R. **Allergies:** Penicillin
    Diagnosis: Acute Psychosis **Medical Records Number:** 874521

Laboratory Report		
Laboratory Test	Client Values	Reference Value
Potassium	4.68	3.5 to 5.3 mEq/L
Sodium	139	135 to 145 mEq/L
Chloride	102	97 to 107 mEq/L

68. The charge nurse responds to an emergency on the psychiatric unit in which the client is angry, yelling, and attempting to hit other clients and the staff. Which interventions should the nurse implement? **Select all that apply.**
    1. Notify the operator to call emergency responders to assist.
    2. Tell the client to sit down and be quiet, or they will lose privileges.
    3. Have the MHW escort the other clients to their rooms.
    4. Ensure the staff speaks loudly and directly to the client.
    5. Request the unit secretary stand by the locked doors to admit emergency responders.

69. The psychiatric nurse is assessing the Abnormal Involuntary Movement Scale (AIMS) for clients on antipsychotic medications.

ABNORMAL INVOLUNTARY MOVEMENT SCALE (AIMS)

Initials: _____ Gender: _____ Date: _____ Interviewer: _____

MOVEMENT RATINGS (Circle One)

0 = None; 1 = Minimal, may be extreme of normal; 2 = Mild; 3 = Moderate; 4 = Severe

Note: 0 = no awareness; 1 = aware, no distress; 2 = aware, mild distress; 3 = aware, moderate distress; 4 = aware, severe distress

Facial and Oral Movements	1. **Muscles of facial expression** (e.g., movement of forehead, eyebrows, periorbital area, cheeks; include frowning, blinking, smiling, grimacing)	0 1 2 3 4
	2. **Lips and perioral area** (e.g., puckering, pouting, smacking)	0 1 2 3 4
	3. **Jaw** (e.g., biting, clenching, chewing, mouth opening, lateral movement)	0 1 2 3 4
	4. **Tongue** (rate only increase in movement both in and out of mouth, NOT inability to sustain movement)	0 1 2 3 4
Extremity Movements	5. **Upper body** (arms, wrists, hands, fingers) (e.g., include **choreic movements** [rapid, objectively purposeless, irregular, spontaneous], **athetoid movements** [slow irregular, complex, serpentine]). Do NOT include tremor (repetitive, regular, and rhythmic).	0 1 2 3 4
	6. **Lower body** (legs, knees, ankles, toes) (e.g., lateral knee movement, foot tapping, and heel dropping, foot squirming, inversion and eversion of foot)	0 1 2 3 4
Trunk Movements	7. **Neck, shoulders, hips**	0 1 2 3 4
Global Judgments	8. **Severity of abnormal movements**	0 1 2 3 4
	9. **Incapacitation due to abnormal movements**	0 1 2 3 4
	10. **Client's awareness of abnormal movements** (rate only client's report; see previous note)	0 1 2 3 4
Dental Status	11. **Current problem with teeth or dentures**	Yes = 1 No = 0
	12. **Does client usually wear dentures?**	Yes = 1 No = 0
	SCORE	

Adapted from Guy, W. (1976). *ECDEU assessment manual for psychopharmacology* (p. 534). National Institute of Mental Health, Department of Health, Education and Welfare.

Which client's scores require **immediate** intervention?
1. The client with a score of 6 on the scale
2. The client with a score of 10 on the scale
3. The client with a score of 15 on the scale
4. The client with a score of 24 on the scale

70. The nurse manager working in the mental health clinic returns a phone call to a client saying, "Voices are telling me to hurt myself, now." Which intervention should the psychiatric nurse implement **first?**
    1. Call 911 and tell the paramedics the client is a danger to themselves or others.
    2. Ask the client whether they have taken their medication this morning.
    3. Notify the HCP of the client's statement.
    4. Keep the client on the phone to discuss the voices they are hearing.

71. The client diagnosed with a panic attack disorder in the clinic waiting room becomes anxious, starts to hyperventilate and tremble, and is diaphoretic. After removing the client from the day room, which intervention should the RN mental health nurse implement next?
    1. Administer alprazolam.
    2. Allow the client to verbalize feelings of anxiety.
    3. Encourage the client to take slow, deep breaths.
    4. Instruct the MHW to obtain the client's pulse oximeter reading.

72. Which client would be **most** appropriate for the RN nurse manager to assign to the LPN in the outpatient psychiatric clinic?
    1. The confused and disoriented client diagnosed with dementia
    2. The client diagnosed with schizophrenia experiencing extrapyramidal side effects
    3. The client diagnosed with bipolar disorder pacing up and down the hallway
    4. The client diagnosed with anorexia nervosa reporting dizziness and is hypotensive

73. The nurse was late to work three times last week. The nurse manager talks to the nurse and finds out they must take the bus to work until their car is fixed, which should be completed in 1 week. Which action should the RN nurse manager implement?
    1. Ask another nurse to give the chronically late nurse a ride to work until the car is fixed.
    2. Document the behavior in writing and place it in the nurse's file.
    3. Tell the nurse they will be placed on administrative leave if they are late again.
    4. Do not take any action now because the nurse has an excellent attendance record.

74. The client has been arrested several times for drunk driving but does not believe he has a problem with alcohol. Which defense mechanism is the client exhibiting?
    1. Isolation
    2. Denial
    3. Projection
    4. Sublimation

75. The client experiences an intense rage but redirects it into playing sports such as boxing and football. Which defense mechanism is the client exhibiting?
    1. Isolation
    2. Rationalization
    3. Projection
    4. Sublimation

76. The client believes cheating on his final examination is acceptable because they studied for all previous examinations in the course. Which defense mechanism is the client exhibiting?
    1. Rationalization
    2. Altruism
    3. Projection
    4. Displacement

77. The client gets mad at their partner, stomps into another room, and pouts. Which defense mechanism is the client exhibiting?
    1. Humor
    2. Isolation
    3. Regression
    4. Suppression

78. The client intensely dislikes someone but buys that person a gift. Which defense mechanism is the client exhibiting?
    1. Undoing
    2. Repression
    3. Altruism
    4. Regression

79. The nurse is caring for a client who is angry at their sister but says nothing and goes outside and kicks the dog. Which defense mechanism is the client exhibiting?
    1. Displacement
    2. Splitting
    3. Undoing
    4. Isolation

80. The client is mad at their doctor but screams that the spouse is angry at the doctor. Which defense mechanism is the client exhibiting?
    1. Splitting
    2. Humor
    3. Projection
    4. Denial

81. The nurse is caring for a client choosing not to discuss their father's funeral details. Which defense mechanism is the client exhibiting?
    1. Regression
    2. Suppression
    3. Denial
    4. Rationalization

82. Which are the phases of group work the clients progress through? **Select all that apply.**
    1. Denial phase
    2. Initial phase
    3. Working phase
    4. Recovery phase
    5. Termination phase

83. The charge nurse is discussing leadership styles for groups. Which leadership style encourages group members to participate and give input?
    1. Autocratic style
    2. Democratic style
    3. Laissez-faire style
    4. Situational style

84. Which clinical manifestations should the nurse expect a client diagnosed with schizophrenia to exhibit? **Select all that apply.**
    1. Auditory and visual hallucinations
    2. Delusions
    3. Amplified emotional expression
    4. Disorganized speech
    5. Disorganized behavior

85. The primary nurse is caring for a client having active hallucinations and thinking they are God. Which interventions should the nurse perform? **Select all that apply.**
    1. Ask the client what the hallucinations are saying.
    2. Pretend to accept what the client is saying about the hallucinations.
    3. Attempt to distract the client from the hallucination.
    4. Pat the client on the hand to show a personal connection.
    5. Provide short, simple directions, displaying a supportive, accepting attitude.

86. Which clinical manifestations should the nurse expect the client diagnosed with bipolar disorder and severe mania to exhibit? **Select all that apply.**
    1. Increased need for sleep
    2. Flight of ideas
    3. Talkative, pressured speech
    4. Easily distracted
    5. Low self-esteem

87. Which interventions can the primary nurse implement when caring for a client diagnosed with bipolar disorder and experiencing a manic state? **Select all that apply.**
    1. Encourage the client to play ping-pong in the recreation room.
    2. Provide the client with protein bars or peanut butter crackers.
    3. Administer a mood stabilizer or antipsychotic medication as ordered.
    4. Remove glass and smoking materials from the client's surroundings.
    5. Set firm limits on intrusive, manipulative behaviors.

88. The primary nurse caring for a 44-year-old female client diagnosed with major depression reports to the team meeting that the client is saying, "I am tired of living. I just need to die, and everyone will be better off." Which interventions should the nurse perform to assess the client's suicide risk? **Select all that apply.**
    1. Ask the client directly if she is thinking about suicide.
    2. Determine whether the client has a specific suicide plan.
    3. Discover whether the client has access to lethal methods to commit suicide.
    4. Question the client about any previous suicide attempts.
    5. Check whether the client has had other family members commit suicide.

89. The charge nurse is teaching the new nurses about the clinical manifestations exhibited by clients diagnosed with major depression. Which findings should the charge nurse include in the teaching? **Select all that apply.**
    1. Change in appetite resulting in weight loss or gain
    2. Grandiose behavior and beliefs
    3. Loss of pleasure in life and usual pursuits
    4. Attentiveness and concentration in activities
    5. Insomnia or excessive sleepiness

90. The HCP determines the client is having alcohol withdrawal and arranges for a transfer to the acute care hospital. Which interventions should the nurse implement for the client experiencing alcohol withdrawal? **Select all that apply.**
    1. Assess the client for delirium tremens (DTs).
    2. Administer benzodiazepines.
    3. Monitor IV fluids.
    4. Reduce environmental stimuli.
    5. Refer to Alcoholics Anonymous.

MENTAL HEALTH CASE STUDY

(1900) The suicide crisis line activated a wellness check on a caller. The dispatch called out a county sheriff to go to the client's home. After multiple attempts to get someone to answer the door, the adult opened the door. The sheriff explained he was at the residence to do a welfare check on a person who had called the crisis line. The telephone conversation had triggered concern with the operator. The person appears disheveled, and their hair is greasy and dirty. They respond slowly to questions, if at all. They only briefly make eye contact with the sheriff. Further inquiry reveals that they recently lost their spouse after a recent diagnosis of metastatic cancer. They spent many days at the hospital during this time, and because of absences from work, they were fired. They report, "There is no reason to keep trying." Additionally, they state, "I do not care if I ever wake up again." The sheriff then asks the person these questions:

1. Have you wished you were dead or wished you could go to sleep and not wake up?
   They responded, "Yes."
2. Have you had any thoughts of killing yourself?
   They responded, "No."
3. Have you ever done anything, started to do anything, or prepared to do anything to end your life?
   They responded, "Yes."
4. The sheriff then asked: Was this within the past 3 months?
   They responded, "Yes."

Based on the person's responses, the sheriff took them into custody and transported them to the nearest medical facility for further evaluation.

(1930) The client arrives at the ED and is triaged by the nurse. The sheriff reports he was dispatched to do a wellness check after a phone call to the Crisis Line. The client told the sheriff about their spouse and recent loss of job. The client's clothes are dirty, they are poorly groomed, and they have bad body odors. The client's speech is clear, and they have a flat affect. When asked why they were brought to the ED, they said, "I do not know. I do not want to be here." They are oriented to person, place, and time. Speech is clear, soft, sometimes whispering, and responses are brief. Skin is warm, dry, pale, and intact, with no visible injuries. Lungs are clear to auscultation bilaterally. Client denies recent history of being sick or sick contacts. Heart rate regular, S_1 and S_2 auscultated. Peripheral pulses present 2+, capillary refill is less than 3 seconds in all four extremities. Client denies smoking, denies alcohol use, and denies recreational drug use. Abdomen is soft, nontender with bowel sounds $\times 4$ quadrants. Reports last bowel movement yesterday. Client reports, "Last meal was a couple of days ago ... I just have not been hungry." Client denies pain. When asked about their sleeping pattern, states "I haven't been sleeping ... maybe a couple of hours here and there." When asked if they wanted to die, client stated, "I would not mind if I did. There really isn't anything to live for anymore." When asked whether they had a plan to take their life, they stated, "I haven't put anything into motion if that is what you mean." Client is placed in an observation room with a one-to-one sitter, asked to change into paper scrubs, and all belongings are cataloged and secured in a locker outside their room per hospital policy. Room safety check was completed per hospital policy. Side rails up $\times 2$. Client was instructed to ask sitter to contact nurse if needs arise and was informed the doctor would come to evaluate them shortly.

Vital Signs	Client Values
Blood pressure	126/88 mm Hg
Heart rate	90 bpm
Respirations	16 breaths/min
Temperature	98.4°F
SpO_2	98% (room air)

1. **Recognize cues. What matters most?** The nurse prepares to call the ED physician. Which priority client data should be reported to the HCP? Select all that apply.
    1. Brought in by police, after Crisis Line notified emergency services of individual in crisis
    2. Police report of Columbia Suicide Severity Rating indicative of possible suicidal thoughts
    3. Recent loss of spouse
    4. Recent loss of job
    5. Not eating
    6. Unkempt physical appearance and body odor
    7. Flat affect with soft speech, abbreviated answers
    8. Says "...would not mind if I died"
    9. Anhedonia—lack of enjoyment in life
    10. Change in sleep pattern.
    11. No plan in place to kill self

2. **Analyze cues. What could it mean?** What at-risk issues should the nurse be concerned about the client developing? Select three answers.
    1. Psychosis
    2. Depression
    3. Grief
    4. Electrolyte imbalance
    5. Suicidal

(1950) The ED provider visits the client and orders a complete blood count (CBC), basic metabolic panel (BMP), thyroid-stimulating hormone (TSH), thyroid panel, urine specimen, and urine drug screen. The client's past medical history and medications are reviewed in the EHR from previous hospitalizations. The physician orders are populated in the chart.

PROVIDER'S ORDERS

Medical hold. Client may not leave. If client attempts to leave, please call security and have client physically detained. Notify provider immediately.
One-to-one sitter at all times, with constant surveillance
Urinalysis
Urine drug screen
Regular diet with safety tray

(2013) Laboratory results reported:

Laboratory Test	Client Values	Reference Values
Hemoglobin (Hgb)	15 g/dL	Male: 14–17.3 g/dL
		Female: 11.7–15.5 g/dL
Hematocrit (Hct)	42%	Male: 42%–52%
		Female: 36%–48%
White blood cell (WBC) count	9.2	4.5 to 11.1 × 10^3/microL
Platelets	173	140 to 400 × 10^3/microL
Creatinine	0.98 mg/dL	Male: 0.61 to 1.21 mg/dL
		Female: 0.51 to 1.11 mg/dL
Glucose	84 mg/dL	Fasting: Less than 100 mg/dL
		Random: Less than 200 mg/dL
Potassium	3.7 mEq/L	3.5 to 5.3 mEq/L
Sodium	137 mEq/L	135 to 145 mEq/L
Blood urea nitrogen (BUN)	14 mg/dL	8 to 21 mg/dL
		Adult over 90 years: 10 to 31 mg/dL

Laboratory Test	Client Values	Reference Values
TSH	1.2 mU/L	0.35 to 5 mU/L
Thyroid Panel		
T$_3$	81.4 ng/dL	80 to 180 ng/dL
T$_4$	7.3 mcg/dL	4.5 to 12 mcg/dL
Free T$_3$	3.1 pmol/L	4 to 7.4 pmol/L
Free T$_4$	1.3 ng/dL	0.7 to 1.9 ng/dL
Reverse T$_3$	11.1 ng/dL	8 to 25 ng/dL
Anti-TPO antibodies	14 IU/mL	Below 35 IU/mL

Urinalysis results showed the following:

Laboratory Test	Client Values	Reference Values
Clarity/Turbidity	Hazy	Clear
Color	Straw	Straw
Foam content	None	None
Odor	None	None to mild
pH	5.9	5 to 8
Specific gravity	1.005	1.001 to 1.030
Red blood cells	2/hpf	<3/hpf
White blood cells	1/hpf	<5/hpf
Proteins	Negative	Negative
Glucose	Negative	Negative
Urobilinogen	0.8 mg/dL	0.2 to 1 mg/dL
Bilirubin	Negative	Negative

Continued

Laboratory Test	Client Values	Reference Values
Ketone bodies	Negative	Negative
Leukocyte esterase	Negative	Negative
Nitrites	Negative	Negative

Urine drug screen was negative:

Laboratory Test	Client Values	Reference Values
Alcohol	Negative	Negative
Amphetamines	Negative	Negative
Benzodiazepines	Negative	Negative
Opioids	Negative	Negative
Marijuana	Negative	Negative
Cocaine	Negative	Negative
Phencyclidine (PCP)	Negative	Negative
Tricyclic antidepressants (TCAs)	Negative	Negative

EHR history:

Medical History	
Cellulitis of the left lower extremity from an insect bite	
Surgical History	
Cholecystectomy	
Allergies	
None	

Medication list:

Medication	Time Taken
Acetaminophen (Tylenol)	1,000 mg every 8 hours PRN pain/fever
Multivitamin (MVI)	1 tablet by mouth every morning

3. **Prioritize hypotheses. Where do I start? Complete the sentence by choosing from the drop-down list of options.** Based on the client's condition at the time, the nurse recognizes that the client is at the highest risk for _____.

> *Select* ▼
> 1. Elopement
> 2. Self-cutting
> 3. Suicide

and will require_____.

> Select ▼
> 1. Medications
> 2. A safe environment
> 3. Restraints

4. **Generate solutions. What can I do?** For each intervention, specify whether the intervention is **indicated** or **not indicated** for the client's care.

Potential Nursing Interventions	Indicated	Not Indicated
Apply bilateral wrist restraints.		
Sit and talk with the patient.		
Establish trust by allowing privacy in the bathroom.		
Ask whether there is anyone the client would like notified.		
Give the client a sandwich and a can of soda.		
Offer a list of community resources for grief.		
Start an IV line to administer IV fluids.		
Tell the patient, "Everything is going to be all right."		
Request a chaplain visit.		

5. **Take action. What will I do?** Which admission orders should the nurse consider a priority action? **Select all that apply.**
   1. Consult psychiatry since the client is medically cleared
   2. Regular diet
   3. Suicide precautions with constant surveillance
   4. Trazodone 50 mg PO PRN at bedtime for sleep; may repeat ×1 if not asleep in 2 hours
   5. Sertraline 50 mg PO daily, first dose now
   6. CBC, BMP, fasting liver panel in a.m.
   7. Social work consult

(2154) Client alert and cooperative. Skin warm, dry, and pale. Client is quiet and withdrawn with flat affect, denies pain or needs. The sitter remains within arm's reach. Informed of consult for a mental health provider to speak with them. Client has no questions and denies having a support person to call to be with them. "There is nobody since my spouse died. I am all alone. My former coworkers are all busy with their own lives. They do not have time for me." It is explained that they are on a medical hold and cannot leave until the provider says they can, or they can be brought back by security and the police. Client received a turkey sandwich and a cup of soda per request, ate about ½ sandwich, and drank 60 mL and has remainder in Styrofoam cup at bedside. Denies suicidal ideation presently. Asks, "How long before I can go home?" Informed the client the psychiatric provider may be better able to answer that. The client closes their eyes and turns their head away.

6. **Evaluate outcomes. Did it help?** For each assessment finding, indicate whether the client's condition has **improved, declined**, or **no change**.

Finding	Improved	Declined	No Change
Safety			
Appetite			
Hygiene			
Elopement risk			
Understanding of discharge plan			
Suicidal thoughts			
Sleep disturbance			
Able to identify two grief community resources			

ANSWERS AND RATIONALES

The correct answer number and rationale are in **boldface purple type.** Rationales for why other answer options are incorrect are also given.

1. 1. The client diagnosed with a histrionic personality has excessive emotionality and seeks attention. Saying "something important" must be understood within this context and would not warrant calling this client first.
   2. **The nurse should contact this client first because the client realizes the voices are telling them to hurt their mother. The nurse should inform this client to come to the clinic immediately and be admitted to a psychiatric unit.**
   3. Because the spouse called the clinic, the client is being watched and should be safe from killing themself. The nurse should call this client immediately but not before a possibly alone client calling about hearing voices.
   4. The nurse should expect the manic client not to sleep; therefore, this behavior is expected. The nurse should call this client immediately, but not before the client hearing voices telling them to hurt their mother.

   CLINICAL JUDGMENT GUIDE: When answering questions in mental health nursing, the test taker should identify safety as a priority intervention. All these situations require intervention by the nurse, but safety is the priority.

2. 1. Oppositional defiant disorder consists of a pattern of uncooperative, defiant, and hostile behavior toward authority figures. Not following the MHW's directions would be expected behavior in a child diagnosed with this disorder and would not require immediate intervention by the RN.
   2. Refusal to talk or make eye contact is a sign of autism, the best known of the pervasive developmental disorders; therefore, this client would not require immediate intervention by the nurse.
   3. **The child diagnosed with conduct disorder is aggressive to people and animals, bullies and threatens others, destroys property, and sets fires. Throwing furniture could endanger the child or other clients. This behavior warrants immediate intervention.**
   4. Eating dirt and sand is pica, which includes ingesting non-nutritive substances such as paint, hair, cloth, leaves, sand, clay, or soil. It is commonly seen in intellectually disabled children, but it is not life-threatening unless a medical complication such as a bowel obstruction, infection, or a toxic condition (e.g., lead poisoning) occurs. This behavior would not require immediate intervention.

   CLINICAL JUDGMENT GUIDE: When deciding which client to assess first, the test taker should determine whether the clinical manifestations the client is exhibiting are normal for the client's situation. After eliminating the expected options, the test taker should determine which situation is more life-threatening.

3. 1. The nurse should discuss how the visit went, but it is not the first intervention.
   2. The nurse should make sure the client took their medications during the weekend pass, but it is not the first intervention.
   3. The client should discuss how the visit went, but it is not the first intervention.
   4. **The nurse's first intervention should be to provide for the client's safety by ensuring the client has no sharps or dangerous objects to hurt themself, because the client is diagnosed with major depression.**

   CLINICAL JUDGMENT GUIDE: When answering questions in mental health nursing, the test taker should identify safety as a priority intervention.

4. 1. The nurse must document the client's behavior that prompted the need for seclusion, but it is not the first intervention.
   2. The day room area should be cleaned up, but it is not the nurse's first intervention.
   3. **The use of restraints and seclusion requires an HCP order every 4 hours for adults and more frequently for children. Additionally, the HCP must perform an evaluation within 1 hour of initiation of restraints or seclusion. The nurse must obtain this order first after placing the client in the seclusion room. The nurse can put the client in seclusion for the safety of the client, staff, and other clients, but the nurse must then immediately obtain an HCP order.**
   4. The charge nurse should ensure the other clients are not injured, but the first intervention is to put the client acting out into seclusion, safely and legally.

   CLINICAL JUDGMENT GUIDE: The NCLEX-RN® test plan includes nursing care ruled by legal requirements. The nurse must be knowledgeable of these issues. The nurse may have to respond first and then follow up with another action.

5. 1. The client may or may not want the police notified, but this is not the triage nurse's first intervention. The triage nurse should first care for the client.
   2. The SANE is a nurse who specializes in caring for raped clients. The SANE can spend time with the client, is knowledgeable of legal issues, and would be an appropriate intervention, but it is not the triage nurse's first intervention.
   3. The triage nurse's first intervention is to address the client's physiological needs, which means to assess for any trauma or injury.
   4. The client can complete the admission form while in the room; the triage nurse's first intervention should be to care for the client, not paperwork.

CLINICAL JUDGMENT GUIDE: When the question asks which intervention to implement first, the test taker should determine whether any of the options concern the physiological needs of the client and then apply Maslow's Hierarchy of Needs to find the correct answer. Remember: Physiological needs take priority over all other needs.

6. 1. The client diagnosed with agoraphobia is afraid to leave the house; therefore, canceling a clinic appointment would be expected of this client. The nurse would not need to return this client's phone call first.
   2. The client diagnosed with a somatoform disorder has physical symptoms without a physiological cause; therefore, reporting numbness in the legs is expected behavior. The nurse would not need to return this client's phone call first.
   3. The client diagnosed with hypochondriasis is preoccupied with the fear that they have or will get a serious disease; fearing breast cancer is then expected behavior. The nurse would not need to return this client's phone call first.
   4. PTSD is an illness that occurs in someone after experiencing a traumatic event. The client feels a numbing of general responsiveness but has outbursts of anger. The nurse should return this call first and assess the situation to determine whether the client should be seen in the clinic.

CLINICAL JUDGMENT GUIDE: When deciding which client to assess first, the test taker should determine whether the clinical manifestations the client is exhibiting are expected for the client's situation. After eliminating the expected options, the test taker should determine which situation is more life-threatening.

7. 1. The depressed client would be expected to look dejected; therefore, the nurse would not need to assess this client first.
   2. This client saying they want to go to heaven to be with their spouse may be suicidal and should be assessed first to see whether they have a plan.
   3. This client needs to be assessed for anorexia but not before a suicidal client.
   4. The nurse should not interrupt a client acting compulsively. The nurse should wait until the client finishes the behavior before talking to the client.

CLINICAL JUDGMENT GUIDE: When deciding which client to assess first, the test taker should determine whether the clinical manifestations the client is exhibiting are expected for the client's situation. After eliminating the expected options, the test taker should determine which situation is more life-threatening.

8. 1. The nurse needs to remove the person from the room so that the nurse can talk to the client and discuss probable abuse. Taking the client to the x-ray department may not arouse suspicion in the person and may allow the client to discuss the situation.
   2. This may be needed but is not the first intervention. This action may cause the person to get angrier or it may cause more problems for the client at home.
   3. The nurse could demand the person leave the room, but this action may cause the person's anger to escalate; therefore, the first intervention is to remove the client from the room.
   4. The nurse should not allow the person to see the nurse discussing a shelter with the client or providing a client with a brochure. This could cause further anger in the person, especially if the client goes home with them.

CLINICAL JUDGMENT GUIDE: The nurse should address the client's needs first and follow the nursing process. Assessment is the first step in the nursing process. The nurse should protect the client's safety when performing an assessment.

9. 1. The therapeutic serum level for lithium is 0.6 to 1.2 mEq/L. Because the client's 1.0 mEq/L level is within normal limits, the charge nurse would not need to notify the psychiatric HCP about the lithium (Eskalith) medication.

2. The WBC count is elevated, which may indicate that the client is experiencing agranulocytosis, a life-threatening complication of clozapine (Clozaril). This laboratory data would warrant notifying the psychiatric HCP.
3. The client's serum potassium level is within normal limits; therefore, this laboratory information does not warrant notifying the psychiatric HCP.
4. This glucose level is slightly elevated for a fasting reading but would not warrant notifying the psychiatric HCP.

CLINICAL JUDGMENT GUIDE: The nurse must know normal laboratory values and be able to determine whether the laboratory value is normal for the client's disease process or the medications the client is taking.

10. 1. The benzodiazepine alprazolam (Xanax) is an appropriate medication for an anxiety attack, but it will take at least 15 to 30 minutes for the medication to treat the physiological clinical manifestations. Therefore, this is not the first intervention.
    2. The nurse should discuss the panic attack and what prompted it, but it is not the nurse's first intervention.
    3. **The first intervention is to remove the client from the busy day room to a quiet area to help decrease the anxiety attack.**
    4. The client's vital signs should be taken, but this is not the nurse's first intervention.

CLINICAL JUDGMENT GUIDE: The nurse should remember that if a client is in distress and the nurse can do something to relieve the distress, that action should be done first before assessment. The test taker should select an option that helps the client's condition directly.

11. 1. The nurse should assess the client's anxiety level, but not before ruling out a physiological reason for the client's reports.
    2. **The nurse should first determine whether the client's vital signs are abnormal, which rules out any physiological reason for the client's symptoms.**
    3. The nurse should discuss techniques to address increased anxiety levels, but a physiological cause of these symptoms should be ruled out first.
    4. The client's HCP will need to be notified if the reports are secondary to a physiological reason but would not if the vital signs are within normal limits.

CLINICAL JUDGMENT GUIDE: If the question asks the nurse, "Which intervention should be implemented first?" then the test taker should apply the nursing process. The psychiatric nurse must first assess to determine whether the client has a physiological problem; because options A and B are assessment interventions, the test taker should select physiological assessment over psychosocial assessment.

12. 1. The nurse should assess the client's weight, but it is not a priority over assessing laboratory values, which may indicate a life-threatening disease process, especially the potassium level.
    2. **The client's laboratory values are the priority, especially potassium, because these reflect the long-term effects of anorexia and possible life-threatening disease processes that must be corrected immediately.**
    3. This is an appropriate intervention, but physiological needs are a priority over problem-solving.
    4. A teaching intervention is not a priority over a physiological need.

CLINICAL JUDGMENT GUIDE: When a question asks, "Which intervention should the nurse implement first?" the test taker should use the nursing process to determine the correct answer. If the client is not in distress, then the nurse should assess. If two options address assessment, select the intervention that addresses a life-threatening complication.

13. 1. This client needs to be assessed, but not before the client diagnosed with chest discomfort. If the client exhibited signs of alcohol withdrawal, then this client would have a physiological need.
    2. **Cocaine causes vasoconstriction of the coronary arteries and can lead to life-threatening cardiovascular problems; therefore, this client should be seen first.**
    3. The client performing compulsive behavior should not be interrupted but should be allowed to finish the behavior.
    4. This client is not exhibiting physiological complications; therefore, this client should not be assessed first.

CLINICAL JUDGMENT GUIDE: The test taker should first determine whether the signs or symptoms are expected for the client's situation. If two or more clients exhibit unexpected signs or symptoms, select the client exhibiting signs or symptoms that are life-threatening, need more assessment, or warrant notifying the HCP.

14. 1. If the nurse does not establish the foundation for a trusting nurse and client relationship, the nurse will not effectively care for this client. This is the first nursing intervention.
    2. Medication is a vital part of the treatment for schizophrenia, but on the initial visit, a trusting relationship is a priority.
    3. Support systems are an essential part of the client's treatment in the community, but the client must trust the nurse when sharing information.
    4. Venting feelings about disease, the current situation, and life is vital to the treatment of a client diagnosed with schizophrenia, but the client must be able to trust the nurse when sharing feelings.

CLINICAL JUDGMENT GUIDE: In mental health nursing, the foundation for all nursing care is having a trusting nurse and client relationship. All the options are possible or plausible for the nurse to implement, but there is only one correct answer.

15. 1. The psychiatric nurse should address the client's feelings, not those of family members.
    2. This comment does not address the client's feelings, and the nurse should not talk about what the doctor believes or doesn't.
    3. The nurse must first calm the client, assess the situation, and ensure a therapeutic nurse and client relationship. This response addresses all these issues.
    4. This response will more than likely further antagonize the client and is not a therapeutic response.

CLINICAL JUDGMENT GUIDE: The psychiatric nurse must de-escalate the client's anger. The nurse's priority intervention is being empathetic and allowing the client to verbalize feelings.

16. 1. Providing phone numbers for the client and family is an intervention that the nurse should discuss with the client and would not warrant intervention by the clinical manager.
    2. Follow-up appointments are essential for the client after being discharged from a psychiatric facility; therefore, this instruction would not warrant intervention by the clinical manager.
    3. The client should be given a 7-day supply of antidepressants because the safety of the client is the priority. As antidepressant medications become more effective, the client is at a higher risk for suicide; therefore, the nurse should ensure that the client cannot take an overdose of medication. This instruction warrants intervention by the clinical manager.
    4. The client should not take OTC medications without talking to the HCP or pharmacist. This instruction would not warrant intervention by the clinical manager.

CLINICAL JUDGMENT GUIDE: When the question asks, "Which warrants immediate intervention?" it is an "except" question. Three of the actions are correct interventions, whereas one is not.

17. 1. The client diagnosed with dementia would be expected to have confusion and disorientation; therefore, the LPN could be assigned to this client. This client is not experiencing any potentially life-threatening complications of dementia.
    2. The client is experiencing tardive dyskinesia, a potentially life-threatening complication of antipsychotic medication. An experienced RN should be assigned to this client.
    3. The therapeutic serum level for lithium is 0.6 to 1.2 mEq/L. The client's level is toxic, and an experienced RN should care for the client.
    4. This client is experiencing a potentially life-threatening complication of alcohol withdrawal. An experienced RN should be assigned to this client.

CLINICAL JUDGMENT GUIDE: The test taker must determine which client is the most stable, which makes this an "except" question. Three clients are either unstable or have potentially life-threatening conditions.

18. 1. Clients are allowed, encouraged, and expected to participate in the multidisciplinary team meeting. This is an appropriate task to delegate to the MHW.
    2. One of the MHW's primary responsibilities is to watch clients in the day room area. This is an appropriate task to delegate.
    3. The MHW can remain with a client on a one-to-one suicide watch. This is an appropriate nursing task to delegate.
    4. The MHW does not draw blood, and this would be an inappropriate task to delegate. The laboratory technician draws the client's blood work.

CLINICAL JUDGMENT GUIDE: The nurse is responsible for knowing the scope of practice for the subordinate healthcare team members.

19. 1. Telling the client to place the letter in the mailbox empowers the client to take responsibility. This action would not warrant intervention by the nurse.
    2. The RN should explain to the MHW that mental health clients retain all the civil rights afforded to all persons, except the right to leave the hospital in the case of involuntary commitments. The client has the right to mail and receive letters.
    3. Mailing the client's letter is an appropriate action; therefore, this would not warrant intervention by the nurse.
    4. Reporting the client mailed a letter to his family at the team meeting may or may not be pertinent to the client's care, but this action would not warrant intervention by the nurse.

CLINICAL JUDGMENT GUIDE: The NCLEX-RN® test plan includes nursing care ruled by legal requirements. The nurse must be knowledgeable of these issues.

20. 1. Whenever the nurse is given information indicating a potentially life-threatening complication, the nurse must assess the client first.
    2. The client is unstable; therefore, the RN should not instruct the UAP to take the client's vital signs.
    3. The nurse should not notify the HCP before assessing the client.
    4. Chlordiazepoxide (Librium) is an antianxiety medication used for alcohol withdrawal, not for heroin withdrawal.

CLINICAL JUDGMENT GUIDE: If the test taker wants to select "notify the HCP" as the correct answer, the test taker must examine the other three options. If the information in any of the other options is data the HCP would need to make a decision, then the test taker should eliminate the "notify the HCP" option.

21. 1. The client diagnosed with lithium toxicity is unstable, and the RN should not delegate this task to an MHW.
    2. Having someone stay with the client after a meal will prevent the client from inducing vomiting and could be delegated to an MHW. The client diagnosed with bulimia needs someone there to prevent vomiting, which is a sign of this mental health problem.
    3. The RN should not delegate teaching. Helping the client with anger management would be the nurse's or the therapy department's responsibility.
    4. The client has a right to talk to his mother on the phone without someone listening.

CLINICAL JUDGMENT GUIDE: An RN cannot delegate assessment, teaching, evaluation, medications, or an unstable client to a UAP or MHW. Tasks that cannot be delegated are nursing interventions requiring nursing clinical judgment.

22. 1. The RN should be assigned to update the individualized care plans.
    2. The MHWs should be assigned to watch the clients in the day area.
    3. The LPNs' scope of practice allows the administration of medication. This is an appropriate assignment.
    4. The LPNs can enter a laboratory order into the EHR, but a unit secretary can also. This would not be the most appropriate assignment for the LPNs.

CLINICAL JUDGMENT GUIDE: The nurse is responsible for knowing the scope of practice for the subordinate healthcare team members.

23. 1. All psychiatric staff members are taught how to "take down" a client physically if the client is a danger to self or others. The RN should assist the MHW in subduing the client so that no one is injured.
    2. The psychiatric staff members are trained to deal with angry and aggressive clients; there is no need to contact hospital security.
    3. The nurse can document the occurrence, but because the nurse observed the "take down," the nurse should assist the MHW. The psychiatric staff members must be able to depend on each other no matter the situation.
    4. The nurse can have other staff members remove clients from the day room area; the RN psychiatric nurse should help the MHW with the "take down."

CLINICAL JUDGMENT GUIDE: When answering questions in mental health nursing, the test taker should identify safety as a priority intervention. The nurse should assist the MHW to promote the safety of the client and the MHW.

24. 1. The nurse should address the behavior with the clients and not delegate this task to the MHW. This inappropriate behavior needs

further investigation to determine whether it is consensual or under duress.
2. The inappropriate behavior should be addressed immediately with both clients.
3. If the behavior does not stop, one of the clients may need to be transferred to another unit, but this is not the appropriate action now.
4. The nurse needs to talk to the clients to determine whether the kissing was consensual or under duress. Either way, the behavior is inappropriate, and the clients should be told there is no kissing or sexual activity allowed between clients while they are hospitalized in the psychiatric unit.

CLINICAL JUDGMENT GUIDE: The nurse should assess the situation to gather information and reinforce the rules of the psychiatric unit.

25. 1. The MHW could walk with the agitated client. This may help decrease the client's agitation and anxiety.
    2. The nurse should not assign a task that is the responsibility of another staff member. The housekeeping or custodial department should be assigned to clean the floor.
    3. The MHW cannot take telephone orders from an HCP. A licensed nurse must do this.
    4. The RN cannot delegate teaching to an MHW. The nurse should explain seizure precautions to staff members.

CLINICAL JUDGMENT GUIDE: The RN cannot delegate assessment, evaluation, teaching, administering medications, or caring for an unstable client to an MHW.

26. 1. This is an example of battery, which is touching a client without consent.
    2. This is an example of false imprisonment, which is the deliberate and unauthorized confinement of a person within fixed limits by using verbal or physical means.
    3. This is an appropriate action by the MHW, which would not require immediate intervention.
    4. This is an example of assault, which is an act that results in a person's genuine fear and apprehension of being touched without consent.

CLINICAL JUDGMENT GUIDE: The nurse must maintain all clients' legal rights, even when in a locked psychiatric unit.

27. 1. When an individual is declared incompetent in a court, a guardian makes decisions for the client. The client loses the right to refuse medication.
    2. Unless a mental health court orders the client to receive medication, the LPN cannot force the client to take the medication. This client voluntarily admitted themself to the unit.
    3. Unless a mental health court orders the client to receive the medication, the LPN cannot force a client to take it, even if the client was involuntarily admitted to the unit.
    4. Charges pending in court do not remove the client's right to refuse medication.

CLINICAL JUDGMENT GUIDE: The charge nurse must know the client's rights in the mental health–nursing arena. The two options addressing a court of law should be included as possible correct options because "force" is in the question's stem.

28. 1. The more experienced psychiatric nurse should be assigned the client who is actively hallucinating and is delusional.
    2. The aggressive client should be assigned to a more experienced psychiatric nurse because this is a safety issue.
    3. The chronically depressed client should be assigned to the surgical nurse floated to the psychiatric unit. The client is not identified as suicidal in the option.
    4. The client diagnosed with antisocial personality disorder is angry, manipulative, and tends to split staff, so this client should be assigned to a more experienced psychiatric nurse.

CLINICAL JUDGMENT GUIDE: The test taker should select the client who is most stable and requires the least amount of psychiatric nursing knowledge. The primary concern in the psychiatric unit is safety, on which client assignments must be based.

29. 1. A client on a one-to-one watch must not be left alone for any reason, and the MHW should always be within arm's length.
    2. The client should not be allowed steel utensils while on suicide watch, so plastic utensils are appropriate.
    3. As long as the client is with a staff member, the client can attend group therapy.
    4. The MHW should remain in constant presence of the client, not observing the client from the porch.

CLINICAL JUDGMENT GUIDE: The RN supervises any task delegated to an MHW (UAP in mental health nursing).

30. 1. The MHW can assist the client with activities of daily living.
    2. The MHW is a vital part of the mental health team and is included in team meetings to discuss the client's psychiatric care.
    3. The MHW cannot administer medication; therefore, this comment warrants intervention.
    4. The MHW should stay in the day room to maintain client safety, so this comment does not warrant intervention.

CLINICAL JUDGMENT GUIDE: The MHW is a UAP. The RN cannot delegate assessment, teaching, evaluation, medication administration, or an unstable client to a UAP.

31. 1. Lorazepam (Ativan) is used to prevent delirium tremens, and an elevated pulse would not warrant questioning the administration of this medication.
    2. Methadone (Methadose) is prescribed to prevent withdrawal symptoms from heroin addiction, and an increased respiratory rate would not warrant questioning the administration of this medication.
    3. Clonidine (Catapres) is administered primarily to treat hypertension but is also used to reduce the symptoms of withdrawal from opioids, nicotine, and alcohol. The nurse would question administering this medication because of the client's low blood pressure, no matter why it is being prescribed.
    4. Thiamine (vitamin B_1) is used to diminish Wernicke-Korsakoff encephalopathy, which is characterized by confusion, memory loss, and loss of cranial nerve function resulting from chronic alcohol abuse. The nurse would not question giving this medication to a client diagnosed with Wernicke-Korsakoff syndrome, and a subnormal temperature would not warrant questioning the administration of this medication.

CLINICAL JUDGMENT GUIDE: The nurse must be aware of the expected actions of medications and assessment data indicating whether the medication should be administered or held. Also, the nurse should be able to determine whether the medication is effective or causing a side effect or an adverse event.

32. 1. This is incorrect information; therefore, the RN should not praise the MHW.
    2. The psychiatric nurse should not correct the MHW in front of the client because it will compromise the MHW's authority with the client.
    3. The RN should explain to the MHW that the mental health client retains all the civil rights afforded to all persons, except the right to leave the hospital in the case of involuntary commitments. The client may have restricted phone calls if included in the care plan—for example, if the client calls and threatens the president.
    4. This situation should not be discussed at the weekly team meeting. The RN psychiatric nurse can discuss this one-on-one with the MHW.

CLINICAL JUDGMENT GUIDE: The nurse is responsible for maintaining client legal rights, even when in a locked psychiatric unit.

33. 1. The client has a chemical imbalance in the brain, and a firm voice will not effectively get the client to sit down. The client cannot sit still.
    2. The mood stabilizer medication lithium (Eskalith) is the medication of choice, but it takes up to 3 weeks to become therapeutic; therefore, this intervention would not help the nurse complete the admission assessment.
    3. Walking or pacing with the client will allow the client to work off energy and may decrease restlessness and agitation. The nurse should implement this intervention to obtain information for the admission assessment.
    4. The nurse must obtain an admission assessment; therefore, the nurse should walk and pace with the client while attempting to get the priority admission assessment.

CLINICAL JUDGMENT GUIDE: In mental health nursing, the foundation for all nursing care is having a trusting nurse and client relationship. The nurse can choose an intervention that supports the client's needs.

34. 1. Evaluating the effectiveness of a client's medication is primarily the role of the psychiatric nurse, psychologist, and psychiatrist, not the social worker.
    2. The recreational therapist helps the client balance work and play and then provides activities that promote constructive leisure or unstructured time.
    3. The vocational therapist helps the client with job-seeking or job-retention skills and pursuing further education if needed and desired.

4. According to the National Council of State Boards of Nursing (NCSBN) referrals area content on the NCLEX-RN® test plan, the psychiatric social worker may conduct therapy and often has the primary responsibility for working with families, community support, and referrals.

CLINICAL JUDGMENT GUIDE: The test taker must know the roles of all members of the multidisciplinary healthcare team as well as appropriate referrals. The nurse must implement a referral to the most appropriate person or agency.

35. 1. The first intervention should be to talk to the client and remove them from the day room to the least restrictive environment. Restraining the client is the most restrictive environment.
    2. The nurse should first attempt to talk to the client and remove the client from the day room area, not try to remove all the other clients.
    3. The client will probably need a PRN medication to calm the behavior, but it is not the nurse's first intervention. An intramuscular medication takes at least 30 minutes to become effective.
    4. The first intervention is to approach the client calmly and attempt to remove them from the day room. Staff members should not approach the agitated client alone but be accompanied by other personnel.

CLINICAL JUDGMENT GUIDE: When answering questions in mental health nursing, the test taker should identify safety as a priority intervention.

36. 1. This child has been abused, and until Child Protective Services has been notified, the nurse should not share any information with the child's father.
    2. The Health Insurance Portability and Accountability Act (HIPAA) considers parents the "personal representative" of the minor child with the right to information. However, there are exceptions to this rule, including when the provider reasonably believes that the minor may be a victim of abuse or neglect by the parent or guardian. This statement is the nurse's best response.
    3. Because the mother is accusing the spouse of the abuse, this is not an appropriate response.
    4. The social worker must adhere to HIPAA regulations; therefore, referring the spouse to the social worker will not help the spouse determine how their son is doing.

CLINICAL JUDGMENT GUIDE: The nurse is responsible for knowing and complying with local, state, and federal standards of care.

37. 1. This client should be instructed to attend the anger management class, but this does not warrant immediate intervention.
    2. The MHW could escort the client outside to smoke, but this does not warrant immediate intervention by the RN.
    3. The nauseated and vomiting client has a physiological problem that should be assessed by the nurse immediately. This client warrants immediate intervention.
    4. A client having menses, or "period," may experience abdominal cramping and would need to be assessed, but not before the client vomiting twice.

CLINICAL JUDGMENT GUIDE: When the question asks, "Which warrants immediate intervention?" it is an "except" question. Physiological problems have the highest priority when deciding on a course of action. If the client is in distress, then the nurse must intervene with a nursing action that attempts to alleviate or control the problem.

38. 1. Because the clinical manager wants to reward the unit for no absences or tardies, the manager must reward all shifts, so providing a thank-you meal to all shifts would be most appropriate. This allows all the staff members to celebrate the unit's accomplishment.
    2. A thank-you note is nice, but knowing the clinical manager took the time to arrange the meal means a lot to staff members. The meal could encourage the staff to try to do the same the next month.
    3. Individually telling the staff "job well done" is a possible action to take, but for the clinical manager to take the time to arrange for the meal on all shifts is above and beyond just saying thank you to each staff member.
    4. Having no absences or tardies for 1 month for an individual employee is the expected behavior. The fact that the entire unit had no absences or tardies is being acknowledged.

CLINICAL JUDGMENT GUIDE: All options in this question are plausible. The test taker must identify the most appropriate intervention. There will be management questions on the NCLEX-RN®. In many instances, there is no test-taking strategy for these questions. The nurse must be knowledgeable of management issues.

39. 1. The nurse must take action to protect the spouse.
    2. The statement can be documented, but this is not the appropriate action for the nurse to implement.
    3. Mental health clinicians have a duty to warn identifiable third parties of threats made by a person, even if these threats were discussed during a therapy session (*Tarasoff v. Regents of the University of California*, 1976). The nurse should notify the client's psychiatric HCP so the spouse can be notified of the threat.
    4. The nurse should not encourage this behavior because it could cause serious harm to the spouse.

CLINICAL JUDGMENT GUIDE: The NCLEX-RN® test plan includes nursing care ruled by legal requirements. The nurse must know these issues.

40. Correct answers are 3 and 4.
    1. Exercise often causes the client to have trouble sleeping. This intervention is not appropriate.
    2. Elopement precautions are implemented for clients at risk of leaving the facility; therefore, this is inappropriate.
    3. Caffeinated beverages are stimulants; therefore, this is an appropriate intervention.
    4. An alarm on the bed would help ensure the safety of the client because the nurse will know immediately when the client leaves the bed.
    5. The one-to-one watches are for suicidal clients; therefore, this is not an appropriate intervention.

CLINICAL JUDGMENT GUIDE: The test taker must select all the correct interventions for "select all that apply" questions. The test taker should read each option and determine whether it is an appropriate intervention.

41. Correct order is 3, 4, 2, 5, 1.
    3. Denial
    4. Anger
    2. Bargaining
    5. Depression
    1. Acceptance

CLINICAL JUDGMENT GUIDE: This is a knowledge-based question, but the test taker must remember many facts that must be applied when taking the NCLEX-RN® examination. This information is the basis for many questions addressing the grieving process. The nurse must know these in the correct order and the appropriate interventions for each stage of grief.

42. 1. Identifying strengths and weaknesses is included in the orientation phase.
    2. **Identifying problem-solving techniques is part of the working phase.**
    3. Evaluating the client's experience is part of the termination phase.
    4. Establishing the meeting rules is part of the orientation phase.

CLINICAL JUDGMENT GUIDE: If the test taker is not familiar with the phases of group dynamics, then the word "middle" may give the test taker an idea of the goals of this part of group dynamics. Evaluation is usually done at the end, and establishing rules is usually done at the beginning.

43. 1. **On the inpatient psychiatric unit, the priority is maintaining client and staff safety.**
    2. Contacting family members is not a priority over safety.
    3. Safety is the priority over a client exhibiting behavior common in an inpatient psychiatric unit.
    4. This client needs to be assessed, but fasting for 2 days is not a safety issue for the inpatient psychiatric unit.

CLINICAL JUDGMENT GUIDE: When answering questions in mental health nursing, the test taker should identify safety as a priority intervention. All these situations require intervention, but safety is the priority.

44. Correct answers are 1 and 3.
    1. **Each member of AA has a sponsor who successfully quit drinking and supports a new member trying to stop drinking.**
    2. AA does not discuss medications used to help prevent drinking alcohol.
    3. **AA is a support group made up of recovering alcoholics helping others to stop drinking based on the 12-step approach.**
    4. AA helps alcoholics realize they are helpless over the addiction. They have no power over the addiction.
    5. Recovering alcoholics speak at the meetings, not professional guest speakers.

CLINICAL JUDGMENT GUIDE: "Select all that apply" questions require the test taker to select multiple options. This is an alternate question type on the NCLEX-RN®.

45. 1. The nurse should determine the lithium level, but it is not the first intervention the nurse should implement.

2. The nurse should assess the behavior that prompted the admission, but this is not the first intervention.
3. The nurse should first assess the client's physiological needs because the client in the manic state may not have slept, bathed, or had anything to eat for days. The client's physiological needs are the priority.
4. Lithium, a mood stabilizer medication, takes 2 to 3 weeks to become therapeutic; therefore, a STAT dose of lithium orally will not help the client's manic state. This is not the nurse's first intervention.

CLINICAL JUDGMENT GUIDE: Assessment is the first step of the nursing process, and the test taker should use the nursing process or some other systematic process to assist in determining priorities.

46. 1. A democratic manager is people-oriented and emphasizes efficient group functioning. The environment is open, and communication flows both ways, including having meetings to discuss concerns.
    2. This statement is that of an autocratic manager using an authoritarian approach to direct the activities of others.
    3. This statement concerns a laissez-faire manager maintaining a permissive climate with little direction or control. Instructing the staff to handle the situation independently does not support the staff.
    4. This statement is taking control of the situation; therefore, this is not a statement indicating a laissez-faire manager.

CLINICAL JUDGMENT GUIDE: There will be management questions on the NCLEX-RN®. In many instances, there is no test-taking strategy for these questions. The nurse must be knowledgeable of management issues.

47. 1. Unless the client is anorexic and there is a court order, the nurse cannot force-feed a client.
    2. This is client abuse, and the charge nurse must investigate the allegation immediately with the nurse. If the allegations are true, they should be documented in writing and reported to the client abuse committee.
    3. The charge nurse should not ask the client about the situation first. The RN and MHW should be involved in investigating the allegation. Then, if needed, the client can be asked about the situation.
    4. The RN charge nurse should investigate the allegations first and then, if needed, have the MHW document details of the situation.

CLINICAL JUDGMENT GUIDE: There will be management questions on the NCLEX-RN®. In many instances, there is no test-taking strategy for these questions. The nurse must be knowledgeable of management issues.

48. Correct answers are 1, 2, and 5.
    1. The nurse should assess the client for any injury, side effects of medication, and general well-being every 2 to 4 hours.
    2. As soon as possible, the nurse must inform the client of what behavior will allow the client to be released from the seclusion room.
    3. According to the Joint Commission Restraint and Seclusion Standards for Behavioral Health, the client's family is notified promptly of initiating restraint or seclusion.
    4. The nurse's goal is to release the client as soon as possible from the seclusion room. When the client has calmed down and can verbalize feelings and concerns rationally, the client should be released. The seclusion order must be renewed every 24 hours, but the client should not be secluded for 24 hours unless necessary.
    5. Clients must be checked at least every 10 to 15 minutes in person and may be continuously monitored on video cameras.

CLINICAL JUDGMENT GUIDE: This is an alternate type of question included in the NCLEX-RN®. The nurse must be able to select all the options that answer the question correctly.

49. 1. The RN should first separate the MHW from the client; therefore, asking the MHW to go to the nurse's station would be the first intervention.
    2. The nurse should not correct the MHW in front of the client and should not use the word "arguing"; therefore, this would not be appropriate.
    3. The psychiatric nurse should handle this situation immediately. If this is a pattern of behavior of the MHW, then the RN clinical manager should be notified.
    4. This behavior may or may not need to be reported to the client abuse committee, but if the RN overhears the MHW and the client arguing, the nurse should stop the behavior.

CLINICAL JUDGMENT GUIDE: In any business, including a healthcare facility, arguments or discussions of confidential information should not occur between staff or clients. In this case, the MHW should be removed from the situation to stop the behavior.

50. 1. The psychiatric social worker can refer clients, but the nurse should assess the client to see what type of help they want.
    2. The psychiatric social worker does not perform or participate in ECT treatment; therefore, this client should not be referred.
    3. The nurse needs to assess the client to determine why the client is having difficulty going to work. For example, is it sedation secondary to medications?
    4. The psychiatric social worker can assist with financial arrangements, referrals, and nonphysiological concerns.

CLINICAL JUDGMENT GUIDE: The test taker must know the roles of all members of the multidisciplinary healthcare team as well as appropriate referrals. The nurse must implement a referral to the most suitable person or agency.

51. 1. Two times in 1 week is becoming a pattern of behavior. The clinical manager should talk informally to the nurse to determine what is happening.
    2. This is only the second time the nurse has taken 45 minutes for lunch and does not warrant formal counseling. The clinical manager should assess the situation before formally documenting the behavior.
    3. This is very punitive behavior for the psychiatric nurse. The clinical manager should talk to the nurse before taking this action.
    4. The clinical manager should talk to the nurse informally and find out what is happening. This behavior cannot continue, but it is not behavior that requires anything more than informally finding out why the nurse has been late.

CLINICAL JUDGMENT GUIDE: There will be management questions on the NCLEX-RN®. In many instances, there is no test-taking strategy for these questions. The nurse must be knowledgeable of management issues.

52. 1. The client diagnosed with Alzheimer's disease would be expected to be confused; therefore, this would not warrant immediate intervention.
    2. The client diagnosed with Alzheimer's disease has difficulty completing simple routine activities of daily living. This would not warrant immediate intervention.
    3. The client diagnosed with Alzheimer's disease should not be difficult to arouse from sleep. This is not a typical symptom of this disease and would warrant immediate intervention from the nurse.
    4. The client diagnosed with Alzheimer's disease has difficulty completing simple routine activities of daily living. This would not warrant immediate intervention.

CLINICAL JUDGMENT GUIDE: When the question asks, "Which warrants immediate intervention?" it is an "except" question. Three of the client scenarios listed are normal or expected symptoms for the client situation. After eliminating the expected options, the test taker should select the one remaining.

53. 1. This is a therapeutic response that helps the client to vent feelings, but this statement does not support the ethical principle of veracity.
    2. Veracity is the ethical principle "to tell the truth." The truth is that schizophrenia is a thought disorder caused by a chemical imbalance of the brain. Antipsychotic medication can control the client's hallucinations and delusions.
    3. This is interviewing the client, and this statement does not support the ethical principle of veracity.
    4. Schizophrenia is a mental illness, but if the client takes antipsychotic medication, the client may be able to work, get married, and live a productive life. This is a false statement.

CLINICAL JUDGMENT GUIDE: The NCLEX-RN® test plan includes nursing care that addresses ethical principles, including autonomy, beneficence, justice, and veracity, to name a few.

54. 1. Carbamazepine (Tegretol), an anticonvulsant, is a medication that is often prescribed for clients diagnosed with bipolar disorder, even though it is classified as an anticonvulsant. A medication with a different classification is often prescribed for another disease process.
    2. Antacids such as aluminum hydroxide magnesium hydroxide (Maalox) neutralize gastric acid and may reduce the effects of antipsychotic medications and lead to medication failure. The client diagnosed with schizophrenia would be on an antipsychotic medication; therefore, the nurse should discuss this client with the psychiatric HCP.

3. The client receiving isoniazid (INH), an antituberculosis medication, must receive it to prevent resistant tuberculosis strains and protect the community. The nurse would not need to discuss this client with the HCP.
4. Amitriptyline (Elavil), a tricyclic antidepressant, has shown efficacy in promoting weight gain in clients diagnosed with anorexia nervosa; therefore, the nurse would not discuss this medication with the HCP.

CLINICAL JUDGMENT GUIDE: The nurse should be aware of medications' expected actions and side effects.

55. 1. The nurse must know the bomb scare policy of the facility, and in many cases, the nurse looks for the bomb but does not touch it if found. Sometimes, the nurse should not attempt to look for a bomb, but because the client is on a psychiatric unit, the nurse should look for a suspicious-looking object before notifying the bomb squad and evacuating the clients.
2. The nurse would implement the bomb scare protocol if there was a bomb or suspicious-looking bag, but the nurse should first investigate the comment because the client is on a psychiatric unit.
3. The nurse would evacuate the clients if a bomb or suspicious-looking bag was under the couch. The nurse should have the clients leave the lobby area, not the unit.
4. Just because the client is in a psychiatric unit does not mean that someone did or did not put a bomb under the couch. The nurse should look under the couch and take appropriate action.

CLINICAL JUDGMENT GUIDE: The nurse must be knowledgeable of emergency preparedness. Employees receive this information in employee orientation and are responsible for implementing procedures correctly. The NCLEX-RN® includes questions on a safe and effective care environment. The protocol may differ in the mental health setting; therefore, the nurse should follow policy.

56. 1. The response is closed and does not allow the new nurse to voice their opinion and be part of the team.
2. The charge nurse should be open to change. Just because something has been done the same way for years does not mean it can't be done another way.
3. The charge nurse should not make the new nurse talk to the other nurses because the shift report is not done how they want.
4. The best response is to allow the new nurse to share ideas with the charge nurse. The charge nurse could then talk to the other staff members and take the change to the clinical manager to determine whether the change should be instituted.

CLINICAL JUDGMENT GUIDE: There will be management questions on the NCLEX-RN®. In many instances, there is no test-taking strategy for these questions. The nurse must be knowledgeable of management issues.

57. 1. The client may eventually be able to go to the activity area. Still, while the client is confined to the unit, the nurse should refer the client to a recreational therapist to be provided with activities to alleviate boredom.
2. Allowing the client to vent feelings will not help alleviate the client's boredom on the unit.
3. According to the NCLEX-RN® test plan, the nurse must know the multidisciplinary team. The recreational therapist helps the client to balance work and play, then provides activities that promote constructive use of leisure or unstructured time.
4. The nurse should acknowledge the client's concern and contact the recreational therapist.

CLINICAL JUDGMENT GUIDE: The test taker must know the roles of all members of the multidisciplinary healthcare team as well as appropriate referrals. The nurse must implement a referral to the most suitable person or agency.

58. 1. A client, after being raped, would be expected to be upset and crying. This client would not require the most experienced nurse.
2. The client diagnosed with bipolar disorder would be agitated in the manic state. This client would not require the most experienced nurse.
3. The client found wandering in a daze and having no diagnosis requires an in-depth assessment. This client should be assigned to the most experienced nurse.
4. The client diagnosed with schizophrenia would have hallucinations if not taking antipsychotic medication. The client would not require the most experienced nurse.

CLINICAL JUDGMENT GUIDE: The test taker must determine which client is the most unstable and would require the most experienced nurse, thus making this type of question an "except" question. Three clients are either stable or have non-life-threatening conditions.

59. 1. When admitted to a psychiatric unit, the client does not lose any rights. The client has a right to refuse treatment, but if the client is a danger to themselves, then the psychiatric team must go to court and obtain an order to force-feed the client. This could be with nasogastric tube feedings or total parenteral nutrition.
    2. The client has a right to refuse treatment, but if the client is a danger to themselves, then the psychiatric team must intervene. If the client does not eat, the client will die.
    3. If the client is discharged and dies, the psychiatric team will be responsible. If a person has a mental illness, the psychiatric team must protect the client.
    4. This is against the client's rights. The nurse cannot restrain a client without a court order.

CLINICAL JUDGMENT GUIDE: The NCLEX-RN® test plan includes nursing care ruled by legal requirements. The nurse must be knowledgeable of these issues.

60. 1. The nurse would notify the police department if the client left the unit.
    2. The nurse's first intervention is to place the unit on high alert, which includes putting signs on the exit doors warning all people coming in and out that a client is threatening to leave the unit.
    3. The nurse should talk to the client, but the first intervention is to prevent the client from making good on the threat of running away.
    4. The client on an involuntary admission loses the right to sign out of the psychiatric unit against medical advice (AMA).

CLINICAL JUDGMENT GUIDE: When answering questions in mental health nursing, the test taker should identify safety as a priority intervention.

61. 1. The nurse does not have a right to ask the caller for their name. Mr. Jones has a right to telephone calls.
    2. Mr. Jones retains all his civil rights when admitted to a psychiatric unit unless phone restriction is part of the individualized care plan.
    3. The access code for client information is requested when the caller is asking questions about the client. It is not used when the caller wants to talk directly to the client.
    4. **The nurse should find Mr. Jones and tell him he has a phone call. The client cannot have rights restricted unless it is a part of** the client's individualized care plan. For example, the client may not be allowed to use the phone to call 911 and make false reports.

CLINICAL JUDGMENT GUIDE: The NCLEX-RN® test plan includes nursing care ruled by legal requirements. The nurse must be knowledgeable of these issues.

62. 1. The psychiatric nurse should not make promises they cannot keep. If the information must be shared with the healthcare team, then the nurse must break a promise to the client. This will compromise the nurse-client relationship.
    2. **This is the nurse's best response. The nurse is honest with the client but will keep the information confidential if it does not affect the client's care.**
    3. The client may need to share information pertinent to the client's care and should be encouraged to communicate with the nurse.
    4. Asking the client "Why?" may put the client on the defensive, thereby being less inclined to share the information.

CLINICAL JUDGMENT GUIDE: In mental health nursing, the foundation for all nursing care is having a trusting nurse and client relationship. The nurse should be honest with the client about the information the nurse can keep confidential and which information must be shared with the healthcare team.

63. 1. The client diagnosed with schizophrenia would be expected to be delusional; therefore, this situation would not warrant immediate intervention.
    2. The charge nurse has the entire shift to arrange for another nurse to cover the LPN; therefore, this situation does not warrant immediate intervention.
    3. **The loss of a unit key card is a priority because the RN must determine when the MHW last had the key card and whether it may be lost on the psychiatric unit. The unit is no longer secure if a client finds the key card.**
    4. Signing the supply order is important but does not warrant immediate intervention.

CLINICAL JUDGMENT GUIDE: When answering questions in mental health nursing, the test taker should identify safety as a priority intervention. The loss of a key card could put the safety of all the clients on the unit at risk.

64. 1. The local police department must be called, but the nurse must first talk to the client and attempt to diffuse the situation. This action tries to ensure the safety of the client, the other clients, and the staff.
    2. Ensuring the safety of the other clients and staff is important, but the nurse should first attempt to contact the client.
    3. The nurse should not encourage the client to talk about feelings until the gun is removed. The anger may cause the client to shoot an innocent person accidentally or on purpose.
    4. The nurse should try to talk to the client and diffuse the situation first. This action attempts to ensure the safety of the client, the other clients, and the staff.

CLINICAL JUDGMENT GUIDE: When answering questions in mental health nursing, the test taker should identify safety as a priority intervention. The nurse could perform all these actions, but safety is the priority.

65. Correct answers are 2 and 5.
    1. This client requires the care of a nurse to make attempts at getting the client to participate in therapy.
    2. The client diagnosed with diabetes can be monitored by the medical-surgical nurse. The option does not state that any unusual situations are occurring with the client's diagnosed illness.
    3. Dissociative identity disorder (DID) was formerly known as multiple personality disorder (MPD). This client may be experiencing a different personality; an experienced psychiatric nurse should assess this situation.
    4. This client is creating a disturbance in the day room by blocking the television and may be at risk from the other clients. This client needs intervention by an experienced psychiatric nurse to diffuse the situation.
    5. A client diagnosed with major depression starting antidepressant medications 2 days ago could be cared for by the medical-surgical nurse. It is expected that this client has not received medication therapy long enough to make a difference in the depression. The medication requires 2 to 3 weeks of administration before showing effectiveness.

CLINICAL JUDGMENT GUIDE: The test taker must evaluate each option individually and decide, based solely on the facts included in the option, to select correctly in a "select all that apply" question. One option does not rule out another option. The test taker must decide whether the medical-surgical nurse has the knowledge required to care for the client.

66. Correct order is 2, 4, 3, 1, 5.
    2. Part of the National Patient Safety Goals is implementing two identifiers when the client is to receive a procedure. The nurse must do this to determine whether the client is correct and what procedure is correct.
    4. The client should have been NPO for several hours before the procedure for safety reasons. If the client were to vomit during the procedure, then aspiration might occur.
    3. The client will require an IV line for medication administration and emergency reasons.
    1. The electric impulses will be administered via electrodes.
    5. The HCP is not notified to begin the procedure until the nurse completes all the required preprocedure steps.

CLINICAL JUDGMENT GUIDE: The test taker should mentally visualize the procedure area and identify which steps to complete. Some steps, such as identifying the correct client, should be taken after washing their hands.

67. 1. This laboratory value is within normal range.
    2. This laboratory value is within normal range.
    3. This client has schizophrenia and also has a low white blood cell count. Many clients diagnosed with schizophrenia are placed on atypical antipsychotic agents such as clozapine (Clozaril); these medications can cause agranulocytosis. This places the client at risk for a life-threatening infection. The nurse should hold the dose of any atypical antipsychotic medication and notify the HCP of the result.
    4. This laboratory value is within normal range.

CLINICAL JUDGMENT GUIDE: The test taker must be aware of complications due to treatments for particular diseases. However, the laboratory data in this question have only one abnormal result. If the test taker is unsure, the abnormal result should be chosen.

68. Correct answers are 1, 3, and 5.
    1. Psychiatric units have emergency codes to request assistance for a "take down" procedure when a client is deemed uncontrollable; the charge nurse should request this assistance.
    2. The client is in an excited state, so telling them they will lose privileges is useless at this time.
    3. **The other clients should be removed from possible harm.**
    4. The staff should speak in a calm, soft tone to assist the client in regaining composure.
    5. **The psychiatric unit is a locked unit. When the notification is made for assistance, someone must open the door so the emergency responders can enter the unit.**

CLINICAL JUDGMENT GUIDE: The test taker must decide on each option individually and cannot choose based on any other option in "select all that apply" questions. A "take down" procedure requires that safety is a significant consideration for the client and staff.

69. 1. This client has some beginnings of tardive dyskinesia but can continue the antipsychotic medications.
    2. This client has some moderate signs of tardive dyskinesia but can continue the antipsychotic medications.
    3. This client has some tardive dyskinesia but can continue the antipsychotic medications with frequent monitoring of the AIMS test. At a score of 20 or above the medications must be discontinued.
    4. **This client is exhibiting severe abnormal behavior, and the antipsychotic medication should be discontinued. The AIMS test was devised to detect extrapyramidal symptoms. If continued, the client will have permanent tardive dyskinesia from the medication.**

CLINICAL JUDGMENT GUIDE: This question can be answered from the chart by recognizing that the higher the number, the more serious the side effects of the medications will be.

70. 1. **The client is a risk to themselves, and Emergency Medical Services (EMS) should be notified to go to the client and ensure that no harm comes to them. The client is not in the outpatient clinic with the nurse; therefore, EMS should be notified to go to the client before the client harms themself.**
    2. This is an assessment question but not the first intervention. The first intervention is to arrange for help to get to the client as soon as possible.
    3. The HCP will be notified, but it is not the first intervention.
    4. The nurse manager should remain on the phone to keep the client occupied until the paramedics arrive.

CLINICAL JUDGMENT GUIDE: When the question asks which intervention should be implemented first, the test taker must know that all options are plausible. Safety is a priority, and the client is not in the nurse's presence; therefore, help should be sent to the client.

71. 1. The benzodiazepine alprazolam (Xanax) is an appropriate medication for an anxiety attack, but it will take at least 15 to 30 minutes for the medication to treat the physiological clinical manifestations. Therefore, this is not the first intervention.
    2. Allowing the client to vent feelings is an appropriate intervention, but not the first intervention, because the client is hyperventilating.
    3. **The first intervention is to address the client's physical discomfort, which is hyperventilating; therefore, encouraging the client to take slow, deep breaths is the next intervention for the nurse.**
    4. The client's pulse oximeter reading can be obtained, but it will not address the client's hyperventilating; therefore, it is not the nurse's first intervention.

CLINICAL JUDGMENT GUIDE: If the client is in distress, then the nurse should intervene with a nursing action that attemps to alleviate or control the problem.

72. 1. **The client diagnosed with dementia would be expected to have confusion and disorientation; therefore, the LPN could be assigned to this client. This client is not experiencing any potentially life-threatening complications of dementia.**
    2. Extrapyramidal side effects are a complication of antipsychotic medication. A more experienced RN should be assigned to this client.
    3. The client pacing up and down the hallway is exhibiting the manic behavior of bipolar disorder. This client needs further assessment and should be assigned to an RN.
    4. This client is experiencing potentially life-threatening complications of anorexia and needs further assessment, so an RN should be assigned to this client.

CLINICAL JUDGMENT GUIDE: The nurse is responsible for knowing the scope of practice for the healthcare team members who are subordinates.

The RN should not delegate an unstable client to an LPN.

73. 1. The nurse manager should not involve other employees in the nurse's situation. A clinical manager should allow the nurse to resolve the problem.
    2. Because the nurse has a reason for being late and the car will be fixed in a week, the behavior does not need to be documented and placed in their file.
    3. This is very punitive behavior for the nurse manager because she is having car trouble and riding the bus to get to work.
    4. The nurse manager needs to work with the employees, and being understanding of situations is an attribute of an effective clinical manager. The nurse has a valid reason for being late, and because the nurse has an excellent attendance record, the nurse manager should be understanding and work with them.

CLINICAL JUDGMENT GUIDE: There will be management questions on the NCLEX-RN®. In many instances, there is no test-taking strategy for these questions.

74. 1. Isolation occurs when the client attempts to avoid a painful thought or feeling by objectifying and emotionally detaching themselves from the feeling.
    2. The client is not accepting reality because it is too painful. The client is exhibiting denial.
    3. Projection is attributing unacceptable thoughts or feelings to someone or something else.
    4. Sublimation occurs when the client redirects unacceptable, instinctual drives into personally and socially acceptable channels.

CLINICAL JUDGMENT GUIDE: The test taker should know defense mechanisms to provide clients with effective coping strategies. This question is knowledge-based.

75. 1. Isolation occurs when the client attempts to avoid a painful thought or feeling by objectifying and emotionally detaching themself from the feeling.
    2. Rationalization occurs when the client justifies their behavior and motivation by substituting acceptable reasons and excuses for these motivations.
    3. Projection is attributing unacceptable thoughts or feelings to someone or something else.
    4. The client is redirecting unacceptable, instinctual drives into personally and socially acceptable channels. This client is exhibiting sublimation.

CLINICAL JUDGMENT GUIDE: The test taker should know defense mechanisms to provide clients with effective coping strategies. This question is knowledge-based.

76. 1. The client is justifying their behavior and motivation by substituting acceptable reasons and excuses for these motivations. This defense mechanism is rationalization.
    2. Altruism is handling and transforming one's pain and uncomfortable thoughts into helping others.
    3. Projection is attributing unacceptable thoughts or feelings to someone or something else.
    4. Displacement is channeling a feeling or thought from its actual source to something or someone else.

CLINICAL JUDGMENT GUIDE: The test taker should know defense mechanisms to provide clients with effective coping strategies. This question is knowledge-based.

77. 1. Humor as a defense mechanism focuses on funny aspects of a painful situation.
    2. Isolation occurs when the client attempts to avoid a painful thought or feeling by objectifying and emotionally detaching themself from the feeling. This client is exhibiting emotion.
    3. The client is exhibiting regression by reverting to an older, less mature way of handling stress and feelings.
    4. Suppression is the voluntary burying of a painful feeling or thought from awareness.

CLINICAL JUDGMENT GUIDE: The test taker should know defense mechanisms to provide clients with effective coping strategies. This question is knowledge-based.

78. 1. The client is exhibiting undoing. The client is trying to reverse or "undo" a thought or feeling by performing an action that signifies an opposite feeling than originally thought or felt.
    2. Repression is the involuntary blocking of a painful feeling or experience from awareness.
    3. Altruism is handling and transforming one's pain and uncomfortable thoughts into helping others.
    4. Regression is reverting to an older, less mature way of handling stress and feelings.

CLINICAL JUDGMENT GUIDE: The test taker should know defense mechanisms to provide clients with effective coping strategies. This question is knowledge-based.

79. 1. The client channels a feeling or thought from its source to something or someone else. This defense mechanism is displacement.
    2. Splitting occurs when the client sees everything in the world as all good or all bad with nothing in between.
    3. Undoing occurs when the client is trying to reverse or "undo" a thought or feeling by performing an action that signifies an opposite feeling than initially thought or felt.
    4. Isolation occurs when the client attempts to avoid a painful thought or feeling by objectifying and emotionally detaching themself from the feeling.

CLINICAL JUDGMENT GUIDE: The test taker should know defense mechanisms to provide clients with effective coping strategies. This question is knowledge-based.

80. 1. Splitting occurs when the client sees everything in the world as all good or all bad with nothing in between.
    2. Humor as a defense mechanism focuses on funny aspects of a painful situation.
    3. The client is attributing unacceptable thoughts or feelings to someone else. This defense mechanism is projection.
    4. Denial occurs when the client does not accept reality because it is too painful.

CLINICAL JUDGMENT GUIDE: The test taker should know defense mechanisms to provide clients with effective coping strategies. This question is knowledge-based.

81. 1. Regression is reverting to an older, less mature way of handling stress and feelings.
    2. The client is exhibiting suppression. Suppression is the voluntary burying of a painful feeling or thought from awareness.
    3. Denial occurs when the client does not accept reality because it is too painful.
    4. Rationalization occurs when the client justifies behavior and motivation by substituting acceptable reasons and excuses for these motivations.

CLINICAL JUDGMENT GUIDE: The test taker should know defense mechanisms to provide clients with effective coping strategies. This question is knowledge-based.

82. Correct answers are 2, 3, and 5.
    1. The client in denial is not working through a group process. This is not an identified phase.
    2. The initial phase is usually the first one or two meetings of a group in which the client's anxiety is high. During these meetings, the nurse leader will address the reason for the group and group rules, establish a trusting relationship with the clients, and implement appropriate interventions with group members.
    3. In the working phase problems are identified, clients begin problem-solving, and the group develops a sense of bonding. These meetings allow for the clients to accomplish goals.
    4. The recovery phase is not an identified phase of the group process.
    5. The termination phase occurs in the last one or two meetings. The clients should evaluate the group experience. Some clients may be anxious about ending the group, while others may be glad to disband.

CLINICAL JUDGMENT GUIDE: The test taker should know the stages of group work. This question is knowledge-based.

83. 1. The leader leads the autocratic style with set goals. This style often lacks member input.
    2. The democratic leadership style encourages members to participate in problem-solving and is best for facilitating member participation and input.
    3. Laissez-faire leadership provides no direction to group members and can limit productivity.
    4. Situational leadership is not suited to this type of group. It does not necessarily promote long-term goals.

CLINICAL JUDGMENT GUIDE: The test taker should know about group work in mental health nursing and different leadership styles. The NCLEX_RN® test plan includes leadership topics.

84. Correct answers are 1, 2, 4, and 5.
    1. Clients diagnosed with schizophrenia often have false perceptions of sound and images.
    2. Clients diagnosed with schizophrenia often have delusions. Delusions are irrational or false beliefs about oneself not supported by the individual's education, culture, or talents.
    3. The client diagnosed with schizophrenia often exhibits negative symptoms such as

diminished emotional expression and reduced motivation to perform purposeful activities.
4. Schizophrenia can be associated with disorganized, incoherent, and illogical speech.
5. Disorganized behavior in the client diagnosed with schizophrenia can include a decline in daily functioning or even a catatonic state.

CLINICAL JUDGMENT GUIDE: This is an alternate type of question included in the NCLEX-RN®. The nurse must be able to select all the options that answer the question correctly.

85. Correct answers are 1, 3, and 5.
    1. The nurse should determine whether the hallucinations are indicating the client could harm themself or others; however, the nurse should not have prolonged discussions about false ideas.
    2. The nurse should not pretend to accept what the client is saying. The client must understand that the nurse does not view the hallucinations as real.
    3. The nurse should use distractions and involve the client in reality-based topics.
    4. The nurse should avoid touching the client without warning, as this could lead to fear and aggression in the client.
    5. The nurse should provide short, simple directions and convey a supportive and accepting attitude toward the client.

CLINICAL JUDGMENT GUIDE: This is an alternate type of question included in the NCLEX-RN®. The nurse must be able to select all the options that answer the question correctly.

86. Correct answers are 2, 3, and 4.
    1. The client experiencing a severe manic episode will display a decreased need for sleep and often exhibit continuous activity.
    2. The client experiencing a severe manic episode will experience a flight of ideas or racing thoughts.
    3. Talkative, pressured speech is commonly noted in the client experiencing a manic episode.
    4. The client experiencing a manic episode is often easily distracted by irrelevant external stimuli.
    5. Delusions of grandeur and inflated self-esteem are noted in a client experiencing a manic episode.

CLINICAL JUDGMENT GUIDE: This is an alternate type of question included in the NCLEX-RN®. The nurse must be able to select all the options that answer the question correctly.

87. Correct answers are 2, 3, 4, and 5.
    1. The nurse should encourage the client to participate in physical activity such as walking, throwing a basketball, etc. The nurse should avoid promoting competitive sports such as ping-pong or cards to minimize anxiety and agitation in the client.
    2. High-protein, high-calorie foods the client can carry around and eat "on the go" are appropriate for nutrition in the manic phase as clients are unlikely to sit at a table.
    3. Mood stabilizers such as lithium are often combined with antipsychotic medications to control mania. This is a correct intervention, although the medication may take 1 to 3 weeks to begin working.
    4. Glass, smoking materials, and all sharp objects should be removed from the client's surroundings to avoid the client using these objects to harm themself or others.
    5. The nurse should set firm limits on intrusive and manipulative behaviors by the client and assist the client in respecting boundaries.

CLINICAL JUDGMENT GUIDE: This is an alternate type of question included in the NCLEX-RN®. The nurse must be able to select all the options that answer the question correctly.

88. Correct answers are 1, 2, 3, and 4.
    1. The nurse should ask the client directly if she is thinking about suicide. This assists the nurse in determining whether the client is a suicide risk.
    2. The client with a specific plan to commit suicide is at high risk. This information will assist the nurse in determining the seriousness of the client's intent.
    3. The nurse should discover how easy it would be for the client to access lethal methods, such as guns or pills, to use in a suicide attempt.
    4. Previous suicide attempts increase the client's risk of attempting to commit suicide.
    5. Suicide is not an inherited family trait.

CLINICAL JUDGMENT GUIDE: This is an alternate type of question included in the NCLEX-RN®. The nurse must be able to select all the options that answer the question correctly.

89. Correct answers are 1, 3, and 5.
    1. The client diagnosed with major depression often exhibits changes in appetite that result in weight loss or weight gain.
    2. Grandiose behaviors and beliefs are common in bipolar disorder or schizophrenia but not in major depressive disorders.
    3. Loss of pleasure in life and usual pursuits is a symptom exhibited by clients diagnosed with major depression.
    4. Clients diagnosed with major depression often have difficulty concentrating and thinking clearly, not attentiveness.
    5. Clients diagnosed with major depression often are either unable to sleep or exhibit excessive sleepiness daily.

    CLINICAL JUDGMENT GUIDE: This is an alternate type of question included in the NCLEX-RN®. The nurse must be able to select all the options that answer the question correctly.

90. Correct answers are 1, 2, 3, and 4.
    1. Delirium tremens (DTs) occurs approximately 3 days after a client stops drinking following heavy alcohol use. The client exhibits anxiety, tremors, disorientation, and hallucinations. The nurse should assess for DTs as this could be life-threatening.
    2. Benzodiazepines should be given as ordered to prevent seizures and delirium.
    3. The nurse should initiate and monitor IV fluids, which normally include vitamins such as thiamine and folic acid, also known as a "banana bag."
    4. The nurse should attempt to keep the environmental stimuli to a minimum.
    5. A referral to Alcoholics Anonymous is appropriate once the client has recovered from the acute symptoms of alcohol withdrawal, but not at this time.

    CLINICAL JUDGMENT GUIDE: This is an alternate type of question included in the NCLEX-RN®. The nurse must be able to select all the options that answer the question correctly.

CASE STUDY ANSWERS

1. Correct answers are 1, 2, 3, 4, 5, 6, 7, 8, 9, 10, and 11.
   The client is brought in by police after Crisis Line notified emergency services of individual in crisis. The client reached out for help, initiating the community activated mental health response. Police report of Columbia Suicide Severity Rating is indicative of possible suicidal thoughts. Police are trained to identify the need for additional medical attention for mental health crises. Loss of support person and grief from loss of life partner constitute a major life stressor along with loss of additional social and financial support. Social isolation also happened from loss of coworkers. Loss of appetite may be physical or psychological and should be reported. Unkempt physical appearance, body odor, and lack of interest in self-care should be reported. Flat affect with soft speech, abbreviated answers should be reported. Saying "...would not mind if I died," statements associated with wanting to die, wanting to go to sleep and never wake up, not being missed if they died, are all statements that should be reported. Anhedonia—lack of enjoyment in life—is indicative of depression and may be due to hormonal or psychological change. Changes in sleep patterns can be indicative of increased stress and hormonal imbalances and are unhealthy. There is no plan in place to kill self. Not having a plan helps the provider determine the severity of the situation. All this information needs to be reported.

2. Correct answers are 2, 3, and 5.
    1. The client is not experiencing auditory or visual hallucinations. No assessment information indicates this client is experiencing psychosis.
    2. Depression. The client is experiencing loss of enjoyment of life activities, or anhedonia.
    3. Grief. The client is experiencing grief from the loss of their spouse. In addition, they may be grieving the loss of their job and the separation from coworkers.

4. No assessment information indicates this client is experiencing an electrolyte imbalance.
5. Suicidal. The client reached out to a crisis line, the sheriff evaluated the client with an evidence-based assessment tool, which indicated the client needed further evaluation for potential suicidal ideation.

3. The correct answers are 3 and 2.
Based on the client's condition at the time, the nurse recognizes that the client is at the highest risk for

| 3. Suicide |

and will require

| 2. A safe environment |

4. Correct answers are marked.

Potential Nursing Interventions	Indicated	Not Indicated
Apply bilateral wrist restraints.		X
Sit and talk with the patient.	X	
Establish trust by allowing privacy in the bathroom.		X
Ask whether there is anyone the client would like notified.	X	
Give the client a sandwich and can of soda.	X	
Offer a list of community resources for grief.	X	
Start an IV line to administer IV fluids.		X
Tell the patient, "Everything is going to be all right."		X
Request a chaplain visit.	X	

5. Correct answers are 1, 3, 4, and 5.
   1. Consult psychiatry since the client is medically cleared. This consult is a priority to meet the ongoing needs of the client best. Psychiatry can assist with grieving, depression, loss, and suicidal ideation. Moving the client to the correct treatment area can help to begin the client's journey back to wellness.
   2. Regular diet is not a priority. The client has been given something to eat and drink, and breakfast will be served in several hours.
   3. Suicide precautions with constant surveillance. Based on the client's presentation and the provider's continued orders, this is a priority for patient safety.
   4. Trazodone 50 mg PO PRN at bedtime for sleep. May repeat ×1 if not asleep in 2 hours. The client has not slept well, and a PRN sleeping medication is ordered for bedtime. Since it is nighttime, this should be administered tonight.
   5. Sertraline 50 mg PO daily, first dose now. This is ordered to start now and is a priority.
   6. CBC, BMP, fasting liver panel in a.m. This is not a priority because the order indicates it is due in the morning.
   7. Social work consult is not a priority but it should be a part of the client's plan of care. Social work consult is indicated for discharge planning to ensure appropriate follow-up and identification of community resources. Additionally, case management might be able to assist with finding funding for financial assistance for the hospital care and follow-up, depending on the client's resources.

6. Correct answers are marked.

Finding	Improved	Declined	No Change
Safety	X		
Appetite			X
Hygiene			X
Elopement risk			X
Understanding of discharge plan	X		
Suicidal thoughts	X		
Sleep disturbance			X
Able to identify two community resources for grief	X		

The client currently denies suicidal ideation, but the nurse and staff should remain vigilant because often, once the client is in a treatment facility, the client starts to feel better and may now have the energy to act on previous thoughts. Another possibility is that the client's desire to go home may override their need for treatment, and they might say what they think the staff wants to hear. Always follow the provider's order for level of safety.

Case Studies 14

The ultimate measure of a man is not where he stands in moments of comfort, but where he stands at times of challenge and controversy.

– Martin Luther King, Jr.

CASE STUDY #1

(1300) A 22-year-old woman presents to the emergency department (ED) escorted by a police officer. The police officer reports to the admitting registered nurse (RN) that the cashier from a local department store called the police when the patient began to act in a hostile and threatening manner. Before arriving to the ED, the client was in a department store for several hours trying on items and then attempted to purchase several hundred dollars worth of clothing. When her credit card was declined, the client became irate, acted irrationally, and threatened to kill the cashier if she was not allowed to purchase the clothing.

(1305) The client is alert and oriented to person, place, and time. She does not understand why she is at the hospital. Her color is adequate, lips pink. Lungs are clear bilaterally in all lobes. Pupils are equal, round at 6 mm bilateral. The client is dressed in clean cut-off shorts, a midriff top, and high heels, exposing a lot of her body. Her makeup is appropriate, and her hair is clean and combed. The client is speaking quickly and loudly in an angry tone. She states, "I do not have time to be here. I need to study. My final exams are tomorrow. I have millions of dollars in my bank account. When my lawyer discovers all this, I will sue you idiots. Don't touch me." Weight per bed scale is 118 lb, with a body mass index (BMI) of 20.

(1308) The client becomes increasingly agitated as the nurse obtains vital signs. She attempts to hit the nurse with her purse and quickly stands up on the stretcher unsteadily with arms held outward, shouting, "I can fly out of here if I want to; get back, or I will." The patient throws her high heel at the nurse and barely misses.

(1310) Hospital security personnel come into the room. The client remains standing on the stretcher, yelling, "There is nothing wrong with me. The last time I was here, the nurse tried to poison me."

Vital Signs	Client Values
Temperature	97.2°F (36.2°C)
Heart rate	105 bpm, regular
Blood pressure	138/84 mm Hg
Respirations	26/min, shallow
SpO_2	100% on room air

(1318) The client's mother arrives at the ED. The client sits on the bed per her mother's request, then begins to pace around the room, rapidly talking nonstop about the need to study and having millions of dollars.

(1320) History is obtained from mother: The mother reports that her daughter was diagnosed with major depressive disorder at age 20. One year ago, she took a large amount of acetaminophen but disclosed it immediately to her mother. Her diagnosis was changed to bipolar last year by her psychiatrist owing to labile emotions and a week-long episode of mania. She is a full-time college student and has been studying nonstop for her finals for the past week. She slept little, if any, in the previous few days. She has had little to eat or drink. Her medications include lithium 300 mg twice daily and lurasidone 20 mg daily. The mother is unsure whether the client has been taking her prescribed medication.

1. **Recognize cues. What matters most?** Which **priority** client data should be reported to the healthcare provider (HCP)? **Select all that apply.**
   1. Rapid, pressured speech
   2. Blood pressure (BP) 138/84 mm Hg
   3. Heart rate (HR) 105 bmp
   4. Alert and oriented ×3
   5. Grooming
   6. Angry, agitated affect
   7. Self-harm behaviors
   8. Delusions of grandeur
   9. Lack of sleep
   10. Refusal of care

2. **Analyze cues. What could it mean?** What at-risk conditions should the nurse be concerned about the client developing? **Select all that apply.**
   1. Full-blown mania
   2. Dysthymia
   3. Major depressive episode
   4. Suicidal intent
   5. Physical exhaustion
   6. Hypertension
   7. Refusal of medications

(1335) The ED physician interviews the client with her mother at her bedside. The client denies ingesting any illicit substances. She denies any current suicidal ideation or plan. She reports that she does not remember the last time she took her medications. "I don't need the medication; it makes me too tired to study." The client cries loudly, "Those people at the store are lying. I have millions to pay for my purchases. They hate me, everybody's fake; wait—I can see in your eyes that you do, too!" She refuses to sit down, walking back and forth in the room. The physician orders are written and populated in the medical record.

PROVIDER ORDERS:

Dx: Bipolar disorder
Lithium level
CBC and CMP
Quantative lurasidone level
Quantitative hCG
Urinalysis, routine
Urine drug screen
Acetaminophen level
Colombia Suicide Scale
Administer olanzapine 10 mg as oral disintegrating tablet ×1. May Administer IM if remains agitated.
Lithium 300 mg PO BID, start now
Lurasidone 20 mg PO daily with food, start now

(1338) Mother remains in the room with the client. Blood is drawn for lab tests. The client continues to be restless, pacing and wringing her hands, crying hysterically.

3. **Prioritize hypotheses. Where do I start?** Complete the sentence by choosing from the drop-down list of options. Based on the client's condition at the time, the nurse recognizes that the patient is at the highest risk for _____

> *Select* ▼
> 1. Self-harm
> 2. Physical exhaustion
> 3. Dehydration

and will require _____.

> *Select* ▼
> 1. Normal saline 0.9% at 50 mL/hr
> 2. Olanzapine 10 mg IM now
> 3. Vest restraint

(1405) Lab results are posted.

Laboratory Test	Client Values	Reference Values
Hemoglobin (Hgb)	12.5	Male: 14 to 17.3 g/dL
		Female: 11.7 to 15.5 g/dL
Hematocrit (Hct)	52	Male: 42% to 52%
		Female: 36% to 48%
White blood cell (WBC) count	13.2	4.5 to 11.1 $\times$ 10^3/microL
Platelets	153	140 to 400 $\times$ 10^3/microL
Creatinine	0.9	Male: 0.61 to 1.21 mg/dL
		Female: 0.59 to 1.04 mg/dL
Glucose	112	Fasting: Less than 100 mg/dL
		Random: Less than 200 mg/dL
Blood urea nitrogen	25	8 to 21 mg/dL
		Adult over 90 years: 10 to 31 mg/dL
Sodium	150	135 to 145 mEq/L or mmol/L
Lithium	0.3	0.6 to 1.2 mEq/L
Urine, routine	Negative	Negative: RBCs, WBCs, protein, glucose, ketones
Specific gravity	1.037	1.005 to 1.030
Urine drug screen	Pending	None detected
Quantitative hCG	0	Nonpregnant: Less than 5 mIU/mL
Acetaminophen	0	Less than 10 to 20 mcg/mL
Lurasidone	20	15 to 40 ng/mL
		Critical: 120 ng/mL

4. **Generate solutions. What can I do?** For each intervention, specify whether the intervention is **indicated** or **not indicated** for the client's care.

Potential Nursing Interventions	Indicated	Not Indicated
Place on one-to-one suicidal precautions		
Apply wrist restraints		
Place in a private room		
Utilize verbal de-escalation techniques		
Administer ordered medications as soon as possible		
Discuss her irrational thinking regarding the money in her bank account		
Decrease environmental stimuli		
Obtain repeat vital signs		
Weigh client		

5. **Take action. What will I do?** Which admission orders should the nurse consider a **priority** action? **Select all that apply.**
    1. Lithium level in a.m.
    2. Safety search of client and belongings
    3. Columbia Suicide Severity Rating Scale
    4. Monitor vital signs every 2 hours while awake
    5. Diet: High-protein, high-calorie finger foods and drinks
    6. Attend all structured activities in the unit
    7. Administer lorazepam 0.5 mg orally (PO) every 4 hours as needed for anxiety/agitation/excessive pacing
    8. Daily weight
    9. Monitor sleep hours
    10. Encourage daily hygiene
    11. Instruct on relaxation techniques

(1445) The client is alert and oriented ×3. T 98.0°F temporal, HR 78 bpm, respirations 22/min, BP 132/78 mm Hg. The client states, "I don't know why I've been admitted. I need to ask my mom to bring my books? I have finals in a few days." Speech is rapid, and loose associations noted. Client denies auditory or visual hallucinations. The client has been slowly walking back and forth on the unit at intervals. She is cooperative and sat with the nurse during the intake procedure. She spent approximately 5 minutes drawing with crayons before getting up and walking back and forth on unit. She drank 240 mL of high-protein shake, voided straw-colored urine, quantity sufficient. Then, she spent approximately 5 minutes drawing with crayons before getting up and walking back and forth on unit. Columbia's Suicide Severity Rating Score indicates moderate risk. A call was placed to the psychiatrist on call.

6. **Evaluate outcomes. Did it help?** For each assessment finding, indicate whether the patient's condition has **improved**, **declined**, or had **no change**.

Finding	Improved	Declined	No Change
Level of consciousness			
Vital signs			
Hydration			
Suicidal ideation			
Content of thought			
Activity/pacing			

CASE STUDY #2

(0900) A 65-year-old male client presents to the ED reporting dizziness, activity intolerance, and chronic fatigue for the last month. The client's daughter describes her father as "almost fainting" during ambulation to the bathroom. "After breakfast, he was unsteady on his feet, and I had to help him walk. It scared me, so I brought him here." Initial vital signs are taken.

Vital Signs	Client Values
Blood pressure	94/56 mm Hg
Heart rate	48 bpm
Respirations	20 breaths/min
O₂ saturation	96% on room air
Temperature	98.4°F (36.9°C)
Pain	4 on a 1 to 10 scale

During the assessment of the client, the triage nurse notices the client is slow to answer the questions and appears confused. PERRLA. Heart rate is regular with no murmurs or adventitious sounds. Lungs are clear bilaterally without wheezing or crackles. Bowel sounds present ×4 quadrants. Skin is warm and dry, without cyanosis, diaphoresis, or rough, flaky skin. No edema noted. Peripheral pulses +1. BMI is 20.5, and no recent weight loss or gain has occurred.

With assistance from his daughter, the client relays a history of hyperlipidemia and gastroesophageal reflux disease (GERD). The client's current medications include omeprazole (Prilosec), atorvastatin (Lipitor), and a daily multivitamin. The daughter shares that her father was a former smoker but quit 10 years ago and likes to have a nightly gin and tonic to relax. The daughter states her father does not have a history of heart problems, but her grandfather, the client's father, had a myocardial infarction at 70 years old and died.

1. **Recognize cues. What matters most?** The ED nurse prepares to give the report to the physician. Which priority client data should be reported to the HCP? **Select all that apply.**
   1. Blood pressure
   2. Heart rate
   3. Respirations
   4. Temperature
   5. Confusion
   6. Current medications
   7. History of smoking
   8. Report of "almost fainting"
   9. Eating breakfast this morning
   10. Activity intolerance for 1 month

2. **Analyze cues. What could it mean?** For each client finding, indicate whether it is consistent with the disease process of hypothyroidism, myocardial infarction (MI), or anemia. Each finding may support more than one condition.

Finding	Hypothyroidism	Myocardial Infarction	Anemia
Hypotension			
Bradycardia			
Activity intolerance/ fatigue			
Confusion			
Edema			
Decreased SpO_2			
Weight gain			
Diaphoresis			
Pain			

(0915) The nurse places the client on continuous cardiac monitoring and records the following telemetry strip.

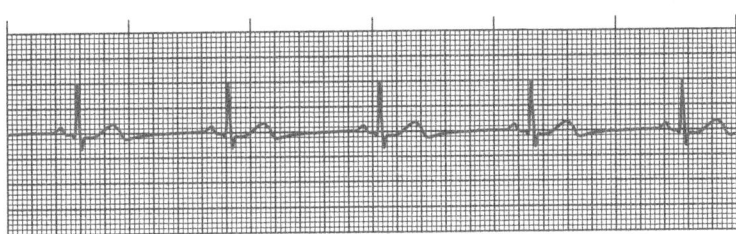

3. **Prioritize hypotheses. Where do I start?** Complete the sentence by choosing from the drop-down list of options. The nurse recognizes that the client is at the highest risk for _____

   Select
   1. Chest pain
   2. Falls
   3. Infection

   and will require _____

   Select
   1. Antiarrhythmic
   2. Anti-infective
   3. Antianginal

(0925) The physician visits the client and provides orders.

PROVIDER ORDERS:

Dx: Symptomatic bradycardia
EKG STAT
Labs: CBC, BMP, TSH, cardiac enzymes STAT
Oxygen at 2 L via nasal cannula
Portable chest x-ray
Echocardiogram STAT
IV NS @ 100 mL/hr
Atropine 0.5 mg IV push per protocol
Cardiology referral

(0945) Oxygen via nasal cannula started at 2 L, blood drawn for lab tests, and portable chest x-ray is completed. Cardiology is notified. Echocardiogram is performed.

(1015) Diagnostic and laboratory results are posted.

EKG: Sinus bradycardia, no ST-T wave changes

Chest x-ray report: No acute findings

Echocardiogram: Ejection fraction 55%, no significant valvular disease

Laboratory Test	Client Values	Reference Values
Hemoglobin (Hgb)	14	Male: 14 to 17.3 g/dL
		Female: 11.7 to 15.5 g/dL
Hematocrit (Hct)	45	Male: 42% to 52%
		Female: 36% to 48%
White blood cell (WBC) count	10.6	4.5 to 11.1 × 10^3/microL
Platelets	210	150 to 450 × 10^3/microL
Creatinine	0.9	Male: 0.61 to 1.21 mg/dL
		Female: 0.59 to 1.04 mg/dL
Glucose	116	Fasting: Less than 100 mg/dL
		Random: Less than 200 mg/dL
Potassium	4.7	0.5 to 5.3 mEq/L or mmol/L
Sodium	136	135 to 145 mEq/L or mmol/L
Blood urea nitrogen	21	8 to 21 mg/dL
		Adult over 90 years: 10 to 31 mg/dL
Thyroid-stimulating hormone (TSH)	2	Adults: 0.4 to 4.2 mIU/mL
Troponin I	< 0.01	Less than 0.03 ng/mL

4. **Generate solutions. What can I do?** For each intervention, specify whether the intervention is **indicated** or **not indicated** for the client's care.

Potential Nursing Intervention	Indicated	Not Indicated
Maintain IV 0.9% NS at 100 mL/hr.		
Administer atropine 0.5 mg IV push.		
Place client on a continuous cardiac monitor.		
Administer morphine sulfate 10 mg IV for pain.		
Restrict the client's fluid intake.		
Administer furosemide 40 mg PO daily.		
Administer atenolol 25 mg PO daily.		
Implement fall precautions.		
Educate the client and family about bradycardia, possible causes, and treatments.		

(1130) The client is admitted to the medical-surgical floor for continued evaluation. The client remains unresponsive to medication administered to treat the symptomatic bradycardia. After further evaluation, the physician determines the client is a candidate for a leadless pacemaker. The client and his daughter consent to the procedure, and the client undergoes it.

5. **Take action. What will I do?** After the leadless pacemaker procedure, the client returned to the medical-surgical floor and had a 2-hour recovery in the postanesthesia care unit (PACU). Which interventions should the nurse perform? **Select all that apply.**
   1. Assist the client to ambulate to the bathroom to measure urine output.
   2. Remove the groin dressing to assess the incision site.
   3. Palpate the pedal pulses distal to the incision site.
   4. Ensure the client remains on continuous cardiac monitoring.
   5. Assess vital signs every 30 minutes for 24 hours after the procedure.

The next day, the nurse performs teaching in preparation for discharge.

6. **Evaluate outcomes. Did it help?** For each statement by the client, indicate whether the discharge teaching was effective or ineffective.

Client Statement	Effective	Ineffective
"I should avoid heavy lifting for 1 week."		
"I can expect the dizziness to last for 2 to 3 days."		
"I will keep all my follow-up appointments with my HCP."		
"I need to assess my radial pulse daily."		
"I will always carry my pacemaker identification card."		
"I need to avoid all airport security screenings."		
"I should avoid ambulating long distances."		
"I should have an exam by my HCP before I travel anywhere."		

CASE STUDY #3

(1000) A 68-year-old female client presents to the ED with her adult son. The son reports his mother has had a productive cough, shortness of breath, and fatigue for the last week. The client appears anxious and states she is short of breath.

Vital Signs	Client Values
Blood pressure	128/76 mm Hg
Heart rate	89 bpm
Respirations	30 breaths/min
O_2 saturation	90%
Temperature	102.9°F (39°C)
Pain	4 on a 1 to 10 scale

The client is alert but is confused about where she is and why she came to the ED. PERRLA. Respirations are labored and the nurse detects the odor of cigarettes. The son states that his mother has smoked 1 pack of cigarettes daily for 40 years. Bilateral crackles are noted in the lower lung lobes. Productive cough with thick, yellow-tinged sputum is noted. Heart rate is regular without adventitious sounds. Capillary refill in all four extremities is less than 3 seconds. Skin is warm, dry, and intact. Peripheral pulses are present, 3+. Bowel sounds hypoactive in 4 quadrants and the client reports having two loose brown stools this morning.

1. **Recognize cues. What matters most?** The nurse prepares to give a report to the ED physician. Which **priority** client data should the nurse report to the HCP? **Select all that apply.**
    1. Sputum, thick and yellow-tinged
    2. Bilateral crackles in lower lung lobes
    3. Capillary refill in fewer than 3 seconds
    4. Loose brown stool ×2
    5. Shortness of breath
    6. Peripheral pulses 3+
    7. Oxygen saturation of 90%
    8. Pain level 4 on a 1 to 10 scale
    9. Blood pressure
    10. Temperature

2. **Analyze cues. What could it mean?** The client is at risk for developing which issues? **Select two answers.**
    1. Decreased oxygenation
    2. Dehydration
    3. Heart failure
    4. Sepsis
    5. Bowel obstruction
    6. Pressure injury

The ED physician assesses the client and writes orders. The client's past medical history and medications are reviewed in the electronic health record (EHR).

PROVIDER ORDERS
Chest x-ray STAT
CBC, CMP, urinalysis
Sputum culture
Oxygen: titrate to maintain SpO_2 >94%
IV 0.9% NS @ 100 mL/hr
STAT EKG

(1030) Diagnostic and partial laboratory results are posted.

EKG: Sinus bradycardia, no ST-T wave changes

Chest x-ray report: Right lower lobe pneumonia without an effusion

Laboratory Test	Client Values	Reference Values
Hemoglobin (Hgb)	14.1	Male: 14 to 17.3 g/dL
		Female: 11.7 to 15.5 g/dL
Hematocrit (Hct)	42.3	Male: 42% to 52%
		Female: 36% to 48%
White blood cell (WBC) count	4.2	4.5 to 11.1 × 10^3/microL
Platelets	180	150 to 450 × 10^3/microL
Creatinine	1.1	Male: 0.61 to 1.21 mg/dL
		Female: 0.59 to 1.04 mg/dL
Glucose	100	Fasting: Less than 100 mg/dL
		Random: Less than 200 mg/dL
Potassium	4.2	0.5 to 5.3 mEq/L or mmol/L
Sodium	138	135 to 145 mEq/L or mmol/L
Blood urea nitrogen	17	8 to 21 mg/dL
		Adult over 90 years: 10 to 31 mg/dL

The physician diagnoses the client with community-acquired pneumonia. The nurse receives orders that follow the Centers for Medicare & Medicaid Services (CMS) and The Joint Commission (TJC) core measures.

3. **Prioritize hypotheses. Where do I start?** Which interventions are required to be performed within the **first 24 hours** according to CMS and TJC Pneumonia Core Measures? **Select all that apply.**
   1. Refer to counseling for substance use disorder.
   2. Administer a broad-spectrum antibiotic.
   3. Provide smoking cessation counseling.
   4. Perform influenza vaccination.
   5. Obtain blood cultures.

4. **Generate solutions. What can I do?** For each intervention, specify whether the intervention is **indicated** or **not indicated** for the client's care.

Potential Nursing Intervention	Indicated	Not Indicated
Maintain IV 0.9% NS at 100 mL/hr.		
Restrict the client's smoking to three cigarettes per day.		
Place the client on oxygen via nasal cannula.		
Allow for periods of rest during activities of daily living.		
Implement fluid restrictions of 1,000 mL/day.		
Monitor the client's oxygen saturation with a pulse oximeter.		
Elevate the head of the bed.		
Stay with the client to attempt to calm her.		
Request the client take slow, deep breaths.		

The physician has ordered the IV administration of levofloxacin, a broad-spectrum antibiotic.

5. **Take action. What will I do?** Which actions are appropriate for the IV administration of levofloxacin? **Drag and drop one correct action from the options listed in the left column into the right column.**

Possible Actions	Correct Actions
Ensure blood cultures are drawn before starting infusion.	
Draw blood culture and review results before starting the infusion.	
Begin the infusion immediately, then draw blood cultures.	
Explain to the client that the route is PO.	
Explain to the client that the route is IV.	
Explain to the client that the route is SQ.	
Administer 250 mg slow IV push.	
Administer 250 mg IVPB over 30 minutes.	
Administer 250 mg IVPB over 60 minutes.	
Instruct the client to finish all the antibiotics completely.	
Instruct the client to notify the nurse if they have thoughts of suicide.	
Instruct the client to inform the nurse if they experience constipation.	

Three days later: The nurse is assessing the client. The client is alert and awake and states her cough has significantly improved. She is eager to return home to see her small dog and asks whether she can take the IV medication in pill form.

Vital Signs	Client Values
Blood pressure	128/76 mm Hg
Heart rate	79 bpm
Respirations	24 breaths/min
O₂ saturation	98%
Temperature	99°F (37.2°C)
Pain	4 on a 1 to 10 scale

6. **Evaluate outcomes. Did it help?** For each assessment finding, indicate whether the client's condition **improved**, **declined**, or had **no change**.

Finding	Improved	Declined	No change
Blood pressure			
Temperature			
Oxygen saturation			
Respirations			
Cough			
Pain			
Heart rate			

CASE STUDY #4

(0200) A 25-year-old gravida 2, para 1 client presents to the childbirth center at 39 weeks', 2 days' gestation. The client began regular prenatal care at 8 weeks' gestation. She states her uterine contractions started about 4 hours ago and are 5 minutes apart and lasting 60 seconds each. She denies leakage of fluid. An external fetal monitor is applied. Fetal heart rate (FHR) baseline is 140 bpm. Accelerations are present, no decelerations noted. A sterile vaginal examination indicates the client is 4 cm dilated, 100% effaced, and at −1 station.

Vital Signs	Client Values
Blood pressure	120/78 mm Hg
Heart rate	85 bpm
Respirations	20 breaths/min
O₂ saturation	99% room air
Temperature	98.7°F (37°C)
Pain	6 on a 1 to 10 scale (with contractions)

(0220) A review of the EHR shows regular prenatal visits, no significant medical history, no known allergies, and group B streptococcus (GBS) positive at 36 weeks. Blood type O+.

1. **Recognize cues. What matters most?** The nurse prepares to call the physician. Which **priority** client data should be reported to the HCP? **Select all that apply.**
   1. 39 weeks', 2 days' gestation
   2. Regular prenatal care
   3. Uterine contractions starting 4 hours ago
   4. Fetal heart rate of 140 bpm
   5. Dilation of 4 cm
   6. Blood pressure
   7. Oxygen saturation
   8. Pain level
   9. GBS positive
   10. Blood type O+

2. **Analyze cues. What could it mean?** Complete the sentence by choosing from the drop-down list of options. Based on the client's condition at the time, the nurse recognizes that the client is at the **highest** risk for _____

Select ▼
1. Gestational hypertension
2. Prolonged labor
3. Neonatal complications

   and will require _____

Select ▼
1. Antibiotics
2. Oxytocin
3. Magnesium sulfate

(0210) The nurse calls a report to the physician and receives orders. The client is requesting an epidural. Anesthesia is notified. The nurse starts an IV infusion of lactated Ringer's solution. Labs are drawn. Penicillin G 5 million units is administered IV piggyback (IVPB).

(0230) Partial lab results are received. Anesthesia arrives to initiate the epidural.

Laboratory Test	Client Values	Reference Values
Hemoglobin (Hgb)	11.5	Male: 14 to 17.3 g/dL
		Female: 11.7 to 15.5 g/dL
Hematocrit (Hct)	35%	Male: 42% to 52%
		Female: 36% to 48%
White blood cell (WBC) count	12	4.5 to 11.1 × 10³/microL
Platelets	140	150 to 450 × 10³/microL

3. **Prioritize hypotheses. Where do I start?** The client has received epidural anesthesia. Which **priority** assessment should the labor and delivery nurse perform?
   1. Assess for paresthesia in the feet and legs.
   2. Assess for a drop in maternal blood pressure.
   3. Assess for an increase in maternal temperature.
   4. Assess for the presence of fetal heart rate accelerations.

(0620) The labor and delivery nurse is evaluating the client's fetal monitor strip

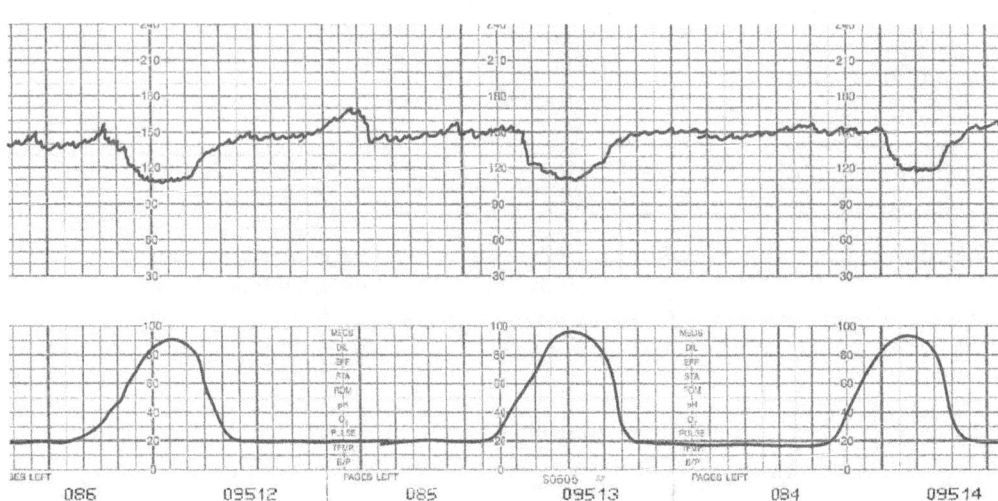

4. **Generate solutions. What can I do?** For each intervention, specify whether the intervention is **indicated** or **not indicated** for the client's care.

Potential Nursing Intervention	Indicated	Not Indicated
Reposition the client on her left side.		
Perform a sterile vaginal examination.		
Increase the IV infusion rate.		
Prepare to administer IV oxytocin.		
Administer pain medication to the client.		

(0630) The client is completely dilated. The HCP arrives and spontaneously delivers a viable male newborn. The amniotic sac ruptured at delivery with clear fluid. The HCP hands the newborn to the nursery nurse, who places the newborn on a prewarmed infant warmer, dries the newborn, and removes the wet linens. The nurse performs the initial assessment:

Assessment	Newborn Finding
Heart rate	110 bpm
Respirations	Slow, weak cry
Muscle tone	Minimal flexion of extremities
Reflex irritability	Grimace with stimulation
Color	Acrocyanosis

5. **Take action. What will I do?** Based on the initial assessment, which interventions should the nurse perform? **Select all that apply.**
   1. Suction the mouth and nose.
   2. Provide oxygen via face mask.
   3. Administer epinephrine endotracheally.
   4. Initiate an IV line of normal saline (NS).
   5. Assess the need to administer naloxone.

(0640) Following interventions provided by the nurse, the newborn has an Apgar score of 10 at 5 minutes. After breastfeeding and bonding with the client, couplet care is assigned.

24 hours later: The baby boy and postpartum client are assessed by the nurse, and teaching is provided to the mother.

6. **Evaluate outcomes. Did it help?** For each statement by the client, indicate whether the discharge teaching was effective or ineffective.

Client Statement	Effective	Ineffective
"I should avoid sexual activity and tampons until my first postpartum visit."		
"I should take a daily laxative to avoid straining and constipation."		
"I should cleanse my perineal area with warm water after urination."		
"I should notify the HCP if I experience heavy bleeding."		
"I should take frequent rest periods, especially when the baby is sleeping."		
"I should apply antibiotic ointment to my baby's cord stump daily."		
"I should avoid vigorous exercise and heavy lifting for several weeks."		

LABORATORY AND DIAGNOSTIC TEST INTENSIVE QUESTIONS

Refer to the Electronic Health Record Order Screen to answer the next set of questions:

Laboratory and Diagnostic Services

Chemistry	Hematology/Coagulation	Microbiology/Cultures
• Albumin • Calcium • Cholesterol, total • Creatinine • Folic acid • Glucose • Glucose tolerance, OB • hCG • Hemoglobin A1C • Hepatitis panel • HIV screen • Iron, total • Potassium • PSA screening • Rubella • Thyroid-stimulating hormone (TSH), thyroid panel	• Platelet count • White blood cell count • Prothrombin time (PT) with INR • PTT, activated **Toxicology** • Blood alcohol • Digoxin • Lithium • Valproic acid **Serology** • Influenza • Mono screen • Rapid plasma reagin (RPR)	• Blood • Sputum • Strep screen • Stool • Urinalysis • Wound, deep • Wound, superficial **Diagnostic Tests** • Audiometry • Electromyography (EMG) • Endoscopy, upper GI • Mammogram • Scratch test • Tensilon test • X-ray, chest

1. The clinic nurse is assessing the client taking prescribed diuretics and reports leg cramps in the calf. Which laboratory or diagnostic test should the nurse expect to be ordered for this client?

2. The client tells the clinic nurse, "I am having burning upon urination." Which laboratory or diagnostic test should the nurse expect to be ordered for this client?

3. The client states, "I am having pain in my right lower abdomen, and I have a low-grade fever." Which laboratory or diagnostic test should the nurse expect to be ordered for this client?

4. The client states, "I am taking warfarin daily." Which laboratory or diagnostic test should the nurse expect to be ordered for this client?

5. The client states, "I am having burning in my chest after I eat, especially if I lie down after I eat." Which laboratory or diagnostic test should the nurse expect to be ordered for this client?

6. The client states, "I have type 2 diabetes and have been taking my medication as directed for the last 3 months." Which laboratory or diagnostic test should the nurse expect to be ordered for this client?

7. The client states, "The last doctor I saw told me I might have a peripheral nerve disease and needed a test, but I can't remember the name of the test." Which laboratory or diagnostic test should the nurse expect to be ordered for this client?

8. The client states, "I am always weak since I became a vegetarian. My family tells me I am pale and have no energy." Which laboratory or diagnostic test should the nurse expect to be ordered for this client?

9. The client states, "I have been a type 2 diabetic for 20 years, and I think I may have diabetic nephropathy." Which laboratory or diagnostic test should the nurse expect to be ordered for this client?

10. The client states, "I think I have myasthenia gravis, similar to my sister. Could you please give me the test to diagnose myasthenia gravis?" Which laboratory or diagnostic test should the nurse expect to be ordered for this client?

11. The client states, "I am hot all the time, I have problems holding my pen when I write, and I am breathing faster." Which laboratory or diagnostic test should the nurse expect to be ordered for this client?

12. The client states, "I think I may have been exposed to syphilis." Which laboratory or diagnostic test should the nurse expect to be ordered for this client?

    [ ]

13. The client states, "I am receiving chemotherapy and have noticed bleeding after I brush my teeth and when I blow my nose." Which laboratory or diagnostic test should the nurse expect to be ordered for this client?

    [ ]

14. The client states, "I have been on a heart-healthy diet for more than 6 months since my heart attack." Which laboratory or diagnostic test should the nurse expect to be ordered for this client?

    [ ]

15. The client states, "My wife says I am having trouble hearing, but I don't think so." Which laboratory or diagnostic test should the nurse expect to be ordered for this client?

    [ ]

16. The client states, "I think I am allergic to dust or mold because my nose gets stuffy, I sneeze all the time, and sometimes I break out in a rash." Which laboratory or diagnostic test should the nurse expect to be ordered for this client?

    [ ]

CLINICAL SKILLS INTENSIVE QUESTIONS

1. The nurse is preparing to perform endotracheal suctioning on a client. Which interventions should the nurse implement? **Rank in order of performance.**
   1. Provide mouth care to the client.
   2. Apply suction while withdrawing the catheter.
   3. Hyperoxygenate the client as needed.
   4. Determine the measurement of length to suction.
   5. Lubricate the catheter tip with saline solution.

2. The clinic nurse must obtain a throat culture from a client who has possible strep throat. Which interventions should the nurse perform? **Rank in order of performance.**
   1. Instruct the client to tilt their head back and open the mouth.
   2. Insert the applicator stick into the specimen tube until the swab is in the culture medium.
   3. Remove the sterile applicator from the culture tube by rotating the cap to break the seal.
   4. Label the specimen tube and send to the laboratory.
   5. Swab the back of the throat along the tonsillar area from left to right.

3. The home health nurse is caring for a female client who needs her indwelling urinary catheter changed. After explaining the procedure to the client and performing hand hygiene, which interventions should the nurse implement? **Rank in order of performance.**
   1. Don sterile gloves.
   2. Insert the lubricated urinary catheter.
   3. Spread the labia and cleanse the urinary meatus.
   4. Inflate the catheter balloon using a prefilled syringe.
   5. Open the sterile catheter set.

4. The nurse is caring for a client with a central venous access device in the subclavian vein. The nurse must perform a central line dressing change. Which interventions should the nurse implement? **Rank in order of performance.**
   1. Don sterile gloves and arrange a sterile field.
   2. Remove the old dressing and assess the needle insertion site.
   3. Allow the area to dry and cover with transparent dressing.
   4. Scrub insertion site using a back-and-forth motion.
   5. Document the date and time of the dressing change.

5. The home health nurse is teaching the home health aide how to perform colostomy irrigation for the client with a sigmoid colostomy. After explaining the procedure to the client and performing hand hygiene, which interventions should the nurse implement? **Rank in order of performance.**
   1. Lubricate the cone tip of the tubing, insert it into the stoma opening, and begin the inflow of water.
   2. Fill the irrigation bag with 1,000 mL of warm tap water and hang it at shoulder height.
   3. Put an irrigation sleeve over the stoma and place the outflow into the toilet above the water line.
   4. Cleanse the stoma site and apply a new colostomy pouch over the stoma.
   5. Allow evacuation of feces and water; may take 30 minutes to 1 hour.

6. The clinic nurse must draw an International Normalized Ratio (INR) for a client taking warfarin daily. Which interventions should the nurse implement? **Rank in order of performance.**
   1. Hold skin taut and insert needle with bevel up at 30-degree angle.
   2. Place tourniquet 4 to 6 inches above the client's elbow.
   3. With the vacutainer system, insert the blood collection tube into the plastic adapter.
   4. Remove the needle from the vein, cover the site with gauze, and apply pressure.
   5. Cleanse the antecubital fossa with an antimicrobial wipe.

7. The nurse must insert a nasogastric (NG) tube for a client receiving tube feedings for 1 month. Which interventions should the nurse implement? **Rank in order of performance.**
   1. Elevate the head of the bed and assess the nares for patency.
   2. Have the client swallow or sip water while inserting the tube to the predetermined mark.
   3. Measure the NG tube from the tip of the client's nose to the earlobe to the xiphoid process.
   4. Have the client extend their head, then insert the tube through the nostril to the back of the throat.
   5. Lubricate the end of the tube with water-soluble lubricant.

8. The nurse is teaching the male client how to collect a midstream urine specimen. Which instructions should the nurse provide? **Rank in order of performance.**
   1. Urinate in the toilet, then place the sterile container under the urine stream.
   2. Replace the cap on the specimen container.
   3. Fill the cup with 30 to 60 mL of urine, then remove before stopping the urine stream.
   4. Open the specimen cup, place the cap inside surface up, do not touch the inside of the container.
   5. Cleanse the penis with an antiseptic wipe using a circular motion from the center out.

9. The nurse must administer a cleansing enema to a client. Which interventions should the nurse implement? **Rank in order of performance.**
   1. Assist the client to the toilet or bedpan to expel the total volume of the enema.
   2. Fill the container with 750 to 1,000 mL of lukewarm water and soap as ordered.
   3. Lubricate the tip, gently spread the client's buttocks, and insert tubing 3 to 4 inches.
   4. Instruct the client to hold fluid for at least 10 to 15 minutes or longer.
   5. Hold the tubing in place and infuse the solution slowly.

10. The home health nurse is teaching the client's spouse how to transfer the client from the bed to the chair. Which instructions should the nurse provide? **Rank in order of performance.**
    1. Assist the client in dangling at the bed's side and apply the gait belt.
    2. Instruct the client to move back in the chair until the client's back is flush with the chair back.
    3. Have the client reach for the arms of the chair, flex hips and knees, and lower slowly.
    4. Position a chair at the side of the bed and apply nonslip footwear on the client.
    5. Have the spouse stand facing the client; the client stands and pivots with their back to the chair.

11. The nurse is teaching the client how to administer 20 units of 70% insulin isophane and 30% regular insulin mixture in a bottle. Which instructions should the nurse provide? **Rank in order of performance.**
    1. Expose the abdomen and identify an area 2 inches from the umbilicus.
    2. Insert 20 units of air into the bottle in upright position, invert, and withdraw 20 units.
    3. Discard the needle safely and do not reuse it.
    4. Holding the syringe like a dart, insert the needle at a 45- or 90-degree angle.
    5. Slowly administer the insulin, then remove the needle from the skin.

12. The wound care nurse must apply a hydrocolloid dressing to a client's wound. Which interventions should the nurse implement? **Rank in order of performance.**
    1. Cut the hydrocolloid dressing to the desired shape with the backing in place.
    2. Cleanse the wound as directed and allow it to dry completely.
    3. Peel the backing from one edge of the dressing and apply it to the skin with a rolling motion.
    4. Apply skin prep to the area around the wound bed, approximately 1 to 2 inches.
    5. Smooth the dressing and hold it in place for several seconds.

13. The HCP has ordered a sputum culture for a client. Which interventions should the nurse implement? **Rank in order of performance.**
    1. Teach the client to expectorate directly into the specimen container.
    2. Instruct the client to rinse their mouth with water.
    3. Have the client take several deep breaths.
    4. Label the specimen container and send it to the laboratory.
    5. Position the client sitting or in a high Fowler's position.

ANSWERS TO CASE STUDIES

The correct answer number and rationale for why it is the correct answer are given in boldface type. Rationales for why the other possible answer options are incorrect also are given, but they are not in boldface type.

CASE STUDY #1

1. **Correct answers are 1, 6, 7, 8, and 9.**
   The correct answers are the clinical manifestations of a manic episode. Delusions of grandeur are apparent in the belief that the client has millions of dollars and can fly. A previous history of suicidal attempts is concerning. Bipolar patients have a 10% to 30% higher rate of suicide than the general population, with 20% to 60% attempting suicide at least one time. Lack of sleep is a known trigger for acute mania. It can lead to physical exhaustion. Although angry and agitated, the client has not refused care. The nurse obtained vital signs. Her heart rate and blood pressure are stable. She is clean and well-groomed despite her revealing clothing.

2. **Correct answers are 1, 4, and 5.**
   In most instances, mania occurs abruptly. Full-blown mania is extremely dangerous because of the physiological toll it brings upon the body. It is a medical emergency. Clients who are manic do not take the time to eat, drink, or sleep. They remain engaged in constant psychomotor activity. Severe exhaustion and lack of adequate sleep and rest, coupled with dehydration, can lead to cardiac collapse. Depressive episodes may come after a manic episode, but the client currently is not displaying the clinical manifestations of depression. Dysthymia is a long-acting persistent low mood lasting at least 2 years, not noted in the history by the mother. The BP of 138/84 mm Hg is not concerning and does not indicate hypertension. Her pulse and blood pressure elevations are a result of her agitation.

3. **Correct answers are 2 and 3.**
   Based on the patient's condition at the time, the nurse recognizes that the patient is at the highest risk for

   | **2. Physical exhaustion** |

   and will require

   | **3. Olanzapine 10 mg IM now.** |

   The Food and Drug Administration (FDA) approves olanzapine (an atypical antipsychotic agent) for use in the treatment of acute mania in adult patients diagnosed with bipolar I disorder. It decreases delusions, hallucinations, and disorganized thoughts and behaviors. It has a sedative effect, which helps the patient to calm down and obtain rest. A vest restraint is not indicated because the client is not threatening to harm herself or others at this time. There is always a danger in using any type of restraint, and it should be used as a last resort. Many institutions do not use vest restraints because of the danger of strangulation. Although the client's lab work does indicate minor dehydration, nonemergent invasive procedures at this time would increase agitation. An IV fluid at a maintenance rate is not indicated.

4. Correct answers are marked.

Potential Nursing Intervention	Indicated	Not Indicated
Place on one-to-one suicidal precautions.		X
Apply wrist restraints.		X
Place in a private room.	X	
Utilize verbal de-escalation techniques.	X	
Administer ordered medications as soon as possible.	X	
Discuss her irrational thinking regarding the money in her bank account.		X
Decrease environmental stimuli.	X	
Obtain repeat vital signs.		X
Weigh patient.		X

452

The client has denied suicidal ideation and has not made any threat that would necessitate placing her on one-to-one suicidal precautions at the current time. She is not displaying aggressive, hostile behavior toward others or herself now. Thus, there is no need for wrist restraints. Upon taking the initial vital signs, the client became increasingly agitated. Her vital signs are not an emergent issue, as they were stable 2 hours ago. Vital signs every 4 hours would be appropriate. The weight has been obtained. Delusions regarding her bank account amounts are fixed false beliefs that cannot be changed, even if proof is provided. Do not focus on false ideas; they can increase delusions. Direct the conversation to the underlying feelings rather than the content of the delusion.

Providing a private room and reducing environmental stimuli are indicated because of her current manic stage. Maintaining a low level of stimuli (dim lighting, few persons, decreased noise levels) reduces anxiety and agitation. Administering psychiatric medication provides relief from agitation and hyperactivity, and it has a sedative effect. The client must rest to avert physical exhaustion, which is a medical emergency.

5. Correct answers are 1, 2, 3, 4, 5, 7, and 9. Safety searches are a priority when arriving at a psychiatric unit. They protect the client, staff, and visitors. It is a priority that the nurse complete the Columbia Suicide Severity Rating Score (C-SSRS). Despite earlier denial of suicidal ideation, after the client is admitted and medicated, her willingness to disclose her thoughts and feelings may be more forthcoming. Her past suicidal attempt and her bipolar diagnosis increase her risk of suicide completion. Lorazepam can be used for acute mania episodes. It aids in reducing manic agitation by promoting rest and sleep. It peaks within 30 minutes. The lithium level is below the normal range at this time. It is a first-line treatment choice for acute mania and maintenance treatment of bipolar disorder. The physician utilizes the levels to regulate dosage. A therapeutic level of lithium between 0.6 and 1.2 mEq/L is needed for effectiveness. Fluids and high-calorie finger foods should be provided. Lack of fluids and nutritious food, lack of sleep, and continual physical activity increase her chance of exhibiting physical exhaustion, which can lead to cardiac collapse. Her vital signs are monitored closely to assess the effects of administered medication and to determine her cardiac status. The nurse should offer fluids and food every hour. Her weight, daily hygiene, and attending the structured unit activities are not a priority. Discharge planning begins upon admission, yet it is not a priority over physiological needs. Teaching will occur when the client can concentrate and is no longer manic.

6. Correct answers are marked.

Findings	Improved	Declined	No Change
Level of consciousness			X
Vital signs	X		
Hydration	X		
Suicidal ideation		X	
Content of thought			X
Activity/pacing	X		

The client remains delusional regarding her monetary status and her lack of understanding why she is being admitted. Her content of thought and level of consciousness have not changed. She continues to exhibit loose associations, rapid speech, and situational disorientation. Her vital signs are within normal ranges. She continued to pace slowly but did spend several minutes sitting and coloring. Thus, her activity level and pacing have slowed. Her hydration has improved. She drank 240 mL of a nutritious shake and her urine output is quantity sufficient. Her Columbia Suicide Severity Risk rating score is moderate. Thus, her suicidal ideation has increased and she is no longer denying suicidal ideation.

CASE STUDY #2

1. **Correct answers are 1, 2, 5, 6, 8, and 10.**
The blood pressure and heart rate are low and should be reported to the HCP. Confusion, report of "almost fainting," and activity intolerance for 1 month are abnormal findings that are concerning to the client and his daughter. Current medication usage is significant because adverse reactions to medications can cause hypotension and bradycardia. Respirations and temperature are normal. A history of smoking would be important, but the client does not exhibit any respiratory issues. The client's last oral intake is important in preparing for a procedure or diagnostic test but is not critical information for the HCP at this time.

2. **Correct answers are marked.**

Finding	Hypothyroidism	Myocardial Infarction	Anemia
Hypotension		X	X
Bradycardia	X		
Activity intolerance/fatigue	X	X	X
Confusion	X	X	
Edema	X		
Decreased SpO₂		X	
Weight gain	X		
Diaphoresis	X	X	
Pain		X	

Hypothyroidism is characterized by a lack of energy and activity intolerance, bradycardia, and memory issues. Hypertension, edema in the face, hands, and feet are present with accompanying weight gain. Clients often present with rough, flaky skin, brittle nails, and thinning hair. Pain is uncommon. For **myocardial infarction**, clients commonly present with pain in the chest, radiating to the shoulders or jaw; tachypnea; shortness of breath; and diaphoresis. Hypertension is common, but hypotension can occur as a result of reduced cardiac output or extensive myocardial damage. Clients often describe fatigue for days or weeks before an MI. Weight gain and edema are not common.

Anemia is characterized by tachycardia (the heart pumps more to compensate for the reduced oxygen-carrying capacity of the blood), hypotension, and tachypnea but normal SpO₂. Clients are often fatigued, feel dizzy, and describe shortness of breath. Weight gain, pain, diaphoresis, and edema are not typical symptoms of anemia.

3. **Correct answers are 2 and 1.**
Based on the client's condition at this time, the nurse recognizes that the client is at the highest risk for

> 2. Falls

and will require an

> 1. Antiarrhythmic.

The syncope, hypotension, and confusion put the client at risk for falls. The nurse should expect the HCP to order the antiarrhythmic atropine, which decreases vagal stimulation and increases the heart rate. It is the medication of choice to treat symptomatic bradycardia. Antibiotics would treat an infection, but the client is not exhibiting signs of an infection. Antianginals, such as the coronary vasodilator nitroglycerin, will increase blood flow to the myocardium and cause the blood pressure to decrease even further.

4. **Correct answers are marked.**

Potential Nursing Intervention	Indicated	Not Indicated
Maintain IV 0.9% NS at 100 mL/hr.	X	
Administer atropine 0.5 mg IV push.	X	
Place client on a continuous cardiac monitor.	X	
Administer morphine sulfate 10 mg IV for pain.		X
Restrict the client's fluid intake.		X
Administer furosemide 40 mg PO daily.		X
Administer atenolol 25 mg PO daily.		X
Implement fall precautions.	X	
Educate the client and family about bradycardia, possible causes, and treatments.	X	

IV fluids, atropine, continuous cardiac monitoring, fall precautions, and education are necessary for the client experiencing symptomatic bradycardia.

Morphine sulfate can depress the cardiovascular system and exacerbate the bradycardia. Furosemide, a diuretic, and atenolol, a beta blocker, are contraindicated. Restricting fluid intake can lead to dehydration and electrolyte imbalances. There is no indication of heart failure or renal impairment, so this is unnecessary.

5. Correct answers are 3 and 4.
   1. The client should be on complete bedrest for 4 to 6 hours after the procedure.
   2. The nurse should not remove the dressing. It is in place to prevent an infection. The nurse can assess and document any drainage noted on the dressing in the EHR.
   3. The nurse should palpate the pulses in the involved extremity to assess circulation distal to the insertion site.
   4. The client should remain on continuous cardiac monitoring until discharge.
   5. The client does not need his vital signs assessed that frequently. The nurse should follow hospital protocol unless assessment data indicate they should be done more frequently.

6. Correct answers are marked.

Client Statement	Effective	Ineffective
"I should avoid heavy lifting for 1 week."	X	
"I can expect the dizziness to last for 2 to 3 days."		X
"I will keep all my follow-up appointments with my HCP."	X	
"I need to assess my radial pulse daily."		X
"I will always carry my pacemaker identification card."	X	
"I need to avoid all airport security screenings."		X
"I should avoid ambulating long distances."		X
"I should have an exam by my HCP before I travel anywhere."		X

The client should avoid heavy lifting and squatting for 1 week after the procedure to allow the groin incision to heal. The client should be instructed to keep all follow-up appointments with the HCP. The client should always carry his pacemaker identification card to inform other HCPs about his leadless pacemaker.

No dizziness is expected after the procedure. The client should notify the HCP if he experiences dizziness, syncope, or activity intolerance, as this could indicate a problem with the pacemaker. The client is not expected to assess his pulse. The client can pass through metal detectors but should avoid the handheld metal detector wands. The client can show security the ID card and request a different security screening. The client has no restrictions on daily activities such as ambulation. The client does not need an examination to fly in an airplane.

CASE STUDY #3

1. Correct answers are 1, 2, 5, 7, 8, and 10. Sputum, thick and yellow-tinged, bilateral crackles in lower lung lobes, shortness of breath, SpO_2 90%, pain level 4, and elevated temperature are abnormal findings and should be reported to the HCP. Capillary refill in less than 3 seconds, loose brown stool ×2, normal peripheral pulses, and blood pressure do not need to be reported at this time.

2. Correct answers are 1 and 4.
   1. Clients experiencing shortness of breath and low oxygen saturation are at risk for decreased oxygenation.
   2. The client is not showing signs of dehydration.
   3. The client is not showing signs of heart failure.
   4. An elevated temperature and infection puts the client at risk for sepsis.
   5. The client is not showing signs of a bowel obstruction.
   6. No assessment data indicate the client is at risk for pressure injuries.

3. Correct answers are 2 and 5.
   1. Clients are to be provided access to substance use disorder counseling, but this is not required to be performed within the first 24 hours of admission or presentation to the ED.
   2. According to the Pneumonia Core Measures for community-acquired pneumonia, clients must have blood cultures performed and appropriate antibiotics administered within 24 hours of admission or presentation to the ED.
   3. Clients are to be provided resources for smoking cessation, but it is not required to be performed within the first 24 hours of admission or presentation to the ED.
   4. Clients are to be provided the influenza vaccine per the Pneumonia Core Measures, but it is not required to be performed within the first 24 hours of admission or presentation to the ED.
   5. According to the Pneumonia Core Measures for community-acquired pneumonia, clients must have blood cultures performed and appropriate antibiotics administered within 24 hours of admission or presentation to the ED.

4. Correct answers are marked.

Potential Nursing Intervention	Indicated	Not Indicated
Maintain IV 0.9% NS at 100 mL/hr.	X	
Restrict the client's smoking to three cigarettes per day.		X
Place the client on oxygen via nasal cannula.	X	
Allow for periods of rest during activities of daily living.	X	
Implement fluid restrictions of 1,000 mL/day.		X
Monitor the client's oxygen saturation with a pulse oximeter.	X	
Elevate the head of the bed.	X	
Stay with the client to attempt to calm her.	X	
Request the client take slow, deep breaths.	X	

Not indicated interventions include restricting smoking and limiting fluids. The client should not smoke any cigarettes because cigarette smoking depresses the action of the cilia in the lungs. Fluids are encouraged to thin secretions.

Indicated interventions include maintaining IV fluids. A client diagnosed with pneumonia has some degree of deficit in gas exchange and should be placed on oxygen. Activities of daily living require energy and increased oxygen consumption. The nurse should allow for rest periods between activities to allow the client to rebuild oxygen reserves. Pulse oximeter assessment gives the nurse an estimate of the oxygenation level in the client's periphery. Elevating the head of the bed, staying with the client, and encouraging slow, deep breaths are appropriate interventions.

5. Correct answers are marked.

Possible Actions	Correct Actions
Ensure blood cultures are drawn before starting infusion.	Ensure blood cultures are drawn before starting infusion.
Draw blood culture and review results before starting the infusion.	
Begin the infusion immediately, then draw blood cultures.	
Explain to the client that the route is PO.	Explain to the client that the route is IV.
Explain to the client that the route is IV.	
Explain to the client that the route is SQ.	
Administer 250 mg slow IV push.	Administer 250 mg IVPB over 60 minutes.
Administer 250 mg IVPB over 30 minutes.	
Administer 250 mg IVPB over 60 minutes.	
Instruct the client to finish all the antibiotics completely.	Instruct the client to notify the nurse if they have thoughts of suicide.
Instruct the client to notify the nurse if they have thoughts of suicide.	
Instruct the client to notify the nurse if they experience constipation.	

Blood cultures should be drawn before administering the broad-spectrum antibiotic. Levofloxacin can be started before the results of the cultures are received. The medication is given IVPB, and 250 mg should be diluted and administered intravenously over at least 60 minutes. The client does not need to be instructed to complete antibiotics because the nurse is administering them. It is critical to assess for suicidal tendencies, depression, or changes in behavior during therapy. Levofloxacin can cause diarrhea, not constipation.

6. Correct answers are marked.

Finding	Improved	Declined	No change
Blood pressure			X
Temperature	X		
Oxygen saturation	X		
Respirations	X		
Cough	X		
Pain			X
Heart rate	X		

The client's blood pressure and pain level have remained the same, but all other values have improved.

CASE STUDY #4

1. Correct answers are 1, 2, 3, 4, 5, 8, and 9.
   Gestational age, regular prenatal care, contraction pattern, FHR, dilation, pain level and GBS positive status should be reported to the HCP. Normal data, such as blood pressure, oxygen status, and an Rh positive blood type are not immediate concerns.

2. Correct answers are 3 and 1.
   Based on the client's condition at the time, the nurse recognizes that the client is at the **highest risk for**

   | 3. Neonatal complications |

   and will require

   | 1. Antibiotics. |

3. 1. Paresthesia in the feet and legs is expected following epidural anesthesia.
   2. **The most common side effect of epidural anesthesia is decreased maternal blood pressure. The client normally receives a bolus of IV fluids before administration of the epidural to prevent this from occurring. This is the priority assessment.**
   3. The nurse should frequently assess maternal temperature, but the maternal blood pressure is the priority assessment.
   4. Fetal heart rate accelerations are a reassuring sign that the fetus has an adequate oxygen supply. This is important but not before the assessment of maternal blood pressure.

4. Correct answers are marked.

Potential Nursing Intervention	Indicated	Not Indicated
Reposition the client on her left side.		X
Perform a sterile vaginal examination.	X	
Increase the IV infusion rate.		X
Prepare to administer IV oxytocin.		X
Administer pain medication to the client		X

The external fetal monitor strip is showing early decelerations of the fetal heart rate, indicating head compression. The nurse should first perform a sterile vaginal examination to determine whether delivery is imminent.

The client can be positioned on her side, but the fetal monitoring strip does not indicate this. No data suggest a need to increase the IV infusion rate. Oxytocin (Pitocin) is often given after delivery, but not at this time. If the nurse suspects the client is close to delivery, pain medications should not be administered.

5. Correct answers are 1, 2, and 5.

Sign	Score = 0	Score = 1	Score = 2
Heart rate	Absent	Below 100 bpm	Above 100 bpm
Respiratory effort	Absent	Weak, irregular, or gasping	Good, crying
Muscle tone	Flaccid	Some flexion of arms and legs	Well flexed, or active movements of extremities
Reflex/irritability	No response	Grimace or weak cry	Good cry
Color	Blue all over, or pale	Body pink, hands and feet blue	Pink all over

The nurse's assessment findings help determine the neonate's Apgar score. A heart rate above 100 bpm is 2 points; a slow, weak cry is 1 point; minimal flexion of extremities is 1 point; grimace with stimulation is 1 point; and acrocyanosis is 1 point. The total Apgar score is 6 points.

1. The mouth and nose should be suctioned to ensure airway patency.
2. The infant is breathing and has a heart rate greater than 100 bpm but is experiencing slow respirations and acrocyanosis, so oxygen should be given via face mask or "blow by."
3. The newborn has a normal heart rate, so epinephrine should not be administered now.
4. An IV line is not indicated at this time.
5. An infant having a normal heart rate and color (acrocyanosis is a normal finding in a newborn), but poor respiratory effort should be assessed for the need for naloxone. If the mother received opiates within 4 hours of delivery, naloxone may need to be administered to the infant to counteract respiratory depression.

6. Correct answers are marked.

Client Statement	Effective	Ineffective
"I should avoid sexual activity and tampons until my first postpartum visit."	X	
"I should take a daily laxative to avoid straining and constipation."		X
"I should cleanse my perineal area with warm water after urination."	X	
"I should notify the HCP if I experience heavy bleeding."	X	
"I should take frequent rest periods, especially when the baby is sleeping."	X	
"I should apply antibiotic ointment to my baby's cord stump daily."		X
"I should avoid vigorous exercise and heavy lifting for several weeks."	X	

The client should be instructed to avoid sexual activity, tampons, and douching until her postpartum visit, around 6 weeks. The client should be instructed to change perineal pads frequently and cleanse with warm water using a "peri" bottle at each change. A sitz bath and perineal wipes can help with discomfort. The client should notify the physician for a temperature above 100°F, severe cramping or abdominal pains with chills and fever, heavy bleeding or passage of large clots, foul-smelling vaginal discharge, and pain or burning on urination. The client should be instructed to rest frequently, especially when the baby sleeps. The client should avoid vigorous exercise or heavy lifting for several weeks.

Daily laxatives are not recommended. The client can avoid constipation by eating a well-balanced diet, including fruits and vegetables, and drinking plenty of fluids. Stool softeners may be ordered. Antibiotic ointment does not need to be applied to the normal newborn's umbilical cord stump.

LABORATORY SKILLS INTENSIVE ANSWERS

1. Potassium
2. Urinalysis
3. White blood cell count
4. Prothrombin time (PT) with INR
5. Endoscopy, upper GI
6. Hemoglobin A1C
7. Electromyography (EMG)
8. Iron, total
9. Creatinine
10. Tensilon test
11. Thyroid-stimulating hormone (TSH), thyroid panel
12. Rapid plasma reagin (RPR)
13. Platelet count
14. Cholesterol, total
15. Audiometry
16. Scratch test

CLINICAL SKILLS INTENSIVE ANSWERS

1. Correct order is 4, 3, 5, 2, 1.
    4. The nurse should premeasure the length of the suction catheter. Length is determined by using the marking on the endotracheal tube and adding the additional space for the adapter, usually 1 to 1.5 cm.
    3. The nurse should hyperoxygenate the client before suctioning by having the client take three or four deep breaths, manually ventilating with a bag-mask device, or activating the hyperoxygenate button on the ventilator.
    5. The nurse should lubricate the catheter tip with saline solution and insert the catheter to the premeasured length.
    2. Suction should be applied only when withdrawing the catheter.
    1. The nurse should provide mouth care for the client's comfort after the procedure is complete.

2. Correct order is 3, 1, 5, 2, 4
   3. After explaining the procedure to the client, gathering equipment, and performing hand hygiene, the nurse should don nonsterile gloves and position the client in the high Fowler's position. The nurse should remove the sterile applicator from the culture tube by rotating the cap to break the seal.
   1. The nurse should have the client tilt their head back and open the mouth.
   5. Then, using a tongue depressor (if desired) to depress the tongue, the nurse should swab the back of the throat along the tonsillar area from left to right.
   2. Return the applicator stick to the tube, ensuring the swab is saturated with culture medium and the cap reaches the black dot.
   4. Label the specimen tube and send it to the laboratory.

3. Correct order is 5, 1, 3, 2, 4.
   5. The nurse should open the sterile catheter set and place the sterile absorbent pad under the client's buttocks.
   1. The next step is to don sterile gloves and arrange the sterile items from the catheter set on the sterile field.
   3. The nurse should use one gloved hand to separate the client's labia and keep them separated during the procedure. Using the sterile gloved hand and sterile applicator or forceps, the nurse should cleanse the meatus and surrounding area in a downward stroke, discard used cleaning materials in a nonsterile area, and then repeat.
   2. Using the sterile gloved hand, the lubricated catheter is inserted approximately 2 to 3 inches until urine enters the tube.
   4. The nurse uses all the contents of the prefilled syringe (10 mL) to inflate the catheter balloon.

4. Correct order is 2, 1, 4, 3, 5.
   2. The nurse performs hand hygiene and dons *nonsterile* gloves and a mask. The old dressing is removed. The needle insertion site and surrounding area are examined for redness, edema, inflammation, tenderness, and exudate.
   1. The nurse performs hand hygiene, dons sterile gloves, and then arranges the sterile field.
   4. The nurse activates the chlorhexidine cleanser and scrubs the insertion site using a back-and-forth motion with friction.
   3. Allow the area to dry. A chlorhexidine-impregnated dressing (Biopatch) and a transparent dressing are applied.
   5. The nurse should document the date and time of the dressing change. A label should be placed near, but not covering, the insertion site.

5. Correct order is 2, 3, 1, 5, 4.
   2. The irrigation bag should be filled with 1,000 mL of warm tap water, and the tubing should be primed. Water that is too cold can cause cramping and discomfort.
   3. The irrigation sleeve should be placed over the stoma, allowing the end to be in the toilet but above the water line.
   1. The cone tip of the irrigation tubing should be lubricated with a water-soluble lubricant, inserted into the stoma opening, and held snugly against the skin. The clamp should be opened to allow the water to flow. If cramping starts, the flow can be stopped briefly and then restarted.
   5. Allow 15 minutes for the initial evacuation of stool from the colostomy; then the sleeve can be clamped, and the client is allowed to ambulate.
   4. After evacuation is complete, cleanse the stoma site with water or a disposable wipe and apply a new colostomy appliance.

6. Correct order is 2, 5, 1, 3, 4.
   2. Explain the procedure, perform hand hygiene, and don *nonsterile* gloves. Place the tourniquet 4 to 6 inches above the client's elbow, and instruct the client to open and close the hand.
   5. Cleanse the antecubital fossa with an antimicrobial wipe starting at the vein site and cleanse in circular motions. Let dry.
   1. Hold the skin taut, then insert the needle with the bevel up at a 30-degree angle. Lower the needle toward the skin and thread the needle along the path of the vein.
   3. When blood is obtained, insert the blood collection tube into the plastic holder while holding the vacutainer system steady. Fill to the desired level.
   4. Remove the needle from the vein, cover the site with gauze, and apply pressure to stop bleeding. Cover with an adhesive bandage or pressure dressing.

7. Correct order is 1, 3, 5, 4, 2.
   1. Explain the procedure, perform hand hygiene, and don *nonsterile* gloves. Elevate the client's head of bed. Ask the client about nose injury or deviated septum. Check the nares for patency.
   3. Measure the NG tube from the tip of the client's nose to the earlobe to the xiphoid process, then mark the tube.
   5. Lubricate the end of the tube with water-soluble lubricant.
   4. Have the client slightly extend their head, then insert the tube through the nostril to the back of the throat.
   2. Ask the client to flex their head forward. Have the client sip water or swallow while inserting the tube until the predetermined mark is reached.

8. Correct order is 4, 5, 1, 3, 2.
   4. Perform hand hygiene and don *nonsterile* gloves. Instruct the client to open the specimen container and place the sterile cap with the inside surface up. Ask client not to touch the inside of the container.
   5. Have the client hold the penis with the foreskin retracted if applicable. Using a circular motion, cleanse the area with the antiseptic wipe from the center out.
   1. Tell the client to urinate in the toilet, then place the sterile container under the urine stream.
   3. Collect 30 to 60 mL of urine in the specimen cup. Remove the specimen container before the flow of urine stops and before releasing the penis.
   2. Replace the specimen cap on the cup and cleanse urine from the external surface of the container.

9. Correct order is 2, 3, 5, 4, 1.
   2. Explain the procedure, perform hand hygiene, and don *nonsterile* gloves. Fill the container with 750 to 1,000 mL of lukewarm water. Add soap if ordered. Prime the tubing with solution.
   3. Lubricate the tip of the tubing with water-soluble lubricant. Gently spread the client's buttocks. Insert the tubing 3 to 4 inches.
   5. Hold the tubing in place and let the client take slow, deep breaths while infusing the solution.
   4. Instruct the client to hold the fluid for at least 10 to 15 minutes or as long as possible.
   1. Assist the client to the toilet or bedpan and provide privacy until the client has expelled the total volume of the enema.

10. Correct order is 4, 1, 5, 3, 2.
    4. A chair with arms should be positioned beside the bed, and nonslip footwear placed on the client to avoid slipping during the transfer.
    1. The client should sit on the side of the bed with legs dangling while a gait belt or transfer belt is applied.
    5. The spouse should stand facing the client with feet closest to the chair and between the client's feet. The client is assisted to a standing position, and the spouse uses the gait belt to assist the client in pivoting with the back to the chair.
    3. The client should reach to place hands on the arms of the chair while slowly lowering onto it.
    2. Tell the client to move back in the chair so the client's back is flush with the back of the chair.

11. Correct order is 2, 1, 4, 5, 3.
    2. The client should pull the plunger down on the syringe to obtain 20 units of air and insert the air into the bottle in the upright position. Then, flip the bottle to a downward position and withdraw 20 units of insulin.
    1. The client should expose the abdomen and identify an area 2 inches from the umbilicus. The nurse should instruct the client to rotate sides.
    4. Have the client hold the syringe similar to a dart between the thumb and forefinger, then insert the needle into the skin at a 45- or 90-degree angle. The client does not have to cleanse the skin or aspirate for blood.
    5. After slowly administering insulin, the client removes the needle and applies a swab to the injection site if needed.
    3. Have the client discard the needle safely so no one else can use it.

12. Correct order is 2, 4, 1, 3, 5.
    2. The nurse should perform hand hygiene and don nonsterile gloves. The wound should be cleansed as directed. Assess the wound.
    4. With clean, nonsterile gloves, apply the skin prep to the area covered by tape, approximately 1 to 2 inches from the wound edge.

1. With the backing intact, trim the hydrocolloid dressing to the desired shape, extending 1 to 2 inches from the wound edge.
3. Peel the backing from one edge of the dressing and center over the wound. Apply to the skin using a rolling motion.
5. Smooth the hydrocolloid dressing and hold it in place for several seconds to improve adhesion.

13. Correct order is 5, 2, 3, 1, 4.
    5. The client should be positioned sitting on the side of the bed or in a high Fowler's position.
    2. The nurse should instruct the client to rinse their mouth with water to avoid contaminating the specimen with bacteria from the mouth.
    3. The nurse should instruct the client to take several deep breaths. This opens the airway and provides force to expel the sputum from the lungs.
    1. The client should cough forcefully and expectorate directly into the middle of the specimen container to avoid contamination from outside organisms. The client should repeat this step until a minimum of 5 mL of sputum is obtained.
    4. The specimen container should be labeled at the bedside and then sent to the laboratory for analysis.

Comprehensive Examination

QUESTIONS

1. The nurse is using the PQRST pain assessment tool to evaluate a client's pain. Which factors are included in the tool? **Select all that apply.**
   1. Precipitating or provoking factors
   2. Quality or intensity of the pain
   3. Risk factors for the pain
   4. Severity of symptoms of the pain
   5. Timing and duration of the pain

2. The intensive care unit (ICU) nurse is caring for a client with tachypnea, intercostal and suprasternal retractions, and a change in mental status. Which **priority** interventions should the nurse perform? **Select all that apply.**
   1. Prepare to place the client on a ventilator.
   2. Administer oxygen using a high-flow system.
   3. Place the client in the supine position.
   4. Address nutritional needs.
   5. Continuously monitor oxygen saturation.

3. The ICU nurse is assisting the provider in the endotracheal intubation of a client. Which **priority** interventions should be performed to determine the correct placement of the endotracheal (ET) tube? **Select all that apply.**
   1. Obtain arterial blood gas readings.
   2. Auscultate the lungs bilaterally.
   3. Perform a chest x-ray.
   4. Check capillary refill.
   5. Suction secretions from the ET tube.

4. The nurse is caring for a client scheduled for an endoscopy this morning. The client has scheduled morning medications, including an IV proton pump inhibitor and an oral angiotensin-converting enzyme (ACE) inhibitor. Which interventions should the primary nurse implement when preparing the client for this diagnostic test? **Select all that apply.**
   1. Ensure the client is NPO (nothing by mouth).
   2. Confirm with the HCP to hold the oral medication.
   3. Administer the IV medication.
   4. Confirm the informed consent is signed.
   5. Insert the indwelling urinary catheter.

5. The nurse is caring for a client who has just returned from an endoscopy procedure. Which **priority** intervention should the nurse perform?
   1. Assess the client's gag reflex.
   2. Administer a.m. medications.
   3. Give the client water to gargle for their sore throat.
   4. Determine whether the client is hungry for breakfast.

6. The nurse is caring for a client with a nasogastric (NG) tube. Which interventions can the nurse delegate to the unlicensed assistive personnel (UAP)? **Select all that apply.**
   1. Determine the amount of NG tube output.
   2. Examine the nares for irritation.
   3. Palpate the abdomen for firmness and tenderness.
   4. Listen to bowel sounds in all four quadrants.
   5. Provide mouth care.

7. The client diagnosed with renal calculus is reporting severe pain. Which interventions should the nurse perform **before** administering IV narcotic pain medication? **Select all that apply.**
   1. Assess the urine for blood and strain for particulates.
   2. Check the MAR to determine the last time pain medicine was given.
   3. Determine whether the medication is compatible with the primary IV solution.
   4. Document the medication administration in the electronic health record (EHR).
   5. Compare the medication administration record (MAR) with the client's ID band.

8. The client reports to the nurse that they just passed a renal stone. Which action should the nurse implement **first?**
   1. Obtain a urine sample for urinalysis.
   2. Send the calculus to the laboratory.
   3. Assess the client with a bladder scanner.
   4. Administer a urinary analgesic.

9. The laboratory determined that the client a nurse is caring for had an oxalate renal calculus. The HCP has ordered a low oxalate diet. Which interventions should the nurse include in the teaching plan? **Select all that apply.**
   1. Drink 8 to 12 cups of fluid a day.
   2. Avoid high doses of vitamin C supplements.
   3. Avoid nuts, soy, and whole wheat bread.
   4. Limit oxalate intake to 100 mg per day.
   5. Increase consumption of berries such as blueberries.

10. The nurse is discharging a client diagnosed with left leg cellulitis. Which information should the nurse include in the discharge instructions? **Select all that apply.**
    1. Elevate your left leg on two pillows.
    2. Eat meals high in protein, vitamins, and minerals.
    3. Apply a topical corticosteroid ointment to the affected area daily.
    4. Take all prescription oral antibiotics as ordered.
    5. Apply warm compresses to the reddened area.

11. Which alternate methods should the nurse use to communicate with the client intubated with an ET tube and on a ventilator? **Select all that apply.**
    1. Usage of an electrolarynx
    2. Communication boards
    3. Hand gestures
    4. Eye blinks for yes or no questions
    5. Augmented communication device

12. Which interventions should the nurse implement when caring for a client on a ventilator? **Select all that apply.**
    1. Collaborate with the respiratory therapist.
    2. Continuously monitor the pulse oximeter reading.
    3. Ensure a manual resuscitation bag is at the bedside.
    4. Assess the ventilator settings throughout the shift.
    5. Confirm ventilator alarms are set to silence.

13. The nurse is assessing a client with suspected spinal shock. Which set of assessment findings indicates the client is experiencing spinal shock?
    1. Decreased reflexes and flaccid paralysis
    2. Hypotension and bradycardia
    3. Dyspnea and constricted airway
    4. Tachycardia and confusion

14. After 5 days in the ICU, a client becomes agitated, very disoriented, and reports "hearing voices." Which interventions should the nurse perform? **Select all that apply.**
    1. Use clocks and calendars to orient the client to time.
    2. Dim lights at night and open window blinds during the day.
    3. Schedule activities frequently throughout the day and night.
    4. Have the family bring familiar objects from home.
    5. Minimize noise from shift change and monitoring equipment.

15. The nurse is assessing a client and notes the client opens their eyes when the nurse calls their name but only moans when questioned. When the nurse applies pressure to the nailbed of the finger, the client slowly pulls their hand away from the nurse. Which rating on the Glasgow Coma Scale should the nurse document?

Glasgow Coma Scale

Appropriate Stimulus	Response	Score
Eye Opening		
Approach to bedside	Spontaneous response	4
Verbal command	Opens eyes to name on command	3
Pain	Lack of opening of eyes to previous stimuli but opens to pain	2
	Lack of opening of eyes to any stimulus	1
	Untestable	0
Best Verbal Response		
Verbal questioning with maximum arousal	Oriented to person, place, time, and events	5
	Confusion, conversant but disoriented	4
	Disorganized use of words	3
	Incomprehensible words, groaning	2
	Lack of sound even with painful stimuli	1
	Untestable	0
Best Motor Response		
Verbal command	Follows verbal command	6
Pain (pressure on proximal nailbed)	Localizes pain, attempts to remove offending stimulus	5
	Flexion withdrawal of arm in response to pain without abnormal posturing	4
	Abnormal flexion, flexing of arm at elbow and pronation, making a fist	3
	Abnormal extension, extension of arm at elbow with adduction, and internal rotation of arm at shoulder	2
	Lack of response	1
	Untestable	0

1. Glasgow Coma Scale rating of 14
2. Glasgow Coma Scale rating of 12
3. Glasgow Coma Scale rating of 9
4. Glasgow Coma Scale rating of 7

16. The nurse is caring for a client with a Glasgow Coma Scale rating of 9. Which interventions should the nurse include in the client's plan of care? **Select all that apply.**
    1. Keep the head of the bed elevated 30 degrees.
    2. Perform active range of motion exercises every 4 hours.
    3. Explain all procedures to the client.
    4. Turn the client every 4 hours.
    5. Maintain normal body temperature.

17. The nurse is caring for a client with suspected disseminated intravascular coagulation (DIC). Which findings by the nurse support the diagnosis of DIC?
    1. Sudden onset of chest pain and frothy sputum
    2. Foul-smelling, concentrated urine
    3. Oozing of blood from the IV site
    4. Fever of unknown origin

18. The HCP has ordered an endoscopy for a client. Which teaching interventions should the nurse include when explaining the procedure to the client? **Select all that apply.**
    1. Explain that the client cannot eat or drink anything 8 hours before the procedure.
    2. Tell the client they will have an IV and be sedated during the procedure.
    3. Inform the client they will have vital signs taken frequently after the procedure.
    4. Instruct the client that they will be given narcotics after the procedure for the pain.
    5. Teach the client to contact the HCP if they have bleeding or vomiting.

19. The HCP has ordered a colonoscopy for a client. Which teaching interventions should the nurse include when explaining the procedure to the client? **Select all that apply.**
    1. Explain the bowel preparation necessary before the procedure.
    2. Teach the client not to eat or drink anything 8 hours before the procedure.
    3. Instruct the client to remain on a clear liquid diet for 24 hours after the procedure.
    4. Inform the client that they must stay overnight in the hospital.
    5. Tell the client to report any rectal bleeding, dizziness, or abdominal pain to the HCP.

20. The clinic nurse is caring for a client with a sprained right ankle. Which interventions should the nurse include in the discharge teaching for the client? **Select all that apply.**
    1. Instruct the client to rest and avoid stress on the right ankle.
    2. Tell the client to apply warm compresses to the injury.
    3. Show the client how to apply an elastic bandage to the ankle.
    4. Recommend the client elevate the right foot above the level of the heart.
    5. Teach the client to alternate acetaminophen and ibuprofen for pain.

21. The clinic nurse is caring for a client diagnosed with a common cold. The client asks the nurse, "Why won't the doctor give me some antibiotics when I feel so bad?" Which response by the nurse is **most** appropriate?
    1. "Over-the-counter (OTC) medications are cheaper than antibiotics for the common cold."
    2. "The doctor will know which antibiotics to give you based on your nasal culture."
    3. "The common cold is caused by a virus; antibiotics only treat bacterial infections."
    4. "You should go to a different doctor so you will get proper treatment."

22. The client diagnosed with the common cold asks the nurse about interventions to help with cold symptoms. Which interventions should the nurse teach the client? **Select all that apply.**
    1. Avoid alcohol, coffee, and caffeinated sodas.
    2. Recommend intranasal zinc for symptoms.
    3. Encourage intake of chicken noodle soup.
    4. Suggest a warm, saltwater gargle.
    5. Avoid saline nasal sprays and drops.

23. The nurse hung the wrong IV antibiotic for the postoperative client. Which intervention should the nurse implement **first?**
    1. Assess the client for any adverse reactions.
    2. Complete the incident or occurrence report.
    3. Administer the correct IV antibiotic medication.
    4. Notify the client's HCP.

24. The RN, licensed practical nurse (LPN), and UAP are caring for clients in a critical care unit. Which task would be **most** appropriate for the RN to assign or delegate?
    1. Instruct the UAP to obtain the client's serum glucose level.
    2. Request the LPN to change the central line dressing.
    3. Ask the LPN to bathe the client and change the bed linens.
    4. Tell the UAP to obtain urine output for the 12-hour shift.

25. Which task should the RN critical care nurse delegate to the UAP?
    1. Check the pulse oximeter reading for the client on a ventilator.
    2. Take the client's sterile urine specimen to the laboratory.
    3. Obtain the vital signs for the client in an Addisonian crisis.
    4. Assist the HCP with performing a paracentesis at the bedside.

26. Which situation would prompt the healthcare team to utilize the client's advance directive when making decisions for the client?
    1. The client diagnosed with a head injury exhibiting decerebrate posturing
    2. The client diagnosed with a C6 spinal cord injury (SCI) and on a ventilator
    3. The client diagnosed with chronic renal disease being placed on dialysis
    4. The client diagnosed with terminal cancer and intellectually disabled

27. The RN is caring for clients in a skilled nursing unit. Which tasks should be delegated to the UAP? **Select all that apply.**
    1. Instruct the UAP to apply sequential compression devices to the client on strict bedrest.
    2. Ask the UAP to assist the radiology tech to position a client for a STAT portable chest x-ray.
    3. Request the UAP to prepare the client for a wound débridement at the bedside.
    4. Tell the UAP to obtain the intakes and outputs (I&Os) for all the clients on the unit.
    5. Ask the UAP to check a client's blood glucose with the glucometer ac and hs.

28. The nurse is assigned to a quality improvement committee to decide on a quality improvement project for the unit. Which issue should the nurse discuss at the committee meetings?
    1. Systems that make it difficult for the nurses to do their job
    2. How unhappy the nurses are with their current pay scale
    3. Collective bargaining activity at a nearby hospital
    4. The number of medication errors committed by an individual nurse

29. The clinic manager is discussing osteoporosis with the clinic staff. Which activity is an example of a secondary nursing intervention when discussing osteoporosis?
    1. Obtain a bone density evaluation test on a female client older than 50.
    2. Perform a spinal screening examination on all female clients.
    3. Encourage the client to walk 30 minutes daily on a hard surface.
    4. Discuss risk factors for developing osteoporosis.

30. The new graduate nurse is assigned to work with a UAP to care for a group of clients. Which action by the nurse is the **best** method to evaluate whether delegated care is being provided?
    1. Check with the clients to see whether they are satisfied.
    2. Ask the RN charge nurse whether the UAP is qualified.
    3. Make rounds to ensure the clients are turned as delegated.
    4. Watch the UAP perform all the delegated tasks.

31. The RN pediatric charge nurse is making assignments on a pediatric unit. Which client should be assigned to the LPN?
    1. The 6-year-old client diagnosed with a sickle cell crisis
    2. The 8-year-old client diagnosed with biliary atresia
    3. The 10-year-old client diagnosed with anaphylaxis
    4. The 11-year-old client diagnosed with pneumonia

32. The nurse is caring for clients on a medical unit. Which client should the nurse assess **first**?
    1. The client diagnosed with disseminated intravascular coagulation (DIC) oozing blood from the IV site and having a seizure
    2. The client diagnosed with benign prostatic hypertrophy (BPH) reporting terminal dribbling and inability to empty bladder
    3. The client diagnosed with renal calculi reporting severe flank pain and hematuria
    4. The client diagnosed with Addison's disease and hypoglycemia, with bronze skin pigmentation

33. The charge nurse is making assignments in the day surgery center. Which client should be assigned to the **most** experienced nurse?
    1. The client being prepared for discharge after surgery for an inguinal hernia
    2. The client in the preoperative area scheduled for laparoscopic cholecystectomy
    3. The client receiving 2 units of blood after scheduled chemotherapy treatment
    4. The client diagnosed with end-stage renal disease after creation of an arteriovenous fistula

34. The RN charge nurse of a critical care unit is making assignments for the night shift. Which client should be assigned to the graduate nurse having completed an internship?
    1. The client diagnosed with a head injury resulting from a motor vehicle accident (MVA) with a Glasgow Coma Scale score of 13
    2. The client diagnosed with inflammatory bowel disease (IBD) having severe diarrhea and a serum K⁺ level of 3.2 mEq/L
    3. The client diagnosed with Addison's disease, lethargic, with a BP of 80/45 mm Hg, P of 124 bpm, and R rate of 28 breaths/min
    4. The client diagnosed with hyperthyroidism having undergone a thyroidectomy and with a positive Trousseau's sign

35. The nurse on a medical unit has just received the evening shift report. Which client should the nurse assess **first**?
    1. The client diagnosed with a deep vein thrombosis (DVT), with a heparin drip infusion, and a PTT of 92 seconds
    2. The client diagnosed with pneumonia with an oral temperature of 100.2°F (37.9°C)
    3. The client diagnosed with cystitis reporting burning on urination
    4. The client diagnosed with pancreatitis reporting pain that is an 8 on a scale of 10

36. The 75-year-old client underwent an open cholecystectomy for cholelithiasis 2 days ago and has a T-tube drain in place. Which intervention should the RN delegate to the UAP? **Select all that apply.**
    1. Explain the procedure for using the patient-controlled analgesia (PCA) pump.
    2. Check the client's abdominal dressing for drainage.
    3. Take and record the client's vital signs.
    4. Empty the client's indwelling catheter bag at the end of the shift.
    5. Assist the client to ambulate three to four times daily in the hallway.

37. The surgical unit has a low census and is overstaffed. Which staff member should the house supervisor notify **first** and request to stay home?
    1. The nurse with the most vacation time
    2. The nurse requesting to be off
    3. The nurse with the least experience in the unit
    4. The nurse having called in sick the previous 2 days

38. The nurse and the UAP are caring for residents in a long-term care facility. Which task should the RN delegate to the UAP?
   1. Apply a sterile dressing to a stage IV pressure wound.
   2. Check the blood glucose level of the weak and shaky resident.
   3. Document the amount of food the residents ate after a meal.
   4. Teach the residents how to play different types of bingo.

39. The RN director of nurses in a long-term care facility observes the LPN charge nurse explaining to a UAP how to calculate the amount of food a resident has eaten from the food tray. Which action should the director of nurses implement?
   1. Ask the charge nurse to teach all the other UAPs.
   2. Encourage the nurse to continue to work with the UAP.
   3. Tell the charge nurse to discuss this in a private area.
   4. Give the UAP a better explanation of the procedure.

40. A long-term care facility's RN wound care nurse asks the UAP for assistance. Which tasks should be delegated to the UAP? **Select all that apply.**
   1. Apply the wound débriding paste to the wound.
   2. Keep the resident's heels off the surface of the bed.
   3. Turn the resident at least every 2 hours.
   4. Encourage the resident to drink a high-protein shake.
   5. Assist the resident to put on a clean shirt.

41. The older adult client becomes confused and wanders in the hallways. Which fall precaution intervention should the nurse implement **first**?
   1. Place a Posey vest restraint on the client.
   2. Move the client to a room near the nurse's station.
   3. Ask the HCP for an antipsychotic medication.
   4. Raise all four side rails on the client's bed.

42. The clinic nurse is caring for a client diagnosed with osteoarthritis. The client tells the nurse, "I am having problems getting in and out of my bathtub." Which intervention should the clinic nurse implement **first**?
   1. Determine whether the client has grab bars in the bathroom.
   2. Encourage the client to take a shower instead of a bath.
   3. Initiate a referral to a physical therapist for the client.
   4. Discuss whether the client takes NSAIDs.

43. The employee health nurse has cared for six clients having similar symptoms. The clients have a fever, nausea, vomiting, and diarrhea. Which action should the nurse implement **first** after assessing the clients?
   1. Have another employee drive the clients home.
   2. Notify the public health department immediately.
   3. Send the clients to the emergency department (ED).
   4. Obtain stool specimens from the clients.

44. The clinic nurse is caring for clients in a pediatric clinic. Which client should the nurse assess **first**?
   1. The 4-year-old child reporting left leg pain after a fall
   2. The 3-year-old child now drooling and not wanting to swallow
   3. The 8-year-old child reporting a headache for 2 days
   4. The 10-year-old child losing weight and thirsty all the time

45. Which statement is an example of community-oriented, population-focused nursing?
   1. The nurse cares for an older adult client with a kidney transplant living in the community.
   2. The nurse develops an educational program for persons with type 2 diabetes in the community.
   3. The nurse refers a client diagnosed with Cushing's syndrome to the registered dietitian.
   4. The nurse provides a pamphlet for the client diagnosed with chronic renal disease.

46. The home health agency director of nursing is making assignments for the nurses. Which client should be assigned to the nurse **new** to home health nursing?
    1. The dyspneic and confused client diagnosed with AIDS
    2. The client without money to get prescriptions filled
    3. The client diagnosed with full-thickness burns on the arm needing a dressing change
    4. The client reporting pain diagnosed with diabetic neuropathy

47. The home health RN and aide are caring for a client 3 weeks postoperative for open reduction and internal fixation of a right hip fracture. Which task would be appropriate for the nurse to delegate to the aide?
    1. Instruct the aide to palpate the right pedal pulse.
    2. Ask the aide to change the right hip dressing.
    3. Tell the aide to elevate the right leg on two pillows.
    4. Request that the aide mop the client's bedroom floor.

48. The charge nurse has received laboratory data for clients in the medical department. Which client would require intervention by the charge nurse?
    1. The client diagnosed with a myocardial infarction (MI) having elevated troponin levels
    2. The client receiving IV heparin with a PTT of 68 seconds
    3. The client diagnosed with end-stage liver failure and elevated ammonia levels
    4. The client receiving phenytoin with levels of 24 mcg/mL

49. Which client would **most** benefit from acupuncture, a traditional Chinese technique considered complementary alternative medicine?
    1. The client diagnosed with deep vein thrombosis
    2. The client diagnosed with Alzheimer's disease
    3. The client diagnosed with reactive airway disease
    4. The client diagnosed with osteoarthritis

50. The home health nurse notes that the 88-year-old client cannot cook for themself and mainly eats frozen foods and sandwiches. Which intervention should the RN implement?
    1. Discuss the situation with the client's family.
    2. Refer the client to the home health occupational therapist.
    3. Request the home health aide to cook all the client's meals.
    4. Contact the community's Meals on Wheels.

51. Which legal intervention should the nurse implement on the **initial** visit when admitting a client to the home healthcare agency?
    1. Discuss the professional boundary-crossing policy with the client.
    2. Provide the client with a copy of the NAHC Bill of Rights.
    3. Tell the client how many visits the client will have while on service.
    4. Explain that the client must be homebound to be eligible for home healthcare.

52. The UAP accidentally pulled the client's chest tube out while assisting the client to the bedside commode. Which intervention should the RN implement **first**?
    1. Securely tape petroleum gauze over the insertion site.
    2. Instruct the UAP on how to move a client with a chest tube.
    3. Assess the client's respirations and lung sounds.
    4. Obtain a chest tube and a chest tube insertion tray.

53. The RN pediatric nurse and LPN have been assigned to care for clients on a pediatric unit. Which nursing task should be assigned to the LPN?
    1. Administer PO (oral) medications to a client diagnosed with gastroenteritis.
    2. Take the routine vital signs for all the clients on the pediatric unit.
    3. Transcribe the HCP's orders into the computer.
    4. Assess the urinary output of a client diagnosed with nephrotic syndrome.

54. The hospital will be implementing a new EHR for documenting medication administration. Which action should the clinical manager take **first** when implementing the new EHR?
    1. Discuss the new EHR with each nurse individually.
    2. Schedule meetings on all shifts to discuss the new EHR.
    3. Require the nurse to read a handout explaining the new EHR.
    4. Ask the nurses to watch a video explaining the new EHR.

55. Which client warrants **immediate** intervention from the nurse on the medical unit?
    1. The client diagnosed with an abdominal aortic aneurysm having an audible bruit
    2. The client diagnosed with pneumonia and bilateral crackles
    3. The client diagnosed with bacterial meningitis, with nucal rigidity and neck pain
    4. The client diagnosed with Crohn's disease having abdominal pain, vomiting, and diarrhea

56. Which assessment data warrant **immediate** intervention by the nurse for the client diagnosed with chronic kidney disease (CKD) on peritoneal dialysis?
    1. The client's serum creatinine level is 2.4 mg/dL.
    2. The client's abdomen is soft to the touch and nontender.
    3. The dialysate being removed from the abdomen is cloudy.
    4. The dialysate instilled was 1,500 mL (50.7 oz) and the amount of output was 2,100 mL (71 oz).

57. The nurse is taking a history on a client in a women's clinic when the client tells the nurse, "I have been trying to get pregnant for 3 years." Which question is the nurse's **best** response?
    1. "How many attempts have you made to get pregnant?"
    2. "What have you tried to help you get pregnant?"
    3. "Does your insurance cover infertility treatments?"
    4. "Have you considered adoption as an option?"

58. The nurse working at the county hospital is admitting an Rh-negative client to the labor and delivery unit. The client is gravida 2, para 0. Which assessment data are **most** important for the nurse to assess?
    1. Why the client did not have a viable baby with the first pregnancy
    2. Whether the mother received Rho(D) immune globulin after the last pregnancy
    3. The period of time between the client's pregnancies
    4. When the mother terminated the previous pregnancy

59. The unconscious 4-year-old child diagnosed with bruises covering the torso in varying stages of healing is brought to the ED by paramedics. The nurse notes small burn marks on the child's genitalia. Which actions should the nurse implement? **Select all that apply.**
    1. Notify Child Protective Services.
    2. Ask the parent how the child was injured.
    3. Perform a thorough examination for more injuries.
    4. Tell the parents that the police have been called.
    5. Prepare the child for skull x-rays or a CT scan.

60. The 24-month-old toddler is admitted to the pediatric unit diagnosed with vomiting and diarrhea. Which interventions should the nurse implement? **Rank in order of performance.**
    1. Teach the parent about weighing diapers to determine output status.
    2. Show the parent the call light and explain safety regimens.
    3. Assess the toddler's tissue turgor.
    4. Place the appropriate size diapers in the room.
    5. Take the toddler's vital signs.

61. The nurse has received the shift report. Which client should the nurse assess **first?**
    1. The client diagnosed with a deep vein thrombosis (DVT) reporting a feeling of doom
    2. The client diagnosed with gallbladder ulcer disease refusing to eat the food served
    3. The client diagnosed with pancreatitis wanting the nasogastric tube removed
    4. The client diagnosed with osteoarthritis reporting stiff joints

62. The home health nurse is planning their rounds for the day. Which client should the nurse plan to see **first?**
    1. The 56-year-old client diagnosed with multiple sclerosis reporting a cough
    2. The 78-year-old client diagnosed with congestive heart failure (CHF) reporting losing 3 lb (1.4 kg)
    3. The 42-year-old client diagnosed with an L5 spinal cord injury having developed a stage 4 pressure injury
    4. The 80-year-old client diagnosed with a cerebrovascular accident (CVA) and right-sided paralysis

63. The nurse is preparing to perform a sterile dressing change on a client diagnosed with full-thickness burns on the right leg. Which intervention should the nurse implement **first?**
    1. Premedicate the client with a narcotic analgesic.
    2. Prepare the equipment and bandages at the bedside.
    3. Remove the old dressing with nonsterile gloves.
    4. Place a sterile glove on the dominant hand.

64. The physical therapist has notified the unit secretary that the client will be ambulated in 45 minutes. After receiving notification from the unit secretary, which task should the RN charge nurse delegate to the UAP?
    1. Administer a pain medication 30 minutes before therapy.
    2. Give the client a washcloth to wash their face before walking.
    3. Check to ensure the client has been offered bathroom use.
    4. Find a walker that is the correct height for the client.

65. The volunteer on a medical unit tells the nurse that one of the clients on the unit is their neighbor and asks about the client's condition. Which information should the nurse discuss with the volunteer?
    1. Determine how well they know the client before talking with the volunteer.
    2. Tell the volunteer the client's condition in layperson's terms.
    3. Ask the client whether it is all right to talk with the volunteer.
    4. Explain that client information is on a need-to-know basis only.

66. The medical unit is governed by a system of shared governance. Which statement **best** describes an advantage of this system?
    1. It guarantees that unions will not be able to come into the hospital.
    2. It makes the manager responsible for sharing information with the staff.
    3. It involves staff nurses in the decision-making process of the unit.
    4. It is a system used to represent the nurses in labor disputes.

67. The visitor on a medical unit is shouting and making threats about harming the staff because of the perceived poor care their loved one received. Which statement is the nurse's **best** initial response?
    1. "If you don't stop shouting, I will have to call security."
    2. "I hear that you are frustrated. Can we discuss the issues calmly?"
    3. "You are disrupting the unit. Calm down or leave the hospital."
    4. "This behavior is uncalled for and will not resolve anything."

68. The experienced nurse has recently taken a position on a medical unit in a community hospital, but after 1 week on the job finds the staffing is not what was discussed during the employment interview. Which approach would be **most** appropriate for the nurse to take when attempting to resolve the issue?
1. Immediately give a 2-week notice and find a different job.
2. Discuss the situation with the interviewing manager.
3. Talk with the other employees about the staffing situation.
4. Tell the charge nurse the staffing is not as explained before.

69. The nurse is preparing to administer the client's **first** IV antibiotic. **Rank in order of priority.**
1. Check the HCP's order in the EHR.
2. Determine whether the client has any known allergies.
3. Hang the secondary IV piggyback (IVPB) higher than the primary IV bag.
4. Set the IV pump at the correct rate.
5. Determine whether the antibiotic is compatible with the primary IV line.

70. At 0830, the day shift nurse is preparing to administer medications to the client.

Client's Name: R.B. Height: 62 in (157.5 cm)	Account Number: 1253456 Weight: 105 lb (47.6 kg)	Allergies: NKDA Date: Today
Medication	1901–0700	0701–1900
Digoxin 0.125 mg PO every day		0900
Furosemide 40 mg PO BID		0900
		1600
Ranitidine 150 mg in 250 mL NS IV continuous infusion every 24 hours	0300 NN@ 11 mL/hr	
Vancomycin 850 mg IVPB every 24 hours		1200
		1800
Signature/Initials	Night Nurse RN/NN	Day Nurse RN/DN

Which action should the nurse take **first**?
1. Check the client's armband against the MAR.
2. Assess the client's IV site for redness and patency.
3. Ask for the client's date of birth.
4. Determine the client's last potassium level.

71. A major disaster has been called, and the charge nurse on a medical unit must recommend to the medical discharge officer on rounds which clients to discharge. Which client should **not** be discharged?
1. The client diagnosed with chronic angina pectoris on new medication for 2 days
2. The client diagnosed with DVT had heparin discontinued and has been on warfarin for 4 days
3. The client diagnosed with an infected leg wound receiving vancomycin IVPB every 24 hours for methicillin-resistant *Staphylococcus aureus* (MRSA) infection
4. The client diagnosed with COPD having arterial blood gas (ABG) levels: pH, 7.34; Pco_2 55 mm Hg; HCO_3 28 mmol/L; Pao_2 89 mm Hg

72. The nurse has been named in a lawsuit concerning the care provided. Which action should the nurse take **first**?
1. Consult with the hospital's attorney.
2. Review the client's EHR.
3. Purchase personal liability insurance.
4. Discuss the case with the supervisor.

73. The nurse has accepted the clinical manager position for a medical-surgical unit. Which role is an important aspect of this management position?
    1. Evaluate the job performance of the staff.
    2. Be the sole decision-maker for the unit.
    3. Take responsibility for the staff nurse's actions.
    4. Attend the medical staff meetings.

74. The charge nurse notices that one of the staff takes frequent breaks, has unpredictable mood swings, and often volunteers to care for clients requiring narcotics. Which **priority** action should the charge nurse implement regarding this employee?
    1. Discuss the nurse's actions with the unit manager.
    2. Confront the nurse about the behavior.
    3. Do not allow the nurse to take breaks alone.
    4. Prepare an occurrence report on the employee.

75. A HCP frequently tells jokes with sexual overtones at the nursing station. Which action should the RN charge nurse implement?
    1. Tell the HCP that the jokes are inappropriate and offensive.
    2. Report the behavior to the medical staff committee.
    3. Discuss the problem with the chief nursing officer.
    4. Call a Code Purple and have the nurses surround the HCP.

76. The night shift nurse is caring for clients on the surgical unit. Which client situation would **warrant immediate** notification of the surgeon?
    1. The client 2 days postoperative for bowel resection refusing to turn, cough, and deep breathe
    2. The client 5 hours postoperative for abdominal hysterectomy reporting feeling a "pop" and then her pain went away
    3. The client 2 hours postoperative for total knee replacement (TKR) with 400 mL in the cell-saver collection device
    4. The client 1 day postoperative for bilateral thyroidectomy and has a negative Chvostek sign

77. Which client should the postanesthesia care unit (PACU) nurse assess **first**?
    1. The client after receiving general anesthesia reporting a sore throat
    2. The client after right knee surgery having a pulse oximeter reading of 90%
    3. The client receiving epidural surgery with a palpable 2+ dorsalis pedal pulse
    4. The client after abdominal surgery having green bile draining from the NG tube

78. The client with a below-the-knee amputation (BKA) has a large amount of bright red blood on the residual limb dressing and the nurse suspects an arterial bleed. Which intervention should the nurse implement **first**?
    1. Increase the client's IV rate.
    2. Assess the client's vital signs.
    3. Apply a tourniquet above the amputation.
    4. Notify the client's HCP.

79. The client after surgery on the right elbow has no right radial pulse and their fingers are cold. The client reports tingling and inability to move the fingers of their right hand. Which intervention should the nurse implement **first**?
    1. Document the findings in the client's EHR.
    2. Elevate the client's right hand.
    3. Assess the radial pulse with the Doppler ultrasound.
    4. Notify the client's HCP.

80. The HCP writes an order for the client diagnosed with a fractured right hip and operative repair to ambulate with a walker four times per day. Which action should the RN implement?
    1. Tell the UAP to ambulate the client with the walker.
    2. Request a referral to the physical therapy department.
    3. Obtain a walker that is appropriate for the client's height.
    4. Notify the social worker of the HCP's order for a walker.

81. The LPN is working in a surgical rehabilitation unit. Which nursing task would be **most** appropriate for the LPN to implement?
    1. Bathe the client experiencing incontinence of urine.
    2. Document the amount of food the client eats.
    3. Conduct the afternoon bingo game in the lobby.
    4. Perform routine dressing changes on assigned clients.

82. The UAP tells the nurse the client 5 hours postoperative for an L3/L4 laminectomy is reporting numbness in both feet. Which intervention should the RN implement?
    1. Ask the UAP to take the client's vital signs.
    2. Request the UAP to log roll the client to the right side.
    3. Complete the neurovascular assessment on the client's legs.
    4. Contact the physical therapist to check the client.

83. The ED nurse is requesting a bed in the ICU. The ICU charge nurse must request a transfer of one client from the ICU to the surgical unit to make room for the client coming into the ICU from the ED. Which client should the ICU charge nurse request to transfer to the surgical unit?
    1. The client diagnosed with flail chest arriving from the operating room with a right-sided chest tube
    2. The client diagnosed with acute diverticulitis 1 day postoperative for creation of a sigmoid colostomy
    3. The client 1 day postoperative for elective total hip replacement with dry and intact incisional dressings
    4. The client 2 days postoperative for repair of a fractured femur with a fat embolism

84. A terrible storm causes the electricity to go out in the hospital and the emergency generator lights come on. Which action should the RN charge nurse implement?
    1. Request all family members to leave the hospital as soon as possible.
    2. Instruct the staff to plug critical electrical equipment into the red outlets.
    3. Have the UAP place a portable flashlight on each bedside table.
    4. Contact the maintenance department to determine how long the electricity will be out.

85. The HCP is angry and yelling in the nurse's station because the client's laboratory data are not available. Which action should the charge nurse implement **first?**
    1. Contact the laboratory for the client's results.
    2. Ask the HCP to step into the nurse's office.
    3. Tell the HCP to discuss the issue with the laboratory.
    4. Report the HCP's behavior to the chief nursing officer.

86. The staff nurse is concerned about possible increasing infection rates among clients with peripherally inserted central catheters (PICCs). The nurse has noticed several clients with problems in the last few months. Which action would be appropriate for the staff nurse to implement **first?**
    1. Discuss the infections with the chief nursing officer.
    2. Contact the infection control nurse to discuss the problem.
    3. Assume the employee health nurse is monitoring the situation.
    4. Volunteer to be on an ad hoc committee to research the infection rate.

87. The RN surgery charge nurse on the 30-bed surgical unit has been told to send one staff member to the medical unit. The surgical unit is full, with multiple clients requiring custodial care. Which staff member would be **most** appropriate to send to the medical unit?
    1. Send the UAP having worked on the surgical unit for 5 years.
    2. Send the RN having worked in the hospital for 8 years in various areas.
    3. Send the LPN with 3 years of experience, which includes 6 months on the medical unit.
    4. Send the new graduate nurse orienting to the surgical unit.

88. The nurse educator is discussing fire safety with new employees. The nurse should teach the actions to ensure the safety of clients and employees in the case of fire on the unit. **Rank in order of performance.**
    1. Extinguish.
    2. Rescue.
    3. Confine.
    4. Alert.
    5. Evacuate.

89. The client tells the surgical nurse, "I am having surgery on my right knee." However, the operative permit is for surgery on the left knee. Which action should the nurse implement **first**?
    1. Notify the operating room team.
    2. Initiate the time-out procedure.
    3. Clarify the correct extremity with the client.
    4. Call the surgeon to discuss the discrepancy.

90. The older adult client fell and fractured their left femur. The nurse finds the client crying and tells the nurse, "I don't want to go to the nursing home, but my child says I have to." Which response would be **most** appropriate by the nurse?
    1. "Let me call a meeting of the healthcare team and your child."
    2. "Has the social worker talked to you about this already?"
    3. "Why are you so upset about going to the nursing home?"
    4. "I can see you are upset. Would you want to talk about it?"

91. The client is confused and pulling at the IV line and indwelling catheter. Which order from the HCP should the nurse clarify concerning restraining the client?
    1. Restrain the client's wrists as needed.
    2. Offer the client fluids every 2 hours.
    3. Apply a hand mitt to the arm opposite the IV site for 12 hours.
    4. Check circulation of the restrained limb every 2 hours.

92. The RN surgery charge nurse on a 20-bed surgical unit has one RN, two LPNs, and two UAPs for a 12-hour shift. Which task would be an **inappropriate** delegation of assignments?
    1. The RN will perform the shift assessments.
    2. The LPN should administer all IV push (IVP) medications.
    3. The UAP will complete all a.m. care.
    4. The RN will monitor laboratory values.

93. The head nurse is completing the yearly performance evaluation on a nurse. Which data regarding the nurse's performance should be included in the evaluation?
    1. The number of times the nurse has been tardy
    2. The attitude of the nurse at the client's bedside
    3. The thank-you notes the nurse received from clients
    4. The EHR audits of the clients the nurse cared for

94. The nurse is discharging the 72-year-old client 5 days postoperative for repair of a fractured hip diagnosed with comorbid medical conditions. At this time, which referral would be the **most** appropriate for the nurse to make for this client?
    1. Home healthcare agency
    2. Senior citizen center
    3. Rehabilitation facility
    4. Outpatient physical therapist

95. The nurse is caring for clients on a 12-bed intermediate care surgical unit. Which task should the nurse implement **first?**
    1. Reinsert the nasogastric tube for the client after they pulled it out.
    2. Complete the preoperative checklist for the client scheduled for surgery.
    3. Instruct the client being discharged home about colostomy care.
    4. Change the client's surgical dressing that has a 2-cm area of drainage.

96. The nurse is preparing to administer medications to clients on a surgical unit. Which medication should the nurse **question** administering?
    1. The clopidogrel to a client scheduled for surgery
    2. The enoxaparin to a client after a TKR
    3. The sliding scale regular insulin to a client after a Whipple procedure
    4. The vancomycin to a client allergic to the antibiotic penicillin

97. The nurse is caring for clients on a surgical ICU. Which client should the nurse assess **first?**
    1. The client 4 hours postoperative for abdominal surgery reporting abdominal pain with hypoactive bowel sounds
    2. The client 1 day postoperative for total hip replacement with 550 mL (18.6 oz) of clear amber urine voided in the last 8 hours
    3. The client 8 hours postoperative for open cholecystectomy with a T-tube draining green bile
    4. The client 12 hours postoperative for total knee replacement (TKR) reporting numbness and tingling in the foot

98. Which situation should the charge nurse in the ICU address **first** after receiving the shift report?
    1. Talk to the irate family member about their loved one's nursing care.
    2. Complete the 90-day probationary evaluation for a new ICU graduate intern.
    3. Call the laboratory concerning the type and crossmatch for a client needing blood.
    4. Arrange for a client to be transferred to the telemetry step-down unit.

99. The critical care unit is having problems with staff members clocking in late and clocking out early from their shifts. Which statement by the charge nurse indicates a democratic leadership style?
    1. "You cannot clock out 1 minute before your shift is complete."
    2. "As long as your work is done, you can clock out whenever you want."
    3. "We will have a meeting to discuss the clocking procedure."
    4. "The clinical manager will take care of anyone clocking out early."

100. The nurse in the burn unit is preparing to perform a wound dressing change at the bedside. **Rank in order of priority.**
    1. Obtain the needed supplies for the procedure.
    2. Explain the procedure to the client.
    3. Remove the old dressing with nonsterile gloves.
    4. Medicate the client with narcotic analgesics.
    5. Assess the client's burned area.

101. Which client should the charge nurse of a long-term care facility see **first** after receiving shift report?
    1. The client being placed in a long-term care facility and is unhappy about it
    2. The client wanting the HCP to order a nightly glass of wine
    3. The upset client because their call light was not answered for 30 minutes
    4. The client with a child being discharged from the hospital after heart surgery

102. The client in a long-term care facility says that the staff does not listen to their reports of symptoms unless a family member also describes the discomfort. Which action should the director of nurses implement?
    1. Call a staff meeting and tell the staff to listen to the resident when talking to them.
    2. Determine which staff member neglected listening to the resident and place them on leave.
    3. Ignore the situation because long-term care residents cannot determine their needs.
    4. Talk with the resident about their concerns and then initiate a plan of action.

103. The newly admitted client in a long-term care facility stays in their room and refuses to participate in client activities. Which statement is a **priority** for the nurse to discuss with the client?
    1. "You have to leave this room, or you will never make friends here."
    2. "It is not so bad living here; you are lucky we care about what happens to you."
    3. "You seem sad; would you want to talk about your feelings about being here?"
    4. "The activities director can arrange for someone to come and visit you in your room."

104. A client's family member in a long-term care facility is unhappy with the care being provided for the loved one. Who would be **most** appropriate to investigate and report the findings during a client care conference?
    1. The ombudsman for the facility
    2. The social worker for the facility
    3. The unhappy family member
    4. The director of nurses

105. The 65-year-old client is being discharged from the hospital following major abdominal surgery and is unable to drive. Which referral should the nurse make to ensure continuity of care?
    1. A church that can provide transportation
    2. A home health agency
    3. An outpatient clinic
    4. The HCP's office

106. The nurse in an assisted living facility notes that the client has several new bruises on both arms and hands. Which intervention should the nurse implement **first**?
    1. File an elder abuse report with the Department of Human Services.
    2. Ask the client whether they fell and hurt themself during the night.
    3. Check the MAR to determine which medications the client is receiving.
    4. Notify the client's family of the bruises so they are not surprised on their visit.

107. The resident in a long-term care facility tells the nurse, "I think my family just put me here to die because they think I am too much trouble." Which statement is the nurse's **best** response?
    1. "Can you tell me more about how you feel since your family placed you here?"
    2. "Your family did what they felt was best for your safety."
    3. "Why would you think that about your family? They care for you."
    4. "Tell me, how much trouble were you when you were at home?"

108. The admitting nurse is subpoenaed to give testimony in a case in which the client fell from the bed and fractured their left hip. The nurse initiated fall precautions on admission but was not on duty when the client fell. Which issue should the nurse be prepared to testify about the incident?
    1. The events preceding the client's fall from the bed
    2. The extent of injuries the client sustained
    3. The client's mental status before the incident
    4. The facility's policy covering fall prevention

109. The RN charge nurse must notify a staff member to stay home because of low census. The unit currently has 35 clients having at least one IV line and multiple IV medications. The unit is staffed with two RNs, three LPNs, and three UAPs. Which nurse should be notified to stay home?
    1. The least experienced RN
    2. The most experienced LPN
    3. The UAP asking to be requested off
    4. The UAP hired 4 weeks ago

110. The charge nurse in an extended care facility notes an elderly resident holding hands with another elderly resident. Which intervention should the charge nurse implement?
    1. Do nothing because this is a natural human need.
    2. Notify the family of the residents about the situation.
    3. Separate the residents for all activities.
    4. Call a care plan meeting with other staff members.

111. An extended care facility's chief nursing officer (CNO) is attending shift report with two charge nurses, and an argument about a resident's care ensues. Which action should the CNO implement **first?**
    1. Ask the two charge nurses to stop arguing and go to a private area.
    2. Listen to both sides of the argument and then implement a plan of care.
    3. Ask the family to join the discussion before deciding how to implement care.
    4. Tell the nurses to stop arguing and continue to give report.

112. Which action by the nurse violates The Joint Commission's Patient Safety Goals?
    1. The surgery nurse calls a time-out when a discrepancy is noted on the surgical permit.
    2. The unit nurse asks the client for their date of birth before administering medications.
    3. The nurse educator gives the orientee the answers to the quiz covering the IV pumps.
    4. The admitting nurse initiates the facility's fall prevention program on an older adult client.

113. The ED nurse is triaging victims at a bus accident. Which client would the nurse categorize as red or immediate priority?
    1. The client diagnosed with head trauma exhibiting fixed and dilated pupils
    2. The client diagnosed with compound fractures of the tibia and fibula
    3. The client diagnosed with a sprained right wrist and a 1-inch (2.5-cm) laceration
    4. The client diagnosed with a piece of metal embedded in the right eye

114. The clinic nurse is reviewing the laboratory data of clients seen in the clinic the previous day. Which client requires **immediate** intervention by the nurse?
    1. The client with white blood cell (WBC) count of 9.5×10^3/microL
    2. The client with cholesterol level of 230 mg/dL
    3. The client with calcium level of 10.1 mg/dL
    4. The client with International Normalized Ratio (INR) of 3.8

115. The community health nurse is triaging victims at the scene of a building collapse. Which intervention should the nurse implement **first**?
    1. Discuss the disaster situation with the media.
    2. Write the client's name clearly in the disaster log.
    3. Place disaster tags securely on the victims.
    4. Identify an area for family members to wait.

116. Which statement **best** describes the role of the parish nurse?
    1. The parish nurse practices holistic healthcare within a faith community.
    2. The parish nurse cares for clients in a religious-based hospital.
    3. The parish nurse practices nursing in a parish clinic.
    4. The parish nurse is an LPN caring for clients in the home.

117. The 32-year-old client diagnosed with a traumatic right above-the-elbow amputation tells the home health nurse they are worried about supporting their family and finding employment because they can't be a mechanic anymore. Which intervention should the nurse implement?
    1. Contact the home health agency's occupational therapist.
    2. Refer the client to the state rehabilitation commission.
    3. Ask the home health agency's social worker about disability.
    4. Suggest talking to their spouse about these concerns.

118. The labor and delivery nurse has assisted in the delivery of a 37-week fetal demise. Which intervention should the nurse implement?
    1. Remove the baby from the delivery area quickly.
    2. Tell the client's partner to arrange to take the infant home.
    3. Wrap the infant in a towel and place it aside.
    4. Obtain a lock of the infant's hair for the parents.

119. The newborn nursery nurse has received report. Which client should the nurse assess **first**?
    1. The 2-hour-old infant with nasal flaring and grunting
    2. The 6-hour-old infant having not passed meconium stool
    3. The 12-hour-old infant refusing to latch onto the breast
    4. The 24-hour-old infant with a positive startle reflex

120. The psychiatric clinic nurse is returning telephone calls. Which telephone call should the nurse return **first**?
    1. The client reporting being slapped by their drunk spouse last night
    2. The client reporting being tired of living because their spouse left after the client's job loss
    3. The client diagnosed with anorexia thinking they cannot stand to eat today
    4. The client diagnosed with Parkinson's disease reporting their hands shaking more than yesterday

121. The psychiatric nurse and mental health worker (MHW) on a psychiatric unit are caring for a group of clients. Which nursing task should the RN delegate to the MHW?
    1. Take the school-age children to the on-campus classroom.
    2. Lead a group therapy session on behavior control.
    3. Explain the purpose of recreation therapy to the client.
    4. Give a bipolar client a bed bath and shampoo their hair.

122. The 36-year-old client in the women's health clinic is being prescribed birth control pills. Which information is important for the nurse to teach the client? **Select all that apply.**
    1. Do not smoke while taking birth control pills.
    2. Take one pill at the same time every day.
    3. If a birth control pill is missed, do not double up.
    4. Stop taking the pill if breakthrough bleeding occurs.
    5. There can be interactions with other medications.

123. The nurse is caring for a female client 3 days post–knee replacement surgery when the client reports vaginal itching. The MAR indicates the client has been receiving calcium carbonate, ceftriaxone, and enoxaparin. Which **priority** intervention should the nurse implement?
    1. Request the dietary department to send yogurt on each tray.
    2. Explain to the client this is the result of the antibiotic therapy.
    3. Notify the HCP on rounds of the client's vaginal itching.
    4. Ask the client whether she is having unprotected sexual activity.

124. The nurse manager of the maternal-child department is developing the budget for the next fiscal year. Which statement **best** explains the **first** step of the budgetary process?
    1. Ask the staff for input about needed equipment.
    2. Assess any new department project for costs.
    3. Review the department's current year budget.
    4. Explain the new budget requirements to the staff.

125. The nurse on the psychiatric unit observes one client shove another client. Which intervention should the nurse implement **first**?
    1. Discuss the aggressive behavior with the client.
    2. Document the occurrence in the client's EHR.
    3. Approach the client with another staff member.
    4. Instruct the client to go to the unit's quiet room.

126. The client in the operating room states, "I don't think I will have this surgery after all." Which intervention should the nurse implement **first**?
    1. Have the surgeon speak with the client.
    2. Ask the client to discuss their concerns.
    3. Continue to prep the client for surgery.
    4. Immediately stop the surgical procedure.

127. Which data indicate therapy has been **effective** for the client diagnosed with bipolar disorder?
    1. The client only has four episodes of mania in 6 months.
    2. The client goes to work every day for 9 months.
    3. The client wears a nightgown to the day room for therapy.
    4. The client has had three motor vehicle accidents.

128. The nurse administered erythropoietin alpha to a client diagnosed with anemia. Which data indicate the client may be experiencing an adverse reaction?
    1. BP 200/124 mm Hg
    2. Apical pulse 54 bpm
    3. Hematocrit 38%
    4. Long bone pain

129. The client diagnosed with sickle cell disease reports joint pain rated 10 on a pain scale of 1 to 10. Which intervention should the nurse implement **first?**
    1. Administer a narcotic analgesic to the client.
    2. Check the ID before administering the medication.
    3. Assess the client to rule out (R/O) complications.
    4. Obtain the medication from the medication administration system.

130. The nurse is caring for a 34-year-old female client telling the nurse, "I have been diagnosed with a human papillomavirus (HPV) infection in my mouth. I don't **understand.** I get cervical smears for that." Which is the nurse's **best** response?
    1. "You must have had oral sex to get the HPV infection in your mouth."
    2. "You should have a smear made of your mouth every 6 months from now on."
    3. "I would have the test repeated; it is not possible to have an HPV infection in the mouth."
    4. "This infection is on the rise from oral contact with a person having the infection."

131. The nurse is teaching a health class for 14- to 18-year-old students. Which information regarding sexually transmitted infections (STIs) should the nurse include in the discussion?
    1. HIV is only transmitted through multiple exposures.
    2. The use of a condom during intercourse ensures that an STI is not passed from one partner to the other.
    3. The more sexual contacts an individual has both for oral sex and intercourse, the greater the probability that individual has of contracting an STI.
    4. Syphilis and gonorrhea are easily treatable, and no lasting effects will be experienced with either of these infections.

132. Which nursing task should the experienced pediatric RN delegate to the UAP?
    1. Escort the child being discharged via wheelchair out to the parent's car.
    2. Determine whether a young child's growth and developmental level are on target.
    3. Explain how to care for the teen's below-the-knee cast to the parents.
    4. Assist the HCP to suture an older child's leg laceration.

133. While making rounds, the charge nurse notices an unattended workstation with the computer screen open to a client's EHR. Which actions should the charge nurse implement? **Select all that apply.**
    1. Ensure automatic locks are functioning for inactive workstations.
    2. Leave the EHR open and find the nurse using the workstation.
    3. Educate the unit staff that an unattended and exposed EHR could violate HIPAA.
    4. Protect the workstation from unauthorized viewing of the EHR.
    5. Notify the Office of Civil Rights about a breach of client health information.

134. The clinical manager is presenting a lecture on collective bargaining. One of the nurse participants asks, "What happens if nurses decide to go on strike?" Which statement is the RN clinical nurse manager's **best** response?
    1. "The UAPs and managers will have to take care of the clients."
    2. "If nurses go on strike, it is considered abandonment of the clients."
    3. "The clients will get better care once the nurses' demands are met."
    4. "The nurses must give a 10-day notice before a strike takes place."

ANSWERS AND RATIONALES

The correct answer number and rationale are in **boldface purple type.** Rationales for why other answer options are incorrect are also given.

1. Correct answers are 1, 2, 4, and 5.
   1. The nurse should assess any activities the client was engaging in that they associate with the onset of the pain.
   2. Quality or intensity of pain should be assessed. The client should be asked to describe the pain, such as crushing, stabbing, aching, and so on.
   3. Risk factors for pain are important to assess but are not part of the pain assessment.
   4. Severity should be assessed using a scale of 1 to 10 with 1 representing no pain and 10 representing the worst pain the client can imagine.
   5. Timing and duration should be assessed. How long does the pain last?

2. Correct answers are 1, 2, and 5.
   1. The client's acute respiratory distress is progressing to respiratory failure. The nurse needs to prepare for immediate intubation and mechanical ventilation.
   2. The client needs a high-flow oxygen delivery system to correct hypoxia.
   3. The upright or prone positions support oxygenation and lung expansion. It can be complicated to utilize the prone position if a client is too sick.
   4. Nutritional needs are important but not a priority over respiratory support.
   5. The client should have continuous monitoring of oxygen saturation levels.

3. Correct answers are 2 and 3.
   1. Arterial blood gas readings are used to assess a client's oxygenation but will not confirm ET tube placement.
   2. Listening to the breath sounds in both lungs will indicate whether both lungs are being ventilated.
   3. A portable chest x-ray will be performed to confirm correct ET tube placement.
   4. Capillary refill assesses the blood flow to the periphery; it will not confirm the correct placement of the ET tube.
   5. Suctioning secretions may be necessary but does not confirm correct ET tube placement.

4. Correct answers are 1, 2, 3, and 4.
   1. The client is sedated during an endoscopy and should avoid eating or drinking for 8 hours before the procedure.
   2. The client should not take oral medications such as ACE inhibitors, diuretics, or oral hypoglycemics immediately before the endoscopy procedure. The nurse should confirm with the HCP concerning whether the oral ACE inhibitor should be administered.
   3. The nurse may administer the IV proton pump inhibitor.
   4. The nurse should confirm the consent for the procedure is signed and in the EHR.
   5. An endoscopy takes about 15 minutes to perform. An indwelling urinary catheter is not indicated.

5.
   1. The nurse should determine the presence or absence of the client's gag reflex before administering any PO fluids or medications.
   2. The nurse will give the client their a.m. medications but should assess the gag reflex first.
   3. The client can be given water to gargle for their sore throat, but the nurse should assess the gag reflex first.
   4. The nurse can assess whether the client is hungry, but the nurse should assess the gag reflex before giving the client anything by mouth.

6. Correct answers are 1 and 5.
   1. The UAP can record the amount of output from the NG tube.
   2. Examining the nares is an assessment. The RN should not delegate assessment to the UAP.
   3. Palpating the abdomen is an aseessment. The RN should not delegate assessment to the UAP.
   4. Listening to the bowel sounds is an assessment. The RN should not delegate assessment to the UAP.
   5. Performing mouth care is within the scope of duties for the UAP.

7. Correct answers are 1, 2, 3, and 5.
   1. The nurse should rule out complications before administering narcotic pain medication, which in this case includes an assessment of the client's urine for blood and straining the urine.
   2. The nurse should determine the last time the client received any form of pain medication.
   3. The medication is to be administered intravenously, so the nurse should determine whether the narcotic medication is compatible with the existing IV solution.

4. The nurse should not document the administration of the medication in the EHR until it has been given.
5. The nurse should identify the client and confirm the correct medication and other safety checks before giving the medication.

8. 1. A urinalysis is not indicated immediately following the passage of a renal stone.
   2. The nurse should place the calculus in a sterile specimen cup, label it with the client's information, and send it to the laboratory for analysis.
   3. The bladder scanner is used to evaluate for urinary retention and prevent unnecessary urinary catheterization. It is not indicated immediately following the passage of a renal stone.
   4. Urinary analgesics such as phenazopyridine (AZO, Pyridium) relieve symptoms caused by urinary tract infections and urinary tract irritation. The nurse should first ensure the calculus is sent to the laboratory for analysis.

9. Correct answers are 1, 2, and 3.
   1. The client should be encouraged to consume 8 to 12 cups of fluid a day.
   2. The body may turn extra vitamin C into oxalate. The client should avoid high doses of vitamin C (more than 2,000 mg of vitamin C daily).
   3. Oxalate is found in many foods. The client should limit foods such as nuts or seeds, soy cheese, soy milk, soy yogurt, cereal (bran or high fiber), fruitcake, pretzels, wheat bran, wheat germ, whole wheat bread, whole wheat flour, dark or "robust" beer, black tea, chocolate milk, cocoa, instant coffee, and hot chocolate.
   4. The client should limit oxalate intake to 40 to 50 mg daily.
   5. Blueberries are high in oxalate and contain more than 10 mg per serving. The client should be instructed to limit the consumption of these and other berries.

10. Correct answers are 1, 2, 4, and 5.
    1. The client should be instructed to elevate their affected leg to reduce edema.
    2. Meals high in protein, vitamins, and minerals promote wound healing.
    3. Cellulitis is not treated with topical ointments; it requires systemic antibiotic therapy.
    4. The client should take all systemic antibiotics ordered by the HCP.
    5. Warm compresses to the affected area can help to decrease pain.

11. Correct answers are 2, 3, 4, and 5.
    1. An electrolarynx is an artificial larynx. It can be successfully used for clients with a tracheostomy.
    2. Communication boards with words, pictures, and dry-erase components are helpful to facilitate communication with an intubated client on a ventilator.
    3. Hand gestures are helpful to facilitate communication with an intubated client on a ventilator.
    4. Eye blinks for yes or no questions facilitate communication with an intubated client on a ventilator.
    5. Augmented and assistive communication devices, such as cell phones or tablets, use icons, pictures, and words to facilitate communication.

12. Correct answers are 1, 2, 3, and 4.
    1. The respiratory therapist is a part of the multidisciplinary team and is responsible for the ventilator.
    2. The client should be on continuous monitoring of oxygen saturation.
    3. A manual resuscitation bag should be at the bedside in case of ventilator failure.
    4. The nurse should assess the ventilator settings frequently throughout the shift.
    5. The ventilator alarms should not be silenced, but attempts should be made to decrease alarms to avoid ICU psychosis.

13. 1. Decreased reflexes, loss of sensation, and flaccid paralysis are signs of spinal shock.
    2. Hypotension and bradycardia are signs of neurogenic shock.
    3. Dyspnea and constricted airway are signs of anaphylactic shock.
    4. Tachycardia and confusion are signs of septic shock.

14. Correct answers are 1, 2, 4, and 5.
    1. The client is experiencing ICU psychosis. Clocks and calendars can be used in the ICU to help orient the client to time and date.
    2. The coordination of the day-night pattern, achieved by dimming the lights at night and opening the window blinds during the day, can alleviate ICU psychosis.
    3. The nurse should attempt to structure sleep by creating a wake cycle, clustering sleep, and scheduling rest periods.

4. The client is experiencing ICU psychosis. Familiar objects from home can decrease anxiety for the client.
5. The client is experiencing ICU psychosis. All attempts should be made to minimize noise from nursing shift changes and from alarms on monitoring equipment.

15.
1. The client's Glasgow Coma Scale rating would be 9.
2. The client's Glasgow Coma Scale rating would be 9.
3. The client receives 3 points for opening her eyes when her name is called, 2 points for moaning but no words used, and 4 points for withdrawing her arm away from the nurse in response to pain. The Glasgow Coma Scale rating would be 9.
4. The client's Glasgow Coma Scale rating would be 9.

16. Correct answers are 1, 3, and 5.
1. The nurse should keep the head of the bed elevated 30 degrees to help the lungs expand and prevent stasis of secretions.
2. Active range of motion exercises require the client to participate. The client's Glasgow Coma Scale rating was 9, indicating moderate severity. The client would not be able to participate in this intervention.
3. The nurse should always explain procedures to the client even when the nurse does not know how much the client is hearing.
4. The client should be turned more frequently than every 4 hours to prevent skin breakdown.
5. Traumatic brain injuries impact temperature regulation in the body. Steps should be taken to maintain normothermia in the client.

17.
1. Sudden onset of chest pain and frothy sputum may indicate a pulmonary embolus.
2. Foul-smelling, concentrated urine may indicate a urinary tract infection.
3. DIC symptoms result from clotting and bleeding. Oozing from the IV site would support this diagnosis.
4. Fever of unknown origin may indicate an infection.

18. Correct answers are 1, 2, 3, and 5.
1. The client should be NPO for 8 hours before the procedure.
2. The client will have an IV and be provided with mild sedation or conscious sedation as determined by the HCP.
3. The client should be informed that the nurse will take vital signs every 15 to 30 minutes after the procedure.
4. The client will only have a mild sore throat and minimal discomfort following the procedure. Saline gargles and OTC medication will be recommended as needed.
5. The client should be instructed to contact the HCP if they have any bleeding, vomiting, or severe pain.

19. Correct answers are 1, 2, and 5.
1. The nurse should explain the bowel preparation required before the procedure. This preparation could include PEG-3350-electrolytes (GoLYTELY). The bowel must be free of feces before the procedure.
2. The client should be on a clear liquid diet 24 hours before the procedure and NPO 8 hours before the procedure.
3. The client will not have diet restrictions after the procedure.
4. If no complications arise, the client can go home shortly after the procedure.
5. The client should be instructed to report any rectal bleeding, dizziness or light-headedness (signs of blood loss), and abdominal pain.

20. Correct answers are 1, 3, 4, and 5.
1. The client should be taught the acronym RICE—rest, ice, compression, and elevation. Rest prevents further injury and avoids stress on the injured ankle. The client may need to be taught how to use crutches so that no weight will be placed on the right ankle.
2. The client should be taught to apply ice to the ankle to help decrease pain and edema. Instruct the client not to apply ice directly to the skin; use a towel and apply the ice for 20 minutes at a time, allowing at least 30 minutes to elapse between applications.
3. The nurse should apply compression to support the ankle and help prevent inflammation. An elastic (ACE) bandage should be applied in a figure 8 wrap. It should not be too tight. Toes should not be cold, turn blue, or tingle.
4. The client should be taught to elevate the foot above the level of the heart.
5. Recommend the client use ibuprofen or alternate ibuprofen with acetaminophen for pain and discomfort.

21.
  1. The common cold is caused by a virus; antibiotics only treat bacterial infections. OTC medications can alleviate some of the discomforts of the common cold.
  2. Nasal cultures are not performed for the common cold. Antibiotics are not effective on the common cold virus.
  3. A virus causes the common cold; antibiotics only treat bacterial infections. This is the correct response.
  4. The nurse should not tell the client to go to a different doctor. Not prescribing antibiotics for a viral infection is an appropriate treatment.

22. Correct answers are 1, 3, and 4.
  1. Alcohol, coffee, and caffeinated sodas will increase the possibility of dehydration in the client and should be avoided.
  2. Intranasal zinc is not recommended. In 2009, the Federal Drug Administration warned against intranasal zinc because of its association with long-term or permanent loss of smell in clients. Oral zinc, echinacea, and large doses of vitamin C have conflicting research about their effectiveness.
  3. Chicken noodle soup and other warm fluids can help loosen congestion and have mucus-thinning effects.
  4. A saltwater gargle made with ½ tsp of salt in 8 oz of warm water can help relieve a scratchy throat.
  5. Saline nasal drops and sprays can help alleviate nasal stuffiness and congestion. These items are safe for use, even in children.

23.
  1. The nurse should first assess the client before taking any other action to determine whether the client is experiencing any untoward reaction.
  2. An incident or occurrence report must be completed by the nurse, but not before taking care of the client.
  3. The nurse should administer the correct medication, but not before assessing the client.
  4. The client's HCP must be notified, but the nurse should be able to provide the HCP with pertinent client information, so this is not the first intervention.

24.
  1. The serum blood glucose level requires a venipuncture, which is not within the scope of the UAP's expertise. The laboratory technician would be responsible for obtaining a venipuncture.
  2. This is a sterile dressing change and requires assessing the insertion site for infection; therefore, this would not be the most appropriate task to assign to the LPN.
  3. The RN should ask the UAP to bathe the client and change bed linens because this is a task the UAP can perform. The LPN could be assigned higher-level tasks.
  4. The UAP can add up the urine output for the 12-hour shift; however, the RN is responsible for evaluating whether the urine output is expected for the client.

25.
  1. The client on the ventilator is unstable; therefore, the RN should not delegate any tasks to the UAP.
  2. The UAP can take specimens to the laboratory; this is within the scope of practice for a UAP.
  3. The client in an Addisonian crisis is unstable; therefore, the RN should not delegate tasks to the UAP.
  4. The UAP cannot assist the HCP with an invasive procedure at the bedside.

26.
  1. The client must have lost decision-making capacity because of a condition that is not reversible or must be in a condition specified under state law, such as a terminal, persistent vegetative state, irreversible coma, or as specified in the advance directive. A client exhibiting decerebrate posturing is unconscious and unable to make decisions.
  2. The client on a ventilator has not lost the ability to make healthcare decisions. The nurse can communicate by asking clients to blink their eyes to yes or no questions.
  3. The client receiving dialysis is alert and does not lose the ability to make decisions; therefore, the advance directive should not be consulted to make decisions for the client.
  4. Being intellectually disabled does not mean the client cannot make decisions unless the client has a legal guardian with a durable power of attorney for healthcare. If the client has a legal guardian, then the client cannot complete an advance directive.

27. Correct answers are 1, 2, 4, and 5.
  1. The UAP can apply sequential compression devices to the client on strict bedrest.
  2. The UAP can assist in positioning the client for a portable STAT chest x-ray.
  3. The client must be premedicated for wound débridement; therefore, this task cannot be delegated to the UAP.

4. The UAP can obtain intake and output for clients.
5. The UAP can check the blood glucose level of stable clients. The designation that the checks are to be performed before meals and at bedtime indicates a routine order.

28. 1. A quality improvement project examines how tasks are performed and attempts to see whether the system can be improved. A medication delivery system in which it takes a long time for the nurse to receive a STAT or "now" medication is an example of a system that needs improvement and should be addressed by a quality improvement committee.
2. Financial staff reimbursement is a management issue, not a quality improvement issue.
3. Collective bargaining is an administrative issue, not a quality improvement issue.
4. The number of medication errors a nurse commits is a management-to-nurse issue. It does not involve a systems issue unless several nurses have committed the same error because the system is not functioning properly.

29. 1. A secondary nursing intervention includes screening for early detection. The bone density evaluation will determine the density of the bone and is diagnostic for osteoporosis.
2. Spinal screening examinations are performed on adolescents to detect scoliosis. This is a secondary nursing intervention, but is not used to detect osteoporosis.
3. Teaching the client is a primary nursing intervention. This is an appropriate intervention to help prevent osteoporosis but is not a secondary intervention.
4. Discussing risk factors is an appropriate intervention but is not a secondary nursing intervention.

30. 1. The clients would not understand the importance of the specific tasks. Clients will tell the RN whether the UAP is pleasant in the room but not whether the delegated tasks have been completed.
2. The nurse retains responsibility for the delegated tasks. The charge nurse may be able to tell the RN that the UAP has been checked off as competent to perform the care but would not know whether the care was provided.

3. The nurse retains responsibility for the care. Making rounds to see that the care has been provided is the best method to evaluate the care.
4. The nurse would not have time to complete the nursing duties if the RN watched the UAP perform all the UAP's work.

31. 1. A client in a crisis should be assigned to the RN.
2. Biliary atresia involves liver failure involving multiple body systems. This client should be assigned to the RN.
3. Anaphylaxis is an emergency. The client should be assigned to the RN.
4. The LPN can administer routine medications and care for clients having no life-threatening conditions.

32. 1. The nurse would expect the client diagnosed with DIC to be oozing blood; however, the presence of a seizure indicates bleeding in the brain. This client should be assessed first.
2. The nurse would expect the client diagnosed with BPH to have urinary findings such as terminal dribbling, so the nurse does not need to assess this client first.
3. The nurse would expect the client diagnosed with renal calculi to have blood in the urine (hematuria) and flank pain; therefore, the nurse does not need to assess this client first.
4. The nurse would expect the client diagnosed with Addison's disease to have bronze pigmentation and hypoglycemia; therefore, the nurse should not need to assess this client first.

33. 1. The most experienced nurse should be assigned to the client who requires teaching and evaluation of knowledge for home healthcare because the client is in the surgery center for less than 1 day.
2. A routine preoperative client does not require the most experienced nurse.
3. Any nurse can administer and monitor a blood transfusion to the client.
4. Although creating an arteriovenous fistula requires assessment and teaching from the most experienced nurse, this client is not being discharged home at this time.

34. 1. The Glasgow Coma Scale ranges from 0 to 15, with 15 indicating the client's neurological status is intact. A Glasgow Coma Scale score of 13 indicates the client is stable and would be the most appropriate client to assign to the graduate nurse.

2. This client's K⁺ level is low, and the client is at risk for developing cardiac dysrhythmias; therefore, the client should be assigned to a more experienced nurse.
3. This client has low blood pressure, evidence of tachycardia, and could go into an Addisonian crisis, which is a potentially life-threatening condition. A more experienced nurse should be assigned to this client.
4. A positive Trousseau sign indicates the client is hypocalcemic and experiencing a surgery complication; therefore, this client should be assigned to a more experienced nurse.

35. 1. The therapeutic PTT should be 1.5 to 2 times the control time. Most control times average 35 seconds, so the therapeutic levels of heparin would place the control between 52 and 70 seconds. With a PTT of 92 seconds, the client is at risk for bleeding, and the heparin drip should be held. The nurse should assess this client first.
    2. A client diagnosed with pneumonia would be expected to have a fever. This client can be seen after the client diagnosed with a DVT.
    3. Cystitis is inflammation of the urinary bladder, and burning on urination is an expected symptom.
    4. Pancreatitis is a very painful condition. Pain is a priority but not over the potential for hemorrhage.

36. Correct answers are 3, 4, and 5.
    1. Teaching is the responsibility of the RN and cannot be delegated to a UAP.
    2. The word "check" indicates a step in the assessment process, and the RN cannot delegate assessing to a UAP.
    3. The client is 2 days postoperative, and vital signs should be stable, so the UAP can take vital signs. The RN must ensure the UAP knows to immediately report vital signs that are not within the guidelines the nurse provides to the UAP.
    4. This action does not require judgment on the part of the UAP. It does not require assessing, teaching, or evaluating. This can be delegated to the UAP.
    5. A client 2 days postoperative should be ambulating frequently. The UAP can perform this task.

37. 1. Staff members will not stay if forced to always use their paid time off for the hospital's convenience.
    2. This nurse wants to take time off. Therefore, it is best to let the nurse desiring to be off from work to take time off if all other situations are equal.
    3. The nurse will not gain experience if always requested not to come to work, and presumably, this nurse would not have benefit time to pay for the time out of work.
    4. This nurse could be allowed to stay home only if the nurse is still ill.

38. 1. An RN, not the UAP, should perform sterile dressing changes.
    2. A nurse should perform this task because this client is unstable.
    3. The UAP can check the amount of food the residents consume and document the information.
    4. This is the job of the activity director and volunteers working with the activities department. Staffing is limited in any nursing area; the UAP should be assigned a nursing task.

39. 1. The LPN charge nurse is not the nurse educator but is responsible for the subordinate UAPs. This is adding additional duties to the charge nurse.
    2. The director of nurses should encourage responsible behavior on the part of all staff. The LPN charge nurse is performing a part of the responsibility of the charge nurse and should be encouraged to work with the UAP.
    3. Because this is not a private conversation about a client, there is no reason for the charge nurse to be told to go to a private area. The LPN charge nurse is not reprimanding the UAP.
    4. The director of nurses should not interfere with a "better explanation." This could intimidate the charge nurse and make it difficult for the charge nurse to perform their duties.

40. Correct answers are 2, 3, 4, and 5.
    1. Wound debriding formulations are medications, and a UAP cannot administer medications.
    2. The UAP can position the resident so that pressure is not placed on the resident's heels.
    3. The UAP can turn the resident.
    4. The UAP can give the resident a protein shake to drink.
    5. The UAP can assist the resident in dressing and changing clothes.

41. 1. The nurse should implement the least restrictive measures to ensure client safety. Restraining a client is one of the last measures implemented.
    2. **Moving the client near the nursing station where the staff can closely observe the client is one of the first measures in most fall prevention policies.**
    3. This is considered medical restraints and one of the last measures to prevent falls.
    4. Four side rails are considered a restraint. Research has shown that having four side rails up does not prevent falls and only gives the client farther to fall when the client climbs over the rails before falling to the floor.

42. 1. The first intervention is for the nurse to ensure the client is safe in the home. Assessing for grab bars in the bathroom is addressing the safety of the client.
    2. Taking a shower in a stall shower may be safer than getting in and out of a bathtub, but the nurse should first determine whether the client has grab bars and safety equipment when taking a shower.
    3. According to the NCLEX-RN® test plan for management of care, the nurse must be knowledgeable of referrals. The physical therapist can help the client with transferring, ambulation, and other lower extremity difficulties and is an appropriate intervention, but it is not the nurse's first intervention. Safety is the priority.
    4. NSAIDs are used to decrease the pain of osteoarthritis, but this intervention will not address safety issues for the client getting into and out of the bathtub.

43. 1. The employee health nurse should keep the clients at the clinic or send them to the ED. The clients should be kept together until the causes of their illnesses are determined. If it is determined that the clients are stable and not contagious, they should be driven home.
    2. **The employee health nurse should be aware that six clients with the same symptoms indicate a potential deliberate or accidental dispersal of toxic or infectious agents. The nurse must notify the public health department so that an investigation of the cause can be initiated and appropriate action to contain the cause can be taken.**
    3. As long as the clients are stable, the nurse should keep the clients in the employee health clinic. These clients should not be exposed to other clients and ED staff. If the clients must be transferred, decontamination procedures may need to be initiated.
    4. The client may need to provide stool specimens, but this would be done at the ED. Employee health clinics do not have laboratory facilities to perform tests on stools.

44. 1. This child needs an x-ray to rule out a fractured left leg, but this is not life-threatening.
    2. **Drooling and not wanting to swallow are the cardinal signs of epiglottitis, which is potentially life-threatening. This child should be assessed first. The nurse should not attempt to visualize the throat area and should allow the HCP to do this in case an emergency tracheostomy is required.**
    3. A child usually does not report a headache, and this child should be assessed, but it is not life-threatening.
    4. This client may have type 1 diabetes mellitus and should be assessed, but this is not life-threatening at this time.

45. 1. This is an example of community-based nursing in which nurses care for a client living in the community.
    2. **Community-oriented, population-focused nursing practice involves the engagement of nursing in promoting and protecting the health of populations, not individuals in the community. Therefore, this is an example of community-oriented, population-focused nursing.**
    3. This is an example of community-based nursing, in which nurses care for a client living in the community.
    4. This is an example of community-based nursing, in which nurses care for a client living in the community.

46. 1. Dyspnea and confusion are not expected in a client diagnosed with AIDS; therefore, this client would warrant a more experienced nurse to assess the reason for the complications.
    2. The client with financial problems should be assigned to a social worker, not a nurse.
    3. A full-thickness (third-degree) burn is the most serious and requires excellent assessment skills to determine whether complications occur. This client should be assigned to a more experienced nurse.

47.
4. The client diagnosed with diabetic neuropathy would be expected to have pain; therefore, this client could be assigned to a nurse new to home health nursing. The client is not exhibiting a complication or an unexpected sign or symptom.

47. 1. The RN cannot delegate assessment to the home health aide.
2. The aide cannot assess the incisional wound, and the wound should be assessed. The RN cannot delegate assessment.
3. The aide can place the right leg on two pillows. This task does not require assessment, teaching, or evaluating, and the client is stable.
4. Mopping the floor is not part of the aide's responsibility. This is not an appropriate task to delegate.

48. 1. The nurse would expect the client diagnosed with an MI to have an elevated troponin level; thus, the nurse would not assess this client first.
2. Because the client's PTT of 68 seconds is 1.5 to 2 times the normal range, the anticoagulant heparin is considered therapeutic and would not warrant the nurse's assessing this client first.
3. The nurse would expect a client diagnosed with end-stage liver failure to have an elevated ammonia level.
4. The therapeutic range for the anticonvulsant phenytoin (Dilantin) is 10 to 20 mcg/mL. This client's higher level warrants intervention because the serum level is above the therapeutic range.

49. 1. This client would not benefit from acupuncture.
2. Mental health issues are not treated with acupuncture. They may be treated with herbal supplements.
3. The client diagnosed with asthma must be treated with a medical regimen.
4. Acupuncture, the most common complementary therapy recommended by HCPs, would benefit a client diagnosed with osteoarthritis.

50. 1. The RN should not make the client dependent on family members to prepare meals. If the family were willing to do this, they would probably already do it.
2. The occupational therapist would teach the client how to cook, but this client is 88 years old and needs meals provided. Therefore, delivering meals through Meals on Wheels is the most appropriate intervention.
3. The aide's duties do not include cooking all three meals for the client.
4. Meals on Wheels delivers a hot, nutritionally balanced meal once a day on weekdays, usually at noon for older people without assistance in the home for food preparation. This intervention would be most helpful to the client.

51. 1. Home healthcare agency employees are responsible for knowing and adhering to the professional boundary-crossing standards. The nurse should not discuss this with the client.
2. Home healthcare agencies are required by law to address the concepts in the National Association for Home Care (NAHC) Bill of Rights with all home health clients on the initial visit. The agencies may also make additions to the NAHC's original Bill of Rights.
3. The nurse should discuss this with the client, but it is not a legal intervention.
4. This is a true statement but not a legal intervention. If the client is not homebound, they are not eligible for home healthcare.

52. 1. Taping petroleum gauze over the chest tube insertion site will prevent air from entering the pleural space. This is the first intervention.
2. The RN should make sure the UAP knows the correct method to assist a client with a chest tube, but the safety of the client is the first priority.
3. This is the second intervention the nurse should implement. Remember, if the client is in distress and the nurse can do something to relieve that distress, then the nurse should not assess first. The nurse should take action to take care of the client.
4. The nurse should obtain the necessary equipment for the HCP to reinsert the chest tube, but the priority intervention is to prevent air from entering the pleural space.

53. 1. The LPN can administer routine medications.
2. The UAP, not the LPN, should be assigned to take the routine vital signs.
3. The unit secretary, not an LPN, should be assigned to transcribe the HCP orders.

4. The RN, not the LPN, should assess the urinary output of the client. The RN should not delegate assessment.

54. 1. The clinical manager may need to discuss the EHR with some nurses individually, but it is not the clinical manager's first intervention.
    2. **The first intervention should be to arrange meetings to explain the new EHR and allow nurses to ask questions to clarify the new policy.**
    3. The clinical manager can provide a written handout explaining the new EHR, but the first intervention should be small discussion groups.
    4. A video is an excellent tool for explaining new procedures, but the first intervention should be small discussion groups so that all questions can be answered.

55. 1. The nurse would expect the client diagnosed with an abdominal aortic aneurysm to have an audible bruit; therefore, this client does not warrant immediate intervention.
    2. The nurse would expect the client diagnosed with pneumonia to have respiratory symptoms; therefore, this client does not warrant immediate intervention.
    3. One of the findings of bacterial meningitis is nuchal rigidity; therefore, this client does not warrant immediate intervention.
    4. **The client diagnosed with Crohn's disease will have pain and diarrhea during an exacerbation. The presence of vomiting, however, could indicate a bowel obstruction, which is a complication of Crohn's disease.**

56. 1. The client diagnosed with CKD would have an elevated creatinine level. The normal creatinine level is 0.61 to 1.21 mg/dL in males and 0.51 to 1.04 mg/dL in females. The data would not warrant immediate intervention.
    2. Peritonitis, inflammation of the peritoneum, is a serious complication resulting in a hard, rigid abdomen; therefore, a soft abdomen would not warrant immediate intervention.
    3. **The dialysate return should be colorless or straw-colored but never be cloudy, indicating an infection; therefore, the data warrant immediate intervention.**
    4. Because the client has end-stage renal disease, fluid must be removed from the body, so the output should be more than the amount instilled; therefore, this indicates that peritoneal dialysis is effective and does not warrant intervention.

57. 1. The nurse could ask this question, but the client has already told the nurse that 3 years have passed, so the client has tried approximately 36 times.
    2. **This is the best question to assess the client. The nurse would not want to suggest a futile intervention.**
    3. Infertility treatments are very expensive, but the nurse should assess the client's attempts.
    4. This question does not help assess the client or address the client's statement.

58. 1. The reason that the first pregnancy did not yield a viable infant is irrelevant now. The relevant information is whether the mother received the Rho(D) immune globulin injection.
    2. **The important information to assess is whether the client received the Rho(D) immune globulin (RhoGAM) injection within 72 hours of losing the first pregnancy. If the client did not receive the injection, the fetus is at risk for erythroblastosis fetalis.**
    3. This is not important information at this time.
    4. This is not important information at this time.

59. Correct answers are 1, 3, and 5.
    1. This child has injuries consistent with child abuse. Child Protective Services and the police should be notified.
    2. This could result in being unable to prosecute the perpetrator if the nurse is not trained in forensic medicine.
    3. The nurse should determine the full extent of the child's injuries.
    4. The nurse should not notify the parent of the potential involvement. The police are fully capable of doing this for themselves. The nurse could instigate an inflammatory situation with this action.
    5. The child needs x-ray studies to determine the extent of internal injuries.

60. Correct order is 5, 3, 2, 4, 1.
    5. Taking the vital signs is part of the assessment and a beginning point for the nurse.
    3. Because the child has been losing fluids, the nurse should assess tissue turgor to determine whether the parents' fluid replacement has been effective.

2. The nurse should make sure that the parents do not leave the child alone in the room; the nurse should make sure the parents are aware of any safety measures used to protect the toddler from abduction, as well as how to call the nurse in case of need.
4. The client will need diapers. They should be available to the parents so the diaper can be changed and the child will not develop skin irritation problems.
1. When the nurse provides the diapers, it is a good opportunity for the nurse to teach the parents about weighing the diapers before and after the child soils them.

61. 1. This client is exhibiting symptoms of a potentially fatal complication of DVT—pulmonary embolism. The nurse should assess this client first.
2. Refusing to eat hospital food should be discussed with the client, but the nurse could ask the unit secretary to have the dietitian see the client.
3. Clients diagnosed with pancreatitis have nasogastric tubes to rest the bowel. However, these tubes are typically uncomfortable. Regardless, the nurse should see this client after the client diagnosed with DVT has been assessed and appropriate interventions initiated. The nurse should discuss the importance of maintaining the tube with the client.
4. This is an expected symptom of osteoarthritis. This client does not need to be assessed first.

62. 1. This client may be developing a complication of immobility, one of which is pneumonia. The nurse should assess this client first.
2. Weight loss in a client diagnosed with CHF indicates the client is responding to therapy. This client does not need to be assessed first.
3. Pressure injuries are a chronic problem frequently in paralyzed clients. This client does not need to be assessed first.
4. Paralysis is expected for a CVA. This client does not need to be assessed first.

63. 1. The nurse should first medicate the client because this procedure is very painful for the client.
2. The nurse should prepare the equipment, but not before medicating the client. This should be done 30 minutes before the procedure starts.
3. The nurse should use nonsterile gloves to remove the old dressing but not before medicating the client.
4. The nurse should don sterile gloves (can put one on the dominant hand), but not before medicating the client.

64. 1. Administering pain medication is the RN's responsibility, not that of the UAP.
2. A washcloth should be provided to the client before a meal but not before ambulating with the physical therapist.
3. The client should be ready to work on therapy when the physical therapist arrives. The UAP should ensure the client has used the bathroom or has not been incontinent before the therapist arrives, thus making the most efficient use of the therapist's time.
4. Obtaining a walker that is the correct height for the client is the physical therapist's responsibility, not that of the UAP.

65. 1. The fact that the client is a neighbor of the volunteer has no bearing on whether or not the nurse can discuss a client's condition with the volunteer. The nurse should inform the volunteer that information obtained inadvertently is still confidential.
2. The nurse cannot release the client's information in layperson's or medical terms; this violates the HIPAA. In many facilities, the client can give a "password" to individuals designated to receive information about the client's condition.
3. The nurse should not discuss the situation with the client. This would alert the client to potential breaches of confidentiality.
4. The nurse should remind the volunteer of the HIPAA and confidentiality rules that govern any information concerning clients in a healthcare setting.

66. 1. Under shared governance, some nurses become so involved with managing facilities that they are no longer eligible for representation by a bargaining agent (union), but there are no guarantees.
2. The manager is responsible for disseminating information under a centralized organization system.
3. Shared governance is an organizational framework in which the nurse has autonomy over the nursing practice. The nurse is given direct input into the workings of the unit.

4. Shared governance is a system in which the nurse represents the nursing practice.

67. 1. This might be the second statement for the nurse to make if the client does not calm down and discuss the problems with the nurse. Because it could escalate the anger, it should not be the first statement.
    2. The nurse should remain calm and allow the client to verbalize their frustrations more acceptably. The nurse should repeat instructions to the client calmly and in a low voice.
    3. This statement will escalate the situation and could cause the visitor to lash out at the nurse.
    4. This statement will escalate the situation and could cause the visitor to lash out at the nurse.

68. 1. The nurse should leave if determining that the staffing is not now nor ever will be as it was relayed in the interview; however, this may be a temporary situation that can be resolved.
    2. The nurse should give the manager a chance to discuss the situation before quitting. A temporary problem, such as illness, may be affecting staffing.
    3. This action could cause the manager to think of the new nurse as a troublemaker.
    4. The nurse should not discuss this with the charge nurse because this may cause a rift between the charge nurse and the new nurse. The nurse should clarify the staffing situation with the unit manager.

69. Correct order is 1, 5, 2, 3, 4.
    1. This is the first intervention the nurse should implement. Checking the HCP's order is the priority.
    5. This is the second intervention; the nurse should not administer the antibiotic if it is incompatible with the primary IV line.
    2. This is the third intervention the nurse should implement. Determining whether the antibiotic is compatible is second because client allergies won't be assessed if the medication is incompatible.
    3. This is the fourth intervention. The secondary IVPB (antibiotic) must be hung above the primary IV bag so the IVPB will infuse.
    4. This is the fifth intervention. Ensuring the right rate is necessary before starting the infusion.

70. 1. Checking the client's armband is done before actually administering the medications, but it is not the first action for the nurse to take.
    2. The nurse should have assessed the client's IV site on first rounds. At this time, all medications to be administered are oral.
    3. This is part of the two-identifier system of medication administration implemented to prevent medication errors, but it is not the first action for the nurse to take.
    4. The nurse should assess the client's last potassium (K^+) level because hypokalemia (abnormally low K^+ level) is the most common cause of dysrhythmias in clients receiving digoxin (Lanoxin) secondary to clients concurrently taking diuretics. Furosemide (Lasix) is a loop diuretic. The nurse should check for digoxin and K^+ levels and apical pulse (AP) before administering digoxin.

71. 1. This client has been on a medication to control the angina for 2 days and could be discharged.
    2. This client is currently completing the care that would be provided in the hospital setting. The client can be taught to continue the warfarin (Coumadin) at home and return to the HCP's office for blood work, or a home health nurse can be assigned to go to the client's home and draw blood for the laboratory work.
    3. This client should remain in the hospital for the required IVPB medication because resistant infections are very difficult to treat.
    4. These blood gases are expected for a client diagnosed with COPD. This client could go home with oxygen and home health follow-up care.

72. 1. The nurse may wish to consult the hospital's attorneys or retain a personal attorney, but this is not the first action for the nurse.
    2. The nurse should be familiar with the EHR and the situation so that details can be remembered. This should be the nurse's first action.
    3. It is too late to purchase liability insurance to cover the current situation. The nurse may wish to purchase insurance for any future litigation.
    4. The nurse should refrain from discussing the case with anyone with the potential to be called as a witness or be named in the lawsuit.

73. 1. One of the many jobs of a manager is to see that performance evaluations are completed on the staff.
    2. The manager should receive input from many sources to make decisions. Some decisions are made for the manager by the administration based on costs or other reasons.
    3. The nurses retain responsibility for their actions because they practice under the state's Nurse Practice Act. The manager maintains responsibility for the functioning of the unit.
    4. The nurse manager attends many meetings on nursing but attends medical committee meetings only when a nursing issue is being discussed.

74. 1. Usually, the charge nurse should attempt to settle a conflict at the lowest level possible, in this case, confronting the nurse. However, the charge nurse does not have the authority to require a drug screen, which is the intervention needed in this situation. The charge nurse should notify the unit manager.
    2. The charge nurse does not have the authority to force the nurse to submit to a drug screening, which is what this behavior will ultimately require. Therefore, the charge nurse should not confront the staff nurse. The charge nurse should notify the supervisor.
    3. Nurses can take breaks with or without their peers. The charge nurse cannot enforce this option.
    4. An occurrence report is not used for this type of situation. This is a management or peer review issue. The nurse can go through the manager or a peer review committee.

75. 1. Telling jokes with sexual innuendos creates a "hostile work environment" and should be addressed with the HCP. This is a courtesy to allow the HCP to correct the behavior without being embarrassed.
    2. If the behavior is not corrected, the nurse should report the HCP to the manager or CNO. The manager or CNO may need to report the behavior to the medical staff committee or president.
    3. The charge nurse should first report the behavior to the manager and then, if the problem is not resolved, to the CNO; in other words, follow the chain of command.
    4. Some facilities have a code for staff to use when an HCP is acting out, but it is rarely, if ever, used.

76. 1. The nurse would not need to notify the surgeon of the client's refusal because this is a situation the nurse should manage.
    2. Feeling a "pop" after an abdominal hysterectomy may indicate possible wound dehiscence, which is a surgical emergency and requires the nurse to notify the surgeon via telephone.
    3. This situation indicates that it is time for the nurse to reinfuse the lost blood.
    4. A negative Chvostek sign is normal and indicates the calcium level is within normal limits.

77. 1. After an endotracheal tube, the client would have a sore throat; therefore, the PACU nurse would not assess this client first.
    2. A pulse oximeter reading lower than 93% indicates an oxygenation problem; therefore, this client should be assessed first.
    3. Epidural surgery affects the lower extremities, so a palpable pedal pulse indicates a sufficient blood supply; this client should not be assessed first.
    4. Drainage of green bile from the NG tube is normal; therefore, this client should not be seen first.

78. 1. After assessing the client's vital signs, the nurse may need to increase the client's IV rate, but it is not the first intervention.
    2. The nurse should assess the client's vital signs, but not before stopping the bleeding.
    3. The nurse should keep a large tourniquet at the client's bedside and should apply it when suspecting arterial bleeding; this is the nurse's first intervention.
    4. The nurse must notify the client's HCP, but the nurse must first address the immediate concern, which is hemorrhaging.

79. 1. The nurse should always document the findings in the EHR, but the first intervention is to get help because the client has neurovascular compromise.
    2. Elevating the client's right hand will not help neurovascular compromise.
    3. The Doppler ultrasound can assess the radial pulse, but this client is experiencing neurovascular compromise, which requires immediate medical intervention.
    4. The client is exhibiting severe neurovascular compromise, which indicates a surgical complication and requires notifying the surgeon immediately.

80. 1. The first time a client ambulates after hip surgery should be with a physical therapist or an RN qualified to evaluate the client's ability to ambulate safely with a walker. The UAP does not have these qualifications.
    2. **According to the National Council of State Boards of Nursing (NCSBN), collaboration with interdisciplinary team members is part of the Management of Care. Physical therapy is responsible for the management of the client's ability to move and transfer.**
    3. The physical therapist will measure the client and obtain the correct walker for the client.
    4. The social worker is not responsible for assisting the client to ambulate but may assist the client on discharge in obtaining needed medical equipment in the home.

81. 1. The LPN can bathe a client, but this should be assigned to the UAP, thereby allowing the LPN to perform a higher-level task.
    2. The LPN can document the amount of food the client eats, but this should be assigned to the UAP, thereby allowing the LPN to perform a higher-level task.
    3. According to the NCLEX-RN® test plan, collaboration with interdisciplinary team members is part of the management of care. The activity director of the long-term care facility would be responsible for this activity.
    4. **The LPN's scope of practice allows routine sterile procedures on stable clients, such as clients in a surgical rehabilitation facility.**

82. 1. The RN should assess the client's neurovascular status when the UAP reports any abnormality.
    2. The client should be repositioned by log rolling, but it is inappropriate when the client has a neurovascular compromise.
    3. **The nurse should assess the client whenever receiving any information from another healthcare team member.**
    4. The nurse should not request another healthcare team member to assess a client exhibiting a possible surgical complication.

83. 1. The client having just returned from surgery should not be transferred from the ICU because the client may not be stable.
    2. A sigmoid colostomy is a surgical procedure that causes major fluid shifts and has the potential for multiple complications; therefore, this client should not be transferred to the surgical unit.
    3. **Although the client is only 1 day postoperative for a total hip replacement, it is an elective procedure, which indicates that the client was stable before the surgery. The incision is also dry and intact. Of the four clients, this client is the most stable and should be transferred to the surgical unit.**
    4. A fat embolism is a potentially life-threatening complication of a fracture; therefore, this client should not be transferred from the ICU.

84. 1. Family members should be asked to stay in the client's room until the lights come back on. This helps ensure the safety of the family members.
    2. **During an electrical failure, the red outlets in the hospital run on the backup generator, and all IV pumps and necessary equipment should be plugged into these outlets.**
    3. The hospital may provide tap bells for contacting the hospital staff but would not provide flashlights to all clients. The hospital staff would need the flashlights.
    4. The charge nurse should not tie up the phone lines during an emergency; the phones may not even work.

85. 1. The charge nurse should contact the laboratory, but the first action should be to address the HCP's behavior in a private area.
    2. **This is the charge nurse's first action because it will diffuse the HCP's anger. Inappropriate behavior at the nurse's station should not occur in an area where visitors, clients, or staff will observe the behavior.**
    3. The HCP can call the laboratory and share concerns, but it is not the first intervention.
    4. The charge nurse can report any HCP's inappropriate behavior, but the immediate situation must be handled first.

86. 1. The staff nurse should go through the chain of command pursuant to investigating a problem.
    2. **Increased infection rates among clients with PICCs fall within the infection control nurse's scope of practice, and the infection control nursing staff will have data from all units in the hospital.**

3. The nurse should follow through with investigating a potential problem, but this problem does not fall within the scope of practice of the employee health nurse.
4. The staff nurse should be a part of the solution to a problem. Volunteering is an excellent action to effect change, but it is not the first action. More information—which the infection control nurse can provide—is necessary first.

87. 1. Because multiple surgical clients require custodial care, the RN charge nurse should not send an experienced UAP to the medical unit.
2. The charge nurse should not send the experienced RN to the medical unit because this nurse represents the strength of the staff.
3. The LPN would be the most appropriate staff to send to the medical unit because the LPN has experience in the unit. The expertise of the LPN is also not required to perform custodial care.
4. A new orientee should not be sent to an unfamiliar area.

88. Correct order is 2, 4, 3, 1, 5. The nurse must remember the acronym RACE(E), a recognized national fire safety standard in healthcare facilities.
2. R is for rescue.
4. A is for alert.
3. C is for confine.
1. E is for extinguish.
5. E is for evacuate.

89. 1. The nurse should notify the operating room team, but according to The Joint Commission, the first intervention is to call a time-out, which stops the surgery until clarification is obtained.
2. According to The Joint Commission, the first intervention is to call a time-out, which stops the surgery until clarification is obtained.
3. The nurse should discuss this with the client but should first initiate the time-out procedure.
4. Calling the surgeon is a part of the time-out procedure, so the first intervention is to call the time-out.

90. 1. The nurse should initiate a client care conference to discuss the client's feelings, but at this time, the most appropriate response is to allow the client to begin the grieving process.
2. The nurse could notify the social worker about the client's situation, but the most appropriate response is to allow the client to begin the grieving process, which the client often goes through when experiencing any loss. In this situation, the client is losing independence and their home.
3. The client does not owe the nurse an explanation for "feelings."
4. According to the NCLEX-RN® test plan, advocacy is part of Management of Care under Safe and Effective Care Environment client needs. Therapeutic communication involves advocating in this situation because sometimes the nurse cannot prevent a perceived "bad" situation from occurring.

91. 1. The client cannot be restrained just as needed. The nurse must have documentation for the need and an HCP's specific order, including the reason for restraint and the time limited to 24 hours. This HCP order should be clarified.
2. The restrained client should be offered fluids at least every 2 hours.
3. Hand mitts are the least restrictive limb restraints and can help prevent the client from pulling out lines.
4. The nurse must ensure that restrained limbs have adequate circulation at least every 2 hours.

92. 1. The RN is responsible for assessing clients; therefore, this assignment is appropriate.
2. The LPN may be allowed to administer IVP medications in some facilities, but the word "all" makes this an inappropriate assignment. Many IVP medications are considered high-risk, and only RNs should administer such IVP medications.
3. This option has the word "all," but it is within the scope of the UAP to complete the a.m. care. The a.m. care can be performed by the RN and LPN but should be assigned to the UAP.
4. The RN should monitor laboratory values because this sometimes requires interpretation, evaluation, and notification of the HCP.

93. 1. Tardiness information is objective data obtained for all employees in the facility, but it does not explicitly provide information about the nurse's performance.
2. The nurse's attitude is very subjective when evaluating, and it does not explicitly provide information about the nurse's performance.

3. Thank-you notes from the clients are nice for the nurse to receive, but they are not taken into consideration during the evaluation process of the nurse.
4. The nurse's ability to document client care directly correlates with the nurse's performance; therefore, this data should be included in the yearly evaluation.

94. 1. The home healthcare agency would not be the best referral because comorbid conditions increase the client's recovery time. The client at home cannot access healthcare 24 hours a day.
 2. A senior citizen center may help the client's psychosocial needs but not the client's rehabilitation needs.
 3. The rehabilitation facility will provide intensive therapy and address the comorbid conditions 24 hours a day. This will assist in the client's recovery.
 4. An outpatient physical therapist is not educated to address and care for the comorbid issues. The physical therapist is focused on the hip fracture only, and the client may have transportation problems going to an outpatient clinic.

95. 1. The NG tube should be replaced, but this task will require more time and require new equipment; therefore, it should not be done first.
 2. The client scheduled for surgery is the priority and must be ready when the operating room calls; therefore, completing the preoperative checklist is the first task the nurse should implement. The preoperative checklist ensures the client's safety.
 3. The client being discharged can wait until the safety needs of the client going to surgery have been addressed.
 4. This is a minimal amount of drainage, which can require a dressing change, but not before making sure the client going to surgery is ready.

96. 1. Antiplatelet medication will increase the client's bleeding time and should be held 5 days before surgery; therefore, clopidogrel (Plavix) should be questioned.
 2. A client with a TKR is at risk for developing DVT; therefore, enoxaparin (Lovenox), an anticoagulant medication, would not be questioned.
 3. The client with a Whipple procedure has had part of the pancreas removed and is placed on insulin; therefore, the nurse would not question administering sliding scale regular insulin.
 4. Vancomycin, an aminoglycoside antibiotic, is not in the penicillin family; therefore, the nurse would not question administering this medication.

97. 1. A client 4 hours postoperative for abdominal surgery would be expected to have abdominal pain and hypoactive bowel sounds secondary to general anesthesia. This client would not be assessed first.
 2. This output indicates the client is voiding at least 30 mL (1 oz) an hour; therefore, the nurse would not assess this client first.
 3. The client with an open cholecystectomy frequently has a T-tube that would typically drain green bile. This client would not be assessed first.
 4. The client is exhibiting signs of compromised circulation; therefore, the nurse should assess this client first. The nurse should assess for the 6 Ps: pain, pulse, paresthesia, paralysis, pallor, and polar (cold).

98. 1. This situation should be addressed first because the charge nurse is responsible for family and client reports of concerns. If the family contacts the administration, the charge nurse must know the situation.
 2. The evaluation needs to be completed, but it does not take priority over handling an angry family member.
 3. The charge nurse could assign this task to another nurse or unit secretary. Dealing appropriately with an angry family member takes priority over calling the laboratory.
 4. The charge nurse could assign this task to another nurse or unit secretary. Dealing appropriately with an irate family member takes priority over transferring a client.

99. 1. Autocratic managers use an authoritarian approach to direct the activities of others.
 2. Laissez-faire managers maintain a permissive climate with little direction or control.
 3. A democratic manager is people-oriented and facilitates efficient group functioning. The environment is open, and communication flows both ways. This includes having meetings to discuss concerns.
 4. This statement reflects shirking of responsibility, thus letting someone else address the problem, and is not characteristic of a democratic manager.

100. Correct order is 2, 4, 1, 3, 5.
    2. The nurse should always explain the procedure to the client, even if the client has had the procedure done before.
    4. This procedure is very painful and the nurse should premedicate the client 30 minutes before performing wound care.
    1. Obtaining the needed supplies can be done after premedicating the client because the nurse should wait 30 minutes after medicating the client.
    3. The nurse should remove the old dressing.
    5. The nurse should assess the burned area for signs of infection, viable tissue, or any eschar.

101. 1. This client will require time to adjust to living in an extended care facility. This would be an expected reaction.
    2. This client may be allowed a glass of wine at night. Some long-term care facilities do allow the client to have a controlled amount of alcohol with an HCP order and the family supplying the alcohol, but this client is not the priority.
    3. This client may or may not have a valid issue. The nurse should investigate whether or not the report is accurate. Failure to answer a call light can result in the client attempting to ambulate without assistance and could be a safety issue. The nurse should speak with this client first.
    4. The nurse is not in control of the client's child and their discharge, but if the child is being discharged, it can be assumed that the child is in stable condition, and it is not a priority for the charge nurse to see this client.

102. 1. The director of nurses must first understand the extent of the report. Telling staff to ignore preconceived ideas about older adult clients does not work. The director of nurses should have valid information to discuss with the staff.
    2. The client has a general concern, and so more than one staff member may have ignored the client's statements. Neglect was not mentioned in the stem of the question. It is implied that the client should not be treated with the dignity that the client deserves.
    3. This is a false statement. Some residents in a long-term care facility may be unable to determine their needs, but this is not true of all residents.
    4. The director of nurses should discuss the resident's concerns with the resident and then determine a plan of action to remedy the situation.

103. 1. This may be a true statement, but this client is exhibiting symptoms of depression. The client may or may not wish to make friends at the facility.
    2. This is not acknowledging the client's feelings.
    3. This client is exhibiting symptoms of depression. Therapeutic conversation is implemented to help the client verbalize feelings. This statement acknowledges the client's feelings and offers help.
    4. This action may get the client to interact with other people but does not acknowledge the client's feelings.

104. 1. An ombudsman is a representative appointed to receive and investigate reports made by individuals of abuses or capricious acts. All Medicare and Medicaid long-term care facilities must have an ombudsman to act as a neutral party in matters of dispute with the facility. This is the best person to investigate a report.
    2. The social worker employed by the facility is not the best person to investigate the report.
    3. The upset family member should attend the conference but have the ombudsman investigate the report.
    4. The director will be biased; the best person to investigate the validity of the issue is the ombudsman.

105. 1. The nurse should not refer the client to a church or volunteer organization to ensure continuity of care. The organization's work may depend on unpaid individuals, and a volunteer may be unavailable to transport the client when needed.
    2. The nurse should refer the client to a home health agency for follow-up care. The nurse will go to the client's home to assess the client and perform dressing changes. The home health agency will also assess the client and the client's home for further needs.
    3. The client cannot drive and could not get to an outpatient clinic.
    4. The client cannot drive and would not be able to get to the HCP's office.

106. 1. The nurse must assess the cause of the bruises before filing a report of abuse. The nurse would file a report of elder abuse only if it is determined that the client has been abused.
   2. **The nurse should ask the client whether there is a reason for the bruises that the nurse should be aware of. This is the first intervention that can be done while the nurse is with the client.**
   3. The nurse should check the client's MAR to see whether they are currently on medication, such as warfarin (Coumadin) or a systemic steroid, that would increase the risk for bruising; however, this would be done after talking with the client because the bruising is "new," and bruising from the medications can take several days to weeks to develop.
   4. The family may need to be notified, but not until the nurse assesses the situation.

107. 1. **The client is feeling negative about being placed in the nursing home. Asking about the client's feelings is a therapeutic response that encourages the client to verbalize feelings.**
   2. This is not acknowledging the client's feelings and is nontherapeutic because it is a judgmental statement.
   3. The client does not owe the nurse an explanation. "Why" is never therapeutic.
   4. This assumes the client is correct in being "trouble at home" and agreeing that the family would punish the client for being a problem.

108. 1. The nurse cannot testify to what preceded the client's fall because the nurse was not on duty then.
   2. The nurse was not on duty to assess the client's injuries, so any information about the injuries received from the fall must be hearsay or obtained from the EHR.
   3. The nurse cannot testify to the client's mental status before the fall because the nurse was not on duty then.
   4. **The nurse initiated a policy designed to prevent falls, and this is all the nurse can testify to.**

109. 1. The RN, experienced or not, can be assigned nursing duties of assessment, planning, teaching, and other duties that cannot be delegated or assigned. The charge nurse has only two RNs for 35 clients. This nurse should not be requested to stay home.
   2. The unit will need an experienced LPN to care for the many IV lines and medications.
   3. **The UAP cannot administer medications or care for IV lines and has requested to be allowed to stay home. This is the best staff member to ask to stay home.**
   4. This UAP may be less experienced on the floor but has not worked long enough to receive any paid time off, which could significantly affect the UAP's pay.

110. 1. **The charge nurse does not have a right to interfere with two consenting adults having a relationship. Doing nothing is the correct action for the charge nurse. If one of the residents involved cannot consent to a relationship, the charge nurse would need to get involved.**
   2. Two consenting adults have a right to form a bond. The family does not have a right to interfere with expressing a basic human need to form an intimate relationship with another human being.
   3. The residents have the right to companionship. They should be allowed to participate in any activity that they wish when they wish.
   4. This situation is normal and requires no care plan meeting.

111. 1. The argument should already be in a private area because the argument ensued during report. Report should always be held in a confidential area.
   2. **The CNO should evaluate each charge nurse's concerns and then decide on a plan of care for the resident. The CNO is the next in command over the charge nurses in an extended care facility.**
   3. This argument does not involve the family. If, after listening to both sides, the CNO thinks there is a need for a family member's input, then the CNO could contact the family, but a decision should be made until this can occur.
   4. The nurses each have a concern over a resident. This situation should be resolved before continuing report.

112. 1. Calling a time-out when a discrepancy is noted on the surgical permit is an appropriate action to prevent an error during a surgical procedure.
   2. The Joint Commission requires two identifiers to be utilized before administering

medications. Most hospitals use the client's date of birth for the second identifier. This is an appropriate action to prevent an error during a medication administration.
3. A quiz during orientation is given to assess whether the new employee understands the information being taught. Answering the quiz completes the required documentation for the employee's files but does not ensure the new hire understands how to utilize the IV pump. This is a violation of the Patient Safety Goals.
4. Initiating a fall prevention program for an older adult client to prevent falls is an appropriate action to attempt to ensure client safety.

113. 1. This client should be tagged as black, which means the injury is extensive and chances of survival are unlikely even with definitive care. Clients should receive comfort measures and be separated from other casualties, but not abandoned.
2. This client should be red tagged (immediate), which means the injury is life-threatening but survivable with intervention. These clients can deteriorate rapidly without treatment.
3. This client should be tagged as green, which means the injury is minor, and treatment can be delayed hours to days. These clients are considered "walking wounded."
4. The client should be tagged as yellow, which means the injury is significant and requires medical care, but the client is not in immediate danger of death. Clients in this category receive treatment after red tagged (immediate) casualties are treated.

114. 1. The normal white blood cell count is 4.5 to 11.1×10^3/microL; therefore, this client does not require immediate intervention.
2. The client's cholesterol level is elevated, but this would not require immediate intervention by the nurse. Elevated cholesterol levels are not life-threatening and can be discussed at the client's next appointment.
3. The client's calcium level is within the normal range of 8.2 to 10.2 mg/dL; therefore, this client does not require an immediate intervention.
4. The therapeutic range for an INR is 2 to 3. This client is at risk for bleeding and requires immediate intervention by the nurse. The nurse should call the client and instruct the client to stop taking warfarin (Coumadin), an anticoagulant.

115. 1. A spokesperson should address the media away from the victim care area as soon as possible. In some situations, this could be a nurse, but it is not the priority intervention when triaging victims.
2. The disaster tag number and the client's name should be recorded in the disaster log book, but it is not the priority intervention. The disaster tag must be attached to the client before logging the client into the disaster log book.
3. Client tracking is a critical component of casualty management. Disaster tags, which include name, address, age, location, description of injuries, and treatments or medications administered, must be securely attached to the client.
4. The disaster workers must care for family and friends arriving at the disaster, but it is not the first intervention for the nurse triaging disaster victims.

116. 1. Parish nursing emphasizes the relationship between spiritual faith and health. A parish nurse (PN) is an RN with a minimum of 2 years' experience working in a faith community to address the health issues of its members and those in the broader community or neighborhood.
2. The parish nurse works in the community, not in an acute care setting.
3. There is no such thing as a parish clinic.
4. The parish nurse can be an RN or an LPN.

117. 1. The occupational therapist assists the client with activities of daily living, not with employment concerns.
2. The NCLEX-RN® test plan lists referrals under Management of Care. After a client has been injured and cannot return to previous employment because of the injury, the rehabilitation commission of each state will help evaluate the client and determine whether the client is eligible to receive training or education for another occupation.
3. The client is not asking about disability but rather about employment. The nurse needs to refer the client to the appropriate agency.
4. The client should discuss these concerns with their spouse, but the nurse should refer them to an agency that can address their concerns about employment.

118. 1. The mother may want to see her infant before the body is removed from the room.
    2. The infant's body will be sent to a funeral home. The parents will not be allowed to take the body home.
    3. The body should be treated with the dignity accorded to any human remains.
    4. **The nurse can give the parents a lock of the infant's hair and footprints. Giving the parents something of the infant helps with the grieving process.**

119. 1. **Nasal flaring and grunting indicate the infant is in respiratory distress. The nurse should assess this infant first.**
    2. The nurse would not worry about the infant not passing meconium until 20 to 24 hours after birth. The nurse would not assess this infant first.
    3. This situation requires teaching the mother and patience, but the infant is not in distress. The nurse would not assess this infant first.
    4. This is normal for a newborn. The nurse would not assess this infant first.

120. 1. Because this client is reporting an incident that occurred hours ago and is not in imminent danger, this client is not the first client the nurse should call.
    2. **The nurse should return this call first because the nurse must determine whether the client has a suicide plan.**
    3. Not wanting to eat is part of the anorexia disease process. The nurse does not need to return this call first.
    4. Hand trembling is part of the Parkinson's disease process. Control of the symptoms of Parkinson's disease is affected by several factors, including the amount of sleep the client had, fatigue, and the development of tolerance to the medications. Because this client is not at risk for suicide, they are not the first client for the nurse to call.

121. 1. **Pediatric clients in a psychiatric facility must keep up with schoolwork. Clients must be escorted from one building to another. The MHW should be assigned to this task.**
    2. The MHW is not qualified for this task to lead a group therapy session.
    3. Explaining the purpose of recreation therapy is teaching, and teaching cannot be delegated to an MHW.
    4. Clients in a psychiatric facility are expected to meet their hygiene needs as part of assuming responsibility for themselves. This is not the best task to assign to the MHW.

122. Correct answers are 1, 2, and 5.
    1. Smoking while taking birth control pills increases the risk of adverse reactions such as the formation of blood clots.
    2. The client should take the pill at approximately the same time each day to maintain a blood hormone level.
    3. The client should be instructed to take a missed pill as soon as realizing the dose was missed during the intervening 24 hours. However, if the client doesn't realize the pill was missed until the next day, they should not take two pills at that time.
    4. Breakthrough bleeding may indicate a change in dose is needed, but the client should not stop taking the pill.
    5. There may be interactions with other medications. Many antibiotics interfere with the action of the birth control pill, and the client should use other contraceptive methods when on an antibiotic.

123. 1. Vaginal itching while receiving antibiotics indicates that the good bacterial flora in the vagina is being destroyed. Yogurt contains these bacteria and can help replace the needed bacteria. However, requesting the dietary department send yogurt daily is not the priority intervention.
    2. **The nurse should first explain to the client that this is a side effect of the antibiotic medication ceftriaxone (Rocephin). Then, the nurse should notify the dietitian and HCP. The antibiotic therapy cannot be discontinued because of the need for antibiotic therapy after knee replacement surgery.**
    3. The HCP should be notified of the vaginal itching, but it is not an emergency and can wait until the HCP makes rounds.
    4. The client's sexual history is not a concern because the vaginal infection is secondary to the antibiotic therapy.

124. 1. The manager should ask for input into the budgetary needs of the staff, but an assessment of the current year's budget is the first step.
    2. An assessment of the costs of any new department projects should be done, but the first step is to assess the present budget.
    3. **The first step in a budgetary process is to assess the current budget.**
    4. Explaining the new budget to the staff is the last step in the process.

125. 1. The nurse should confront the client with the behavior, but this is not the first intervention.
2. The nurse should document the behavior in the client's EHR, but this is not the first intervention.
3. The nurse should intervene to stop the behavior first before one of the clients is injured. Approaching the client with another staff member shows strength and allows the nurse to perform a safe "take down."
4. The client should be told to return to their room, but stopping the behavior is the first intervention.

126. 1. This surgeon should speak with the client, but the first intervention is to stop the procedure.
2. Asking the client to discuss concerns should be done, but the first intervention is to stop the procedure.
3. Continuing to prep the client for the surgery can be done, but is inappropriate when the client no longer is giving consent.
4. Stopping the surgical procedure is the first intervention for the nurse to implement.

127. 1. Four episodes of mania in 6 months do not indicate therapy has been effective.
2. The ability to hold a job for 9 months indicates the client is responding to therapy.
3. Wearing a nightgown to the day room does not indicate the client is responding to treatment.
4. Three motor vehicle accidents do not indicate the client is responding to treatment.

128. 1. Erythropoietin alpha (Epogen), a biological response modifier, stimulates the bone marrow to produce red blood cells. An adverse reaction to Epogen is hypertension, which this client has, with a BP of 200/124 mm Hg. Hypertension can cause the dosage of erythropoietin to be decreased or discontinued.
2. Erythropoietin alpha (Epogen), a biological response modifier, does not affect the pulse.
3. A hematocrit of 38% would indicate the medication is effective.
4. A side effect of the medication is long bone pain. This can be treated with a non-narcotic analgesic. This is not an adverse reaction.

129. 1. The nurse should assess the client for complications before administering the medication.
2. This should occur, but not before assessing the client for complications.
3. The first step in administering a PRN pain medication is to assess the client for a complication that may require the nurse to notify the HCP or implement an independent nursing intervention.
4. This is not the first intervention.

130. 1. The infection can come from kissing someone having the infection in their mouth as well as from oral sex. This is not the best statement.
2. Smear of oral tissue is not done routinely.
3. HPV can be transferred from mucous membranes to mucous membranes via oral sex or kissing; the infection is the fastest rising cause of head and neck cancers.
4. Human papillomavirus (HPV) infections are increasing exponentially, and many younger persons are developing mouth infections and cancers from HPV.

131. 1. HIV can be transmitted during its first exposure. The class should be taught that no exposure is safe.
2. The use of condoms is somewhat protective, but it does not guarantee protection from a sexually transmitted disease.
3. The more exposure to blood or body fluids from other individuals (more partners), the greater the chance of developing an STI.
4. Both syphilis and gonorrhea are usually treatable, but long-lasting health problems can result. For example, pelvic inflammatory disease can scar the fallopian tube and cause fertility issues.

132. 1. The child is stable, and the UAP can escort the child to the car. The RN can delegate this task.
2. This is assessment, and the RN cannot delegate assessment, teaching, evaluation, medications, or an unstable client to a UAP.
3. This is teaching, and the nurse cannot delegate teaching.
4. The UAP may be able to assist the HCP with this task, but of the four options, the test taker should select the least invasive or the task that will require the least amount of nursing knowledge.

133. Correct answers are 1, 3, and 4.
    1. The charge nurse should notify the unit manager and information technology to ensure automatic locks are set on workstations. Typically, the workstations should be set to lock after 10 minutes of inactivity.
    2. The charge nurse should immediately secure the EHR, leaving it inaccessible to unauthorized viewing.
    3. The staff should be informed that this could violate HIPAA if an unauthorized person read the client's health information in the EHR.
    4. Protection of the workstation from unauthorized viewing is a priority. The charge nurse should lock the screen or remain with the workstation.
    5. The Health and Human Services Office for Civil Rights is responsible for enforcing Privacy and Security rules, but the question does not indicate a breach of personal health information.

134.
    1. The UAPs may or may not cross the picket line, and the managers cannot provide care to all the clients. This is not the best response.
    2. Abandonment is leaving the shift without notifying the supervisor after accepting the assignment. Going on strike with a 10-day notice is not abandonment.
    3. This may or may not be a true statement; therefore, it is not the best response.
    4. Federal law requires that there must be a 10-day notice before going on strike. This allows the hospital to prepare for the strike and make changes to ensure client safety.

Bibliography

Bulger-Noto, J. (2018). Leadless pacemakers: A new technology in cardiac pacing. *American Nurse Today, 13*(10), 18–21.

Hoffman, J., & Sullivan, N. (2024). *Davis advantage for medical-surgical nursing: Making connections to practice* (3rd ed.). F.A. Davis.

National Council of State Boards of Nursing. (2018). *Strategic practice analysis.* NCSBN Research Brief, Vol. 71. Author. https://www.ncsbn.org/public-files/18-Strategic-Practice-Analysis.pdf

National Council of State Boards of Nursing. (2023). *2023 NCLEX-RN test plan.* https://www.ncsbn.org/publications/2023-nclex-rn-test-plan

Nugent, P., & Vitale, B. (2023). *Fundamentals success: NCLEX®-Style Q&A Review* (6th ed.). F.A. Davis.

The Joint Commission. (2024). *2024 Nursing care center national patient safety goals.* https://www.jointcommission.org/-/media/tjc/documents/standards/national-patient-safety-goals/2024

Treas, L. S., Barnett, K. L., & Smith, M. H. (2022). *Davis advantage for basic nursing: Thinking, doing, and caring* (3rd ed.). F.A. Davis.

Vallerand, A. H., & Sanoski, C. A. (2025). *Davis's drug guide for nurses* (19th ed.). F.A. Davis.

Van Leeuwen, A. M., & Bladh, M. L. (2023). *Davis's comprehensive manual of laboratory and diagnostic tests with nursing implications* (10th ed.). F.A. Davis.

Appendix A: Normal Laboratory Values

These values are obtained from *Davis's Comprehensive Manual of Laboratory and Diagnostic Tests with Nursing Implications* (10th ed.). Laboratory reference values may differ slightly depending on the resource manual or the specific laboratory.

Arterial Blood Gas	Adult
pH	7.35 to 7.45
Pco_2	35 to 45 mm Hg
HCO_3	22 to 26 mmol/L
Po_2	80 to 95 mm Hg
O_2 saturation	95% to 99%

Chemistry	Adult
Cholesterol	Less than 200 mg/dL
High-density lipoprotein cholesterol (HDLC)	Male: ≥40 mg/dL
	Female: ≥50 mg/dL
Low-density lipoprotein cholesterol (LDLC)	Less than 100 mg/dL
Creatinine	Male: 0.61 to 1.21 mg/dL
	Female: 0.51 to 1.04 mg/dL
Glucose	Fasting: Less than 100 mg/dL
	Random: Less than 200 mg/dL
Potassium	3.5 to 5.3 mEq/L or mmol/L
Sodium	135 to 145 mEq/L or mmol/L
Calcium	9 to 10.5 mg/dL
Triglycerides	Less than 150 mg/dL
Blood urea nitrogen (BUN)	8 to 21 mg/dL
	Adult over 90 years: 10 to 31 mg/dL

Appendix A: Normal Laboratory Values

Blood Count	Adult
Hematocrit (Hct)	Male: 42% to 52%
	Female: 36% to 48%
Hemoglobin (Hgb)	Male: 14 to 17.3 g/dL
	Female: 11.7 to 15.5 g/dL
Prothrombin time (PT)	10 to 13 seconds
Partial thromboplastin time, activated (aPTT)	25 to 35 seconds
Red blood cell (RBC) count	Male: 4.51 to 6.01 $\times 10^6$ cells/microL
	Female: 4.01 to 5.51 $\times 10^6$ cells/microL
White blood cell (WBC) count	4.5 to 11.1 $\times 10^3$/microL
Platelets	150 to 450 $\times 10^3$/microL
Erythrocyte sedimentation rate (ESR)	Adult younger than 50 years: 0 to 15 mm/hr
	Adult 50 years and older: 0 to 20 mm/hr

Drug Levels	Adult
Digoxin	0.5 to 2.0 ng/mL
International Normalized Ratio (INR)	0.9 to 1.1 without anticoagulation therapy
	2 to 3 with therapy
	2.5 to 3.5 with intensive therapy with warfarin
Lithium	0.6 to 1.2 mEq/L
Phenytoin	10 to 20 mcg/mL
Valproic acid	50 to 125 mcg/mL
Vancomycin (trough level)	5 to 15 mcg/mL

Urinalysis	Adult
pH	4.5 to 8
Specific gravity	1.005 to 1.03
Glucose	Negative
Protein	
Ketones	
Hemoglobin	
Bilirubin	
Nitrite	
Leukocyte esterase	
Urobilinogen	Up to 1 mg/dL
Microscopic	
RBCs	Less than 5/hpf (high-power field)
WBCs	Less than 5/hpf (high-power field)
Bacteria	None seen

Appendix B: Common Abbreviations

Abnormal Involuntary Movement Scale (AIMS)
Absolute neutrophil count (ANC)
Acquired immune deficiency syndrome (AIDS)
Activity of daily living (ADL)
Acute respiratory distress syndrome (ARDS)
Advance directive (AD)
Against medical advice (AMA)
American Cancer Society (ACS)
American Heart Association (AHA)
Americans with Disabilities Act (ADA)
Amyotrophic lateral sclerosis (ALS)
Angiotensin-converting enzyme (ACE)
Antidiuretic hormone (ADH)
Apical pulse (AP)
Arterial blood gas (ABG)
Aspartate aminotransferase (AST)
Attention deficit-hyperactivity disorder (ADHD)
Below-the-knee amputation (BKA)
Benign prostatic hypertrophy (BPH)
Blood pressure (BP)
Blood urea nitrogen (BUN)
Body mass index (BMI)
Cardiopulmonary resuscitation (CPR)
Cerebrospinal fluid (CSF)
Cerebrovascular accident (CVA)
Chief nursing officer (CNO)
Child Protective Services (CPS)
Chronic kidney disease (CKD)
Chronic obstructive pulmonary disease (COPD)
Complementary alternative medicine (CAM)
Complete blood count (CBC)
Computed tomography (CT)
Congestive heart failure (CHF)
Continuous bladder irrigation (CBI)
Continuous glucose monitoring (CGM)
Continuous passive motion (CPM)
Coronary artery bypass graft (CABG)
Coronary artery disease (CAD)

Critical care unit (CCU)
Culture and sensitivity (C&S)
Cystic fibrosis (CF)
Cytomegalovirus (CMV)
Deep vein thrombosis (DVT)
Diabetes insipidus (DI)
Diabetes mellitus (DM)
Diabetic ketoacidosis (DKA)
Disseminated intravascular coagulation (DIC)
Dissociative identity disorder (DID)
Do not resuscitate (DNR)
Durable medical equipment (DME)
Electronic health record (EHR)
Electronic medication administration record (eMAR)
Emergency department (ED)
End-of-life (EOL)
Endotracheal (ET)
End-stage renal disease (ESRD)
Esophagogastroduodenoscopy (EGD)
Evidence-based practice (EBP)
Glomerular filtration rate (GFR)
Graduate nurse (GN)
Group B streptococcus (GBS)
Healthcare provider (HCP)
Health Insurance Portability and Accountability Act (HIPAA)
Hematocrit (Hct)
Hemoglobin (Hgb)
Hemoglobin and hematocrit (H&H)
Hemolysis elevated liver enzymes and low platelet count (HELLP)
Highly active antiretroviral therapy (HAART)
Human immunodeficiency virus (HIV)
Human papillomavirus (HPV)
Hyperglycemic hyperosmolar nonketotic coma (HHNC)
Hypertension (HTN)
Ideal body weight (IBW)
Inflammatory bowel disease (IBD)

Intake and output (I&O)
Intensive care unit (ICU)
International Normalized Ratio (INR)
Intimate partner violence (IPV)
Intracranial pressure (ICP)
Intramuscular (IM)
Intravenous (IV)
Intravenous piggyback (IVPB)
Intravenous push (IVP)
Jackson-Pratt (JP)
Kidney, ureter, bladder (KUB)
Licensed practical nurse (LPN)
Magnetic resonance imaging (MRI)
Medication administration record (MAR)
Mental health worker (MHW)
Methicillin-resistant *Staphylococcus aureus* (MRSA)
Motor vehicle accident (MVA)
Myasthenia gravis (MG)
Myocardial infarction (MI)
Narcissistic personality disorder (NPD)
Nasogastric (NG)
Nasogastric tube (NGT)
National Association for Home Care (NAHC)
National Council Licensure Examination (NCLEX-RN®)
National Council of State Boards of Nursing (NCSBN)
Neonatal intensive care unit (NICU)
Nitroglycerin (NTG)
Nonsteroidal anti-inflammatory drug (NSAID)
Nurse practitioner (NP)
Obstetric (OB)
Occupational Health and Safety Administration (OSHA)
Open reduction and internal fixation (ORIF)
Operating room (OR)
Over the counter (OTC)
Packed red blood cell (PRBC)
Parish nurse (PN)
Parkinson's disease (PD)
Partial thromboplastin time (PTT)
Patient-controlled analgesia (PCA)

Percutaneous endoscopic gastrostomy (PEG)
Peripheral arterial disease (PAD)
Peripherally inserted central catheter (PICC)
Phenylketonuria (PKU)
Physical therapist (PT)
Physician assistant (PA)
Physicians' Desk Reference (PDR)
Postanesthesia care unit (PACU)
Post-traumatic stress disorder (PTSD)
Premature ventricular contractions (PVC)
Pulmonary embolism (PE)
Pupils equal, round, reactive to light and accommodation (PERRLA)
Purified protein derivative (PPD)
Range of motion (ROM)
Rapid Response Team (RRT)
Red blood cell (RBC)
Registered nurse (RN)
Rheumatoid arthritis (RA)
Rheumatoid factor (RF)
Rule out (R/O)
Sequential compression device (SCD)
Sexual assault nurse examiner (SANE)
Sexually transmitted infection (STI)
Significant other (SO)
Spinal cord injury (SCI)
Sudden infant death syndrome (SIDS)
Syndrome of inappropriate antidiuretic hormone secretion (SIADH)
Systemic lupus erythematosus (SLE)
Tetralogy of Fallot (TOF)
To keep open (TKO)
Total hip replacement (THR)
Total knee replacement (TKR)
Total parenteral nutrition (TPN)
Transient ischemic attack (TIA)
Transurethral resection of the prostate (TURP)
Traumatic brain injury (TBI)
Unlicensed assistive personnel (UAP)
Urinary tract infection (UTI)
White blood cell (WBC)

Glossary of English Words Commonly Encountered on Nursing Examinations

Abnormality – defect, irregularity, anomaly, oddity
Absence – nonappearance, lack, nonattendance
Abundant – plentiful, rich, profuse
Accelerate – go faster, speed up, increase, hasten
Accumulate – build up, collect, gather
Accurate – precise, correct, exact
Achievement – accomplishment, success, reaching, attainment
Acknowledge – admit, recognize, accept, reply
Activate – start, turn on, stimulate
Adequate – sufficient, ample, plenty, enough
Angle – slant, approach, direction, point of view
Application – use, treatment, request, claim
Approximately – about, around, in the region of, more or less, roughly
Arrange – position, place, organize, display
Associated – linked, related
Attention – notice, concentration, awareness, thought
Authority – power, right, influence, clout, expert
Avoid – keep away from, evade, let alone
Balanced – stable, neutral, steady, fair, impartial
Barrier – barricade, blockage, obstruction, obstacle
Best – most excellent, most important, greatest
Capable – able, competent, accomplished
Capacity – ability, capability, aptitude, role, power, size
Central – middle, mid, innermost, vital
Challenge – confront, dare, dispute, test, trial, defy, competition
Characteristic – trait, feature, attribute, quality, typical
Circular – round, spherical, globular
Collect – gather, assemble, amass, accumulate, bring together
Commitment – promise, vow, dedication, obligation, pledge, assurance
Commonly – usually, normally, frequently, generally, universally
Compare – contrast, evaluate, match up to, weigh or judge
Compartment – section, part, cubicle, booth, stall
Complex – difficult, multifaceted, compound, multipart, intricate
Complexity – difficulty, intricacy, complication
Component – part, element, factor, section, constituent
Comprehensive – complete, inclusive, broad, thorough
Conceal – hide, cover up, obscure, mask, suppress, secrete
Conceptualize – to form an idea
Concern – worry, anxiety, fear, alarm, distress, unease, trepidation
Concisely – briefly, in a few words, succinctly
Conclude – make a judgment based on reason, finish
Confidence – self-assurance, certainty, poise, self-reliance
Congruent – matching, fitting, going together well
Consequence – result, effect, outcome
Constituents – elements, components, parts that make up a whole
Contain – hold, enclose, surround, include, control, limit
Continual – repeated, constant, persistent, recurrent, frequent
Continuous – constant, incessant, nonstop, unremitting, permanent
Contribute – be a factor, add, give
Convene – assemble, call together, summon, organize, arrange
Convenience – expediency, handiness, ease
Coordinate – organize, direct, manage, bring together
Create – make, invent, establish, generate, produce, fashion, build, construct
Creative – imaginative, original, inspired, inventive, resourceful, productive, innovative
Critical – serious, grave, significant, dangerous, life threatening
Cue – signal, reminder, prompt, sign, indication
Curiosity – inquisitiveness, interest, nosiness, snooping
Damage – injure, harm, hurt, break, wound
Deduct – subtract, take away, remove, withhold
Deficient – lacking, wanting, underprovided, scarce, faulty
Defining – important, crucial, major, essential, significant, central
Defuse – resolve, calm, soothe, neutralize, rescue, mollify
Delay – hold up, wait, hinder, postpone, slow down, hesitate, linger

Demand – insist, claim, require, command, stipulate, ask
Describe – explain, tell, express, illustrate, depict, portray
Design – plan, invent, intend, aim, propose, devise
Desirable – wanted, pleasing, enviable, popular, sought after, attractive, advantageous
Detail – feature, aspect, element, factor, facet
Deteriorate – worsen, decline, weaken
Determine – decide, conclude, resolve, agree on
Dexterity – skillfulness, handiness, agility, deftness
Dignity – self-respect, self-esteem, decorum, formality, poise
Dimension – aspect, measurement
Diminish – reduce, lessen, weaken, detract, moderate
Discharge – release, dismiss, set free
Discontinue – stop, cease, halt, suspend, terminate, withdraw
Disorder – complaint, problem, confusion, chaos
Display – show, exhibit, demonstrate, present, put on view
Dispose – to get rid of, arrange, order, set out
Dissatisfaction – displeasure, discontent, unhappiness, disappointment
Distinguish – to separate and classify, recognize
Distract – divert, sidetrack, entertain
Distress – suffering, trouble, anguish, misery, agony, concern, sorrow
Distribute – deliver, spread out, hand out, issue, dispense
Disturbed – troubled, unstable, concerned, worried, distressed, anxious, uneasy
Diversional – serving to distract
Don – put on, dress oneself in
Dramatic – spectacular, pronounced, substantial, noticeable
Drape – cover, wrap, dress, swathe
Dysfunction – abnormality, impairment
Edge – perimeter, boundary, periphery, brink, border, rim
Effective – successful, useful, helpful, valuable
Efficient – not wasteful, effective, competent, resourceful, capable
Elasticity – stretch, spring, suppleness, flexibility
Eliminate – get rid of, eradicate, abolish, remove, purge
Embarrass – make uncomfortable, make self-conscious, humiliate, mortify
Emerge – appear, come, materialize, become known
Emphasize – call attention to, accentuate, stress, highlight
Ensure – make certain, guarantee
Environment – setting, surroundings, location, atmosphere, milieu, situation
Episode – event, incident, occurrence, experience
Essential – necessary, fundamental, vital, important, crucial, critical, indispensable
Etiology – assigned cause, origin
Exaggerate – overstate, inflate

Excel – to stand out, shine, surpass, outclass
Excessive – extreme, too much, unwarranted
Exertion – intense or prolonged physical effort
Exhibit – show signs of, reveal, display
Expand – get bigger, enlarge, spread out, increase, swell, inflate
Expect – wait for, anticipate, imagine
Expectation – hope, anticipation, belief, prospect, probability
Experience – knowledge, skill, occurrence, know-how
Expose – lay open, leave unprotected, allow to be seen, reveal, disclose, exhibit
External – outside, exterior, outer
Facilitate – make easy, make possible, help, assist
Factor – part, feature, reason, cause, think, issue
Focus – center, focal point, hub
Fragment – piece, portion, section, part, splinter, chip
Function – purpose, role, job, task
Furnish – supply, provide, give, deliver, equip
Further – additional, more, extra, added, supplementary
Generalize – to take a broad view, simplify, to make inferences
Generate – make, produce, create
Gentle – mild, calm, tender
Girth – circumference, bulk, weight
Highest – uppermost, maximum, peak, main
Hinder – hold back, delay, hamper, obstruct, impede
Humane – caring, kind, gentle, compassionate, benevolent, civilized
Ignore – pay no attention to, disregard, overlook, discount
Imbalance – unevenness, inequality, disparity
Immediate – insistent, urgent, direct
Impair – damage, harm, weaken
Implantation – attachment of the early embryo to the maternal uterine wall, to put in
Impotent – powerless, weak, incapable, ineffective, unable
Inadvertent – unintentional, chance, unplanned, accidental
Include – comprise, take in, contain
Indicate – point out, be a sign of, designate, specify, show
Ineffective – unproductive, unsuccessful, useless, vain, futile
Inevitable – predictable, to be expected, unavoidable, foreseeable
Influence – power, pressure, sway, manipulate, affect, effect
Initiate – start, begin, open, commence, instigate
Insert – put in, add, supplement, introduce
Inspect – look over, check, examine
Inspire – motivate, energize, encourage, enthuse
Institute – implement, initiate, institution
Institutionalize – to place in a facility for treatment
Integrate – put together, mix, add, combine, assimilate

Integrity – honesty, honor
Interfere – get in the way, hinder, obstruct, impede, hamper
Interpret – explain the meaning of, to make understandable
Intervention – action, activity, intercession
Intolerance – bigotry, prejudice, narrow-mindedness
Involuntary – instinctive, reflex, unintentional, automatic, uncontrolled
Irreversible – permanent, irrevocable, irreparable, unalterable
Irritability – sensitivity to stimuli, fretful, quick excitability
Justify – explain in accordance with reason, defend
Likely – probably, possible, expected
Liquefy – to change into or make more fluid
Logical – using reason, rational, analytical
Longevity – long life, durability, endurance
Lowest – inferior in rank, least, base
Maintain – continue, uphold, preserve, sustain, retain
Majority – the greater part, more than half, most
Mention – talk about, refer to, state, cite, declare, point out
Minimal – least, smallest, nominal, negligible, token
Minimize – reduce, diminish, lessen, curtail, decrease to smallest possible
Mobilize – activate, organize, assemble, gather, rally
Modify – change, adapt, adjust, revise, alter
Moist – slightly wet, damp
Multiple – many, numerous, several, various
Natural – normal, ordinary, unaffected
Negative – no, harmful, downbeat, pessimistic
Negotiate – bargain, talk, discuss, consult, cooperate, settle
Notice – become aware of, see, observe, discern, detect
Notify – inform, tell, alert, advise, warn, report
Nurture – care for, raise, rear, foster
Obsess – preoccupy, consume, beset
Occupy – live in, inhabit, reside in, engage in
Occurrence – event, incident, happening
Odorous – scented, stinking, aromatic
Offensive – unpleasant, distasteful, nasty, disgusting
Opportunity – chance, prospect, break
Organize – put in order, arrange, sort out, categorize, classify
Origin – source, starting point, cause, beginning, derivation
Pace – speed, rhythm, tempo, rate
Parameter – limit, factor, limitation, issue
Participant – member, contributor, partaker, applicant
Perspective – viewpoint, view, perception
Position – place, location, point, spot, situation
Practice – do, carry out, perform, apply, follow
Precipitate – to cause to happen, to bring on, hasten, abrupt, sudden
Predetermine – fix or set beforehand

Predictable – expected, knowable
Preference – favorite, liking, first choice
Prepare – get ready, plan, make, train, arrange, organize
Prescribe – set down, stipulate, order, recommend, impose
Previous – earlier, prior, before, preceding
Primarily – first, above all, mainly, mostly, largely, principally, predominantly
Primary – first, main, basic, chief, most important, key, prime, major, crucial
Priority – main concern, giving first attention to, higher order of importance
Production – making, creation, construction, assembly
Profuse – a lot of, plentiful, copious, abundant, generous, prolific, bountiful
Prolong – extend, delay, put off, lengthen, draw out
Promote – encourage, support, endorse, sponsor
Proportion – ratio, amount, quantity, part of, percentage, section of
Provide – give, offer, supply, make available
Rationalize – explain, reason
Realistic – practical, sensible, reasonable
Receive – get, accept, take delivery of, obtain
Recognize – acknowledge, appreciate, identify, aware of
Recovery – healing, mending, improvement, recuperation, renewal
Reduce – decrease, lessen, ease, moderate, diminish
Reestablish – reinstate, restore, return, bring back
Regard – consider, look upon, relate to, respect
Regular – usual, normal, ordinary, standard, expected, conventional
Relative – comparative, family member
Relevance – importance of, pertinence, apropos
Reluctant – unwilling, hesitant, disinclined, indisposed, adverse
Reminisce – to recall and review remembered experiences
Remove – take away, get rid of, eliminate, eradicate
Reposition – move, relocate, change position
Require – need, want, necessitate
Resist – oppose, defend against, keep from, refuse to go along, defy
Resolution – decree, solution, decision, ruling, promise
Resolve – make up your mind, solve, determine, decide
Response – reply, answer, reaction, retort
Restore – reinstate, reestablish, bring back, return to, refurbish
Restrict – limit, confine, curb, control, contain, hold back, hamper
Retract – take back, draw in, withdraw, apologize
Reveal – make known, disclose, divulge, expose, tell, make public
Review – appraisal, reconsider, evaluation, assessment, examination, analysis

Ritual – custom, ceremony, formal procedure
Rotate – turn, go around, spin, swivel
Routine – usual, habit, custom, practice
Satisfaction – approval, fulfillment, pleasure, happiness
Satisfy – please, convince, fulfill, make happy, gratify
Secure – safe, protected, fixed firmly, sheltered, confident, obtain
Sequential – chronological, in order of occurrence
Significant – important, major, considerable, noteworthy, momentous
Slight – small, slim, minor, unimportant, insignificant, insult, snub
Source – basis, foundation, starting place, cause
Specific – exact, particular, detail, explicit, definite
Stable – steady, even, constant
Statistics – figures, data, information
Subtract – take away, deduct
Success – achievement, victory, accomplishment
Surround – enclose, encircle, contain
Suspect – think, believe, suppose, guess, deduce, infer, distrust, doubtful
Sustain – maintain, carry on, prolong, continue, nourish, suffer
Synonymous – same as, identical, equal, tantamount

Systemic – affecting the entire organism, pervasive
Thorough – careful, detailed, methodical, systematic, meticulous, comprehensive, exhaustive
Tilt – tip, slant, slope, lean, angle, incline
Translucent – see-through, transparent, clear
Unique – one and only, sole, exclusive, distinctive
Universal – general, widespread, common, worldwide
Unoccupied – vacant, not busy, empty
Unrelated – unconnected, unlinked, distinct, dissimilar, irrelevant
Unresolved – unsettled, uncertain, unsolved, unclear, in doubt
Untoward – adverse, unexpected, inappropriate, inconvenient, unforeseen
Utilize – make use of, employ
Various – numerous, variety, range of, mixture of, assortment of
Verbalize – express, voice, speak, articulate
Verify – confirm, make sure, prove, attest to, validate, substantiate, corroborate, authenticate
Vigorous – forceful, strong, brisk, energetic
Volume – quantity, amount, size
Withdraw – remove, pull out, take out, extract

Index

A

AAA. *See* Abdominal aortic aneurysm
Abandonment, 387
Abdominal aortic aneurysm (AAA), 52, 54
    bruit and, 75
    death from, 50
    discharge teaching for, 56, 73
    low back pain with, 75
    packed red blood cells for, 47
    pneumonia and, 61
    renal failure with, 77
    stethoscope for, 55
Abdominal pain, 128
    with cholecystectomy, 127
    nasogastric tube and, 83
    in pediatric health management, 368
Abductor pillow, for total hip replacement, 283
ABGs. *See* Arterial blood gases
Abnormal Involuntary Movement Scale (AIMS), 403, 427
Absolute neutrophil count, 326
Abuse
    child (*See* Child abuse)
    elder, 50, 68
    intimate partner violence, 323
        orthopedic unit and, 304
        in pediatric health management, 368
        in pregnancy, 333
    in mental health management, 422
ACE-I. *See* Angiotensin-converting enzyme inhibitor
Acetaminophen (Tylenol), 36, 40, 185, 485
Acquired immunodeficiency syndrome (AIDS)
    dementia, 298
    malnutrition with, 304
Acrocyanosis, 458
Activated partial thromboplastin time (aPTT)
    in cardiac management, 21
    for deep vein thrombosis, 40
Activities of daily living (ADLs), 37, 210, 213, 268
    in integumentary management, 288
Acupressure, 248
Acupuncture, 247, 289, 470, 490
Acute bronchitis, 102
Acute respiratory distress syndrome (ARDS), 111
    arterial blood gases for, 89, 109
    oxygen for, 100, 113
    in renal/genitourinary management, 182
    respiratory failure and, 113
    ventilator for, 82
AD. *See* Advance directive
Addison's disease, 225, 239–240, 256–257
ADLs. *See* Activities of daily living
Adrenalectomy, 251
Adult Protective Services, 50, 68
Advance directive (AD), 467, 486
    in gastrointestinal management, 122, 142
    in hematological and immunological management, 298, 315, 327
    for pancreatic cancer, 306

Agranulocytosis, 415, 426
AHA. *See* American Heart Association
AIDS. *See* Acquired immunodeficiency syndrome
Air hunger, 99
Airway management, 44, 378
    in integumentary management, 271, 291
    in neurological management, 220
    in pediatric health management, 390
Albuterol, 44
Alcohol, 211
    in cardiac management, 35
    dehydration and, 486
    in gastrointestinal management, 143
    in hematological and immunological management, 295
    in mental health management, 404, 406
    in postpartum unit, 333
Alcoholics Anonymous (AA), 399, 421
Alcoholism, 399, 421, 431
Alendronate (Fosamax), 156, 173
Allergic contact dermatitis, 287
Allergies, 262
    to iodine, 213
    to latex, 297
    to penicillin, 300, 318–319
Allow natural death (AND), 36
Alport syndrome, 156
Alternate-format questions, 4
Aluminum hydroxide magnesium hydroxide (Maalox), 423
Alzheimer's disease, 188, 190, 209, 270, 290
    in mental health management, 400, 423
American Heart Association (AHA), 104
    on cardiopulmonary resuscitation, 31
    on chest pain, 33
    on unresponsive client, 12
American Nephrology Nurses Association, 177
Americans with Disabilities Act (ADA), 282
Aminoglycoside antibiotics, 112, 171
Ampicillin, 185
Amputations, 50, 69, 264
    above-the-knee, 262, 263
    below-the-knee, 260
    bleeding from, 474
    home health nurse and, 480
    from motor vehicle accident, 266
    right upper extremity, 265
    sexual activity and, 284
Amyotrophic lateral sclerosis (ALS), 195, 220
Anencephaly, 354
Anesthesia
    epidural, 330, 337–338, 352, 356
        blood pressure and, 457
    postanesthesia care unit, 474
        gastrointestinal management and, 147
        pulse oximetry and, 80
    pregnancy and, 345
Angina. *See also* Chest pain
    with aortic valve stenosis, 38
    from atherosclerosis, 43
    discharge teaching for, 22

515

Angiotensin-converting enzyme inhibitor (ACE-I), 62, 463, 483
    for hypertension, 13
Anhedonia, 431
Ankle fracture, 264
Anorexia, 394, 401
Antacids
    for antipsychotic medications, 423
    apical pulse and, 30
    for gastroesophageal reflux disease, 148
Antibiotics, 55, 473. *See also specific drugs*
    aminoglycoside (*See* Aminoglycoside antibiotics)
    in cardiac management, 38
    for cellulitis, 288
    in hematological and immunological management, 297, 313
    for impetigo, 284
    in integumentary management, 286
    medication errors with, 467
    in respiratory management, 101
    sputum culture and, 110, 111
    super-infections from, 285
    for urinary tract infection, 246
Anticholinesterase, 205
Anticoagulants. *See* Aspirin; Heparin; Warfarin
Antidepressants, 416
Antihistamines, 278
Antihypertensive medications, 67
Anti-inflammatory medications, 146
Antineoplastic agents, 380
Antioxidant, 146
Antiplatelet medications, 38, 497. *See also* Ticlopidine
Antipsychotics, 423, 426, 427, 430
Aortic aneurysm
    abdominal (*See* Abdominal aortic aneurysm)
    with bruit, 46
    meperidine for, 47
    packed red blood cells for, 51
Aortic valve stenosis, 38
Apical pulse (AP), 89
    antacids and, 30
    bleeding and, 178
    digoxin and, 27, 38
    grapefruit juice and, 30, 33
    with nephrectomy, 160
    with pneumonectomy, 80
Appendectomy
    emergency department and, 121, 330, 366
    in pediatric health management, 365
aPTT. *See* Activated partial thromboplastin time
Arterial blood gases (ABGs), 29
    for acute respiratory distress syndrome, 89, 109
    for burns, 274
    in endocrine management, 243
    for lymphedema, 52
    for metabolic alkalosis, 101
    respiratory acidosis and, 72
    in respiratory management, 81, 99
    unlicensed assistive personnel and, 39
Arterial hypertension
    antihypertensive medications for, 67
    nifedipine for, 52
    stroke and, 212
Arterial occlusive disease, 49, 53, 56
    heating pad for, 68
    intermittent claudication for, 27
    pulse with, 277
Aspartate aminotransferase (AST), 35
Aspiration
    of bone marrow, 368
    of meconium, 344
    in mental health management, 426
    in pediatric health management, 379
    pneumonia, 136

Aspirin, 38, 43
    for atherosclerosis, 76
    baby, for chest pain, 33
    blood and, 62, 68
Assault, 396, 418, 481
Assisted living facility, 478
Asthma, 88
    gastroesophageal reflux disease and, 144
Atenolol (Tenormin), 289
Atherosclerosis, 56
    aspirin for, 76
    calcium channel blocker and, 46
    from sedentary lifestyle, 43
Atrial fibrillation, 30
    in cardiac management, 13
    with long COVID, 44
    in long-term care, 12
    warfarin for, 31, 32
Augmented and assistive communication devices, 113
Autocratic leadership style, 370, 388
Autonomic dysreflexia, 205, 207, 219
Autonomy
    in long-term care, 52
    in renal/genitourinary management, 176
    in respiratory management, 105
    in women's health management, 348

B

Baby aspirin, for chest pain, 33
Back pain
    from fall, 191
        with abdominal aortic aneurysm, 75
Baclofen, 196
Bacterial meningitis
    lumbar puncture for, 192, 200
    in pediatric health management, 390
Bag-valve-mask device, 104, 113
Bariatric clinic, 126
Barium enema, 118
Barium study, 117, 135
Basal cell carcinoma, 267
Basic metabolic panel (BMP), 58, 94
    for burns, 274
    for COVID-19, 308
    in endocrine management, 237
Bedrest, 85
    for deep vein thrombosis, 74, 78
    in pediatric health management, 364
    pressure injury from, 268
    for varicose veins, 77
Bedside commodes, 178
Benign prostatic hypertrophy (BPH), 156, 176
    disseminated intravascular coagulation and, 169
Bereavement counseling, 142
Beta blockers, 252
    orthostatic hypotension with, 289
Betadine. *See* Povidone iodine
Biological response modifiers, 325
Biopsy, for cancer, 287
    breast, 313
Bipolar disorder, 399, 406, 430, 452, 481
Birth control pills, 481, 501
Bisacodyl (Dulcolax), 178
Bisphosphonates, 173
Bladder
    continuous bladder irrigation, 180
        for transurethral resection of prostate, 163
    cystectomy of, 154, 163, 171
    flaccid, 157
    fundus displacement and, 352, 357
    kidney, ureter, bladder imaging for, 162
    transurethral insection of prostate and, 156

Bleeding (hemorrhage)
    from amputation, 474
    apical pulse and, 178
    blood pressure and, 178
    in cephalohematoma, 358
    with disseminated intravascular coagulation, 487
    from duodenal ulcer, 126, 129
    hypovolemia and, 145
    with indwelling catheters, 298
    International Normalized Ratio and, 277
    after liver biopsy, 149
    liver failure and, 146
    partial thromboplastin time for, 103
    in postpartum unit, 359–360
    from sigmoid resection, 127
    from thyroidectomy, 244
    vital signs for, 325
    in women's health management, 343, 346, 350
Blood (administration)
    aspirin and, 62, 68
    in cardiac management, 10, 29, 40
    for congestive heart failure, 39
    in endocrine management, 248
    in gastrointestinal management, 118
    in hematological and immunological management, 324
    in mental health management, 415
    pneumothorax and, 112
    reactions to, 63
    in renal/genitourinary management, 155
    in urine, gestational hypertension and, 352
    vital signs for, 71
Blood-borne diseases, 65, 75
Blood glucose, 34, 241, 253, 254
    unlicensed assistive personnel and, 487
Blood pressure (BP), 65, 89. *See also* Hypertension; Hypotension
    angiotensin-converting inhibitors and, 39
    biological response modifiers and, 325
    bleeding and, 178
    for burns, 274
    calcium-channel blockers and, 27
    in cardiac management, 11, 29
    epidural anesthesia and, 457
    with long COVID, 44
    with pneumonectomy, 80
    unlicensed assistive personnel and, 48
Blood transfusions
    informed consent for, 64
    packed red blood cells and, 47, 64–65
Blood urea nitrogen (BUN), 274
BMP. *See* Basic metabolic panel
Body fluid contamination, 141
Bomb scare emergency plan, 295, 312, 400, 424
Bone density evaluation, 487
    for osteoporosis, 318
Bone marrow aspiration, 368
Botulism, 213
Bowtie items, 6
BP. *See* Blood pressure
Brain tumor, 189
BRCA gene, 295
Breast cancer, 295
    biopsy for, 313
Breastfeeding, 334, 351
Breath sounds, 107, 483
    with endotracheal tube, 113
Bronchiolitis, 110
Bronchoscopy, 113
Brudzinki's sign, 372
Bruit, 46, 75
Buerger's disease, 46
Bulimia, 125, 417
Bumetanide (Bumex), 87, 107
Buretrol. *See* Volume-controlled device

Burns/burn unit, 267, 269
    to chest, 270, 271
    dressings for, 472, 477
    edema with, 271
    education on, 272
    in emergency department, 272–278, 292–294
    hypovolemic shock with, 289
    pain from, 290–291
    shift reports in, 272

C

CABG. *See* Coronary artery bypass graft
Caffeine, 421, 486
Calcium channel blocker (CCB)
    atherosclerosis and, 46
    blood pressure and, 27
    grapefruit juice and, 29–30, 33
    for hypertension, 13
Calcium gluconate, 356
Call light, 498
    in pediatric health management, 381
    in vascular management, 47
Cancer. *See also* Oncology unit
    biopsy for, 287
    breast, 295
        biopsy for, 313
    colon, 301
    laryngeal, 296
    liver, 124
    lung, 83, 85, 296
        do not resuscitate order for, 301
    ovarian, 306
    pancreatic, 226
        advance directive for, 306
    prostate, 306
    skin of, 326–327
    surgery for, 299
    testicular, 297
    therapeutic communication with, 326
    thyroid, 227
Canes, 287
Captopril (Capoten), 39
Carafate, 38
Carbohydrate-counting diet, 34
Carbon monoxide, 274
Cardiac arrest, 16, 18
Cardiac catheterization, 20
Cardiac dysrhythmias. *See also specific types*
    cardiac monitoring for, 288
    hypokalemia and, 144, 492
Cardiac management, 9–44
    antibiotics in, 38
    blood administration in, 29, 40
    case management in, 10, 13, 28, 32
    case studies for, 23–26, 437–441, 454–455
    chest pain in, 14, 22, 38, 40, 41, 46
    Code Blue in, 28
    conflict resolution in, 13
    critical care unit in, 10
    delegation of care (*See* Float nurse; Graduate nurse; Unlicensed assistive personnel)
    discharge teaching in, 22, 31–32
    do not resuscitate order in, 12
    electronic health record in, 18, 22, 31, 38, 39, 41
    emergency department and, 16, 23–25, 27, 28
    Health Insurance Portability and Accountability Act in, 28, 32, 34, 35, 36, 37, 40
    informed consent in, 29
    intensive care unit in, 11, 25–26
    laboratory tests in, 14, 19, 22, 34, 35–36
    medication administration in, 15, 17, 29, 33
    medication administration records in, 17, 31, 38–39, 42–43

Cardiac management (*continued*)
    mental health management and, 415
    multidisciplinary health-care team and, 32, 34, 36
    postmortem care in, 36, 46
    shift assignments in, 12, 18
    shift reports in, 9, 17, 68
    telemetry in, 10, 16, 19, 21, 29, 42
    triage in, 13, 15
    unresponsive client in, 12
Cardiac rehabilitation, 34
Cardiomyopathy, 15
Cardiopulmonary resuscitation (CPR), 36, 85. *See also* Do not resuscitate (DNR) order
    advance directive for, 122, 306
    American Hospital Association on, 31
Cardiovascular accident (CVA). *See* Stroke
Cardioversion, 44
Care pairs, 353
Car safety seats, 347
Carver, George Washington, 9
Case management
    in cardiac management, 10, 13, 28, 32
    in endocrine management, 229, 246
    in integumentary management, 284
    in pediatric health management, 383
    in rehabilitation unit, 266
    responsibilities of, 283
Case studies, 6, 433–462
    for cardiac management, 23–26, 437–441, 454–455
    in endocrine management, 237–240, 256–257
    for gastrointestinal management, 130–134, 150–151
    in hematological and immunological management, 307–311, 327–328
    in integumentary management, 272–278, 292–294
    in mental health management, 407–412, 431–437, 452–453
    for neurological management, 201–204, 221–222
    in pediatric health management, 373–376, 391–392
    in postpartum unit, 340–342, 359–360
    for renal/genitourinary management, 164–168, 184–185
    for respiratory management, 93–96, 114–115, 441–444, 456–457
    for vascular management, 57–60, 78
    in women's health management, 444–447, 457–459
Catapres. *See* Clonidine
Cataracts, 209
CCB. *See* Calcium channel blocker
Ceftriaxone (Rocephin), 37, 111, 501
Cellulitis, 268, 288, 464
Cephalohematoma, 350, 358
Cerebral palsy, 363
Cerebrospinal fluid (CSF), 246
Cerebrovascular accident (CVA). *See* Stroke
Certified nurse midwife, 334, 351
Cervical dilation, 352
Chaplain
    in endocrine management, 244
    in women's health management, 349
Charge nurse
    in burn unit, 272
    in cardiac management, 22, 29
    conflict resolution by, 494
    in critical care unit, 468, 477
    electronic health record and, 482
    in endocrine management, 231, 232, 233
    family and, 497
    in gastrointestinal management, 120, 125, 128, 129, 143, 149
    in hematological and immunological management, 295, 297, 298, 299, 303, 312, 314
    in integumentary management, 266, 267, 271, 272, 286
    in intensive care unit, 50, 51, 475, 477
    laboratory tests and, 470
    in long-term care, 53, 478, 479
    in mental health management, 393, 394, 396, 400, 401, 403, 405, 424
    narcotics and, 474

    in neurological management, 187, 188, 189, 190, 200, 218, 220
    in oncology unit, 305
    in pediatric health management, 363, 365, 367, 369, 371, 372, 390, 391
    in postpartum unit, 332, 339
    in rehabilitation unit, 263
    in renal/genitourinary management, 154, 158, 164, 171
    in respiratory management, 81, 83, 89, 91
    in surgical unit, 467, 476
    in vascular management, 45, 47, 61, 71
    in women's health management, 330, 331
Chemotherapy, 302
    food taste and, 299
    for ovarian cancer, 305
    in pediatric health management, 380
    urinary tract infection with, 317
Chest
    burns to, 270, 271
    in pediatric health management, 392
    wound, 211
Chest pain
    American Hospital Association on, 33
    baby aspirin for, 33
    in cardiac management, 14, 22, 38, 40, 41, 46
    with deep vein thrombosis, 47
    in emergency department, 16
    from exercise, 41
    morphine for, 41
    with myocardial infarction, 18, 21, 27
    nitroglycerin for, 40, 41
    with pericarditis, 30
    with pulmonary embolism, 72
    telemetry for, 19
    in vascular management, 53
Chest tube, 100, 490
    drainage system for, 106, 112
    for flail chest, 82
    for hemothorax, 90, 110
    pain with, 91
    for pneumothorax, 82, 87, 91
    unlicensed assistive personnel and, 470
    urinary output and, 90, 110
Chest x-ray, 94
    for endotracheal tube, 483
    in hematological and immunological management, 317
    for pneumonia, 83
    pregnancy and, 101, 182, 352
    unlicensed assistive personnel and, 486
    in women's health management, 335
CHF. *See* Congestive heart failure
Chicken noodle soup, 486
Chief nursing officer (CNO), 479, 499
Child abuse, 371, 389, 471, 491
    mental health management and, 398
    pediatric health management and, 385
    women's health management and, 348
Child developmental specialist, 366, 367, 384, 385
Child Protective Services, 389, 491
Cholecystectomy, 126, 144, 468
    abdominal pain with, 127
    smoking and, 137–138
Cholesterol. *See also* Low-fat, low-cholesterol diet
    statins for, 38
Chronic kidney disease (CKD)
    fluids and, 161
    type 2 diabetes and, 230
Chronic obstructive pulmonary disease (COPD), 86
    end-stage, 85, 104
    from smoking, 91
    steroids for, 290
Cinnamon, 247
Circumcision, 336
Civil rights, in mental health management, 417, 419, 425
CKD. *See* Chronic kidney disease

Clinical Judgment Guide, 2
Clinical Judgment Measurement Model (CJMM), 2, 3, 6
Clinical manager
	on collective bargaining, 482
	in integumentary management, 281
	in mental health management, 399, 400, 420, 423, 424
	in pediatric health management, 369
	in postpartum unit, 335, 336, 355
	in surgical unit, 474
	in women's health management, 336
Clonidine (Catapres), 419
Clopidogrel (Plavix), 497
Clozapine (Clozaril), 415, 426
CLOZE questions, 6
Cocaine, 415
Code Blue, in cardiac management, 28
Code Pink
	in nursery, 382
	in pediatric health management, 365
	in women's health management, 349
Coffee ground emesis, 145
Colectomy, 120
Collective bargaining, 482
Colon cancer, 301
Colonoscopy, 122, 466
Colostomy
	bag for, 123, 146
	in pediatric health management, 365
	sigmoid (See Sigmoid colostomy)
Common cold, 466, 486
Communication boards, 113
Community-acquired pneumonia, 90, 441–444
Community health clinic, gastrointestinal management and, 125
Community health nurse, triage by, 480
Community-oriented nursing, 469, 489
	in endocrine management, 229, 247
Compartment syndrome, pain with, 280
Complementary alternative medicine (CAM), 289, 470
	in endocrine management, 229, 230, 247
	in rehabilitation unit, 269
Complete blood count (CBC), 58, 94
	for burns, 274
	for COVID-19, 308
	in endocrine management, 237
Comprehensive exam questions, 463–503
Compression stockings, 263
	leg elevation and, 280
	for pulmonary embolism, 49, 67
Computed tomography (CT), 213, 221
Conduct disorder, 413
Confidentiality
	in cardiac management, 32
	in Health Insurance Portability and Accountability Act, 175, 286
	in hematological and immunological management, 320
	in mental health management, 425
	in renal/genitourinary management, 175
	in volunteer care, 492
Conflict resolution
	in cardiac management, 11, 13
	by charge nurse, 494
	in endocrine management, 248
Congenital heart defects, 370
Congestive heart failure (CHF), 38
	blood administration for, 39
	digoxin IV push for, 10
	do not resuscitate order for, 14
	edematous feet with, 33
	fluid restriction for, 39
	furosemide for, 39
	home health nurse and, 14
	in long-term care, 12
	low-sodium diet for, 12
	packed red blood cells for, 18, 66

	in pediatric health management, 388
	pulmonary edema with, 27, 41
Consent form, in respiratory management, 98
Continuous bladder irrigation (CBI), 180
	for transurethral resection of prostate, 163
Continuous glucose monitoring (CGM), 255
	for type 1 diabetes, 236
Coronary artery bypass graft (CABG), 13, 19
	unlicensed assistive personnel and, 59
Coumadin. See Warfarin
COVID-19, 93, 114–115, 308
CPR. See Cardiopulmonary resuscitation
Cranberries, 246
Crash cart, 12, 21, 31, 41
Creatinine, 35
	for burns, 274
Credés maneuver, 173
Crepitus, 111
Critical care unit (CCU)
	in cardiac management, 10, 11
	charge nurse in, 477
	endocrine management and, 226
	gastrointestinal management and, 122
	hematological and immunological management and, 297, 298
	licensed practical nurse in, 467
	neurological management and, 189
	renal/genitourinary management and, 156, 171
	respiratory management and, 82, 88
	shift assignments in, 468
	unlicensed assistive personnel in, 467
Crohn's disease, 491
Crutch walking, 264, 282
C-section, 346, 357
Culture and sensitivity (C&S), 72, 216
	in respiratory management, 85, 104
Cystectomy, 154, 163, 171
Cystic fibrosis (CF), 88, 106, 108, 343

D

Dabigatran (Pradaxa), 41
D-dimer, 58
Death
	from abdominal aortic aneurysm, 50
	in cardiac management, 34
	distress with, 302
	in endocrine management, 227
	family and, 34, 51, 69, 177, 215
	in hematological and immunological management, 302, 303
	from refusing food and liquids, 105
	of stillborn infant, 333, 336, 354, 480, 501
	from stroke, 206
	unlicensed assistive personnel and, 50, 69
Débridement
	in hematological and immunological management, 317
	for venous ulcer, chronic, 57
Decerebrate posturing, 207, 315
Decorticate posturing, 189
Deep tendon reflexes, 338, 349
Deep vein thrombosis (DVT), 27, 492
	bedrest for, 74, 78
	calf pain with, 61
	chest pain with, 47
	dyspnea with, 46
	edema from, 71
	enoxaparin for, 39
	heparin for, 40, 47, 66, 78
	partial thromboplastin time for, 45
	pulmonary embolism and, 61, 62, 78, 110
	in right leg, 50
	warfarin for, 68
Defense mechanisms, in mental health management, 404–405, 428–429

Dehiscence, of wounds, 138, 147
Dehydration, 104, 148
   alcohol and, 486
   with long COVID, 44
   in pediatric health management, 378
   pyelonephritis and, 172
   in renal/genitourinary management, 159
   serum sodium level and, 146
Delegation of care. *See* Float nurse; Graduate nurse; Licensed practical nurse; Unlicensed assistive personnel
Delirium tremens (DTs), 431
Dementia, 416, 427
   acquired immunodeficiency syndrome, 298
Demerol. *See* Meperidine
Democratic leadership style, 250, 497
Dentures, 289
Dermatological clinic, 267
Descartes, Rene, 1
Diabetes
   mental health management and, 426
   type 1 (*See* Type 1 diabetes)
   type 2 (*See* Type 2 diabetes)
Diabetes insipidus (DI), 227, 244, 251
Diabetic ketoacidosis (DKA), 233
   blood glucose in, 253, 254
   insulin for, 254, 255
   obesity and, 235
   type 1 diabetes and, 236
Diabetic neuropathy, 490
   pain with, 249
Dialysis, 161, 182
Diarrhea
   with Crohn's disease, 135
   in pediatric health management, 371, 378, 471
   potassium and, 125, 285
DIC. *See* Disseminated intravascular coagulation
Dietitian
   in gastrointestinal management, 144
   in hematological and immunological management, 324
Digoxin (Lanoxin)
   apical pulse and, 27, 38
   endoscopy and, 136
   International Normalized Ratio for, 34, 35, 42
   IV push of, 10
   in pediatric health management, 389
   potassium and, 38
   therapeutic level for, 65
Dilantin. *See* Phenytoin
Disasters, 155, 172
   client tracking in, 500
   discharges in, 473
   endocrine management and, 233
   medication administration in, 176
   neurological management and, 192, 211–212
Discharges/discharge teaching
   for abdominal aortic aneurysm, 56, 73
   for angina, 22
   in cardiac management, 22, 31–32
   for cellulitis, 464
   in disasters, 473
   in endocrine management, 248
   for hip fracture, 477
   in mental health management, 395, 453
   in neurological management, 190, 195, 209
   in renal/genitourinary management, 170
Disseminated intravascular coagulation (DIC), 315, 466, 485, 487
   benign prostatic hypertrophy and, 169
Diuretics, 44, 483
   loop (*See* Loop diuretics)
Diverticulitis, 129, 141
Diverticulosis, 124, 130, 149
Documentation. *See also* Electronic health record (EHR); Medication administration records (MARs)
   in endocrine management, 245
   in gastrointestinal management, 118
   in renal/genitourinary management, 177

Dog bite, 49, 67
Do not resuscitate (DNR) order
   in cardiac management, 12
   for congestive heart failure, 14
   on electronic health record, 31
   in gastrointestinal management, 139
   in hematological and immunological management, 327
   for infective endocarditis, 15
   for lung cancer, 301
   in neurological management, 195
   Rapid Response Team and, 36
   telemetry and, 31
Dopamine, 29
Down syndrome, 365, 366, 383
Drag-and-drop questions, 6
Dressings
   for burns, 472, 477
   for pressure injury, 278
Drooling, 30, 378, 384, 489
Dr. Seuss, 295
Drucker, Peter, 79
Drug impairment, 211
   in gastrointestinal management, 143
Duchenne's muscular dystrophy, 366
Dulcolax. *See* Bisacodyl
Duodenal ulcer, 126, 129
Durable medical equipment (DME), 251
Durable power of attorney for health care, 142
DVT. *See* Deep vein thrombosis
Dysphagia, 208
Dyspnea, 40
   with aortic valve stenosis, 38
   with deep vein thrombosis, 46
   with spinal cord injury, 206

E

Eclampsia, 338
ED. *See* Emergency department
Edema, 76, 249
   with burns, 271
   in cephalohematoma, 358
   cool water for, 292
   from deep vein thrombosis, 71
   in gestational hypertension, 351
   in premenstrual syndrome, 355
   pulmonary (*See* Pulmonary edema)
   with thyroidectomy, 244
Einstein, Albert, 45, 393
EKG. *See* Electrocardiogram
Elder abuse, 50, 68
Electrical burns, in emergency department, 268
Electrical failure protocol, 475, 495
Electrocardiogram (EKG), 40
   for long COVID, 44
Electroconvulsive therapy, 402
Electronic health record (EHR), 471, 491, 493
   in cardiac management, 18, 22, 31, 38, 39, 41
   charge nurse and, 482
   do not resuscitate order on, 31
   in gastrointestinal management, 118, 139
   Health Insurance Portability and Accountability Act and, 503
   in hematological and immunological management, 312
   incident reports in, 39
   for myocardial infarction, 22
   in pediatric health management, 381
   in renal/genitourinary management, 180
   in respiratory management, 87, 94
   time-out with, 38
   in vascular management, 47, 49, 57
E-mail communication, in respiratory management, 86, 106
Emergency department (ED)
   appendectomy and, 121, 330, 366
   burns in, 272–278, 292–294

cardiac management and, 16, 23–25, 27, 28
chest pain in, 16
electrical burns in, 268
endocrine management and, 235, 237–240
gastrointestinal management and, 121, 130–134
hematological and immunological management and, 307–311
integumentary management and, 263, 269, 280–281
mental health management and, 394, 400, 427
motor vehicle accident and, 479
neurological management and, 188, 192, 193, 195, 198
payment for, 37
pediatric health management and, 361, 366, 372, 390
renal/genitourinary management and, 155
respiratory management and, 87, 89, 90, 93–96
triage in, 479
vascular management and, 57–60
women's health management and, 338
Employee health nurse, 192, 211, 469, 489
Enalapril (Vasotec), 46, 62
Endarterectomy, 224
Endocarditis, 15, 38
Endocrine management, 223–257
case studies in, 237–240, 256–257
delegation of care (See Float nurse; Graduate nurse; Licensed practical nurse; Unlicensed assistive personnel)
laboratory tests in, 228, 232, 234
medication administration in, 226, 228, 232–233, 241, 243, 244, 254
medication administration records in, 223, 228, 245
shift reports in, 228
End-of-life (EOL) care
in cardiac management, 15
in gastrointestinal management, 124, 142
Endoscopy, 136, 463, 466
Endotracheal tube (ET), 464
breath sounds with, 113
chest x-ray for, 483
in intensive care unit, 463
ventilator with, 88, 92
End-stage Alzheimer's disease, 190, 209
End-stage chronic obstructive pulmonary disease (COPD), 85, 104
End-stage heart failure, in hematological and immunological management, 301
End-stage renal disease (ESRD), 159
for COVID-19, 308
hemodialysis for, 163
Enemas, in vascular management, 46
Enhanced hot spots, 6
Enoxaparin (Lovenox), 39
Epidural anesthesia, 330, 337–338, 352, 356
blood pressure and, 457
Epidural hematoma, 213
Epiglottitis, 489
Epinephrine autoinjector (EpiPen), 290
Epogen. See Erythropoietin alpha
Erikson's Stages of Psychosocial Development, 370
Erythropoietin alpha (Epogen), 179, 481
Escherichia coli, 351
Esophageal bleeding, 122
Esophagus
barium study of, 117, 135
bisphosphonates and, 173
Ethics
in endocrine management, 243
in gastrointestinal management, 139
in mental health management, 423
in pediatric health management, 383
in vascular management, 67
in women's health management, 336, 354
Evidence-based practice (EBP)
in gastrointestinal management, 124, 143
in vascular management, 46
Exercise
for cardiac rehabilitation, 34
chest pain from, 41
in endocrine management, 250
for eye, 250
isotonic, 35
for atherosclerosis, 76
Exophthalmos, 231
Extended multiple responses, 6
Eyes
cataracts of, 209
enucleation of, 195, 215
exercises for, 250
glaucoma of, 215
irrigation of, 216
in pediatric health management, 372, 391
prosthetic, 217
ventilator and, 484

F

Falls, 260, 499
back pain from, 191
after femoral-popliteal bypass, 55
femur fracture from, 476
hip fracture from, 479
neurological management and, 194, 198
in orthopedic unit, 262
Family
cardiac arrest and, 16
in cardiac management, 37
charge nurse and, 497
death and, 34, 51, 69, 177, 215
grieving process of, 215
hematological and immunological management and, 321
hospice care by, 142
long-term care and, 478
low-sodium diet and, 30
mental health management and, 420
Family practice clinic
neurological management and, 191
renal/genitourinary management and, 157
Fat embolism, 287
Femoral-popliteal bypass
fall after, 55
pain after, 54
unlicensed assistive personnel and, 56
Femur fracture, 268
from fall, 476
Fetal monitor, 329
in labor, 339
late decelerations on, 346
Fidelity, in hematological and immunological management, 299, 317
Filgrastim (Neupogen), 290
Fill-in-the-blank questions, 6
Fire alarm, 48, 66
in endocrine management, 252
in pediatric health management, 368
Flaccid bladder, 157
Flail chest, 82
Float nurse
in cardiac management, 10, 28
in hematological and immunological management, 325
in mental health management, 418
in postpartum unit, 339, 346
in respiratory management, 83, 101
in women's health management, 330, 358
Fluid and electrolyte imbalance, 255
in pediatric health management, 387
shock and, 291
Fluids, 104–105. *See also* Dehydration
chronic kidney disease and, 161
for diabetic ketoacidosis, 255
in endocrine management, 249
gastrostomy tube and, 140
heart failure and, 178

Fluids (continued)
  hypertensive crisis and, 53, 73
  lack of, death from, 105
  restriction of, for CHF, 39
  weight and, 179
    gain of, 249
Fontanels, bulging, 379
Food and Drug Administration, 388
Food intake
  lack of, death from, 105
  in mental health management, 399, 401, 417
  by newborns, 350
  in pediatric health management, 363, 380
  unlicensed assistive personnel and, 488
Food poisoning, 213
Food taste, chemotherapy and, 299
Fosamax. *See* Alendronate
Fowler's position, 91, 112, 136
Fracture
  of ankle, 264
  compartment syndrome with, 280
  of femur, 268, 476
  of hip, 475, 477, 479
  of pelvis, 264
Full-thickness burn, 269
Fulminant pulmonary edema, 30
Fundamentals Success (Nugent and Vitale), 7
Fundus, displacement of, 335, 352, 357
Furosemide (Lasix), 3, 38, 48, 290
  for congestive heart failure, 39
  endoscopy and, 136
  for heart failure, 270

G

Gait belt, 287
Gait training, 282
Gangrene, peripheral occlusive disease and, 50
Gastric bypass surgery, 120
  for morbidly obese, 128
Gastric lap banding, 137
Gastroenteritis, 127
Gastroesophageal reflux disease (GERD), 438
  asthma and, 144
  pyrosis with, 148
Gastrointestinal (GI) management, 117–151. *See also specific diseases and procedures*
  case studies for, 130–134, 150–151
  delegation of care (*See* Graduate nurse; Licensed practical nurse; Unlicensed assistive personnel)
  electronic health record in, 139
  laboratory tests in, 119–121, 127, 145
  medication administration in, 118–119, 126
  shift reports in, 119, 128
Gastrostomy tube, fluids and, 140
Genitourinary management. *See* Renal/genitourinary management
Gestational hypertension, 103
  blood in urine and, 352
  edema in, 351
  labor and, 333
Glasgow Coma Scale, 198, 219, 465, 466, 485
  graduate nurse and, 487
  in pediatric health management, 391
Glaucoma, 215
Glomerular filtration rate (GFR), 183
Glomerulonephritis, chronic, 163
Gloves
  for blood-borne diseases, 65, 75
  for body fluid contamination, 141
  in endocrine management, 256
  in hematological and immunological management, 319
  for impetigo, 284
Glucometer, 224, 247, 248
  for type 1 diabetes, 66
  for type 2 diabetes, 229

Glucophage. *See* Metformin
Glucose level. *See also* Blood glucose
  for burns, 274
  in women's health management, 344
Glycosylated hemoglobin, 34
Gonorrhea, 338
Grade 0, 288
Graduate nurse (GN), 467
  in cardiac management, 9
  in endocrine management, 224, 231, 241
  in gastrointestinal management, 129
  Glasgow Coma Scale and, 487
  in hematological and immunological management, 295, 296, 313
  in intensive care unit, 364, 381
  in neurological management, 195, 218
  in pediatric health management, 367, 384
  in postpartum unit, 38
  in renal/genitourinary management, 155
  in respiratory management, 79, 87, 90, 91, 97, 100
  in women's health management, 356
Grapefruit juice
  apical pulse and, 30, 33
  calcium channel blocker and, 29–30, 33
Grieving process
  of family, 215
  in mental health management, 398, 431
  with ovarian cancer, 306
  stages of, 124, 142
  for stillborn infants, 354, 501
  therapeutic communication with, 326
Guided imagery, 289
Guillain-Barré syndrome, 191
Guns, 401

H

Handwashing, 291
  breastfeeding and, 351
Headache
  in pediatric health management, 377
  with spinal cord injury, 188, 199
  with stroke, 192, 199, 212
  tension-type, 194, 214–215
  with transient ischemic attack, 193
  with type 1 diabetes, 227
  with vaso-occlusive sickle cell crisis, 361
Health Insurance Portability and Accountability Act (HIPAA), 61, 104
  in cardiac management, 28, 32, 34, 35, 36, 37, 40
  confidentiality in, 175, 286
  electronic health record and, 503
  in mental health management, 420
  in pediatric health management, 386
  protected health information in, 285, 286, 323
  on sexually transmitted diseases, 170
  volunteer care and, 492
Heart failure
  congestive (*See* Congestive heart failure (CHF))
  fluids and, 178
  furosemide for, 270
  packed red blood cells and, 160
  with type 2 diabetes, 226
Heart murmur, 20, 40, 312
Heating pad, for arterial occlusive disease, 68
Hematocrit (Hct), 103, 278
  for burns, 274
Hematological and immunological management, 295–328
  case studies in, 307–311
  delegation of care (*See* Float nurse; Graduate nurse; Licensed practical nurse; Unlicensed assistive personnel)
  laboratory tests in, 299, 300, 313, 315
Hematuria, 171
  kidney stones and, 181
Hemiparalysis, with stroke, 199

Hemiparesis, stroke and, 188
Hemodialysis, 159, 182
　for end-stage renal disease, 163
　for type 2 diabetes, 231
Hemoglobin (Hgb), 103, 278
　for burns, 274
Hemoglobin A1C
　hyperglycemia and, 253
　type 2 diabetes and, 233
Hemolysis, elevated liver enzymes, low platelet count (HELLP syndrome), 357
Hemorrhage. *See* Bleeding
Hemothorax, chest tube for, 90, 110
Heparin, 77, 488. *See also* Warfarin
　in cardiac management, 21
　for deep vein thrombosis, 40, 47, 66, 78
　partial thromboplastin time and, 38, 52, 54, 56, 61, 78, 173
Hepatitis
　herbal products for, 137
　needlestick injury and, 149
Herbal products. *See also specific types*
　for hepatitis, 137
　in pediatric health management, 388
Herbal remedies, in endocrine management, 247
Hernias, truss for, 76
Highly active antiretroviral therapy (HAART), 325
Hip. *See also* Total hip replacement
　dysplasia, 347
　fracture, 475
　　discharge teaching for, 477
　　from fall, 479
　pain, in women's health management, 333, 349
HIPAA. *See* Health Insurance Portability and Accountability Act (HIPAA)
Hirschsprung's disease, 343
Hives (urticaria), 278
Home health agency, 301, 470, 490, 498
　endocrine management and, 231, 232
Home health aide
　in cardiac management, 18, 39
　in hematological and immunological management, 300, 301, 319
　in integumentary management, 270, 290
　in neurological management, 193
　open reduction and internal fixation and, 470
　in renal/genitourinary management, 159
Home health nurse, 470
　amputations and, 480
　in cardiac management, 14, 15, 34, 35
　congestive heart failure and, 14
　in endocrine management, 230, 248, 249
　in gastrointestinal management, 123
　in hematological and immunological management, 301
　in integumentary management, 270, 271, 281, 284
　in neurological management, 192, 193
　rehabilitation commission and, 283
　in renal/genitourinary management, 159
　in respiratory management, 85, 86
　in vascular management, 49, 77
Hospice care
　in cardiac management, 15, 46
　in endocrine management, 233
　by family, 142
　in gastrointestinal management, 124
　in hematological and immunological management, 301, 320, 322
　in renal/genitourinary management, 159, 177
　in respiratory management, 86
　in vascular management, 50, 69
HTN. *See* Hypertension
Human immunodeficiency virus (HIV). *See also* Acquired immunodeficiency syndrome
　pregnancy and, 315, 325
Human papillomavirus (HPV), 481, 502
Humulin N. *See* Insulin isophane
Hydrochloric acid, 101
Hydrocodone (Vicodin), 51, 70, 386

Hyperglycemia, 246
　hemoglobin A1C and, 253
Hyperglycemic hyperosmolar nonketotic coma, 228
Hypertension (HTN), 419
　arterial (*See* Arterial hypertension)
　in cardiac management, 13, 14, 33
　erythropoietin for, 179
　stroke and, 49
　triglycerides and, 45
Hypertensive crisis, 53, 73
Hyperthyroidism, 231, 251, 252, 254
Hypnosis, 247
Hypochondriasis, 395
Hypoglycemia, 245
　insulin and, 241
　in newborns, 344, 386
Hypokalemia, 35, 285, 492
　cardiac dysrhythmias and, 144
　with diabetic ketoacidosis, 255
Hypopharyngeal obstruction, 98
Hypophysectomy, 252–253
Hypotension
　bleeding and, 325
　with long COVID, 44
　from magnesium sulfate, 356
　with malignant hyperthermia, 242
　with myxedema coma, 248
　orthostatic, 32, 102
　　with beta blockers, 289
　　BP and, 148
　vasovagal response and, 180
Hypothermia
　from magnesium sulfate, 356
　of newborns, 344
Hypothyroidism, 226, 232, 252, 254
　herbal remedies for, 247
Hypovolemia, 4, 278
　bleeding and, 145
Hypovolemic shock, 140
　with burns, 289
Hypoxemia, 243
Hypoxia, 287
　in pediatric health management, 377
Hysterectomy, 494

I

Ibuprofen, 51, 348, 485
ICU. *See* Intensive care unit
Ileal conduit
　for cystectomy, 171
　urinary output and, 183
Immunizations. *See* Vaccinations
Immunological management. *See* Hematological and immunological management
Imperforate anus, 343
Impetigo, 267, 284
Incentive spirometer, 147
Incontinence, 123
Inderal. *See* Propranolol
Indwelling catheters, 63, 163, 172
　bleeding with, 298
　povidone-iodine with, 169
　in renal/genitourinary management, 156
　after transurethral resection of prostate, 164
　urinary tract infection and, 182
　in women's health management, 347, 360
Infection control nurse, 303, 322
Infective endocarditis, 15
Infertility, 351
Inflammatory bowel disease, 129
Influenza, 84
　vaccination for, 103, 172
　in pediatric health management, 371
　veganism and, 350

Informed consent
    for blood transfusions, 64
    in cardiac management, 29
    in gastrointestinal management, 138
    in neurological management, 230
    in pediatric health management, 368, 384, 385
    in renal/genitourinary management, 176
    in respiratory management, 80, 98
    in women's health management, 354
INR. *See* International Normalized Ratio
Insulin, 38, 251, 253
    for diabetic ketoacidosis, 254, 255
    hypoglycemia and, 241
    before meals, 243
    in pediatric health management, 377, 384
    pump, 236, 256
    for type 1 diabetes, 66
Insulin isophane (Humulin N, NPH), 244
    in pediatric health management, 384
Insurance coverage. *See also* Health Insurance Portability and Accountability Act
    for pregnancy, 336, 354
Integumentary management, 259–294
    case studies in, 272–278, 292–294
    delegation of care (*See* Float nurse; Graduate nurse; Licensed practical nurse; Unlicensed assistive personnel)
    laboratory tests in, 266
    medication administration in, 260, 269, 270, 282
    shift reports in, 259, 261
    wheelchair in, 268, 288
Intensive care unit (ICU)
    in cardiac management, 11, 25–26
    charge nurse in, 50, 475, 477
    endocrine management and, 233, 235, 236, 239–240
    endotracheal tube in, 463
    hematological and immunological management and, 298, 316
    management decisions in, 6
    neonatal (*See* Neonatal intensive care unit)
    neurological management and, 189
    psychosis, 484–485
    respiratory management and, 80, 83, 109
    shift report in, 477
    tachypnea in, 463
Intermittent claudication
    for arterial occlusive disease, 27
    Buerger's disease and, 46
    pentoxifylline for, 66
International Normalized Ratio (INR)
    bleeding and, 277
    for digoxin, 34, 35, 42
    for vitamin K, 46
    for warfarin, 30, 31, 32, 35, 38, 49, 61, 67
Intimate partner violence (IPV), 323
    orthopedic unit and, 304
    in pediatric health management, 368
    in pregnancy, 333
Intracranial pressure (ICP), 207, 217
    in pediatric health management, 379
Iodine allergy, 213
Iron deficiency anemia, 66
Isotonic exercise, 35
    for atherosclerosis, 76
IV piggyback (IVPB), 27, 37, 90, 138, 243, 445
IV push (IVP), 27
    of digoxin, 10
    in neurological management, 216
    in vascular management, 48

J

Jackson-Pratt (JP) drain, 64, 128, 147, 326
Jaundice, after liver biopsy, 129
Jehovah's Witness, 333, 350
The Joint Commission (TJC), 29, 87, 98, 107, 347, 479, 496
Justice, in pediatric health management, 383

K

Katz Index of Activities of Daily Living, 268
Kernig's sign, 372
Ketones, 254
Key card, in mental health management, 425
Kidney. *See also* Renal
    transplant, 159
Kidney stones (nephrolithiasis), 162, 171, 464
    hematuria and, 181
Kidney, ureter, bladder (KUB) imaging, 162
King, Martin Luther, Jr., 433
Kübler-Ross, Elisabeth, 361, 398

L

Labor
    cervical dilation in, 352
    fetal monitor in, 329, 339
    gestational hypertension and, 333
Labor and delivery nurse, 330, 331
    epidural anesthesia and, 337–338
    shift reports for, 335
Laboratory tests. *See also specific tests*
    in cardiac management, 14, 19, 22, 34, 35–36
    charge nurse and, 470
    in endocrine management, 228, 232, 234
    in gastrointestinal management, 119–121, 127, 145
    in hematological and immunological management, 299, 300, 313, 315
    in integumentary management, 266
    in mental health management, 402, 415
    normal values in, 505–506
    in postpartum unit, 330, 339, 360
    test questions for, 447–449, 459
    in vascular management, 48, 58, 61
Laissez-faire leadership style, 422
Laminectomy, 475
Lanoxin. *See* Digoxin
Lao Tzu, 329
Laparotomy, 121
Laryngeal cancer, 296
Laryngectomy, 296
Lasix. *See* Furosemide
Latex allergy, 297
Laxative, 178
Legal issues and responsibilities, 2, 6. *See also* Abuse; Do not resuscitate order; Restraints; Safety
    of The Joint Commission, 29, 87, 98, 107, 347, 479, 496
    sexual harassment, 66, 82, 264, 474, 494
Legs
    cramps in, from loop diuretics, 107
    numbness in, 277
    pain in, 48
Leukemia, 368
Licensed practical nurse (LPN), 3–5, 496
    in cardiac management, 10, 13, 27, 32, 42, 46
    in critical care unit, 467
    in endocrine management, 224, 232, 241, 242, 251
    in gastrointestinal management, 123, 128, 148
    in hematological and immunological management, 296, 297, 299, 304, 313, 316, 324, 325
    in integumentary management, 262, 269, 279
    IV piggyback and, 27, 37
    in long-term care, 469
    medication administration by, 487, 490, 496
    in mental health management, 395, 396, 404, 416, 417, 427
    in neurological management, 188, 196, 206, 217
    in nursery, 332
    in oncology unit, 304, 305
    in pediatric health management, 365, 381, 470
    in postpartum unit, 332
    in rehabilitation unit, 475, 495
    in renal/genitourinary management, 154, 155, 156, 157, 164, 170, 173, 174, 175, 183
    in respiratory management, 79, 84, 91, 92, 97, 102, 111, 113

in vascular management, 46, 48, 63, 65, 66, 71
in women's health management, 347, 348
Life expectancy
do not resuscitate order and, 31
respiratory management and, 86, 105
Lifts, 268
Lipohypertrophy, 236, 256
Lithium, 399, 430, 453
Lithotripsy, 162
Liver biopsy, 137
bleeding after, 149
jaundice after, 129
Liver cancer, 124
Liver failure, 146
pruritus and, 137
Liver function tests, 35
Living will, 267
Logrolling, 281
Long COVID, 23, 43–44
Long-term care
atrial fibrillation in, 12
autonomy in, 52
charge nurse in, 53, 478, 479
endocrine management and, 228, 246
family and, 478
gastrointestinal management and, 123
hematological and immunological management and, 298, 299, 300
licensed practical nurse in, 469
neurological management and, 190
renal/genitourinary management and, 160
unlicensed assistive personnel in, 12, 469
vascular management and, 48
Loop diuretics, 32. *See also* Furosemide
for hypertension, 13
leg cramps from, 107
serum sodium level and, 27
for weight gain, 35
Lou Gehrig's disease. *See* Amyotrophic lateral sclerosis
Lovenox. *See* Enoxaparin
Low back pain, with abdominal aortic aneurysm, 75
Low-fat, low-cholesterol diet, 34, 41
for atherosclerosis, 76
Low-sodium diet, 32, 35
for congestive heart failure, 12
family and, 30
LPN. *See* Licensed practical nurse
Lumbar puncture, 220
for bacterial meningitis, 192, 200
Lung
cancer, 83, 85, 296
do not resuscitate order for, 301
sounds, 3, 99
in women's health management, 360
Lymphedema, 52

M

Maalox. *See* Aluminum hydroxide magnesium hydroxide
Macrosomia, 359
Magnesium hydroxide, simethicone, aluminum hydroxide (Mylanta), endoscopy and, 136
Magnesium sulfate, 338, 348, 356
Magnetic resonance imaging (MRI), 227, 245
Major depression, 393, 395, 406, 431
Malignant hyperthermia, 242
Marfan syndrome, 30
MARs. *See* Medication administration records
Maslow's Hierarchy of Needs, 2, 4, 5f, 36, 38, 210, 220, 244
for acute respiratory distress syndrome, 100
for cardiac arrhythmias, 144
in integumentary management, 292
in pediatric health management, 389
Massage
of fundus, 360
for tension-type headaches, 214–215

Masseter rigidity, 242
Mastitis, 334, 351
Matrix items, 6
Meals on Wheels, 490
Mechanical ventilation. *See* Ventilator
Meconium, 343
aspiration of, 344
Medication administration, 473, 483–484. *See also specific drugs*
in cardiac management, 15, 17, 29, 33
in disasters, 176
in endocrine management, 226, 228, 232–233, 241, 243, 244, 254
in gastrointestinal management, 118–119, 126
in integumentary management, 260, 269, 270, 282
by licensed practical nurse, 487, 490, 496
in mental health management, 396, 417, 419
in neurological management, 187, 190, 195, 217
in oncology unit, 302
in pediatric health management, 362, 370, 389, 390
in postpartum unit, 330, 334, 339
in renal/genitourinary management, 154, 169
in respiratory management, 88, 91, 102
in surgical unit, 477
unlicensed assistive personnel and, 36, 499
in vascular management, 46, 52, 63
in women's health management, 348, 358
Medication administration records (MARs), 4–5
in cardiac management, 17, 31, 38–39, 42–43
in endocrine management, 223, 228, 245
in neurological management, 196
in orthopedic unit, 259
in vascular management, 47
Medication errors
with antibiotics, 467
in hematological and immunological management, 297
in women's health management, 352
Melanoma, 278
Meningitis, bacterial, 192
Mental health management, 393–432
in cardiac management, 11, 15
case studies in, 407–412, 431–437, 452–453
defined, 381
delegation of care (*See* Float nurse; Graduate nurse; Licensed practical nurse; Unlicensed assistive personnel)
discharge teaching in, 395, 453
laboratory tests in, 402, 415
medication administration in, 396, 417, 419
pediatric health management and, 369
shift assignments in, 401, 420
shift reports in, 401
Mental health worker (MHW), 395, 396, 397, 399, 415, 417, 480
Meperidine (Demerol), 47, 64
Metabolic alkalosis, 101
Metformin (Glucophage), 251
Methotrexate, 305, 325
Methylergonovine maleate, 360
Methylprednisolone (Solu-Medrol), 246
MHW, 418, 419, 422, 425
Milk thistle, 146
Mitral valve
prolapse, 41
regurgitation, 30
stenosis, 27, 30
Modular nursing, 353
Mood stabilizers, 430
Morbidly obese
gastric bypass surgery for, 128
incentive spirometer and, 147
Mormons, 52, 72
Morphine, 40, 41, 51
Morphine sulfate (MS Contin), 218
Motor vehicle accident (MVA), 87, 122
amputations from, 266
emergency department and, 479
neurological management and, 189, 191, 194
pediatric health management and, 377

Motor vehicle accident (MVA) (*continued*)
    pelvic fracture from, 264
    pregnancy and, 38, 356
    renal/genitourinary management and, 155, 156
MS Contin. *See* Morphine sulfate
Mucolytics, 38
Multidisciplinary healthcare team, 495
    cardiac management and, 32, 34, 36
    integumentary management and, 281
    in mental health management, 424
    in neurological management, 193
    respiratory management and, 79
    respiratory therapist in, 484
Multiple sclerosis (MS), 193, 194, 196
Music therapy, 289
MVA. *See* Motor vehicle accident
Myasthenia gravis (MG), 189, 193, 205, 208, 213
Mylanta. *See* Magnesium hydroxide, simethicone, aluminum hydroxide
Myocardial infarction
    in cardiac management, 14
    chest pain with, 18, 21, 27
    electronic health record for, 22
    rule out (*See* Rule out myocardial infarction)
Myxedema coma, 226, 248

N

Naloxone, 458
Narcotics, 483, 502. *See also specific drugs*
    in cardiac management, 29, 38
    charge nurse and, 474
    in hematological and immunological management, 300, 312, 318
    in integumentary management, 277
    in neurological management, 216
    in pediatric health management, 386
    in renal/genitourinary management, 153, 183
    theft of, 300, 312, 318
    in women's health management, 458
Nasogastric tube (NGT), 83, 464
    after cystectomy, 163
    unlicensed assistive personnel and, 483
The National Council of State Boards of Nursing (NCSBN), 1–2
National Patient Safety Goals, 38, 426
Needle recapping, 125
Needlestick injury, 84, 129
    hepatitis and, 149
    in neurological management, 208
Neonatal intensive care unit (NICU), 264, 282
    graduate nurse in, 364, 381
Neostigmine (Prostigmin), 209
Nephrectomy, 160
Nephrolithiasis. *See* Kidney stones
Nephrotic syndrome, 390
Neulasta. *See* Pegfilgrastim
Neupogen. *See* Filgrastim
Neurological management, 187–222
    case studies for, 201–204, 221–222
    delegation of care (*See* Float nurse; Graduate nurse; Licensed practical nurse; Unlicensed assistive personnel)
    in gastrointestinal management, 140
    medication administration in, 187, 190, 195, 217
    shift reports in, 187, 188
Newborns, 329, 338. *See also* Nursery
    bracelets for, 333, 343, 386
    circumcision of, 336
    with Down syndrome, 365
    evaluation of, 343
    food intake by, 350
    hypoglycemia in, 344, 386
    hypothermia of, 344
    oxygen for, 458
    respiratory rate of, 357
    soap and, 346
New graduate nurse. *See* Graduate nurse
Next-generation NCLEX (NGN), 6
Nifedipine (Procardia XL), 46, 52, 62, 71
Nightingale, Florence, 117, 187
Nitroglycerin (NTG), 38, 40, 41, 43
Nocturia, 35
Nonmaleficence, 87, 282, 335, 353
NPH. *See* Insulin isophane
Nugent, Patricia, 7
Nurse Practice Act, 5
Nursery, 335, 368, 480
    Code Pink in, 382
    endocrine management and, 225, 242
    newborn in, 329, 330, 331
    shift report in, 334, 339
    surgical unit and, 369

O

Obesity
    in cardiac management, 14
    diabetic ketoacidosis and, 235
    lipohypertrophy and, 236
    morbid
        gastric bypass surgery for, 128
        incentive spirometer and, 147
    in women's health management, 359
Occupational Safety and Health Administration (OSHA), 33, 208
Occupational nurse, 48
Occupational therapy, 213, 230
Oliguria, 242
Ombudsman, 498
Omeprazole (Prilosec), 438
Oncology unit, 304
    licensed practical nurse in, 305
    medication administration in, 302
    pediatric health management and, 364, 380
    shift assignments in, 304
Open reduction and internal fixation (ORIF)
    home health aide and, 470
    osteoarthritis and, 301
Ophthalmology clinic, 194
Orchiectomy, 297, 314
Orthopedic unit
    falls in, 262
    intimate partner violence and, 304, 323
    medication administration record in, 259
    stroke in, 259
Orthopneic position, 111
Orthostatic hypotension, 32, 102
    with beta blockers, 289
    BP and, 148
Ortolani maneuver, 347
Osmotic diuretic, 217
Osteoarthritis, 301, 469
Osteomyelitis, 212
Osteoporosis, 300, 467
    alendronate for, 156
    bone density evaluation for, 318, 487
Ostomy care, 121
Otalgia, 216
Outpatient clinic
    endocrine management and, 235
    for mental health management, 395, 398, 400, 402
Ovarian cancer, 306
Overdose accident, 254
Over-the-counter (OTC) medications, 254, 486
Oxalate, 464, 484
Oxycodone, 40, 112
Oxygen, 101, 108
    for acute respiratory distress syndrome, 100, 113
    for deep vein thrombosis, 47

in endocrine management, 248
in hematological and immunological management, 320
for hypoxia, 287
for long COVID, 44
for newborn, 458
pneumonia and, 97
Oxytocin, 360

P

Packed red blood cells (PRBCs), 324
    for abdominal aortic aneurysm, 47
    for aortic aneurysm, 51
    blood transfusion and, 47, 64–65
    for congestive heart failure, 18, 66
    heart failure and, 160
Pain, 112, 463, 483. *See also specific types and locations*
    back, from fall, 191
    from burns, 290–291
    with chest tube, 91
    with compartment syndrome, 280
    control of (*See* Anesthesia)
    cool water for, 292
    with Crohn's disease, 135
    with diabetic neuropathy, 249
    in endocrine management, 242
    after femoral-popliteal bypass, 54
    in gastrointestinal management, 124, 139, 147
    in hematological and immunological management, 319, 321
    with kidney stones, 171
    with renal calculi, 153, 464
    in renal/genitourinary management, 169
    with sickle cell disease, 482
    from varicose veins, 70
    in vascular management, 50
    in women's health management, 348, 355
Pancreatic cancer, 226, 306
Panic attack disorder, 394, 404, 415
Paralysis, 219
Paranoid schizophrenia, 98, 399
Parenteral nutrition, 206
Paresthesia, 61
Parish nurse (PN), 480, 500
    in endocrine management, 229, 247
Parkinson's disease, 208
Partial thromboplastin time (PTT)
    activated (*See* Activated partial thromboplastin time)
    for bleeding, 103
    for deep vein thrombosis, 45
    heparin and, 38, 52, 54, 56, 61, 78, 173
    warfarin, 108
Patient-controlled analgesia (PCA) pump, 48
    in women's health management, 348
Pedal pulses, 96
Pediatric health management, 361–392, 470. *See also* Newborns
    case studies in, 373–376, 391–392
    delegation of care (*See* Float nurse; Graduate nurse; Unlicensed assistive personnel)
    diarrhea in, 471
    medication administration in, 362, 370, 389, 390
    mental health management in, 398, 413
    motor vehicle accident and, 377
    neurological management and, 199
    shift reports in, 362, 363, 377
    stroke in, 377
Pegfilgrastim (Neulasta), 326
Pelvic fracture, 264
Penicillin
    allergy to, 300, 318–319
    intramuscular administration of, 300
Pentoxifylline (Trental), 66
Peptic ulcer disease, 4, 126
Pericarditis, 30
Perineal care
    in gastrointestinal management, 140
    in vascular management, 63
Peripherally inserted central catheters (PICCs), 475, 495
Peripheral occlusive disease, 50
Peripheral vascular management. *See* Vascular management
Peritoneal dialysis, 179
Peritonitis, 137, 150, 326
Personal protective equipment
    in COVID-19 pandemic, 114, 115
    in hematological and immunological management, 322
Phantom pain, 71
Phenytoin (Dilantin), 205, 490
Pheochromocytoma, 243
Phlebitis, 180
Phonophobia, 214
Photophobia, 214
Physical therapist, 176
    in integumentary management, 281, 282, 296
    for mobility, 214
    in rehabilitation unit, 264, 267
    unit secretary and, 472
Pica (eating dirt), in pregnancy, 336, 353–354
Placenta, 343
Platelet count
    in hematological and immunological management, 318
    thrombocytopenia and, 64
Plavix. *See* Clopidogrel
Pneumonectomy, 80
Pneumonia, 85, 90, 327–328, 492
    abdominal aortic aneurysm and, 61
    aspiration, 136
    chest x-ray for, 83
    community-acquired (*See* Community-acquired pneumonia)
    oxygen and, 97
    in renal/genitourinary management, 182
Pneumothorax
    blood and, 112
    chest tube for, 82, 87, 91
Podiatrist, 74
Poison Control, 391
Poisoning
    food, 213
    in pediatric health management, 372, 386, 391
Polymerase chain reaction (PCR), 94
Polysporin, 286
Postanesthesia care unit (PACU), 474
    gastrointestinal management and, 147
    pulse oximetry and, 80
Postmortem care
    in cardiac management, 36, 46
    in hematological and immunological management, 303, 322
    in vascular management, 51
Postpartum unit, 331
    bleeding in, 359–360
    breastfeeding in, 334
    case studies in, 340–342, 359–360
    clinical manager in, 335, 336
    laboratory tests in, 330, 339, 360
    medication administration in, 330, 334, 339
    nonmaleficence in, 335, 353
    shift assignments in, 337
    shift report for, 329
    in women's health management, 330
Posttraumatic stress disorder (PTSD), 414
Potassium, 148, 492
    for burns, 274
    diarrhea and, 125, 285
    digoxin and, 38
    serum (*See* Serum potassium)
Povidone iodine (Betadine), 169
Pradaxa. *See* Dabigatran

PRBCs. *See* Packed red blood cells
Prednisone, 262
Preeclampsia, 333, 343–344
Pregnancy. *See also specific topics*
    anesthesia and, 345
    chest x-rays and, 101, 182, 352
    eating dirt in, 336
    in endocrine management, 226, 243
    gestational hypertension in, 103
    hematological and immunological management and, 297
    human immunodeficiency virus and, 315, 325
    insurance coverage for, 336, 354
    intimate partner violence in, 333
    motor vehicle accident and, 38, 356
    pica in, 336, 353–354
    x-ray and, 180
Premature ventricular contractions (PVCs), 29, 41
Premenstrual syndrome (PMS), 336, 355
Pressure injury, 260, 268
    dressings for, 278
    in hematological and immunological management, 319–320, 323
Prilosec. *See* Omeprazole
Primigravida, 334
Procardia XL. *See* Nifedipine
Prochlorperazine (Compazine), 322
Prolapsed cord, 330, 344
Promethazine, 51
Propranolol (Inderal), 46, 62, 252
Prostate cancer, 306
Prosthetic limbs, 284
Prostigmin. *See* Neostigmine
Protected health information, in Health Insurance Portability and Accountability Act, 285, 286, 323
Prothrombin time (PT), 48
Proton pump inhibitors, 463
Pruritus, 278
    liver failure and, 137
Psychiatric unit. *See* Mental health management
Psychosis, intensive care unit, 484–485
Public health nurse, 338
Puerperal infection, 359
Pulmonary edema
    bumetanide for, 87
    with congestive heart failure, 27, 41
Pulmonary embolism, 492
    chest pain with, 72
    compression stockings for, 49, 67
    deep vein thrombosis and, 61, 62, 78, 110
    thrombophlebitis and, 65
Pulse
    apical (*See* Apical pulse)
    with arterial occlusive disease, 277
    in pediatric health management, 378
    ventricular tachycardia and, 43
Pulse oximetry, 494
    for hypovolemia, 4
    for long COVID, 44
    in pediatric health management, 377
    postanesthesia care unit and, 80
    respiratory distress and, 291
Purified protein derivative (PPD), 84
Pyelogram, intravenous (IV), 158
Pyelonephritis, 172
Pyrosis (heartburn), 148

Q

Quadriplegia, 199
Quality improvement, 467, 487
    in hematological and immunological management, 299, 317
    in respiratory management, 89

R

Rales, 80
Rapid Response Team (RRT)
    cardiac management and, 36, 41
    respiratory management and, 98
Raynaud's phenomenon, 45, 52
Registered nurse (RN). *See specific topics*
Rehabilitation commission, 283
Rehabilitation unit, 497
    case management in, 266
    charge nurse in, 263
    complementary alternative medicine in, 269
    integumentary management and, 261, 269
    licensed practical nurse in, 475, 495
    neurological management and, 191, 195, 196, 206, 210, 217
    physical therapist in, 264, 267
    shift assignments in, 266
    for stroke, 191
    unlicensed assistive personnel in, 262, 263, 265
Renal calculi, 158, 162
    pain with, 153, 464
Renal cell carcinoma, 163
Renal failure
    with abdominal aortic aneurysm, 77
    urinary output with, 137
Renal/genitourinary management, 153–185
    case studies for, 164–168, 184–185
    electronic health record in, 180
    medical alert bracelet in, 174
    medication administration in, 154, 169
    shift reports in, 156, 157
Renal trauma, 156
Respiratory acidosis, 72, 243
Respiratory distress, 483
    acute (*See* Acute respiratory distress syndrome)
    pulse oximetry and, 291
    with ventilator, 99
Respiratory failure, 113
Respiratory management, 79–115. *See also specific diseases*
    case studies for, 93–96, 114–115, 441–444, 456–457
    delegation of care (*See* Float nurse; Graduate nurse; Licensed practical nurse; Unlicensed assistive personnel)
    electronic health record in, 87, 94
    medication administration in, 88, 91, 102
    multidisciplinary healthcare team and, 79
    quality improvement in, 89
    shift assignments in, 90
    shift reports in, 80, 90, 96
Respiratory syncytial virus (RSV), 392
Respiratory therapist (RT), 37, 97
    for burns, 274
    in multidisciplinary healthcare team, 484
Rest, ice, compression, and elevation (RICE), 485
Restraints, 496
    in endocrine management, 250–251
    in hematological and immunological management, 316
    in integumentary management, 279
    in pediatric health management, 381
Rheumatic heart disease, 29, 379
Rheumatoid arthritis (RA), 305, 325
Rho(D) immune globulin (RhoGAM), 333, 350, 471, 491
Rifampin, 97
Rocephin. *See* Ceftriaxone
Roosevelt, Theodore, 259
RT. *See* Respiratory therapist
Rule out (R/O) myocardial infarction, 22, 42

S

Safety, 476, 489
    in hematological and immunological management, 314, 316
    in integumentary management, 286, 287
    in mental health management, 413, 416, 421, 426

in pediatric health management, 385
in women's health management, 347, 349
Saltwater gargle, 486
Saw palmetto, 170, 176
Schizophrenia, 158, 176, 395, 399, 400, 405, 423, 426, 429–430
School nurse, 159, 267
SCI. *See* Spinal cord injury
Seizures, 210
    injury during, 214
    magnesium sulfate for, 348
    tonic-clonic (*See* Tonic-clonic seizures)
    in women's health management, 344, 348
Sengstaken-Blackmore tube, 145
Sequential compression devices (SCDs), 46, 63
Serum amiodarone, 38
Serum potassium, 34
    inflammatory bowel disease and, 129
Serum sodium, 103, 249
    dehydration and, 146
    loop diuretics and, 27
Sexual activity, 13, 31–32
    amputations and, 284
    in mental health management, 418
Sexual harassment, 66, 82, 264, 474, 494
Sexually transmitted infections (STIs), 482, 502
    Health Insurance Portability and Accountability Act on, 170
    in women's health management, 338, 356
Shared governance, 472, 492
Sharps containers
    in cardiac management, 14, 33
    in neurological management, 189, 208
    in pediatric health management, 390
Shift assignments
    in cardiac management, 12, 18
    in critical care unit, 468
    in mental health management, 396, 401, 420
    in neurological management, 200
    in oncology unit, 304
    in pediatric health management, 364
    in postpartum unit, 337
    in rehabilitation unit, 266
    in renal/genitourinary management, 155
    in respiratory management, 90
    in surgical unit, 467
Shift reports
    in burn unit, 272
    in cardiac management, 9, 17, 68
    in endocrine management, 228
    in gastrointestinal management, 119, 128
    in integumentary management, 259, 261
    in intensive care unit, 477
    for labor and delivery nurse, 335
    in mental health management, 401
    in neurological management, 187, 188
    in nursery, 334, 339
    in pediatric health management, 362, 363, 377
    for postpartum care, 329
    in renal/genitourinary management, 156, 157
    in respiratory management, 80, 90, 96
    in vascular management, 48, 52, 53, 54, 55
Shock, 109, 320
    fluid and electrolyte imbalance and, 291
    hypovolemic (*See* Hypovolemic shock)
    spinal (*See* Spinal shock)
Shoulder
    contracture, 210
    dislocation, 205
    pain, cholecystectomy and, 126, 144
Sickle cell disease, 482
Sigmoid colostomy, 121, 123, 129, 149, 301
    stoma and, 124
Sigmoidoscopy, 149
Sigmoid resection, bleeding from, 127

Sinus bradycardia, 30
Skin. *See also* Integumentary management
    cancer, 326–327
    liver failure and, 146
    wheelchairs and, 210
Sleep disturbances
    in endocrine management, 250
    in premenstrual syndrome, 355
Sleepwalking, 398
Smoke detectors, 49, 68
Smoking, 43
    birth control pills and, 501
    cholecystectomy and, 137–138
    chronic obstructive pulmonary disease from, 91
Social worker, 101
    in mental health management, 399, 420, 423
Sodium. *See also* Low-sodium diet
    for burns, 274
    diarrhea and, 285
    serum (*See* Serum sodium)
Solu-Medrol. *See* Methylprednisolone
Somatization disorder, 394
Speech, slurred, 30
Speech therapist, 208, 313
Sperm banking, 314
Spinal cord injury (SCI), 188, 192, 195
    autonomic dysreflexia with, 205
    dyspnea with, 206
    headache with, 199
    osteomyelitis with, 212
    quadriplegia from, 199
Spinal shock, 220, 465
Spinal surgery, 263
Spiritual care, 176
    in endocrine management, 244
    in hematological and immunological management, 321
    in women's health management, 349
Staphylococcus aureus, 351
Stasis venous ulcer, 45
Statins, 38
Steroids, 290
Stethoscope, 55
Stillborn infants, 333, 336, 480, 501
    grieving process for, 354
Stoma, 124
Stomach
    barium study of, 117, 135
    pain in, 124
Strikes, 503
Stroke (cerebrovascular accident, CVA), 93, 189, 196
    arterial hypertension and, 212
    death from, 206
    headache with, 192, 199, 212
    hemiparalysis with, 199
    hemiparesis and, 188
    hypertension and, 49
    in orthopedic unit, 259
    paralysis with, 219
    in pediatric health management, 377
    rehabilitation unit for, 191
    slurred speech with, 30
    swallowing and, 209
    wheelchair for, 190
Subarachnoid hemorrhage, 195
Sucralfate (Carafate), 137
Suicide, 414, 418, 432, 433–437, 452–453
    attempt, 395
    major depression and, 406
    mental health worker and, 397
    plan for, 430, 501
    wellness check for, 407–412
Support groups
    Alcoholics Anonymous, 399, 421
    in pediatric health management, 382

Surgery. *See also specific types*
    for cancer, 299
    in pediatric health management, 384
Surgical unit
    charge nurse in, 476
    clinical manager in, 474
    endocrine management and, 225
    gastrointestinal management and, 117, 121, 122, 125, 128
    hematological and immunological management and, 296, 303
    infection control nurse in, 303
    medication administration in, 477
    mental health management and, 396
    nursery and, 369
    pediatric healthcare and, 363
    postpartum unit and, 331
    shift assignments in, 467
Swallowing, 123
    in pediatric health management, 378
    speech therapists for, 208
    stroke and, 209
Syncope
    with aortic valve stenosis, 38
    with long COVID, 44
    vasovagal response and, 180
Syndrome of inappropriate antidiuretic hormone (SIADH), 230
Syphilis, 155
Systemic lupus erythematosus (SLE), 304, 308

T

Tachycardia
    bleeding and, 325
    with long COVID, 23, 43
    with malignant hyperthermia, 242
    ventricular (*See* Ventricular tachycardia)
Tachypnea, 92, 463
Take down procedure, 427
Telemetry
    in cardiac management, 10, 16, 19, 21, 29, 42
    for chest pain, 19
    do not resuscitate order and, 31
    flat line with, 21
Tenormin. *See* Atenolol
Tension-type headaches, 194, 214–215
Terminal illness. *See also* End-of-life care
    in endocrine management, 231, 252
Terminations, 285
Testicular cancer, 297
Therapeutic communication, 326
Thrombocytopenia, 64
Thromboembolic disease, 359
Thrombophlebitis, 65
Thyroid cancer, 227
Thyroidectomy, 227, 244
Thyrotoxicosis, 251, 252
Ticlopidine (Ticlid), 39
Time-out, with electronic health record, 38
TJC. *See* The Joint Commission
Tonic-clonic seizures, 191, 199
Tonic-neck reflex, 353, 358
Tonsillectomy, 84
Tornado preparedness, 265, 284
Total hip replacement (THR), 263, 265, 495
    abductor pillow for, 283
Total parenteral nutrition (TPN), 127, 161, 179
    in hematological and immunological management, 316
    in integumentary management, 292
    rate for, 129
Tourniquets, 494
Tracheostomy, 99
    in pediatric health management, 378
    ventilator and, 108
Traditional Chinese medicine, 229, 247, 289, 470
Transient ischemic attack (TIA), 193

Transplant
    kidney, 159
    rejection of, 246
Transsphenoidal hypophysectomy, 233
Transurethral resection of prostate (TURP), 156
    continuous bladder irrigation for, 163
    indwelling catheters, 164
    urine output after, 161
Traumatic brain injury (TBI), 194, 195, 196
Trazodone, 432
Trendelenburg position, 344
Trend items, 6
Trental. *See* Pentoxifylline
Triage
    in cardiac management, 13, 15
    by community health nurse, 480
    in dermatological clinic, 267
    in emergency department, 479
    in endocrine management, 228, 235
    in mental health management, 394, 414
    in neurological management, 192, 193
    in pediatric health management, 362
    in respiratory management, 93–96
    in vascular management, 57
Triglycerides, 45
Troponin, 40
Trough lab, 112
Truss, for hernias, 76
Tubal ligation, 366
Tuberculosis, 102
TURP. *See* Transurethral resection of prostate
Tylenol. *See* Acetaminophen
Type 1 diabetes
    blood glucose in, 253
    in cardiac management, 14
    continuous glucose monitoring for, 236
    diabetic ketoacidosis and, 236
    glucometer for, 66
    headache with, 227
    insulin for, 66
    in pediatric health management, 367
Type 2 diabetes, 223, 224
    chronic kidney disease and, 230
    glucometer for, 229
    heart failure with, 226
    hemodialysis for, 231
    hemoglobin A1C and, 233
    hospice care for, 233
    urinary tract infection and, 228

U

UAP. *See* Unlicensed assistive personnel
Unit secretary
    in pediatric health management, 380
    physical therapist and, 472
    in vascular management, 45
Unlicensed assistive personnel (UAP), 5
    arterial blood gases and, 39
    blood glucose and, 487
    in burn unit, 269
    in cardiac management, 10, 11, 12, 13, 14, 21, 27, 28, 29, 31, 32, 33, 36, 37, 39, 42, 46, 59, 129
    chest tube and, 470
    chest x-ray and, 486
    coronary artery bypass graft and, 59
    in critical care unit, 467
    in endocrine management, 224, 227, 230, 231, 232, 235, 236, 241, 244, 247, 249, 250–251, 254
    food intake and, 488
    in gastrointestinal management, 117–118, 120, 122, 123, 125, 127, 128, 135–136, 137, 138–139, 140, 141, 143, 144, 146, 148, 149
    in hematological and immunological management, 296, 297, 298, 299, 303, 313, 314, 315, 316, 317, 322, 326

in integumentary management, 77, 262, 268, 269, 271, 279–280, 281, 283, 285, 288, 289, 291, 292
in long-term care facility, 12, 469
medication administration and, 36, 499
in mental health management, 395
nasogastric tube and, 483
in neurological management, 187, 188, 189, 190, 191, 194, 196, 199, 206, 208, 211, 215–216, 218, 220
in nursery, 331
in oncology unit, 305, 306
in pediatric health management, 362, 364, 365, 369, 370, 371, 372, 379, 380, 381, 386, 390
in postpartum unit, 331, 332, 339
in rehabilitation unit, 262, 263, 265
in renal/genitourinary management, 154, 155, 157–158, 160, 161, 162, 163, 169–171, 174, 175, 177, 178, 180, 181, 182
in respiratory management, 79, 82, 84, 85, 86, 88, 91, 97, 100, 102, 104, 105, 108
urine output and, 486
in vascular management, 45, 46, 48, 49, 50, 52, 53, 54, 56, 63, 65, 66, 67, 69, 71, 72, 73, 74, 76
vital signs and, 488
in women's health management, 331, 346, 347, 357
Unresponsive client, in cardiac management, 12
Unstable angina, 27
Urinalysis
  in hematological and immunological management, 317
  saving urine from, 181
  for urinary tract infection, 174, 175
Urinary catheter. *See* Indwelling catheters
Urinary incontinence, 140, 162, 181
Urinary tract infection (UTI), 93, 245–246
  with chemotherapy, 317
  indwelling catheters and, 182
  type 2 diabetes and, 228
  urinalysis for, 174, 175
Urine
  blood in, gestational hypertension and, 352
  in pediatric health management, 364
Urine output, 73, 315
  chest tube and, 90, 110
  with diabetic ketoacidosis, 255
  ileal conduit and, 183
  in pediatric health management, 378
  with renal failure, 137
  after transurethral resection of prostate, 161
  unlicensed assistive personnel and, 486
Urticaria (hives), 278
UTI. *See* Urinary tract infection

V

Vaccinations
  for influenza, 103, 172
    in pediatric health management, 371
    veganism and, 350
  in pediatric health management, 378
Vaginal delivery, 334, 348
Vaginal discharge, 351
Vaginal dryness, 156, 173
Vaginal examination, prolapsed cord and, 330
Vaginal itching, 481, 501
Vancomycin, 171, 290
Varicose veins
  bedrest for, 77
  neurovascular compromise with, 73
  pain from, 70
Vascular management, 45–78
  case studies for, 57–60, 78
  delegation of care (*See* Graduate nurse; Licensed practical nurse; Unlicensed assistive personnel)
  electronic health record in, 47, 49, 57
  evidence-based practice in, 46
  laboratory tests in, 45, 48, 58, 61
  long-term care and, 48
  medication administration in, 46, 52, 63
  medication administration record in, 47
  shift reports in, 48, 52, 53, 54, 55
Vaso-occlusive sickle cell crisis, 361
Vasotec. *See* Enalapril
Vasovagal response, 180
Veganism, 337, 350, 355
Venous insufficiency, chronic, 54, 56
Venous ulcer, chronic, 57
Ventilator, 80, 464
  for acute respiratory distress syndrome, 82
  alarm for, 89, 109
  augmented and assistive communication devices for, 113
  for burns, 274
  communication boards and, 113
  with endotracheal tube, 88, 92
  eyes and, 484
  in intensive care unit, 82
  in neurological management, 207
  respiratory distress with, 99
  settings for, 100, 114
  tracheostomy and, 108
Ventricular fibrillation, 27
Ventricular tachycardia, 22
  pulse and, 43
  telemetry for, 16
Veracity, 139, 243, 423
Vicodin. *See* Hydrocodone
Vitale, Barbara, 7
Vital signs, 485
  for blood, 71
  for chest pain, 41
  in gastrointestinal management, 131–132
  in hematological and immunological management, 297, 314, 325
  for hypovolemia, 4
  for long COVID, 44
  in mental health management, 415
  in neurological management, 206
  in pediatric health management, 389
  in renal/genitourinary management, 174, 178
  in respiratory management, 84, 96
  unlicensed assistive personnel and, 488
  in vascular management, 45
  in women's health management, 347
Vitamin C, 484
Vitamin K
  International Normalized Ratio for, 46
  liver failure and, 146
  warfarin and, 61
Vocational counselor, 269, 289
Volume-controlled device (Buretrol), 387
Volunteer care
  in cardiac management, 15
  confidentiality in, 492

W

Walkers, 282
Warfarin (Coumadin), 500
  for atrial fibrillation, 31, 32
  for deep vein thrombosis, 68
  International Normalized Ratio for, 30, 31, 32, 35, 38, 49, 61, 67
  partial thromboplastin time and, 108
  vitamin K and, 61
WBC. *See* White blood cell count
Weight
  fluids and, 179
  gain of
    in cardiac management, 13, 35
    fluids and, 249
    in hematological and immunological management, 317, 324
  loss of, for cardiac rehabilitation, 34

Wheelchairs, 216
    in gastrointestinal management, 140
    in hematological and immunological management, 300
    in integumentary management, 268, 288
    skin and, 210
    for stroke, 190
White blood cell (WBC) count
    for burns, 274
    in endocrine management, 253
    filgrastim and, 290
    with gastric lap banding, 137
    in mental health management, 415, 426
    for stasis venous ulcer, 45
Win-lose strategy, 33
Win-win strategy, 11, 30, 33
Women's health management, 329–360, 471.
        See also Postpartum unit; Pregnancy
    birth control pills in, 481, 501
    case studies in, 444–447
    delegation of care (*See* Float nurse; Graduate nurse; Licensed practical nurse; Unlicensed assistive personnel)
    medication administration in, 348, 358
Workers' compensation, 211
Wounds
    chest, 211
    dehiscence of, 138, 147
    from electrical burn, 268
    in gastrointestinal management, 121, 138

X

X-ray
    chest (*See* Chest x-ray)
    for child abuse, 389
    in pediatric health management, 391
    pregnancy and, 180